The Science of Mental Health

Volume 6

Depression

Series Content

Volume 1
BIPOLAR DISORDER

Volume 2
AUTISM

Volume 3
SCHIZOPHRENIA

Volume 4
ATTENTION-DEFICIT HYPERACTIVITY DISORDERS

Volume 5
ADDICTION

Volume 6
DEPRESSION

Volume 7
PERSONALITY AND PERSONALITY DISORDER

Volume 8
COMPULSIVE DISORDER AND TOURETTE'S SYNDROME

Volume 9
STRESS AND THE BRAIN

Volume 10
FEAR AND ANXIETY

The Science of Mental Health

Volume 6
Depression

Edited with introductions by

Steven Hyman
National Institute of Mental Health

ROUTLEDGE
New York/London

Published in 2001 by

Routledge
29 West 35th Street
New York, NY 10001

Published in Great Britain by
Routledge
11 New Fetter Lane
London EC4P 4EE

Routledge is an Imprint of Taylor & Francis Books, Inc.

Printed in the United States of America on acid-free paper.

10 9 8 7 6 5 4 3 2 1

Library of Congress Cataloging-in-Publication Data

The science of mental health / edited with introductions by Steven Hyman.
p. cm.
Includes bibliographical references.
ISBN 0-8153-3743-4 (set)
1. Mental health. I. Hyman, Steven E.
RA790 .S435 2002
616.89--dc21

2001048491

ISBN 0-8153-3743-4 (set)
ISBN 0-8153-3744-2 (v.1)
ISBN 0-8153-3745-0 (v.2)
ISBN 0-8153-3746-9 (v.3)
ISBN 0-8153-3747-7 (v.4)
ISBN 0-8153-3748-5 (v.5)
ISBN 0-8153-3749-3 (v.6)
ISBN 0-8153-3750-7 (v.7)
ISBN 0-8153-3751-5 (v.8)
ISBN 0-8153-3752-3 (v.9)
ISBN 0-8153-3753-1 (v.10)

Contents

Treatment Outcomes

Introduction

In common usage, the term "depression" can refer to the state of being sad or blue, but it also signifies a serious clinical syndrome that affects approximately 10 percent of people at some point in their lives. This clinical syndrome may occur as a primary illness or as a complication of ("secondary to") another mental disorder such as schizophrenia, a medical condition such as hypothyroidism, or the effects of a drug. Based on studies of clinical courses and outcomes, treatment responses, and familial patterns of depression, primary depressive illness is dichotomized into unipolar (depressions only) and bipolar. In bipolar disorder, or manic-depressive illness, depressions are interspersed with manias— periods of elevated mood, high energy, and lack of sleep. Bipolar disorder is described in a separate volume.

"Major depression" is the term used in the *Diagnostic and Statistical Manual of Mental Disorders*, 4th edition (DSM-IV),[1] of the American Psychiatric Association to describe primary unipolar depressive illness of significant severity and duration. Characteristic symptoms include a disturbance of mood, general sadness (often accompanied by irritability), loss of interest in one's usual pursuits, and inability to experience pleasure (anhedonia). Major depression is also characterized by bodily symptoms, including sleep disturbance, generally insomnia (but occasionally excessive sleeping), change in appetite (usually loss of appetite but occasionally overeating), decreased energy, and, when the depression is severe, a slowing of thought, speech, and movement (psychomotor retardation). Cognitively, patients often complain of difficulty concentrating, ruminations on negative thoughts, guilt, a loss of hope, and suicidal thoughts. In a small percentage of severe cases, people may develop psychotic symptoms (most commonly delusions— fixed, culturally inappropriate false beliefs that are congruent with their depressed mood). Grief and bereavement may have many symptoms similar to those of depression. Grief should not be medicalized, but major losses may also trigger major depression. It is a difficult matter of judgment to determine when grieving has slipped into depression, but the diagnosis must be based on the duration, trajectory, and severity of the symptoms.

The course of major depression is often episodic, but recurrences are the rule, especially when the illness begins early in life. Between episodes of major depression many individuals— even with treatment— do not recover fully and may experience chronic low-level symptoms of depression. In perhaps 20 percent of people with major depression, severe symptoms become chronic and relatively unremitting. The term "dysthymia" is applied by the DSM-IV to chronic depression in which symptoms are not severe enough to quality for the diagnosis of a major depressive episode. We have learned, however, that despite diminished severity of symptoms, dysthymia can lead to substantial impairments, perhaps related to the chronicity of the symptoms that may wear people down.

The most serious complication of both major depression (unipolar) and bipolar depression is suicide. It has been estimated that 10 to 15 percent of people with recurrent depression commit suicide, and the most common reason for suicide is depression. Other disorders commonly associated with suicide are schizophrenia and alcoholism. Suicide is currently the eighth leading cause of death in the United States and the third leading cause of death among young people between the ages of 15 and 24.

In all its forms depression causes serious impairments in life roles. Based on a systematic review of data, the World Health Organization ranked major depression as the leading cause of disability in the developed world and the fifth leading cause of disease burden worldwide (defined as years of healthy life lost to premature mortality or disability).[2]

As in all of the volumes in this series, articles are included that cover a diverse range of issues needed to understand depression. The studies included here are derived from the scientific literature, but several books provide poignant personal accounts of the experience of depression that supplement this list.[3] The organization of this volume includes the subjects of epidemiology, genetics, the natural history of depression (for example, the course of depressive illness over a lifetime), examples of the relationship of depression to general medical disorders, an evolutionary view of depression, the neurobiology and behavioral science of depression, and, finally, the treatment of depression.

The epidemiological studies included here reveal that depression is an extremely common illness (Blazer et al., 1994) that creates a substantial economic burden. The negative socioeconomic impact of depression extends even to its less severe forms (Judd et al., 1996). An article in the section on natural history complements the epidemiological findings, demonstrating a potent negative impact of depression on educational attainment (Berndt et al., 2000). An entry on the epidemiology of suicide attempts is also included (Kessler et al., 1999). This article discusses the important role of epidemiology beyond tallying the incidence (new occurrences) and prevalence (total number of cases during a defined period) of a condition and goes into the identification of possible risk factors contributing to illness or mortality, in this case suicide attempts.

The major current controversy in the epidemiology of depression is the question of whether the age of onset of major depression is getting progressively younger in Western countries and whether the rates of depression are increasing. This unsettled question (Murphy et al., 2000) has important implications. Based on the known natural history of depression, if onsets are indeed getting earlier in life, there would be a greater number of recurrences and, likely, increased levels of disability. Such findings would also suggest important public health efforts to find the reasons for such a change combined with increased attention to case finding in children. The central question is whether the findings of Klerman and Weissman and several later investigators reflect real trends or result from artifacts of recent versus distant recall, decreasing stigma associated with talking about depression in younger generations, and an increased awareness of depression in the general population.

Another active area of research represented in this collection is the impact of stress on depression (Kessler, 1997). Fixing the relationship of stress to depression is difficult because different individuals perceive and respond to stress in different ways. Moreover, there is an important chicken-and-egg question that remains unsettled. Do negative life events independently create a risk of depression, or do individuals at risk for depression or who are already depressed have a greater liability— as a result of their symptoms— of putting themselves in harm's way?

The negative impact of depression on functioning is illustrated by its effects on cognitive functioning with aging (Bassuk et al., 1998) and on overall mortality (Schulz et al., 2000). Until recently the interaction among depression, medical illness, and mortality was conceptualized in a rather simplistic manner. It was thought that a medical illness such as a stroke, a heart attack, or diabetes was a serious life stressor (which of course it is) and thus caused depression. Depression would then have a negative impact on overall recovery by diminishing the motivation of the affected person to adhere to medical treatments and engage in self-care and rehabilitation. The situation, however, appears to be far more complex. First, there is good evidence that certain strokes (primarily in the dominant hemisphere) can directly trigger depression independently of the degree of disability. More recently, data have been brought forward to suggest depression that appears later in life may result from cerebrovascular disease (Krishnan et al., 1997). If this hypothesis is corroborated, prevention strategies for depression might come to include diet, exercise, and cardiovascular medications.

Even more unexpected, research has shown that the negative impact of depression on the outcome of cardiovascular disease extends far beyond issues of self-care and motivation. Musselman et al. (1998) review some of the data that establish biological effects of depression that can influence the outcome of cardiovascular disease. There is increasing evidence that depression may be the most potent modifiable risk factor for mortality in individuals who have had a heart attack or who suffer from congestive heart failure.

The origins of depression are to be found neither in genes alone nor in life events alone but in an interaction among multiple genes, developmental events, and stressful environmental triggers. These complex issues are addressed in articles by Kendler et al. (1987, 1995). One of the major emerging developmental risk factors for depression in women is a history of childhood sexual abuse (Weiss et al., 1999). No one would doubt that early abuse is a profound stressor, but further research on the mechanisms by which it leads to later illness is very much in need if we are to develop better preventive interventions for abused children. A history of childhood abuse, including sexual abuse, is also a potential risk factor for other mental disorders, for example, borderline personality disorder. Thus we must also learn the mediators by which this more general risk factor leads down one path or another, and we must learn about the resilience of those who do not develop a subsequent disorder.

Genes exert a less powerful effect in major depression than they do in autism, schizophrenia, or bipolar disorder; yet genes still play a significant role in the risk of depression, at about the same level that they do in risk of type II (adult onset) diabetes. As with all mental illnesses, however, the genetic risks of major depression are not straightforward. The evidence from family studies and from current attempts at gene discovery (for example, by linkage analysis) indicates that risk of depression is the result of the impact of multiple genes that interact with each other and with nongenetic factors. Pinning down the genetic variations that confer risk of depression is made more difficult by the almost certain likelihood that depression is heterogeneous, with multiple and different genetic and environmental pathways of risk. Overall, there may be no one gene or no one type of environmental event that is both necessary and sufficient to cause depression. This complexity is reviewed in Malhi et al. (2000). The high frequency of depression in the population suggests that the genetic variations that produce risk are also very common in the population. This raises the question of whether those genes have some adaptive value; one view of this evolutionary question is addressed by Nesse (2000).

Emotions such as fear or happiness represent transient responses to specific stimuli; mood represents the predominant long-term emotional state. It has been far easier to study emotion (short-term and stimulus-induced) than mood, partly because there are convincing animal models for some emotions, such as fear, and partly because certain emotions can be reliably induced in human research volunteers (see volumes on Fear, Anxiety, and the Brain). In contrast, although there is strong indirect evidence that animals have moods, such states have proven very difficult to measure or study. There are animal models that the pharmaceutical industry has used to identify drugs that may act as antidepressants, but these drug-discovery paradigms are not satisfactory models of the state of depression. Despite these challenges, there has been steady progress during the last decade in the investigation of the neural substrates of depression. For example, studies using noninvasive neuroimaging technologies such as positron emission tomography (PET) to study brain activity and studies using postmortem brain tissue have begun to identify brain structures that might be involved in depression (Drevets et al., 1997; Mayberg et al., 1999) and suicide.

Another important clue as to what goes wrong in the brain in depression is the long-standing observation that approximately half the people with serious major depression have excessive secretion of cortisol, the major stress hormone. Cortisol is the end product of activation of a stress-response system called the hypothalamic-pituitary-adrenal (HPA) axis. Heim and Nemeroff (1999) address the role of stress, including the role of early stress, in risk of depression. This biological and behavioral investigation complements the more epidemiologically oriented studies reviewed by Kessler (1997). Holsboer (2000) has argued that the HPA axis may play a central role in the pathogenesis of depression. His views yield several hypotheses that must be tested in the coming years. One hypothesized effect of long-term disruption of the HPA axis by depression includes atrophy of the hippocampus, a brain structure that plays a central role in explicit (conscious) memory. (See volume on Stress and the Brain.) While much more needs to be done, including longitudinal studies correlating hippocampal volumes with stress, depression, and cortisol measurements, as well as with cognitive function, initial work suggests that depression may indeed produce hippocampal atrophy (Sheline et al., 1999).

Treatment of depression involves certain well-tested psychotherapies, medications, or their combination. Treatment issues are addressed by a review from Frank and Thase (1999) and by Keller et al. (2000), who have developed a combination treatment for chronic depression. The benefits of treatment for functioning are addressed by Wells and Sherbourne (1999). The overall value of treatment must be kept front and center because, unfortunately, many individuals with serious depression still do not receive an appropriate diagnosis and, even if they do, may not get adequate treatment.

References

1. American Psychiatric Association. *Diagnostic and Statistical Manual of Mental Disorders*, 4th ed. Washington, D.C.: American Psychiatric Press, 1994.
2. C. J. L. Murray and A. D. Lopez. *The Global Burden of Disease*. Cambridge, Mass.: Harvard University Press, 1996.
3. William Styron. *Darkness Visible: A Memoir of Madness*. New York: Vintage, 1992; Andrew Solomon. *The Noonday Demon*. New York: Scribner, 2001.

The Prevalence and Distribution of Major Depression in a National Community Sample: The National Comorbidity Survey

Dan G. Blazer, M.D., Ph.D., Ronald C. Kessler, Ph.D.,
Katherine A. McGonagle, Ph.D., and Marvin S. Swartz, M.D.

Objective: Major depression is a frequent and disabling psychiatric disorder in the United States. This report examines the prevalence and risk factor profile of both pure and comorbid major depression according to data from the National Comorbidity Survey. Method: To estimate the prevalence of psychiatric comorbidity in the United States, a national sample of 8,098 persons 15–54 years of age from the 48 conterminous states was surveyed with a modified version of the Composite International Diagnostic Interview. Results: From the survey data the prevalence of current (30-day) major depression was estimated to be 4.9%, with a relatively higher prevalence in females, young adults, and persons with less than a college education. The prevalence estimate for lifetime major depression was 17.1%, with a similar demographic distribution. Both 30-day and lifetime prevalence estimates were higher than estimates from the earlier Epidemiologic Catchment Area study. When pure major depression was compared with major depression co-occurring with other psychiatric disorders, the risk factor profiles exhibited clear differences. Conclusions: These findings suggest a greater burden of major depression in community-dwelling persons than has been estimated from previous community samples. The risk factor profile showed significant differences between persons with pure and combined major depression.

(Am J Psychiatry 1994; 151:979–986)

Depression is considered a major public health problem (1–3). Community-based epidemiologic studies of DSM-III-defined major depression have yielded varying prevalence estimates, primarily because of varying methods of case ascertainment (4–6). By far the most ambitious effort to estimate the prevalence of major depression was the Epidemiologic Catchment Area (ECA) study in five U.S. communities (7). The prevalence estimates of major depression from the ECA study were criticized for at least two reasons. First, a true national estimate could not be abstracted because the investigators sampled only five communities. Second, the prevalence estimates of major depression were much lower than those from previous studies. The 1-month prevalence estimate for the United States, based on data on depression according to the DSM-III criteria from the five sites of the ECA study, was 1.6% for men and 2.9% for women. In contrast, in a retrospective analysis of the Sterling County study (8), the rate was estimated to be 5.3%, and in the New Haven, Conn., study (4), which used the Research Diagnostic Criteria, the rates were 3.2% for men and 5.2% for women. Es-

Received March 22, 1993; revision received Oct. 21, 1993; accepted Nov. 18, 1993. From Duke University Medical Center and the Survey Research Center, University of Michigan, Ann Arbor. Address reprint requests to Dr. Blazer, Duke University Medical Center, Box 3005, Durham, NC 27710.

The National Comorbidity Survey is supported by grant MH-46376 from the U.S. Alcohol, Drug Abuse, and Mental Health Administration, with supplemental support from the W.T. Grant Foundation. Preparation of this report was also supported by Research Scientist Development Award MH-00507 from NIMH to Dr. Blazer.

TABLE 1. Demographic Characteristics of the Subjects in the National Comorbidity Survey and in the U.S. Population

Characteristic	National Comorbidity Survey (N=8,098) (%)[a]	U.S. Population (%)[b]
Age (years)		
15–24	24.7	25.5
25–34	30.1	30.8
35–44	27.1	25.9
45–54	18.1	17.8
Sex		
Male	49.5	49.1
Female	50.5	50.9
Race/ethnicity		
White	75.3	75.0
Black	11.5	11.9
Hispanic	9.7	8.6
Other	3.5	4.5
Education (years)		
0–11	22.3	22.5
12	37.4	36.8
13–15	21.7	21.2
16 or more	18.6	19.5
Marital status		
Married	62.9	59.8
Separated/widowed/divorced	10.6	10.1
Never married	27.1	30.1
Region		
Northeast	20.2	20.0
Midwest	23.8	24.6
South	36.4	33.7
West	19.6	21.7
Urbanicity		
Large metropolitan area	67.8	71.2
Small metropolitan area	7.5	8.1
Rural area	24.7	20.7

[a]Weighted to the population.
[b]From the National Health Interview Survey, U.S. Department of Health and Human Services, National Center for Health Statistics, 1989.

timates of lifetime prevalence from the ECA study were also lower than those found in previous studies (9).

The general methodology applied in the ECA study has been transported to studies throughout the world. For example, studies using case-finding methods similar to that of the ECA study (the National Institute of Mental Health Diagnostic Interview Schedule) and studies that apply DSM-III and DSM-III-R criteria have been conducted in a number of other countries, including Canada (10), Puerto Rico (11), Italy (12), New Zealand (13), and Taiwan (14).

The National Comorbidity Survey represents the first epidemiologic data from a national sample of community residents from which estimates of prevalence distribution and risk factors for selected DSM-III-R psychiatric disorders in the United States can be derived. In this article, prevalence estimates for both current (30-day) and lifetime major depression are presented. Also, a risk factor profile is presented for both "pure" major depression and major depression occurring with other psychiatric disorders, a presentation not emphasized in most community-based epidemiologic studies of major depression. The case ascertainment methods of the National Comorbidity Survey were similar but not identical to those used in the ECA study. The different approach to case ascertainment for lifetime major depression in the National Comorbidity Survey was expected to lead to higher national estimates than those from the ECA study, and the estimates presented here confirm this assumption.

METHOD

The National Comorbidity Survey is a nationwide study of the U.S. population, ages 15–54 years, that was designed to estimate the prevalence, risk factors, and consequences of psychiatric morbidity and comorbidity. It is based on a stratified, multistage area probability sample of the noninstitutionalized civilian population in the 48 conterminous states, with a supplemental sample of students living in campus group housing. The survey was administered by the field staff of the Survey Research Center at the University of Michigan between Sept. 14, 1990, and Feb. 6, 1992. The 158 National Comorbidity Survey interviewers were experienced interviewers who completed a rigorous program of training to administer the Composite International Diagnostic Interview reliably.

Several special design features of the National Comorbidity Survey are noteworthy. A nonresponse survey was carried out in which a sample of persons who did not respond initially to the survey were offered a substantial financial incentive to complete a short form of the diagnostic interview. Significantly higher prevalence of both lifetime and current psychiatric disorders was found among these initial nonrespondents than among respondents in the main survey. This result is consistent with previous research showing that persons with histories of psychiatric disorder are underrepresented in cross-national surveys as well as in reinterview surveys of the general population (15, 16). The survey data were weighted to compensate for this nonresponse. The data were also weighted to adjust for variation in probabilities of selection across and within households and were poststratified by means of an interactive procedure to approximate the national population distribution of the cross-classification of age, sex, race/ethnicity, marital status, education, living arrangements, region, and urbanicity as defined by the 1989 U.S. National Health Interview Survey (17). A more detailed discussion of the National Comorbidity Survey sampling, designing, and weighting procedures is presented in the overview of the survey by Kessler et al. (18).

The overall response rate for the survey was 82.4%. The distribution of demographic characteristics in the sample of 8,098 respondents and in the U.S. population in the same age groups, according to the National Health Interview Survey, is presented in table 1.

The control variables presented in this analysis are primarily demographic variables. Age represents the range of the overall sample, 15–54 years. Two questions were asked to determine race/ethnicity. The first asked about Hispanic background and the second about the self-perception of race/ethnicity (white, black, or other). Respondents who reported a Hispanic background in response to the first question were coded as such regardless of their answer to the second question. Level of education was determined by asking the respondent the number of years of formal schooling she or he had completed. A hierarchy of coding rules was used to determine employment status: all respondents who reported that they were students were coded as student regardless of other reported categories; nonstudent respondents who reported being employed were coded as working regardless of other reported categories; and nonstudent, unemployed respondents who reported being homemakers were coded as homemaker regardless of other reported categories. Income represents total family income before taxes during the year before the interview, including salaries, wages, Social Security, welfare, and any other income.

Religious affiliations were grouped into Protestant, Catholic, and "other" categories. The Catholic category included Roman Catholic, Catholic, Orthodox, Eastern Orthodox, and Greek/Russian Orthodox. "Other" included Christian Science, Jehovah's Witnesses, Latter-Day Saints, Quaker, and Unitarian, as well as Jewish, Muslim, and Eastern religions such as Buddhist and Hindu. For determining ur-

TABLE 2. Prevalence of Current (30-Day) and Lifetime Major Depressive Episode, by Race/Ethnicity, Sex, and Age, From the National Comorbidity Survey (N=8,098)

Race/Ethnicity and Age	Males				Females				Total			
	30-Day		Lifetime		30-Day		Lifetime		30-Day		Lifetime	
	%[a]	SE	%[a]	SE	%[a]	SE	%[a]	SE	%[a]	SE	%[a]	SE
All												
15–24 years	4.3	1.1	11.0	1.8	8.2	1.3	20.8	1.9	6.1	0.9	15.7	1.3
25–34 years	4.0	0.9	13.1	1.3	4.3	0.8	19.4	1.3	4.2	0.6	16.5	0.9
35–44 years	4.2	1.0	14.7	1.6	6.4	1.1	23.8	1.9	5.3	0.8	19.2	1.4
45–54 years	2.3	0.8	11.8	1.9	5.0	1.0	21.8	2.3	3.6	0.7	16.7	1.5
Total	3.8	0.5	12.7	0.9	5.9	0.6	21.3	0.9	4.9	0.4	17.1	0.7
White												
15–24 years	4.1	1.2	11.6	2.1	8.6	1.6	23.1	2.3	6.2	1.0	16.9	1.5
25–34 years	4.3	1.0	14.0	1.4	3.5	0.5	19.6	1.5	3.9	0.6	17.0	1.1
35–44 years	4.7	1.2	15.2	2.0	5.7	1.1	24.2	2.4	5.2	0.9	19.5	1.8
45–54 years	2.6	1.0	12.7	2.0	4.8	1.1	23.1	2.9	3.7	0.8	17.9	1.6
Total	4.0	0.5	13.5	1.0	5.4	0.6	22.3	1.0	4.7	0.4	17.9	0.8
Black												
15–24 years	1.5[b]	1.1	4.7	2.2	4.5	2.0	9.2	2.7	3.1	1.2	7.1	1.8
25–34 years	1.0[b]	0.9	9.0	4.1	5.6[b]	3.6	18.6	4.4	3.8[b]	2.3	14.5	3.3
35–44 years	2.1[b]	1.1	5.9	1.8	9.7	3.1	21.1	4.5	6.4	1.9	14.9	3.3
45–54 years	0.0	0.0	10.2	6.2	1.0[b]	0.7	9.0	3.9	0.5[b]	0.3	9.6	4.1
Total	1.2	0.5	7.2	1.9	5.7	1.7	15.5	2.2	3.8	1.0	11.9	1.6
Hispanic												
15–24 years	8.5[b]	5.1	10.8	5.1	12.7	4.4	22.6	5.7	10.5	3.4	16.5	3.6
25–34 years	3.7	1.6	10.0	3.2	7.5	3.2	19.8	4.2	5.7	1.8	15.1	2.2
35–44 years	3.0[b]	1.8	17.6	6.7	11.2[b]	6.1	30.2	9.0	7.3	3.5	24.2	6.0
45–54 years	3.1[b]	2.3	9.3	5.0	19.6[b]	11.4	30.2	11.7	8.4[b]	5.5	16.0	6.6
Total	5.3	1.9	11.7	2.4	11.1	2.4	23.9	3.6	8.1	1.6	17.7	1.9

[a]Weighted to the population.
[b]Low precision; no prevalence reported.

banicity, persons were categorized as living in a large metropolitan area if they were part of the core of a standard metropolitan statistical area of 250,000 persons or more or on the fringe of such a metropolitan area. Small metropolitan area included individuals who were in the core or on the fringe of areas of fewer than 250,000 persons. Rural area included individuals who lived in nonmetropolitan counties having fewer than 20,000 persons.

The one variable with a substantial amount of missing data was income. A complex, regression-based scheme was developed to assign estimated values of income for cases in which data were missing. Missing data for other variables were few but were estimated as well when necessary.

DSM-III-R diagnoses were based on a modified version of the Composite International Diagnostic Interview (19). This structured interview was developed in a collaborative project of the World Health Organization and the Alcohol, Drug Abuse, and Mental Health Administration (20) to foster epidemiologic and cross-cultural comparative research by producing diagnoses according to both the definitions and criteria of DSM-III-R and the diagnostic criteria for research of ICD-10. Diagnoses were generated by the Composite International Diagnostic Interview computer program. "Pure major depressive episode," derived from the interview, is major depression without current generalized anxiety disorder, panic disorder, phobia, substance abuse or dependence, manic episode, or nonaffective psychosis. "Comorbid major depressive episode" is major depression that is diagnosed concurrent with any of the diagnoses just mentioned. Dysthymia was not included as a comorbid diagnosis, since "double depression" is a unique condition that will be explored in separate analyses.

The approach to case ascertainment in the National Comorbidity Survey, as compared to the use of the Diagnostic Interview Schedule (DIS) in the ECA study (21), is critical to interpreting the results reported in this article. First, there are three stem questions in the Composite International Diagnostic Interview, compared to one question in the DIS, to elicit a positive response that can be used in determining lifetime rates of major depression. These three questions were placed early in the interview, embedded in a series of questions about lifetime symptoms so as to facilitate recall of previous depressive episodes. Fifty-six percent of the total sample reported at least one "yes" to these stem questions. In contrast, approximately 32% of the ECA study respondents gave a positive response to the stem question (22). In addition, the probability of identifying a case among individuals who gave a positive answer to a stem question was higher in the National Comorbidity Survey than in the ECA study. In the survey, 30% of persons giving a positive answer to a stem question received a diagnosis of major depression, compared to approximately 20% in the ECA study. Although the ECA study used DSM-III rather than DSM-III-R criteria, the criteria for major depression in these two versions of DSM are virtually identical. Therefore, use of the revised edition of DSM-III in the National Comorbidity Survey should have had no effect on differences in prevalence estimates.

Data analyzed in this article were obtained from a stratified, multistage sample and were subsequently weighted to adjust for differential probabilities of selection and nonresponse. As a result of this complex sample design and weighting, estimates of standard error based on the usual assumption of equal-probability simple random sampling would be biased. Since more complex methods of analysis were required to obtain appropriate standard errors, estimates of standard errors of proportions were obtained by the Taylor Series linearization method (23). Adjusted rates were developed by using multiple logistic regression, controlling for the demographic factors that were significant in the crude analyses.

RESULTS

A total of 394 of the 8,098 subjects (weighted numbers) included in the sample were diagnosed as having a current (30-day) episode of major depression, a prevalence of 4.9%. One hundred seventy-two respondents experienced a pure episode of major depression,

TABLE 3. Crude and Adjusted Odds Ratios for Prevalence of Current (30-Day) Major Depressive Episode, by Selected Demographic Characteristics, From the National Comorbidity Survey

	Crude		Adjusted[a]	
Characteristic	Odds Ratio	95% Confidence Interval	Odds Ratio	95% Confidence Interval
Age (years)				
15–24	1.74[b]	1.08–2.78	—	—
25–34	1.16	0.72–1.86	—	—
35–44	1.48	0.89–2.48	—	—
45–54	1.00	—	—	—
Sex				
Male	1.00	—	1.00	—
Female	1.57[b]	1.19–2.08	1.36[b]	1.01–1.84
Race/ethnicity				
White	1.00	—	—	—
Black	0.80	0.41–1.51	—	—
Hispanic	1.79[b]	1.16–2.76	—	—
Other	0.56	0.10–3.14	—	—
Education (years)				
0–11	3.30[b]	1.95–5.58	1.93[b]	1.14–3.25
12	1.83[b]	1.07–3.13	1.93[b]	1.14–3.25
13–15	1.94[b]	1.05–3.58	1.93[b]	1.14–3.25
16 or more	1.00	—	1.00	—
Income (household, per year) (dollars)				
0–19,999	2.04[b]	1.08–3.88	—	—
20,000–34,999	1.58	0.83–3.01	—	—
35,000–69,999	1.10	0.64–1.89	—	—
70,000 or more	1.00	—	—	—
Marital status				
Married	0.39[b]	0.27–0.56	0.42[b]	0.28–0.61
Separated/widowed/divorced	1.00	—	1.00	—
Never married	0.52[b]	0.35–0.79	0.58[b]	0.38–0.88
Employment				
Working	1.00	—	1.00	—
Student	1.49	0.89–2.51	1.00	—
Homemaker	2.81[b]	1.80–4.38	2.40[b]	1.54–3.75
Other	3.04[b]	1.90–4.87	2.54[b]	1.51–4.28
Religious affiliation				
Protestant	1.01	0.69–1.47	—	—
Catholic	1.00	—	—	—
No preference	1.12	0.62–2.00	—	—
Other	0.70	0.36–1.38	—	—
Household composition				
Lives alone	1.22	0.79–1.87	—	—
Lives with spouse	1.00	—	—	—
Lives with other	2.06[b]	1.47–2.88	—	—
Lives with parent	1.44	0.97–2.15	—	—
Region				
Northeast	1.22	0.61–2.47	—	—
Midwest	1.06	0.58–1.92	—	—
South	1.26	0.71–2.24	—	—
West	1.00	—	—	—
Urbanicity				
Large metropolitan area	1.07	0.61–1.87	—	—
Small metropolitan area	0.91	0.51–1.62	—	—
Rural area	1.00	—	—	—

[a]Adjusted models were derived after several iterations of predicting major depressive episodes from all of the predictors that were significant in the crude analysis (sex, education, income, marital status, employment, and household composition). Absence of an estimate means low precision and no accurate estimate possible.
[b]$p<0.05$.

and 222 had comorbid major depression. The distribution of current and lifetime major depression by race/ethnicity, sex, and age is presented in table 2. The counterintuitive finding of higher lifetime prevalence in the younger age groups is similar to findings in the ECA study and may represent recall bias as well as a possible cohort effect.

As in other community-based epidemiologic studies, the prevalence of current major depression was higher in females than in males, at a ratio of approximately 2:1. This pattern holds for each of the racial/ethnic groups but appears more prominent among blacks and Hispanics than among whites. Although estimates by age were not precise, the overall prevalence among black males was by far the lowest of any sex and racial/ethnic group. As found in other studies, current major depression was more prevalent among persons less than 45 years of age than in those 45–54 years old. The most dramatic difference in the prevalence of depression by age in previous studies has been the lower prevalence for persons in late life (over 65 years of age), an age group not included in this study. This trend appears to hold for all sex and racial/ethnic groups for whom estimates are available. The estimated prevalence of depression, regardless of age, among all Hispanics was twice the prevalence for blacks.

The overall prevalence of lifetime major depression was estimated as 17.1% in this study. The estimated prevalence by age seems to be relatively constant across age groups. Once again, the estimated prevalence of lifetime major depression was approximately twice as great among females as among males. The estimated prevalence of lifetime major depression was lower overall among blacks (except for blacks 35–44 years of age) than among other race/ethnicity groups. The highest lifetime prevalence, however, appeared in black females 35–44 years of age.

Both crude and adjusted odds ratios (estimates of relative risk) for current (30-day) major depression, by selected demographic characteristics, are presented in table 3. In each case, the odds ratio was set at 1.00 for one of the categorical variables, and other variables within the category were compared to this variable. The adjusted model reports the odds ratios from predictions that remained significant (at the 0.05 level) in the final multivariate model. Female sex, lower level of education, separated/widowed/divorced and never married status, and employment classification as homemaker or "other" were found to be significant correlates for major depression in both the crude and adjusted models. In addition, age 15–24 years, Hispanic ethnic background, low income (an income of less than $20,000 per year), and living with someone other than a spouse were significant in the crude determinations of odds ratios. No significant association was found in adjusted odds ratios for age, race/ethnicity, household income, religious affiliation, household composition, region of the country, or urbanicity.

Crude odds ratios for the same demographic characteristics are presented for both pure and comorbid ma-

TABLE 4. Crude Odds Ratios for Prevalence of Current (30-Day) Pure and Comorbid Major Depressive Episode, by Selected Demographic Characteristics, From the National Comorbidity Survey[a]

	Pure Depressive Episode		Comorbid Depressive Episode		Comorbid Versus Pure	
Characteristic	Odds Ratio	95% Confidence Interval	Odds Ratio	95% Confidence Interval	Odds Ratio[b]	95% Confidence Interval
Age (years)						
15–24	1.03	0.46–2.26	3.00[c]	1.43–6.30	2.86	0.85–9.60
25–34	0.85	0.47–1.56	1.71	0.72–4.05	1.98	0.66–5.94
35–44	0.76	0.35–1.66	2.80[c]	1.21–6.45	3.57[c]	1.06–12.01
45–54	1.00	—	1.00	—	1.00	—
Sex						
Male	1.00	—	1.00	—	1.00	—
Female	1.56[c]	1.09–2.22	1.56[c]	1.03–2.35	1.00	0.58–1.70
Race/ethnicity						
White	1.00	—	1.00	—	1.00	—
Black	0.36[c]	0.21–0.63	1.22	0.56–2.65	3.32[c]	1.51–7.31
Hispanic	1.19	0.68–2.08	2.31[c]	1.29–4.15	1.90	0.85–4.25
Other	0.25[c]	0.07–0.88	0.86	0.10–7.66	3.40	0.19–6.26
Education (years)						
0–11	1.69	0.75–3.77	6.82[c]	2.71–17.19	3.93[c]	1.10–14.02
12	1.12	0.56–2.22	3.45[c]	1.50–7.95	3.04[c]	1.12–8.20
13–15	1.13	0.56–2.26	3.79[c]	1.51–9.53	3.30[c]	1.18–9.17
16 or more	1.00	—	1.00	—	1.00	—
Income (household, per year) (dollars)						
0–19,999	1.60	0.62–4.17	2.48	0.80–7.68	1.53	0.33–6.99
20,000–34,999	1.30	0.49–3.45	1.87	0.58–6.03	1.43	0.29–7.06
35,000–69,999	0.82	0.35–1.92	1.43	0.53–3.85	1.73	0.44–6.82
70,000 or more	1.00	—	1.00	—	1.00	—
Marital status						
Married	0.42[c]	0.22–0.79	0.39[c]	0.23–0.65	0.94	0.40–2.21
Separated/widowed/divorced	1.00	—	1.00	—	1.00	—
Never married	0.51[c]	0.28–0.93	0.56[c]	0.31–1.00	1.11	0.47–2.59
Employment						
Working	1.00	—	1.00	—	1.00	—
Student	1.17	0.57–2.42	1.75	0.88–3.45	1.48	0.58–3.74
Homemaker	2.83[c]	1.26–6.35	2.61[c]	1.55–4.39	0.92	0.35–2.40
Other	1.76	0.93–3.33	4.03[c]	2.09–7.77	2.19	0.87–5.47
Religious affiliation						
Protestant	1.06	0.64–1.77	0.96	0.55–1.69	0.91	0.43–1.93
Catholic	1.00	—	1.00	—	1.00	—
No preference	1.50	0.57–3.99	0.84	0.43–1.64	0.57	0.18–1.85
Other	0.63	0.26–1.52	0.76	0.28–2.08	1.20	0.32–4.56
Household composition						
Lives alone	1.48	0.55–4.02	1.00	0.63–1.58	0.68	0.20–2.32
Lives with spouse	1.00	—	1.00	—	1.00	—
Lives with other	1.83[c]	1.07–3.12	2.16[c]	1.27–3.69	1.17	0.52–2.66
Lives with parent	1.26	0.71–2.23	1.57	0.91–2.73	1.24	0.57–2.70
Region						
Northeast	0.81	0.46–1.44	1.60	0.47–5.39	1.93	0.53–7.04
Midwest	0.93	0.55–1.56	1.18	0.40–3.48	1.27	0.40–4.03
South	1.25	0.83–1.89	1.25	0.43–3.63	1.00	0.34–2.95
West	1.00	—	1.00	—	1.00	—
Urbanicity						
Large metropolitan area	1.05	0.52–2.11	1.08	0.57–2.02	1.02	0.50–2.09
Small metropolitan area	0.86	0.40–1.87	0.95	0.51–1.77	1.10	0.52–2.34
Rural area	1.00	—	1.00	—	1.00	—

[a]All odds ratios are adjusted estimates.
[b]Odds ratio of the odds ratios for comorbid and pure major depressive episode.
[c]$p<0.05$.

jor depression in table 4. The last column represents the ratio of the odds ratios for comorbid versus pure major depression by these same categories and shows whether this ratio of ratios is significant. The pattern of crude odds ratios for pure versus comorbid major depression exhibits substantial variability. Although the prevalence estimates for both pure and comorbid depression were higher for females than for males, for the other factors the estimates were less likely to coincide. Blacks were less likely to be depressed in general, but during a single episode they were more likely to have a comorbid disorder. Hispanics had higher crude rates of comorbid depression than other racial/ethnic groups, and among themselves they demonstrated a trend toward higher rates of comorbid than pure depression. A lower level of education was a risk factor for comorbid depression, and at the level of less than 16 years, the odds ratio for comorbid depression was significantly higher than for pure depression. Homemaker status was significantly related to both pure and comorbid depression, although neither type of depression predominated among homemakers. Living with another person was a significant correlate of comorbid as well as pure depression, but this association disappeared in the adjusted analyses, where factors such as marital status confounded the association, since the prevalence of depression was high among women living with children but not for women living with their spouses. The 15–24 and 35–44 age groups were more likely than older individuals to have comorbid depression; in the 35–44 age group, comorbid depression predominated.

DISCUSSION

Prevalence estimates for current and lifetime major depression in the National Comorbidity Survey were higher than those in the ECA study but similar to those found with the Schedule for Affective Disorders and Schizophrenia/Research Diagnostic Criteria approach to case finding in a community survey of New Haven, Conn. (4, 6): 4.9% versus 4.3% for current prevalence and 17.1% versus 20.0% for lifetime prevalence in the National Comorbidity Survey versus the New Haven study.

To place in context these prevalence estimates of major depression from a large national sample (which used case-identification procedures that are somewhat but not dramatically different from those used in previous large surveys within the United States), three topics should be addressed. First, the higher prevalence estimates of current and lifetime major depression in the National Comorbidity Survey, compared to the ECA study, should be explored. Second, the risk factor profile from the National Comorbidity Survey overall should be compared with the existing literature on major depression regarding risk factors. Third, the difference in the risk factor profiles of pure major depression and comorbid major depression should be addressed.

A number of factors may have contributed to the higher prevalence of major depression in the National Comorbidity Survey as compared to the ECA study. One possibility is that the approach to probing for an episode of major depression led to a higher proportion of true lifetime cases being reported in the survey. This could have occurred because each respondent was given three chances to respond to a stem question for major depression (questions asking about episodes of feeling "sad, blue, or depressed," feeling "down in the dumps and gloomy," and "losing interest in things you usually enjoy") rather than the one question in the DIS. A second possibility is that this more detailed probing caused overreporting and false positives. In an effort to investigate this possibility, a brief Composite International Diagnostic Interview/major depressive episode validation was performed in the National Comorbidity Survey. Thirty persons from the survey—20 who reported a lifetime history of major depression according to the structured interview and 10 who gave a positive answer to a stem question for major depression but failed to meet the DSM-III-R criteria—were reinterviewed. These validating interviews were performed by clinicians, blind to the Composite International Diagnostic Interview diagnosis, who used the Structured Clinical Interview for DSM-III-R (SCID) (24). Fourteen (70%) of the 20 subjects who had lifetime major depression according to the Composite International Diagnostic Interview were classified as having lifetime major depression according to the SCID, while eight (80%) of the 10 classified as not having lifetime major depression by the interview were classified the same way by the SCID. These validation results are similar to those found for major depression according to the DIS in the ECA study, in which findings from a structured questionnaire were compared with those from a standardized diagnostic interview. Differences in prevalence between the ECA study and the National Comorbidity Survey therefore may result from the use of a different validation instrument, the SCID, in the National Comorbidity Survey. In addition, the results of the ECA validation studies varied widely (25, 26).

There may be additional reasons for the greater prevalence of major depression in the National Comorbidity Survey. First, individuals in the sample were younger, and therefore the overall rates would be expected to be higher, given that the lowest rates for major depression were among the over-65 age group in the ECA sample (1). Second, secular trends could also account for these differences, as the National Comorbidity Survey was conducted approximately 10 years after the ECA study (3). This explanation, however, is more difficult to defend, since the interval of 10 years is very short for observing historical trends. Therefore, the best explanation is a methodological one, namely, that the Composite International Diagnostic Interview is a more sensitive instrument than the DIS in community population studies. A third possible reason for the discrepancy between the prevalence estimates of the two studies is that a national sample may yield a higher prevalence than adjusted rates from local surveys, which were used in the ECA study.

Another issue to be addressed is the overall risk factor profile of major depression in this study compared to other studies of major depression. The consensus from most community-based epidemiologic studies is that 1) younger persons are at greater risk for major depression than older persons; 2) blacks are somewhat less at risk than whites; 3) women are at greater risk for major depression than men; 4) persons of a lower socioeconomic status are at greater risk than those who are more well-off economically; 5) persons who are separated or divorced have higher rates of major depression than persons who are married or have never married; and 6) persons in urban areas are at greater risk than persons in rural areas (3, 4, 6, 27–30). The risk factor profile for 1-month prevalence could vary from the profile for 6-month or 1-year prevalence. However, it is probable that comorbidity would be even greater for the latter. Therefore, the 1-month estimate of comorbidity is a lower-boundary estimate of the percentage of persons with comorbid depression.

In general, the risk factor profile from the National Comorbidity Survey does not vary from the profile found in other epidemiologic studies. There are, however, two exceptions. First, the lower prevalence of major depression in rural areas compared to urban areas that was reported from the ECA study (27) was not replicated in this study. The reason for this difference may be that in the ECA study, urban-rural differences were compared in areas where the urban and rural counties are conterminous, as opposed to comparisons from a nationwide sample. Urban versus rural factors vary considerably by region of the country. Unless urban-rural comparisons are made in the same geographic area, urban-rural differences may be obscured by other geographic and demographic factors such as region of the country. Second, the finding of a much higher prevalence of major depression among homemakers than among persons in other categories of employment has not been reported in most major surveys but accords with the work of Brown and Harris in England. These investigators, in a much smaller study (31), found an exceptionally high prevalence of depression among homemakers with small children as compared to other women.

The final topic to be discussed relates specifically to the purpose of the National Comorbidity Survey, namely, to determine the comorbidity of psychiatric [illegible] files for pure versus comorbid expressions of those disorders. Therefore, the National Comorbidity Survey breaks new ground in considering risk factor profiles of pure versus comorbid major depression. The findings are striking. Many risk factors that have been associated with major depression, i.e., younger age, lower level of education, and lower income, were associated with major depression only among persons with comorbid, as opposed to pure, major depression. In contrast, one potential risk for major depression, nonblack race/ethnicity, was found for pure but not comorbid depression. Could it be that comorbid major depression is a more environmentally driven disorder (even though the symptoms of major depression in this circumstance are similar to those of pure major depression)? Stressors in the environment that lead to the symptoms of major depression may also lead to symptoms of anxiety and other psychiatric disorders, such as substance and alcohol abuse, suggesting a major etiologic role for psychosocial adversity in many of the more prevalent disorders. In contrast, individuals with pure major depression may be expressing a disorder less affected by psychosocial stress or perhaps a unique profile of psychosocial correlates. The higher prevalence of depression in females and among homemakers is apparent for both pure and comorbid depression.

ACKNOWLEDGMENTS

The National Comorbidity Survey (Ronald G. Kessler, Principal Investigator) is a collaborative epidemiologic investigation of the prevalence, causes, and consequences of psychiatric morbidity and comorbidity in the United States. Collaborating National Comorbidity Survey sites and investigators are: The Addiction Research Foundation (Robin Room); Duke University Medical Center (Dan Blazer, Marvin Swartz); Johns Hopkins University (James Anthony, William Eaton, Philip Leaf); the Max Planck Institute of Psychiatry (Hans-Ulrich Wittchen); the Medical College of Virginia (Kenneth Kendler); the University of Michigan (Lloyd Johnston, Ronald Kessler); NIMH (Darrell Kirsch, Darrel Regier); New York University (Patrick Shrout); State University of New York at Stony Brook (Evelyn Bromet); University of Toronto (R. Jay Turner); and Washington University School of Medicine (Linda Cottler).

REFERENCES

1. Regier DA, Boyd JH, Burke JD Jr, Rae DS, Myers JK, Kramer M, Robins LN, George LK, Karno M, Locke BZ: One-month prevalence of mental disorders in the United States: based on five Epidemiologic Catchment Area sites. Arch Gen Psychiatry 1988; 45: 977–986
2. Wells KB, Stewart A, Hays RD, Burnam MA, Rogers W, Daniels M, Berry S, Greenfield S, Ware J: The functioning and well-being of depressed patients: results from the Medical Outcomes Study. JAMA 1989; 262:914–919
3. Cross-National Collaborative Group: The changing rate of major depression: cross-national comparisons. JAMA 1992; 268: 3098–3105
4. Weissman MM, Myers JK: Affective disorders in a US urban community: the use of Research Diagnostic Criteria in an epidemiologic survey. Arch Gen Psychiatry 1978; 35:1304–1311
5. Blazer D, Williams CD: Epidemiology of dysphoria and depression in an elderly population. Am J Psychiatry 1980; 137:439–444
6. Myers JK, Weissman MM, Tischler GL, Holzer CE III, Leaf PJ, [illegible] Stoltzman R: Six-month prevalence of psychiatric disorders in three communities: 1980 to 1982. Arch Gen Psychiatry 1984; 41:959–967
7. Regier DA, Myers JK, Kramer M, Robins LN, Blazer DG, Hough RL, Eaton WW, Locke BZ: The NIMH Epidemiologic Catchment Area program: historical context, major objectives, and study population characteristics. Arch Gen Psychiatry 1984; 41: 934–941
8. Murphy JM, Sobol AM, Neff RK, Olivier DC, Leighton AH: Stability of prevalence: depression and anxiety disorders. Arch Gen Psychiatry 1984; 41:990–997
9. Robins LN, Helzer JE, Weissman MM, Orvaschel H, Gruenberg E, Burke JD Jr, Regier DA: Lifetime prevalence of specific psychiatric disorders in three sites. Arch Gen Psychiatry 1984; 41: 949–958
10. Orn H, Newman SC, Bland RC: Design and field methods of the Edmonton Survey of Psychiatric Disorders. Acta Psychiatr Scand (Suppl) 1988; 38:17–23
11. Canino GJ, Bird HR, Shrout PE: The prevalence of specific psychiatric disorders in Puerto Rico. Arch Gen Psychiatry 1987; 44: 727–735
12. Faravelli C, Degl'Innocenti BG, Aiazzi L, Incerpi G, Pallanti S: Epidemiology of mood disorders: a community survey in Florence. J Affect Disord 1990; 20:135–141
13. Wells JE, Bushnell JA, Hornblow AR, Joyce PR, Oakley-Browne MA: Christchurch Psychiatric Epidemiology Study, part I: methodology and lifetime prevalence for specific psychiatric disorders. Aust NZ J Psychiatry 1989; 23:315–326

14. Hwu HG, Yeh EK, Chang LY: Prevalence of psychiatric disorders in Taiwan defined by the Chinese Diagnostic Interview Schedule. Acta Psychiatr Scand 1989; 79:136–147
15. Allgulander C: Psychoactive drug use in a general population sample, Sweden: correlates with perceived health, psychiatric diagnoses, and mortality in an automated record-linkage study. Am J Public Health 1989; 79:1006–1010
16. Eaton WW, Anthony JC, Tepper S, Dryman A: Psychopathology and attrition in the Epidemiologic Catchment Area Study. Am J Epidemiol 1992; 135:1051–1059
17. US Department of Health and Human Services: National Health Interview Survey, 1989 (computer file). Hyattsville, Md, National Center for Health Statistics, 1992
18. Kessler RC, McGonagle KA, Zhao S, Nelson CB, Hughes M, Eshleman S, Wittchen H, Kendler KS: Lifetime and 12-month prevalence of DSM-III-R psychiatric disorders in the United States: results from the National Comorbidity Survey. Arch Gen Psychiatry 1994; 51:8–19
19. World Health Organization: Composite International Diagnostic Interview (CIDI, Version 1.0). Geneva, WHO, 1990
20. Robins LN, Wing J, Wittchen HU, Holzer JE: The Composite International Diagnostic Interview: an epidemiologic instrument suitable for use in conjunction with different diagnostic systems and in different cultures. Arch Gen Psychiatry 1988; 45:1069–1077
21. Robins LN, Helzer JE, Croughan J, Ratcliff KS: The National Institute of Mental Health Diagnostic Interview Schedule: its history, characteristics, and validity. Arch Gen Psychiatry 1981; 38: 381–389
22. Weissman MM, Bruce ML, Leaf PJ, Florio LP, Holzer C: Affective disorders, in Psychiatric Disorders in America. Edited by Regier DA, Robins LN. New York, Free Press, 1991
23. Woodruff RS, Causey BD: Computerized method for approximating the variance of a complicated estimate. J Am Statistical Assoc 1976; 71:315–321
24. Spitzer RL, Williams JBW, Gibbon M, First MB: The Structured Clinical Interview for DSM-III-R (SCID), I: history, rationale, and description. Arch Gen Psychiatry 1992; 49:624–629
25. Helzer JE, Robins LN, McEvoy LJ, Spitznagel EL, Stoltzman RK, Farmer A, Brockington IF: A comparison of clinical and Diagnostic Interview Schedule diagnoses: physician reexamination of lay-interviewed cases in the general population. Arch Gen Psychiatry 1985; 42:657–666
26. Anthony JC, Folstein M, Romanoski AJ, Von Korff MR, Nestadt GR, Chahal R, Merchant A, Brown CH, Shapiro S, Kramer M, Gruenberg EM: Comparison of the lay Diagnostic Interview Schedule and a standardized psychiatric diagnosis: experience in eastern Baltimore. Arch Gen Psychiatry 1985; 42:667–675
27. Blazer D, George LK, Landerman R, Pennybacker M, Melville ML, Woodbury M, Manton KG, Jordan K, Locke B: Psychiatric disorders: a rural/urban comparison. Arch Gen Psychiatry 1985; 42:651–656
28. Somervell PD, Leaf PJ, Weissman MM, Blazer DG, Bruce ML: The prevalence of major depression in black and white adults in five United States communities. Am J Epidemiol 1989; 130:725–735
29. Tennant C: Female vulnerability to depression. Psychol Med 1985; 15:733–737
30. Jorm AF: Sex and age differences in depression: a quantitative synthesis of published research. Aust NZ J Psychiatry 1987; 21: 46–53
31. Brown GW, Harris T: Social Origins of Depression: A Study of Psychiatric Disorder in Women. New York, Free Press, 1978

Comparing Age at Onset of Major Depression and Other Psychiatric Disorders by Birth Cohorts in Five US Community Populations

Kimberly Christie Burke, MS; Jack D. Burke, Jr, MD, MPH; Donald S. Rae, MS; Darrel A. Regier, MD, MPH

• Using data collected in the National Institute of Mental Health (Rockville, Md) Epidemiologic Catchment Area Program, we examined the proposed hypothesis that there has been a shift in major depression to younger ages at onset, or increased prevalence in younger age periods, for recent birth cohorts. Life-table survival methods were used to examine the hazard rates for major depression as well as for other specific mental disorders. The findings are consistent with a gradual shift to increased rates for major depression between the ages of 15 and 19 years for Epidemiologic Catchment Area respondents born more recently. The findings also suggest a similar shift for drug abuse/dependence; similar but less pronounced changes were found for alcohol abuse/dependence and obsessive-compulsive disorder. However, in this study, bipolar disorder, panic disorder, and phobias did not exhibit a consistent increase in onset at younger ages. Further research is required to determine if the shifts in major depression, drug abuse/dependence, and possibly alcohol abuse/dependence are linked. It is important to note that these shifts to adolescent onset are occurring when nearly half the 31 million Americans without health insurance are aged 24 years or younger.

(*Arch Gen Psychiatry.* 1991;48:789-795)

A recent life-table analysis of the age at onset of mental disorders among respondents from the National Institute of Mental Health (NIMH, Rockville, Md) Epidemiologic Catchment Area (ECA) Program[1-6] suggested the importance of onset in adolescence and early adulthood for several specific mental disorders, including major depression.[7] This finding is consistent with the suggestion by Klerman et al[8-11] and others[12-17] that members of recent generations are displaying higher rates and/or younger ages at onset for major depression compared with members of older generations.

Klerman and Weissman[11] recently reviewed evidence suggesting an increase in the rate of major depression among people born since World War II. In 1976, Klerman[8] hypothesized that western societies were entering an "Age of Melancholy" and reported that clinical depression was increasing in adolescence and young adulthood. Later, results from a longitudinal study conducted between 1947 and 1972 in Lundby, Sweden, demonstrated that the probability of suffering a mild or moderate case of depression increased during that 25-year period for both sexes.[13] More recent studies examining relatives of patients have also reported evidence in support of increased rates of major depression,[9] earlier onset of major depression in successive birth cohorts,[14] and a statistically significant difference between the hazard rates for major depression developing for patients born before 1940 and patients born after 1940.[15] Similarly, a study examining hospital records in Zurich, Switzerland, reported that the number of admissions for major depression increased substantially from 1920 to 1982.[16] Most recently, Wickramaratne et al[12] examined birth cohort trends among a subsample of NIMH ECA respondents. For the 10 640 white ECA respondents, they reported increased rates of major depressive episode for both men and women born after 1935, with evidence of a period effect on respondents of all ages after 1960.

Three studies have also examined data relative to bipolar disorders. Angst's[16] study of Zurich admission records also showed increases for bipolar disorder since 1920, and two reports examining relatives in family studies have suggested increases for bipolar I disorder[17] or a category combining bipolar and schizoaffective disorders.[15]

Although findings from these recent investigations suggest a temporal change in recent generations, with major depression and possibly bipolar disorder having earlier ages at onset and/or higher rates than had been true in older generations, the studies have to varying degrees been subject to two limitations. First, these studies generally have not examined other nonaffective disorders to investigate whether the shift to earlier ages at onset is a general phenomenon displayed in all disorders or perhaps a methodologic artifact. Second, these studies typically have not used large, representative general population samples.

To address these problems, this analysis examines selected Diagnostic Interview Schedule (DIS)–*DSM-III* psychiatric disorders, in addition to major depression, in the

Accepted for publication September 20, 1990.

From the Office of the Institute Director (Ms Burke), Division of Applied and Services Research (Dr Burke), and Division of Clinical [illegible] Health, Rockville, Md. Ms Burke is now with Scott and White Clinic, Temple, Tex.

Reprint requests to Scott and White Clinic, 2401 S 31st St, Alexander Bldg, Temple, TX 76508 (Ms Burke).

total NIMH ECA sample of community and institutional residents in terms of two questions. (1) For major depression, has there been a shift to younger ages at onset in more recent birth cohorts? (2) Has any such shift for major depression been matched by similar shifts for other disorders, including drug or alcohol abuse/dependence, the anxiety disorders, or bipolar disorder? In this analysis, self-reported onset experience for the first 30 years of life will be compared for all NIMH ECA respondents grouped into four birth cohorts over the past century.

SUBJECTS AND METHODS

NIMH ECA Program

The data used to analyze the hypothesized shift in the age at onset and/or the increase in rates for major depression were collected as part of the NIMH ECA Program. The NIMH ECA Program was a combined household and institutional survey of mental disorders conducted in five sites throughout the United States, and it has been described in detail elsewhere.[1-7,18] This analysis is based on data from 20 745 household and institutional respondents who were aged 18 years and older at time of entry into the study. Data were excluded for an additional 116 respondents for whom year of birth was missing.

Diagnoses of specific mental disorders were made using the DIS.[19] Designed for use by nonclinicians in epidemiologic studies, this instrument uses self-reported information about symptoms to make diagnoses of specific mental disorders based on *DSM-III* criteria.[20] If a positive diagnosis can be made based on the symptoms reported, an inquiry is made to determine the age at first occurrence of the symptoms. Although it is possible that this first occurrence may not have been severe enough to pass the threshold for a *DSM-III* diagnosis, that initial episode is generally used as the one for dating onset of the disorder in the NIMH ECA data set and appears to be most relevant for dating onset in general.[7,11,12]

The NIMH ECA Program involved complex multistage sampling procedures[21]; therefore, the respondents have been weighted to reflect their probability of selection and then have been weighted to the 1980 US Census on the basis of age, sex, and race/ethnicity as described previously.[18,21]

Life-Table Survival Methods

Life-table survival methods, similar to those used in a recent examination of the age at onset of mental disorders in the NIMH ECA,[7] were used to compare the age at onset of selected mental disorders by birth cohorts. Survival methods were used to examine average yearly hazard rates for specific 5-year age intervals. A hazard rate gives the probability that a disorder will develop during a time interval in a respondent who enters that interval and who is free of a disorder at the beginning of that interval.[7,22,23] In this analysis, the time interval was defined as a range of 5 years during which age at onset could occur, for example, 15 to 19 years or 20 to 24 years.

Using the Statistical Package for the Social Sciences (SPSS) Survival program,[24] hazard rates to age 30 years were examined across four birth cohorts. The birth cohorts examined were those born before 1917 (unweighted n = 6566), between 1917 and 1936 (n = 4432), between 1937 and 1952 (n = 4981), and between 1953 and 1966 (n = 4766). Using an observation period from birth to 30 years of age allowed the comparison of each birth cohort for equivalent periods of risk; 30 years was the oldest age possible for a respondent born in the youngest birth cohort (1953 to 1966) at the time of interview. The youngest birth cohort is the only one whose members may have been less than 30 years of age, but life tables have the advantage of adjusting for the fact that subjects have different ages, or, in analogy to treatment outcome studies, that they have been followed up for different periods.[25]

For each disorder, the hazard rates of the four birth cohorts were compared using the Lee-Desu[26] statistic, which follows a χ^2 distribution with $g-1$ *df*, where g is the number of groups under comparison. This approach tests whether the distributions of onset in the first 30 years of life for the four birth cohorts were drawn from the same population or were significantly different. It compares the probabilities in the cohorts in all age intervals simultaneously[27] and is similar to other analyses of the cohort effect.[15,28] However, there is no method (eg, based on proportional hazards models) to test specifically for shifts in the peak age at onset while applying the complex weights of the ECA data.[12] Rather than using unweighted data, which would be inappropriate for the total ECA sample, we have relied on a graphic approach to identify apparent shifts in peak age at onset.[29] However, these apparent shifts cannot be tested for statistical significance by this approach.[29]

The SPSS software program appropriately weighted the data based on the sampling procedures to produce estimates of hazard rates. However, the program cannot accurately determine the variance associated with complex sampling designs like that used in the NIMH ECA Program. Therefore, two adjustments were necessary before tests of significance could be performed to determine if the onset experience differed by birth cohorts.[7] First, to assure that the sampling weights did not inflate the statistical power of comparisons, the weighted sample was adjusted to the same size as the total actual sample; to accomplish this, the sampling weight used for the five sites was multiplied by the number of respondents in the NIMH ECA sample and then divided by the 1980 US Census population. Second, the χ^2 test statistics were divided by the estimated sample design effect before calculation of P values. This conservative adjustment was done based on repeated estimates of the design effect for prevalences in these conditions that ranged from 1.5 to 2.0[7,30]; these design effect estimates were produced by the program SESUDAAN[31] developed for analyzing such complex surveys. These adjustments are equivalent to reducing the sample size by the design effect.[32]

RESULTS

Hazard rates were plotted and compared for statistically significant differences. The four cohorts examined will be referred to as cohort 1 (respondents born between 1953 and 1966), cohort 2 (respondents born between 1937 and 1952), cohort 3 (respondents born between 1917 and 1936), and cohort 4 (respondents born before 1917). These cohorts were similar to those used by Weissman et al[28] in the initial analysis of NIMH ECA data from New Haven (Conn) respondents. Since the five NIMH ECA sites entered the field at different times in the early 1980s, the end point for cohort 1 is shown as 1966, which is the latest year of birth of any NIMH ECA respondent and applies to the Los Angeles (Calif) site.

Mood Disorders

Unipolar Major Depressive Episode.—For the first 30 years of life in each cohort, Fig 1 plots the hazard rates for development of unipolar major depressive episode (with no lifetime history of manic episodes). For those NIMH ECA respondents born between 1953 and 1966, the hazard rates for unipolar major depression developing peak during two age intervals: 15 to 19 and 25 to 29 years of age. In the age interval 15 to 19 years, there also appears to be an increase in the magnitude of the hazard rate for respondents in cohort 1 compared with those respondents in cohort 2, and similarly for cohort 2 compared with cohort 3. This trend is made apparent by examining the ratio of the hazard rate for ages 15 to 19 years to the hazard rate for ages 25 to 29 years: cohort 1, 0.0055/0.0064 = 0.86; cohort 2, 0.0032/0.0062 = 0.52; and cohort 3, 0.0005/0.0019 = 0.26. The ratio for cohort 4 goes against this trend, but it is based on much smaller hazard rates (0.0003/0.0002 = 1.50).

The hazard rates for major depression developing for respondents born in cohort 1 and for those respondents born in cohort 2 are significantly different ($\chi^2 = 14.2$, $df = 1$, $P = .0002$). The hazard rates for major depression developing for respondents in cohort 2 compared with cohort 3 are also significantly different ($\chi^2 = 85.3$, $df = 1$, $P < .0001$).

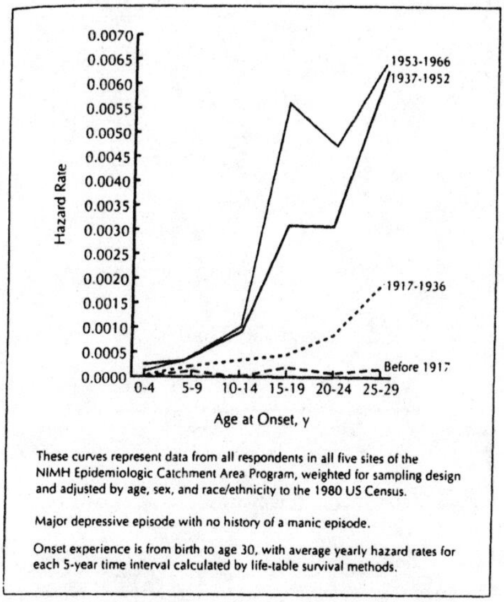

Fig 1.—*Hazard rate by year of birth for unipolar major depression (with no history of a manic episode), by Diagnostic Interview Schedule–DSM-III criteria, for cohorts born before 1917 (dashed line), from 1917 to 1936 (broken line), from 1937 to 1952 (solid line), and from 1953 to 1966 (lightly shaded line). NIMH indicates National Institute of Mental Health.*

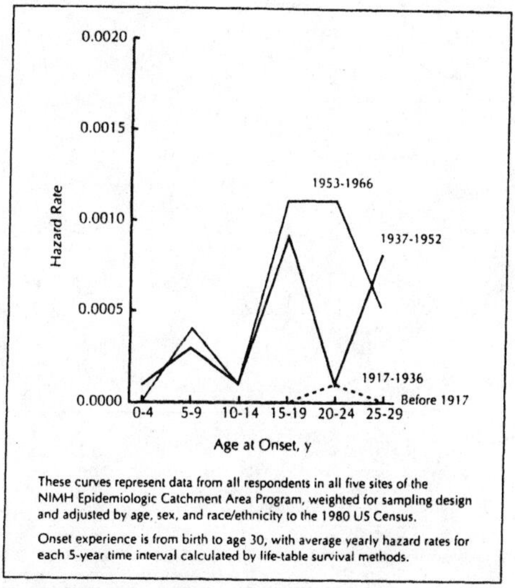

Fig 2.—*Hazard rate by year of birth for mania by same criteria and for same cohorts as in Fig 1. NIMH indicates National Institute of Mental Health.*

Bipolar Disorder.—For those respondents with a diagnosis of mania, there is no apparent shift to an earlier age at onset for the manic episode for those born most recently (Fig 2). The hazard rates for respondents born in cohort 1 compared with the hazard rates for those born in cohort 2 are not significantly different ($\chi^2=1.4$, $df=1$, $P=.240$). However, for those respondents born in cohort 2 compared with those born in cohort 3, the hazard rates are significantly different ($\chi^2=24.0$, $df=1$, $P<.0001$).

In Fig 3, additional information on bipolar disorder is presented. For those ECA respondents with a lifetime diagnosis of mania, the age at onset information presented is the youngest age at which either a major depressive or manic episode occurred, using the age for whichever episode came first. As with manic episode alone (Fig 2), there does not appear to have been a change in age at onset for respondents born in cohort 1 compared with those born in cohort 2 ($\chi^2=0.18$, $df=1$, $P=.6705$). The hazard rates for respondents born in cohort 2 compared with those born in cohort 3 are significantly different ($\chi^2=27.2$, $df=1$, $P<.0001$).

Anxiety Disorders

Panic Disorder.—For ECA respondents, there has been no apparent shift in the age at onset for panic disorder (Fig 4). The peak hazard occurs in the age interval 25 to 29 years for birth cohorts 1, 2, and 3. There is no significant difference between the hazard rates for respondents born after 1953 compared with the hazard rates for respondents born in cohort 2 ($\chi^2=0.5$, $df=1$, $P=.5$). However, the rates for birth cohort 2 are significantly different from the rates for respondents born in cohort 3 ($\chi^2=20.2$, $df=1$, $P<.0001$).

Obsessive-Compulsive Disorder.—For obsessive-compulsive disorder, there appears to have been a shift to a younger age at onset for the most recent birth cohort (cohort 1). Figure 5, a plot of the hazard rates by birth cohorts, shows that the peak hazard rate for cohort 1 occurs during the age interval 20 to 24 years, while the peak hazards for cohorts 2 and 3 both occur in the age interval 25 to 29 years. The hazard rates for respondents born in cohort 1 compared with the rates for respondents born in cohort 2 are significantly different ($\chi^2=9.5$, $df=1$, $P=.002$). The hazard rates for respondents born in cohort 2 and respondents born in cohort 3 ($\chi^2=16.3$, $df=1$, $P<.0001$) are also significantly different.

Phobias.—Figure 6 demonstrates that the hazard rate for development of phobias is highest for cohort 1 in the age interval 10 to 14 years, while the peak hazard for cohorts 2, 3, and 4 occurs in the interval 5 to 9 years. The difference between cohort 1 and cohort 2 just reaches statistical significance ($\chi^2=4.3$, $df=1$, $P=.04$). A significant difference in developing phobias for those respondents born in cohort 2 and those respondents born in cohort 3 is found ($\chi^2=21.1$, $df=1$, $P<.0001$).

Drug and Alcohol Use Disorders

Drug Abuse/Dependence.—In addition to the much higher rates in the youngest cohort, which may be observed by the need to break the vertical axis of the graph, there also appears to be a shift to a younger age at onset for respondents born in cohort 1 compared with cohort 2 for drug abuse/dependence (Fig 7). The peak hazard occurs between the ages of 15 and 19 years for cohort 1 and between the ages of 20 and 24 years for cohort 2; the difference between the hazard rates for respondents born in cohort 1 and for respondents born in cohort 2 is significant ($\chi^2=179.4$, $df=1$, $P<.0001$). There is also a significant difference between the hazard rates for respondents born in cohort 2 and respondents born in cohort 3 ($\chi^2=159.1$, $df=1$, $P<.0001$).

Alcohol Abuse/Dependence.—Like drug abuse/dependence, the hazard rates for alcohol abuse/dependence are highest for those NIMH ECA respondents born between 1953 and 1966 (Fig 8). The difference between the hazard rates for cohort 1 compared with cohort 2 ($\chi^2=58.0$, $df=1$, $P<.0001$) is significant. A significant difference is also found between the hazard rates for respondents born in cohort 2 and rates for respondents born in cohort 3 ($\chi^2=62.3$, $df=1$, $P<.0001$). As with major depression, a trend toward increasing importance of the 15- to 19-year age interval is also seen in Fig 8 across the four cohorts.

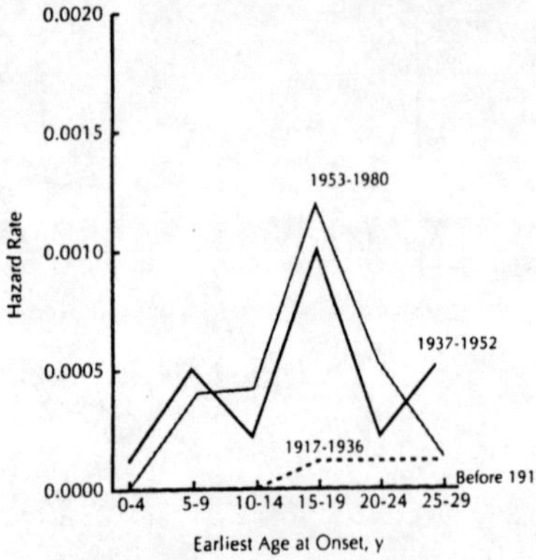

These curves represent data from all respondents in all five sites of the NIMH Epidemiologic Catchment Area Program, weighted for sampling design and adjusted by age, sex, and race/ethnicity to the 1980 US Census.

Mania with or without major depressive episode; onset is for mania unless major depressive episode occurred earlier.

Onset experience is from birth to age 30, with average yearly hazard rates for each 5-year time interval calculated by life-table survival methods.

Fig 3.—*Hazard rate by year of birth for mania (with or without a major depressive episode; onset is for mania unless major depressive episode occurred earlier) by same criteria and for same cohorts as in Fig 1. NIMH indicates National Institute of Mental Health.*

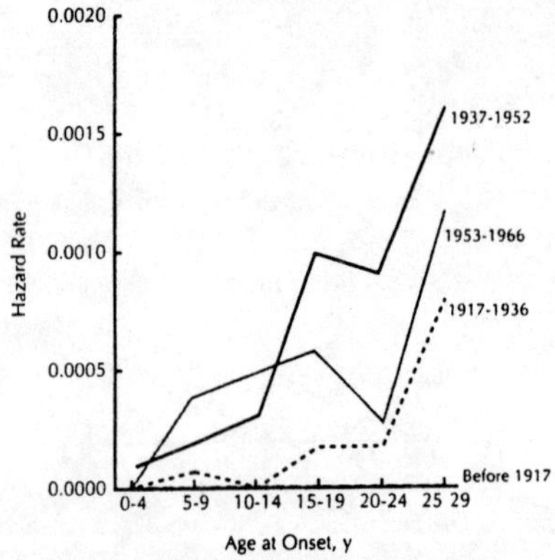

These curves represent data from all respondents in all five sites of the NIMH Epidemiologic Catchment Area Program, weighted for sampling design and adjusted by age, sex, and race/ethnicity to the 1980 US Census.

Onset experience is from birth to age 30, with average yearly hazard rates for each 5-year time interval calculated by life-table survival methods.

Fig 4.—*Hazard rate by year of birth for panic disorder by same criteria and for same cohorts as in Fig 1. NIMH indicates National Institute of Mental Health.*

Fig 5.—*Hazard rate by year of birth for obsessive-compulsive disorder by same criteria and for same cohorts as in Fig 1. NIMH indicates National Institute of Mental Health.*

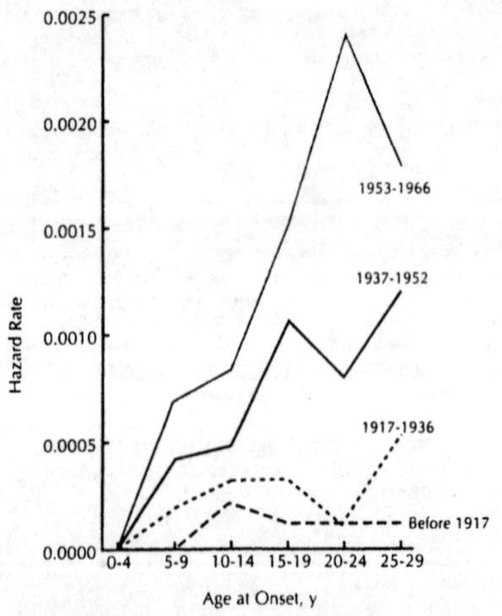

These curves represent data from all respondents in all five sites of the NIMH Epidemiologic Catchment Area Program, weighted for sampling design and adjusted by age, sex, and race/ethnicity to the 1980 US Census.

Onset experience is from birth to age 30, with average yearly hazard rates for each 5-year time interval calculated by life-table survival methods.

Fig 6.—*Hazard rate by year of birth for phobias (agoraphobia, simple phobia, or social phobia) by same criteria and for same cohorts as in Fig 1. NIMH indicates National Institute of Mental Health.*

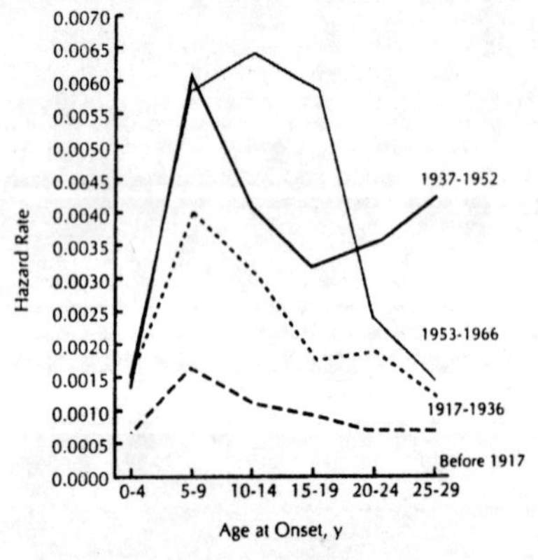

These curves represent data from all respondents in all five sites of the NIMH Epidemiologic Catchment Area Program, weighted for sampling design and adjusted by age, sex, and race/ethnicity to the 1980 US Census.

Agoraphobia, simple phobia, or social phobia.

Onset experience is from birth to age 30, with average yearly hazard rates for each 5-year time interval calculated by life-table survival methods.

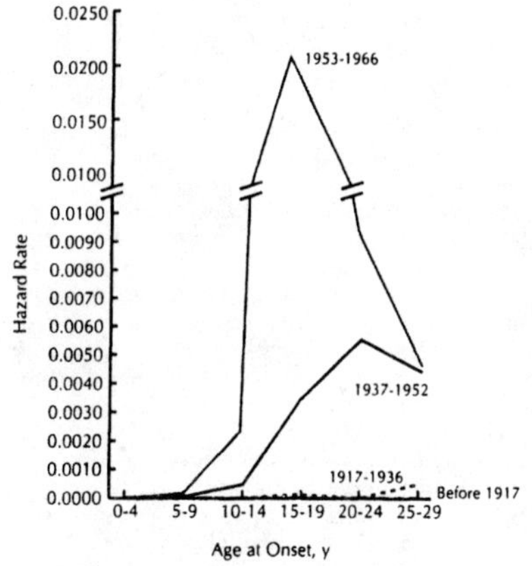

These curves represent data from all respondents in all five sites of the NIMH Epidemiologic Catchment Area Program, weighted for sampling design and adjusted by age, sex, and race/ethnicity to the 1980 US Census.

Onset experience is from birth to age 30, with average yearly hazard rates for each 5-year time interval calculated by life-table survival methods.

Fig 7.—*Hazard rate by year of birth for drug abuse/dependence by same criteria and for same cohorts as in Fig 1. NIMH indicates National Institute of Mental Health.*

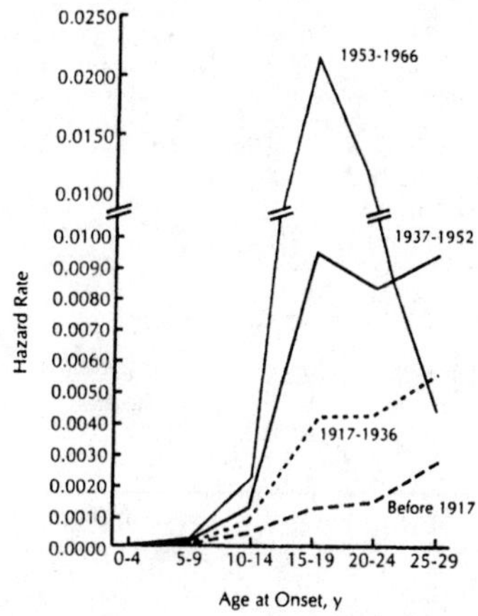

These curves represent data from all respondents in all five sites of the NIMH Epidemiologic Catchment Area Program, weighted for sampling design and adjusted by age, sex, and race/ethnicity to the 1980 US Census.

Onset experience is from birth to age 30, with average yearly hazard rates for each 5-year time interval calculated by life-table survival methods.

Fig 8.—*Hazard rate by year of birth for alcohol abuse/dependence by same criteria and for same cohorts as in Fig 1. NIMH indicates National Institute of Mental Health.*

COMMENT

For unipolar major depression, there appears to have been a gradual increase in the hazard rate for the interval 15 to 19 years of age across the three cohorts born since 1917. These findings are consistent with Klerman's hypothesis[8-11] and the findings of other studies[12-16] that members of recent birth cohorts have a higher risk of having a major depressive episode. One interesting but unexplained finding is the apparent importance of the 15- to 19-year age interval for the oldest cohort, born before 1917. Gershon et al[15] reported a similar, unexplainable increase in hazard rates for relatives born from 1910 to 1919 in an earlier family study, compared with other decades of birth before 1940. That study, and the current findings from the ECA, depend on retrospective recall from respondents for documenting lifetime history and age at onset, but the similarity may suggest the need to examine possible commonalities between that cohort and the more recent ones that appear to experience higher onset rates in adolescence.

For bipolar disorder, these results are not able to corroborate suggestions of a cohort effect shown in some earlier studies.[15-17] Whether this difference is caused by differences in sampling, as those studies used either relatives of probands or admission rates to a psychiatric hospital, or by differences in diagnostic assessment is not clear. It is also possible that a small effect that could be detected in a sample of high-risk family members could not be demonstrated in a general population study for a relatively uncommon disorder such as bipolar disorder.

For drug abuse/dependence, there has been a shift to a younger age at onset for the most recent cohort as well as an increase in the magnitude of the hazard rate for those respondents born between 1953 and 1966. For alcohol abuse/dependence, there has not been a shift in the peak age at onset, since the age period 15 to 19 years was also of predominant importance for cohort 2, but there has been a progressive increase in the magnitude and predominance of the hazard rate in the 15- to 19-year age interval.

Earlier Studies

These findings are interesting for several reasons. They corroborate earlier analyses of a subsample of ECA respondents and findings from other, more targeted, samples for major depression. It is noteworthy that the earlier results can be shown in a large general population sample that includes both sexes, multiple racial and ethnic groups, and five different community sites. They also demonstrate that some disorders, particularly drug abuse/dependence, exhibit the same changes. The demonstration of widely different patterns of onset across the two most recent birth cohorts for the specific disorders examined herein suggests that the shifts observed for major depression and drug abuse/dependence are not the result of a simple methodologic artifact.

The evidence of increasing onset from 15 to 19 years of age for major depression, drug abuse/dependence, and possibly alcohol abuse/dependence raises important questions about the possible association of these conditions. Prior analyses of a subset of ECA respondents in the 18- to 30-year age range have shown that an earlier major depressive or anxiety disorder approximately doubles the risk of subsequent drug abuse/dependence for both men and women (but not alcohol abuse/dependence).[33] Findings from the Yale University (New Haven) Family Study have also shown that major depression occurring before the age of 30 years is linked with panic and drug use disorders.[34] Klerman and Weissman[11] have discussed environmental factors that may contribute to the apparent shift to earlier onset for depression and higher rates in younger cohorts, such as changing family structure and increasing urbanization. In this analysis of ECA data, the youngest cohort also appears to have increased onset of drug abuse/dependence in adolescence. While it has been known that first use of drugs typically occurs in this age period, it is not clear whether the earlier occurrence of major depression somehow contributes to an earlier onset of clinical disorders of drug abuse/dependence in adolescents who may have only experimented with drug use in earlier cohorts. If so, the shift to an earlier age at onset for major depression could be one of the factors leading to increased drug abuse/dependence in the same period of late adolescence.

For obsessive-compulsive disorder, the peak hazard has shifted to a somewhat younger age at onset for the most recently born cohort (respondents born between 1953 and 1966). The onset has shifted from 25 to 29 years of age to 20 to 24 years of age. This demonstration of an apparent shift in onset of an anxiety disorder, if it is found in other studies, may raise the possibility of studying whether onset of the disorder is also possibly linked to the shifts in depression and drug abuse/dependence, or at least whether it results from similar factors.

By restricting analysis to the first 30 years of life for each cohort, this approach does not permit identification of period effects like those shown by Lavori et al[14] for the 1970s and Wickramaratne et al[12] for the 1960s and 1970s. A period effect would operate uniformly on respondents without regard to their age at a particular time in history. The analysis is restricted herein to life before the age of 30 years to allow meaningful tests of significance of any differences observed between cohorts. For that reason, there is no adequate basis for examining the effects of particular calendar years to determine if all respondents show increased rates (period effect) or only those born more recently (cohort effect).

For all disorders examined, a significant difference was found in onset between cohorts 3 and 2. This finding is consistent with earlier reports of the cohort effect for major depression for persons born after 1940. However, the uniform finding for all disorders may represent either a profound effect or a methodologic limitation resulting from retrospective reporting. Further efforts to understand the basis of this apparently uniform effect would be of great importance, especially if methodologic limitations can be ruled out.

Limitations

Findings from epidemiologic studies must be interpreted cautiously, especially when they are early and information is available from only a few other similar studies. In addition to this general caution, there are two possible limitations in this specific analysis that deserve further consideration.

First, test-retest reliability of age-at-onset questions from the DIS suggests that agreement is adequate for all disorders examined herein, with the possible exception of phobias, where agreement with independent clinical examiners was weaker.[35] However, the test-retest agreement has not been good enough to justify use of narrow, 3-year age intervals, so this analysis has used 5-year intervals; onset patterns cannot be determined as precisely as desired in this retrospective analysis. For that reason, the apparent shift for obsessive-compulsive disorder (from 25 to 29 years to 20 to 24 years) and for drug abuse/dependence (from 20 to 24 years to 15 to 19 years) may be less robust than the larger shifts for major depression (from 25 to 29 years to 15 to 19 years).

Second, poor recall or poor reporting by older respondents of either symptom or onset data, or earlier mortality of those respondents with psychiatric disorders in the older cohorts, are also of concern in this retrospective analysis of cross-sectional data.[3,36] Recent evidence from one study that examined the reliability of recall for self-reported age at onset for specific mental disorders demonstrated a tendency for older respondents to increase their reported age at onset for major depression by a few years across interviews[37]; another more recent study found the opposite, that older subjects tend to lower rather than raise their estimated age at onset.[38] If older subjects do increase their reported age at onset, our finding of a uniform significant difference in the risk of developing disorders for respondents in cohort 2 (born between 1937 and 1952) and for respondents in cohort 3 (born from 1917 to 1936) for all disorders may be explained by this tendency. This finding may also support the cautious recommendation by Lavori et al[14] not to rely on age-at-onset reports for subjects older than 50 years. In the NIMH ECA study, there are no data that allow evaluation of recall problems in older subjects or the differential mortality problems in aging cohorts. However, the consistent demonstration of differences between cohorts 2 and 3 may indicate methodologic problems rather than a cohort effect applying to every disorder examined herein. While the shift around World War II was found in earlier studies for major depression, its considerably strong showing for every disorder may raise skepticism about the validity of such retrospective reporting for the oldest respondents (eg, >50 years).

CONCLUSION

With the apparent shift to earlier ages at onset, and with the general demonstration that childhood and adolescence are important periods for development of mental disorders, both research and policy issues arise. Ideally, research on the age at onset of psychiatric disorders should be conducted prospectively to improve accuracy of the onset data and to distinguish cohort and period effects more directly. However, prospective studies to examine the proposed shift for recent birth cohorts have not been reported. As a result, increased study of the onset of disorders in adolescence and early adulthood appears to be of great importance, especially to examine patterns of co-occurrence of depressive and drug use disorders. As noted by Klerman and Weissman,[11] research that is cross-cultural would be especially important in examining how different genetic and environmental factors interact to produce these changes in age at onset.[39]

In terms of policy implications, it should be noted that of the estimated 31 million Americans with no health insurance coverage in 1987, almost half (46%) were 24 years old or younger.[40] As a result, the general problem of ensuring adequate access to mental health services in this country is even more serious for the age group most likely to experience onset of these disorders.

The ECA is a series of five epidemiologic research studies performed by independent research teams in collaboration with staff of the NIMH.

NIMH Principal Collaborators.—Darrel A. Regier, MD, MPH, Ben Z. Locke, MSPH, and Jack D. Burke, Jr, MD, MPH.

NIMH Project Officer.—Carl A. Taube, PhD (1978-1985), and is now William Huber.

Principal Investigators and Coinvestigators.—Jerome K. Myers, PhD, Myrna M. Weissman, PhD, and Gary L. Tischler, MD, Yale University (grant U01 MH-34224); Morton Kramer, DSc, Ernest Gruenberg, MD, and Sam Shapiro, MS, The Johns Hopkins University, Baltimore, Md (grant U01 MH-33870); Lee N. Robins, PhD, and John Helzer, MD, Washington University, St Louis, Mo (grant U01 MH-33883); Linda George, PhD, and Dan Blazer, MD, Duke University, Durham, NC (grant U01 MH 35386); and Marvin Karno, MD, Richard L. Hough, PhD, Javier I. Escobar, MD, M. Audrey Burnam, PhD, and Dianne Timbers, PhD, UCLA (grant U01 MH-35865).

Helpful comments on earlier drafts of the manuscript by Susan Ahmed, PhD, are gratefully acknowledged.

References

1. Regier DA, Myers JK, Kramer M, Robins LN, Blazer DG, Hough RL, Eaton WW, Locke, BZ. The NIMH Epidemiologic Catchment Area program. *Arch Gen Psychiatry*. 1984;41:934-941.

2. Eaton WW, Holzer CE, Von Korff M, Anthony JC, Helzer JE, George L, Burnam A, Boyd JH, Kessler LG, Locke BZ. The design of the Epidemiologic Catchment Area surveys. *Arch Gen Psychiatry*. 1984;41:942-948.

3. Robins LN, Helzer JE, Weissman MM, Orvaschel H, Gruenberg E, Burke JD, Regier DA. Lifetime prevalence of specific psychiatric disorders in three sites. *Arch Gen Psychiatry*. 1984;41:949-958.

4. Myers JK, Weissman MM, Tischler GL, Holzer CE, Leaf PJ, Orvaschel H, Anthony JC, Boyd JH, Burke JD, Kramer M, Stoltzman R. Six-month prevalence of psychiatric disorders in three communities. *Arch Gen Psychiatry*. 1984;41:959-967.

5. Shapiro S, Skinner EA, Kessler LG, Von Korff M, German PS, Tischler GL, Leaf PJ, Benham L, Cottler L, Regier DA. Utilization of health and mental health services. *Arch Gen Psychiatry*. 1984;41:971-982.

6. Boyd JH, Burke JD, Gruenberg E, Holzer CE, Rae DS, George LK, Karno M, Stoltzman R, McEvoy L, Nestadt G. Exclusion criteria of *DSM-III*. *Arch Gen Psychiatry*. 1984;41:983-989.

7. Burke KC, Burke JD, Regier DA, Rae DS. Age at onset of selected mental disorders in five community populations. *Arch Gen Psychiatry*. 1990;47:511-518.

8. Klerman GL. Age and clinical depression: today's youth in the twenty-first century. *J Gerontol*. 1976;31:318-323.

9. Klerman GL, Lavori PW, Rice J, Reich T, Endicott J, Andreasen NC, Keller MB, Hirschfeld RMA. Birth-cohort trends in rates of major depressive disorder among relatives of patients with affective disorder. *Arch Gen Psychiatry*. 1985;42:689-693.

10. Klerman GL. The current age of youthful melancholia. *Br J Psychiatry*. 1988;152:4-14.

11. Klerman GL, Weissman MM. Increasing rates of depression. *JAMA*. 1989;261:2229-2235.

12. Wickramaratne PJ, Weissman MM, Leaf PJ, Holford TR. Age, period, and cohort effects on the risk of major depression. *J Clin Epidemiol*. 1989;42:333-343.

13. Hagnell O, Lanke J, Rorsman B, Ojesjo L. Are we entering an age of melancholy? depressive illness in a prospective epidemiological study over 25 years: the Lundby study, Sweden. *Psychol Med*. 1982;12:279-282.

14. Lavori PW, Klerman GL, Keller MB, Reich T, Rice J, Endicott J. Age-period-cohort analysis of secular trends in onset of major depression. *J Psychiatr Res*. 1987;21:23-35.

15. Gershon ES, Hamovit JH, Guroff JJ, Nurnberger JI. Birth-cohort changes in manic and depressive disorders in relatives of bipolar and schizoaffective patients. *Arch Gen Psychiatry*. 1987;44:314-319.

16. Angst J. Switch from depression to mania. *Psychopathology*. 1985;18:140-154.

17. Price RA, Kidd KK, Paul DL, Gershon ES, Prusoff BA, Weissman MM, Goldin LR. Multiple threshold models for the affective disorders. *J Psychiatr Res*. 1985;19:533-546.

18. Regier DA, Boyd JH, Burke JD, Rae DS, Myers JK, Kramer M, Robins LN, George LK, Karno M, Locke BZ. One-month prevalence of mental disorders in the U.S.: based on five epidemiologic catchment sites. *Arch Gen Psychiatry*. 1988;45:977-986.

19. Robins LN, Helzer JE, Croughan J, Ratcliff KS. NIMH DIS: its history, characteristics, and validity. *Arch Gen Psychiatry*. 1981;38:381-389.

20. American Psychiatric Association, Committee on Nomenclature and Statistics. *Diagnostic and Statistical Manual of Mental Disorders, Third Edition*. Washington, DC: American Psychiatric Association; 1980:215.

21. Eaton WW, Kessler LG, eds. *Epidemiologic Field Methods in Psychiatry*. Orlando, Fla: Academic Press Inc; 1985.

22. Gross A, Clark V. *Survival Distribution: Reliability Applications With Biomedical Science*. New York, NY: John Wiley & Sons Inc; 1975.

23. Kalbfleisch JD, Prentice RL. *The Statistical Analysis of Failure Time Data*. New York, NY: John Wiley & Sons Inc; 1980.

24. *SPSS User's Guide*. 2nd ed. New York, NY: McGraw-Hill International Book Co; 1986:875-887.

25. Fleiss JL, Dunner DL, Stallone F, Fieve RR. The life table. *Arch Gen Psychiatry*. 1976;33:107-112.

26. Lee ET, Desu MM. A computer program for comparing K samples with right censored data. *Comput Methods Programs Biomed*. 1972;2:315-321.

27. Robertson CO, Gehan EA. A computer sub-program for calculating the generalized Wilcoxon test. *Comput Methods Programs Biomed*. 1972;2:315-321.

28. Weissman MM, Leaf PJ, Holzer CE, Myers JK, Tischler GL. The epidemiology of depression: an update on sex differences in rates. *J Affective Disord*. 1984;7:179-188.

29. Wickramaratne PJ, Prusoff BA, Merikangas KR, Weissman MM. The use of survival time models with nonproportional hazard functions to investigate age of onset in family studies. *J Chronic Dis*. 1986;39:389-397.

30. Kessler LG, Folsom R, Royall R, Forsythe A, McEvoy L, Holzer CE, Rae DS, Woodbury M. Parameter and variance estimation. In: Eaton WW, Kessler LG, eds. *Epidemiologic Field Methods in Psychiatry*. Orlando, Fla: Academic Press Inc; 1985:327-349.

31. Shah BV. *SESUDAAN: Standard Errors Program for Computing of Standardized Rates from Sample Survey Data*. Research Triangle Park, NC: Research Triangle Institute; 1981.

32. Kish L. *Survey Sampling*. New York, NY: John Wiley & Sons Inc; 1965:575-577.

33. Christie KA, Burke JD, Regier DA, Rae DS, Boyd JH, Locke BZ. Epidemiologic evidence for early onset of mental disorders and higher risk of drug abuse in young adults. *Am J Psychiatry*. 1988;145:971-975.

34. Price RA, Kidd KK, Weissman MM. Early onset (under age 30 years) and panic disorder as markers for etiologic homogeneity in major depression. *Arch Gen Psychiatry*. 1987;44:434-440.

35. Wittchen HU, Burke JD, Semlar G, Pfister H, Von Cranach M, Zaudig M. Recall and dating of psychiatric symptoms. *Arch Gen Psychiatry*. 1989;46:437-443.

36. Hasin D, Link B. Age and recognition of depression. *Psychol Med*. 1988;18:683-688.

37. Prusoff BA, Merikangas KR, Weissman MM. Lifetime prevalence and age of onset of psychiatric disorders: recall 4 years later. *J Psychiatr Res*. 1988;22:107-117.

38. Farrer LA, Florio LP, Bruce ML, Leaf PJ, Weissman MM. Reliability of self-reported age at onset of major depression. *J Psychiatr Res*. 1989;23:35-47.

39. Sartorius N, Nielsen JA, Stromgren E. Changes in frequency of mental disorder over time. *Acta Psychiatr Scand*. 1989;79:suppl 348.

40. Moyer ME. A revised look at the number of uninsured Americans. *Health Affairs*. 1989(summer);8:102-110.

Socioeconomic Burden of Subsyndromal Depressive Symptoms and Major Depression in a Sample of the General Population

Lewis L. Judd, M.D., Martin P. Paulus, M.D.,
Kenneth B. Wells, M.D., M.P.H., and Mark H. Rapaport, M.D.

Objective: The authors' goal was to evaluate the association between impairment in daily function and subsyndromal depressive symptoms as well as major depression to determine the economic and societal significance of these conditions. Method: Using 12-month prevalence data gathered by the National Institute of Mental Health (NIMH) Epidemiologic Catchment Area Program (ECA), based on responses to the NIMH Diagnostic Interview Schedule, the authors divided the 2,393 subjects from the Los Angeles ECA site into three groups: subjects with subsyndromal depressive symptoms (N=270), major depression (N=102), and no depressive disorder or symptoms (N=2,021). The groups were compared on 10 domains of functional outcome and well-being. Results: Significantly more subjects with depressive symptoms than subjects who had no disorder reported high levels of household strain, social irritability, and financial strain as well as limitations in physical or job functioning, restricted activity days, bed days, and poor health status. Significantly more subjects with major depression than subjects with no disorder reported major financial losses, bed days, high levels of financial strain, limitations in physical or job functioning, and poor health status. Except for lower self-ratings of health status, no significant differences were found between subjects with subsyndromal symptoms and those with major depression. Conclusions: Significantly more people with subsyndromal depressive symptoms or major depression reported impairment in eight of 10 functional domains than did subjects with no disorder. The high 1-year prevalence of subsyndromal depressive symptoms, combined with the associated functional impairment, emphasizes the clinical and public health importance and need for additional investigations into these symptoms.

(Am J Psychiatry 1996; 153:1411–1417)

Interest in subthreshold depression has increased since the report of Wells et al. (1) that subthreshold depressive symptoms in medical and psychiatric outpatients were associated with significant levels of psychosocial dysfunction. Epidemiologic studies have confirmed that, compared with no depressive symptoms, subthreshold depressions, variously defined, are associated with more disability and work days lost (1–3), greater use of services for mental health problems (3), poor self-ratings of emotional health (1, 3, 4), and more lifetime suicide attempts (5).

To clarify the clinical significance of subthreshold depressive symptoms, we defined a more restrictive condition, subsyndromal depressive symptoms, as at least two or more current depressive symptoms, present for most or all of the time, lasting for at least 2 weeks, in individuals who did not meet criteria for major depression or dysthymia. Using this definition, we found that 11.8% of 9,160 community residents in the National Institute of Mental Health (NIMH) Epidemiologic Catchment Area Program (ECA) met criteria for subsyndromal depressive symptoms during a 1-year period (6). Two-thirds of the subjects with subsyndromal depressive symptoms were women; the most common depressive symptoms were insomnia, fatigue, and recurrent thoughts of death. Significantly more subjects with subsyndromal depressive symptoms than other subjects reported lifetime disability benefits, raising the question of whether subsyndromal depressive symptoms are associated with sufficient disruption in the domains of

Received July 12, 1995; revisions received Jan. 11 and April 16, 1996; accepted June 3, 1996. From the Department of Psychiatry, University of California, San Diego; the Psychiatry Service, San Diego VA Medical Center; the Department of Psychiatry and Biobehavioral Sciences, University of California, Los Angeles; and the Rand Corporation, Santa Monica, Calif. Address reprint requests to Dr. Judd, UCSD Department of Psychiatry, 9500 Gilman Dr., La Jolla, CA 92093-0603.

Supported by NIMH Clinical Research Center grant MH-30914 and the Rohrer Fund.

The authors thank Bernadette Benjamin of the Rand Corporation for her assistance in conducting the statistical analysis.

everyday function to have demonstrable public health, societal, and economic impact.

To address this question, we analyzed the database from the Los Angeles site of the ECA, where the investigators systematically probed domains of daily function not obtained at other ECA sites. Results of respondents with subsyndromal depressive symptoms were compared with those of respondents who had no depressive disorder or symptoms. Because the severe impairment associated with major depression has been established unequivocally (1–4, 7), subjects with major depression were included for reference comparison of disability. Two a priori hypotheses were tested: 1) Significantly more subjects with subsyndromal depressive symptoms than subjects with no depressive disorder or symptoms will report functional impairment. 2) Significantly more subjects with major depression than subjects with subsyndromal depressive symptoms or no depressive disorder or symptoms will report functional impairment. Militating against hypothesis 2 are empirical reports that subjects with subsyndromal depressive symptoms, even though significantly less impaired, are relatively comparable in impairment to subjects with major depression (1–4).

METHOD

The sampling methodology, human subject consent procedures, study design, survey methods, and demographic characteristics of the ECA sample have been reported elsewhere (8–10). ECA DSM-III diagnoses were developed from responses to the NIMH Diagnostic Interview Schedule (DIS), previously described in the literature (11, 12). A Spanish-language version of the DIS was also used at the Los Angeles site of the ECA (13, 14).

At three ECA sites, including Los Angeles, data were collected for each individual mental symptom probed by the DIS and the time frames when symptoms occurred (i.e., 1 month, 6 months, 1 year, or lifetime). The DIS specifies a standardized threshold to determine if a symptom is clinically significant. For example, depressive symptoms must have been present for at least 2 weeks and substantial enough that the respondent had either talked to a health professional or had taken medications because of it or felt the symptom had interfered substantially with his or her everyday activities. Depressive symptoms identified by the DIS are clinically substantial in severity and duration, extending well beyond normal mood vicissitudes. The DIS requires that depressive or other mental symptoms should not be associated with current medical illnesses and should not be side effects of drug or alcohol consumption or problems; symptoms associated with these conditions are excluded.

The Los Angeles ECA interviews included questions probing 10 domains of functional outcomes and well-being. Details of the content and methodology of these measures have been reported elsewhere (15–18) but will be summarized here.

Domains of Daily Function

1. High or low social irritability in previous 6 months. Respondents were asked how often over the last 6 months they had felt upset, irritated, or angry in six types of social relationships: with friends, with spouse, with other adults in the household, with family members and relatives not living with the respondent, with boss or supervisor at work, and with co-workers. Response categories were not at all, less than once a month, once a month, a few times a month, and once a week or more. Responses were averaged for each respondent across all applicable categories and then, due to high skewness, were dichotomized into 1) being irritable less than once a month or 2) being irritable more than once a month.

2. High or low household strain. This domain of function is based on the employment strain scale of Pearlin and Lieberman (19) but applied to household responsibilities by Golding (20). Respondents were asked to answer yes or no to four items: "I have more home (and family) duties than I am able to do," "I spend too many hours taking care of my home (and family)," "I do more work around the house than I should have to do," and "Household and family responsibilities keep me from doing things I would really like to do." Dichotomous scoring recommended by Golding (20) was used, in which responses were scored as high when any of the four items was endorsed.

3. High or low social contacts in previous month. Number of contacts (visits or telephone calls) during the last month with friends, family members, or other adults (but not including any persons living in household) were summed. Skewed response distribution required dichotomized scoring: a rating of high was given to reports of 13 or more contacts in the last month, and a rating of low was given to reports of fewer than 13 in the last month.

4. Major financial loss in previous 6 months. This domain was scored present if one or more of the following five items occurred during the last 6 months: job loss, someone important to the respondent was out of work for 1 month or more, loss of home or anything else important, or the financial situation of someone the respondent depended on got much worse.

5. High or low financial strain. In this functional domain, developed by Pearlin and Lieberman (19) and Golding (20), respondents were asked to answer yes or no to five negative or positive items. The negative items were "It is difficult for me to afford the kind of medical care I should have," "It is difficult for me to pay all the monthly bills," and "It is difficult to afford needed furniture or household appliances." The positive items were "I have enough money to pay for the kind of food I should have" and "I have enough money to pay for the kind of clothes I should have." As described by Golding (20), low financial strain was present if any positive item was endorsed and high financial strain was present if any negative item was endorsed.

6. Talked to someone about most personal problems, fears, and hopes in previous 6 months. Respondents were asked to answer yes or no to the question, "In the last 6 months, is there someone you have talked to about your most personal problems, hopes, or fears?"

7. Any day with restricted activity due to physical illness in previous 2 weeks. Respondents were asked, "During the last 2 weeks, how many days did physical illness or your physical condition make you cut down on things you would like to do, such as getting around or having visitors?" Scores were dichotomized as present or absent.

8. Any day in bed due to physical illness in previous 2 weeks. Respondents were asked, "During the last 2 weeks, how many days did you stay in bed all or most of the day because of feeling physical pain or illness?" Scoring was dichotomized as present or absent.

9. Any chronic limitation in physical or job functioning due to physical illness. Respondents were asked to answer yes or no to seven items, similar to the Hispanic Health and Nutrition Examination Survey (17, 18): "Does your physical health or physical condition make it difficult for you to carry out your daily activities?" "Does your physical health or physical condition keep you from taking the kind of job you would like?" "Does your physical health or physical condition limit the work you can do on your job?" "Does your physical health or physical condition make it difficult for you to get around (outside the home, in this place)?" "Does your physical health or physical condition prevent you from getting the kind of job you would like?" "Are you able to dress yourself completely, or do you need help?" and "Do you have any problems going to the bathroom, like not being able to get there in time, or needing help to get there?" Due to skewing of responses, scoring was dichotomized as present if one or more items were endorsed or absent if no items were endorsed.

10. General health status. Respondents were asked one item from the Rand Health Insurance Experiment: "Would you say that your health is excellent, good, fair, or poor?" This item was scored as 1=excellent, 2=good, 3=fair, or 4=poor.

TABLE 1. Demographic Characteristics of 2,393 Subjects in the Los Angeles Site of the NIMH Epidemiologic Catchment Area Survey Divided by Depression Status Into Three Mutually Exclusive Groups

Characteristic	Subjects With No Depressive Disorder or Symptoms (N=2,021)		Subjects With Subsyndromal Depressive Symptoms (N=270)		Subjects With Major Depression (N=102)	
	N	%	*N*	%	*N*	%
Gender						
Male	1,014	50.2	96	35.6	35	34.3
Female	1,007	49.8	174	64.4	67	65.7
Marital status						
Married with children	575	28.5	52	19.3	14	13.7
Married without children	467	23.1	51	18.9	12	11.8
Single with children	242	12.0	43	15.9	24	23.5
Single without children	718	35.5	122	45.2	52	51.0
Ethnicity						
Native Hispanic	433	21.4	78	28.9	27	26.5
Immigrant Hispanic	643	31.8	48	17.8	15	14.7
Non-Hispanic white	945	46.8	144	53.3	60	58.8
	Mean	*SD*	*Mean*	*SD*	*Mean*	*SD*
Age (years)	41.33	17.06	37.29	14.88	36.18	11.00
Education (total years)	11.34	4.58	12.14	3.83	12.53	3.84

Description of Sample

Demographic characteristics of the Los Angeles ECA site sample have been described in greater detail elsewhere (15, 16). Using the 12-month DIS data, we divided the 2,393 subjects into three mutually exclusive subgroups: those with subsyndromal symptomatic depression, defined by the presence of at least two or more depressive symptoms in respondents not meeting criteria for major depression or dysthymia; those with major depression as defined by DSM-III; and those with no depressive disorder or symptoms.

During a 12-month period, 270 subjects met criteria for subsyndromal depressive symptoms, 102 met DSM-III criteria for major depression, and 2,021 were assigned to the subgroup subjects with no depressive disorder or symptoms. The demographic characteristics of the three groups are given in table 1. The groups with subsyndromal depressive symptoms and major depression had approximately a two-to-one preponderance of women to men, and the group with no depressive disorder or symptoms had a balanced sex distribution. Compared with the group with no depressive disorder or symptoms, the group with subsyndromal depressive symptoms had fewer married people and the group with major depression even fewer. The groups with subsyndromal depressive symptoms and major depression were, on the average, younger and better educated. There was a slightly higher prevalence of non-Hispanic whites and native Hispanics and fewer immigrant Hispanics in the groups with subsyndromal depressive symptoms and major depression than in the group with no depressive disorder or symptoms.

TABLE 2. Effect of Depression Status[a] on 10 Domains of Function and Well-Being in 2,393 Subjects in the Los Angeles Site of the NIMH Epidemiologic Catchment Area Survey

Domain of Function	Effect of Depression Status (MANOVA) F (df=2, 2255)	p
High social irritability[b]	22.32	<0.0001
High household strain[b]	10.72	<0.0001
High social contacts	1.52	n.s.
Talked to someone about most personal problems, fears, and hopes in last 6 months[b]	13.67	<0.0001
Major financial loss in last 6 months[b]	27.46	<0.0001
High financial strain[b]	21.95	<0.0001
Any day with restricted activity due to physical illness in previous 2 weeks[b]	28.39	<0.0001
Any day in bed due to physical illness in previous 2 weeks[b]	19.95	<0.0001
Any chronic limitation in physical or job functioning due to physical illness[b]	31.93	<0.0001
General health status[b]	21.16	<0.0001

[a]No depressive disorder or symptoms (N=2,021), subsyndromal depressive symptoms (N=270), or major depression (N=102).

[b]The scores of subjects with subsyndromal depressive symptoms and subjects with major depression were significantly higher (indicating greater impairment) than the scores of subjects with no depressive disorder or symptoms ($p<0.05$, Tukey's Studentized Range test).

Statistical Methods

Due to the complex sampling design and the multiple comparisons involved, two distinct statistical approaches were used to determine the effects of depression on functional status. First, a multiple analysis of variance (MANOVA) (SAS) was carried out that included all variables characterizing functional status as dependent measures and depression status (i.e., no depressive disorder or symptoms, subsyndromal depressive symptoms, or major depression) as the independent measure to determine whether depression status had a significant effect on functional status. This analysis included one-way ANOVAs and Tukey's Studentized Range post hoc comparisons to determine the effect of depression status on the individual variables characterizing functional status. Second, a multinomial logistic regression analysis adapted for the multistate sampling design was used to obtain predictions for the prevalence of disturbances in functional status due to the effect of depression status (21, 22). The STATA statistical package, which enables the adjustment of standard error calculations by means of Taylor linearization, was used for this regression analysis. For each dependent variable, a separate Huber regression analysis was calculated (22). Candidate variables included education, age, marital status, ethnicity, gender, current chronic medical condition, comorbid mental disorder, comorbid alcohol use disorder (12-month and lifetime), comorbid drug use disorder (12-month and lifetime), and the three diagnostic groups (no depressive disorder or symptoms, subsyndromal depressive symptoms, and major depression). The comorbid mental disorder variable included manic episode, dysthymia (lifetime only), bipolar disorder (lifetime only), atypical bipolar disorder (lifetime only), cannabis abuse or dependence, schizophrenia,

TABLE 3. Adjusted Percentages[a] of Subjects in the Los Angeles Site of the NIMH Epidemiologic Catchment Area Survey, Divided by Depression Status, Who Reported Impairment in Social, Financial, and Physical or Role Function

Category of Function	Subjects With No Depressive Disorder or Symptoms (N=2,021) %	SE	Subjects With Subsyndromal Depressive Symptoms (N=270) %	SE	Subjects With Major Depression (N=102) %	SE	Significant Difference
Social function							
High social contact (≥13 contacts per month)	50	1	41	3	37	5	None
Talked to someone about your most personal problems, fears, and hopes in last 6 months	64	1	69	3	73	5	None
Financial status							
Major financial loss in last 6 months	14	1	17	3	25	4	Between subjects with major depression and those with no depressive disorder or symptoms (t=3.1, df=2289, p=0.002)[b]
High financial strain	53	1	61	3	69	6	Between subjects with subsyndromal depressive symptoms and those with no depressive disorder or symptoms (t=2.2, df=2253, p=0.03)[b] and between subjects with major depression and those with no depressive disorder or symptoms (t=2.3, df=2253, p=0.02)[b]
Physical or role limitations							
Any chronic limitations in physical or job functioning due to physical illness	9	1	18	2	24	3	Between subjects with subsyndromal depressive symptoms and those with no depressive disorder or symptoms (t=4.3, df=2305, p<0.0001)[b] and between subjects with major depression and those with no depressive disorder or symptoms (t=6.2, df=2305, p<0.0001)
Any restricted activity day due to physical illness in last 2 weeks	10	1	18	2	16	3	Between subjects with subsyndromal depressive symptoms and those with no depressive disorder or symptoms (t=3.7, df=2296, p<0.0001)
Any bed day due to physical illness in previous 2 weeks	5	1	11	2	11	3	Between subjects with subsyndromal depressive symptoms and those with no depressive disorder or symptoms (t=2.9, df=2300, p<0.004)[b] and between subjects with major depression and those with no depressive disorder or symptoms (t=2.3, df=2300, p=0.03)[b]

[a]Percentages are adjusted for education, age, marital status, ethnicity, gender, current chronic medical conditions, comorbid mental disorders, comorbid alcohol use disorder (12-month and lifetime), and comorbid drug use disorder (12-month and lifetime).
[b]Confirmed by Tukey's Studentized Range test (p<0.05). In all cases, the scores of subjects with subsyndromal depressive symptoms and subjects with major depression were higher (indicating greater impairment) than those of subjects with no depressive disorder or symptoms.

schizophreniform disorder, obsessive-compulsive disorder, phobias, somatization disorder, panic disorder, antisocial personality disorder (lifetime only), and anorexia nervosa (lifetime only).

Based on the calculated logistic regression model, predicted prevalences for the following dependent variables were obtained: social irritability (high versus low), household strain (high versus low), social contacts (high [≥13] versus low [≤12]), talking to someone about personal problems, financial loss, financial strain, restricted activity days due to physical illness, bed days due to physical illness, chronic limitations in physical or job functioning, and general health status (excellent, good, fair, poor). Three different statistical analyses were used to address the two hypotheses.

The hypotheses advanced here were tested by using the two statistical approaches already described here. Specifically, the hypothesis that depression status significantly affects domains of function was tested by a MANOVA followed by post hoc comparisons using Tukey's Studentized Range tests for alpha <0.05. Moreover, specific predictions of prevalence rates of disturbances in domains of function were obtained for the groups with no depressive disorder or symptoms, subsyndromal depressive symptoms, and major depression. The average predictions and the standard errors were subjected to a t score comparison. Only those comparisons which were found to be significant by using Tukey's test *and* the t score differences obtained from the regression analysis are reported as significant in this investigation.

RESULTS

The MANOVA for effects of depression status on domains of function revealed that significant effects were present for nine of the 10 domains of everyday function (table 2).

Table 3 includes results of regression analyses for seven of the 10 functional domains. Subjects with major depression differed significantly from those with no depressive disorder or symptoms on two financial status domains and from the group with subsyndromal depressive symptoms on one financial status domain. Significantly more of the subjects with subsyndromal depressive symptoms than of those with no depressive disorder or symptoms reported impairment in three physical or role limitation domains; significantly more of the subjects with major depression than of those with no depressive disorder or symptoms reported disability in two of these domains. There were no significant differences between the subjects with major depression and those with subsyndromal depressive symptoms in these domains of function.

Figure 1 compares the results of the regression analyses on the domains of household strain and social irritability. Compared with the subjects who had no depressive disorder or symptoms, significantly more of the subjects with subsyndromal depressive symptoms reported high levels of household strain and social irritability. No significant differences were found between the subjects with major depression and those with no depressive disorder or those with subsyndromal depressive symptoms.

Estimates of general health status. On the 4-point health scale (1=poor to 4=excellent), the subjects with subsyndromal depressive symptoms gave themselves a significantly poorer mean health rating (mean=2.91, SE=0.05) than did the subjects with no depressive disorder or symptoms (mean=3.13, SE=0.02) ($t=4.5$, $df=2289$, $p<0.001$). Respondents with major depression also gave themselves a significantly poorer mean health rating (mean=2.67, SE=0.09) than did those with no depressive disorder or symptoms ($t=5.03$, $df=2289$, $p<0.0001$). The respondents with major depression gave themselves a significantly poorer mean health rating than did the subjects with subsyndromal depressive symptoms ($t=4.6$, $df=2305$, $p=0.05$).

DISCUSSION

The full Los Angeles ECA sample included approximately equal numbers of Hispanic and non-Hispanic whites, which differs from the general U.S. population (15, 16). Our conclusions here, therefore, should be tested in more representative samples; however, the reported findings apply for both Hispanic and non-Hispanic groups, and ethnicity was controlled for in the analysis.

Significantly more subjects with subsyndromal depressive symptoms than subjects with no depressive disorder or symptoms reported disability on seven of 10 domains of function: high social irritability (62%), high household strain (45%), high financial strain (63%), restricted activity days due to physical illness (18%), bed days due to physical illness (11%), chronic limitation in physical or job functioning (18%), and self-rating of health as poor.

Although one primary study goal was to evaluate associations between "pure" subsyndromal depression and major depression and functional impairment, some identified impairment could be associated with other conditions. The logistic regression analysis was designed to control for the comorbid effects of lifetime and current (12-month) alcohol and drug use disorders,

FIGURE 1. Adjusted Percentages of Subjects With No Depressive Disorder or Symptoms, Subsyndromal Depressive Symptoms, or Major Depression Reporting High Levels of Household Strain or Social Irritability[a]

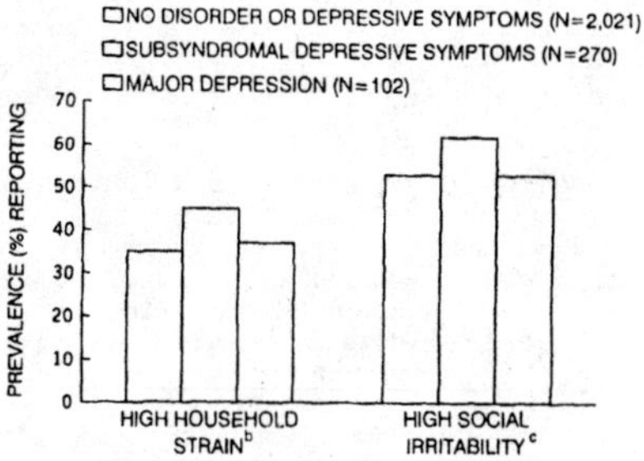

[a]Percentages are adjusted for education, age, marital status, ethnicity, gender, current chronic comorbid medical condition, comorbid mental disorder, comorbid alcohol use disorder (12-month and lifetime) and comorbid drug use disorder (12-month and lifetime).

[b]Significant difference between the group with subsyndromal depressive symptoms and the other two groups ($t=3.1$, $df=2270$, $p<0.002$) (significant according to Tukey's Studentized Range test, $p<0.05$).

[c]Significant difference between the group with subsyndromal depressive symptoms and the other two groups ($t=3.3$, $df=2274$, $p<0.001$) (significant according to Tukey's Studentized Range test, $p<0.05$).

mental disorders, and current chronic medical conditions. An additional control in reducing the influence of comorbid conditions was provided by the DIS itself, which requires that when a depressive symptom is recorded it not be associated with a medical illness or be a side effect from alcohol or drug use or disorders. These data support and extend findings from six previous studies reporting significant associations between subthreshold depressive symptoms and greater impairment in everyday function (1–6). There is now strong evidence that subsyndromal depressive symptoms are associated with substantial disability in many spheres of human activity, placing notable burdens on individuals and the society.

Compared with respondents who had no depressive disorder or symptoms, individuals with major depression reported impairment in five of 10 functional domains. Significantly more subjects with major depression reported major financial loss in the last 6 months (25%), more suffered from high financial strain (69%), more reported physical or job limitations due to illness (24%), more reported bed days (11%), and their self-ratings of health were poorest. These data strengthen the confluence of scientific evidence that major depression is associated unquestionably with severe pervasive disability in many aspects of daily functioning, which has a palpable impact on society and the economy (1, 2, 4, 7, 23). For example, 24% of the subjects with major depression reported limitations in physical or job functioning, and this is consistent with annual cost estimates for mood disorders, which found that the two largest cost categories were increased absenteeism and reduced worker productivity (23).

No large consistent differences in impairment in the domains of function emerged between the subjects with subsyndromal depressive symptoms and those with major depression, apart from their self-ratings of their health status, which could have occurred by chance alone. This does not support one of our a priori hypotheses—that more subjects with major depression than those with subsyndromal depressive symptoms will report impairment. However, every other study using different outcome measures than those reported here, such as absenteeism, use of health services, use of public assistance, and suicide attempts, have found significantly more adverse outcome associated with major depression than subsyndromal depressive symptoms (1–6). We did find that higher absolute percentages of subjects with major depression than of subjects with subsyndromal depressive symptoms reported impairment in five of 10 functional domains, but the differences were not sufficiently robust to survive formal testing. Further, the functional measurements used in this study were primarily dichotomous; it is apparent that there are differences between subsyndromal depressive symptoms and major depression that we did not have the power to detect. It should be noted that our findings are also consistent with those of previous investigations (1–4), which found that the impairments in subjects with subsyndromal depressive symptoms and those with major depression are qualitatively comparable and more similar to each other than they are to any impairment found in subjects without subsyndromal depressive symptoms or major depression.

It is not fully clear what subsyndromal symptomatic depression represents clinically, but we do know from the studies of Broadhead et al. (2) and Howarth et al. (5) that subthreshold depressive symptoms are associated with greater risk for future major depressive episodes. In a large sample of medical and psychiatric outpatients (24), we found that the demographic and clinical characteristics of subjects with subsyndromal depressive symptoms significantly more closely resembled those of subjects with major depression than those of nondepressed medical outpatients. For example, we found that 41% of outpatients with subsyndromal depressive symptoms had family histories of depression, a rate nearly as high as that for subjects with major depression (59%). We have proposed that subsyndromal depressive symptoms represent, respectively, either prodromal manifestations or residual depressive symptoms from impending or incompletely resolved major depression or dysthymia (25). Subsyndromal depressive symptoms may also be a low-grade chronic condition, placing patients at higher risk for future major depressive episodes (25). This has led us to conclude that subsyndromal depressive symptoms are a clinically meaningful, subthreshold variant of unipolar major depression.

The fact that approximately one in 10 people in this community sample met criteria for subsyndromal depressive symptoms during 1 year, when combined with the associated functional impairment reported by us and others (1–6), supports the conclusion that subsyndromal depressive symptoms are a clinical condition of public health significance. Prospective, controlled studies of subsyndromal depressive symptoms in unipolar major depression are needed, especially treatment investigations, because no data are available indicating that subsyndromal depressive symptoms respond to treatment or if they should be treated at all. It is possible that effective treatment of subsyndromal depressive symptoms may not only reduce the associated functional disability identified but also prevent more severely disabling future episodes of major depression or dysthymia.

REFERENCES

1. Wells KB, Stewart A, Hays RD, Burnam MA, Rogers W, Daniels M, Berry S, Greenfield S, Ware J: The functioning and well-being of depressed patients: results from the Medical Outcomes Study. JAMA 1989; 262:914–919
2. Broadhead WE, Blazer DG, George LK, Tse LK: Depression, disability days and days lost from work in a prospective epidemiologic survey. JAMA 1990; 264:2524–2528
3. Johnson J, Weissman MM, Klerman GL: Service utilization and social morbidity associated with depressive symptoms in the community. JAMA 1992; 267:1478–1483
4. Spitzer RL, Kroenke K, Linzer M, Hahn SR, Williams JB, deGruy FV III, Brody D, Davies M: Health-related quality of life in primary care patients with mental disorders: results from the PRIME-MD 1000 study. JAMA 1995; 274:1511–1517
5. Howarth E, Johnson J, Klerman GL, Weissman M: Depressive symptoms as relative and attributable risk factors for first-onset major depression. Arch Gen Psychiatry 1992; 49:817–823
6. Judd LL, Rapaport M, Paulus M, Brown J: Subsyndromal Symptomatic Depression. J Clin Psychiatry 1994; 55(April suppl)
7. Mintz J, Mintz TH, Aruda MJ, Hwang SS: Treatment of depression and functional capacity to work. Arch Gen Psychiatry 1992; 49:761–768
8. Regier DA, Myers JK, Kramer M, Robins LN, Blazer DG, Hough RL, Eaton WW, Locke BZ: The NIMH Epidemiologic Catchment Area Program: historical context, major objectives, and study population characteristics. Arch Gen Psychiatry 1984; 41:934–941
9. Eaton WW, Holzer CE III, Von Korff M, Anthony JC, Helzer JE, George L, Burnam A, Boyd JH, Kessler LG, Locke BZ: The design of the Epidemiologic Catchment Area surveys: the control and measurement of error. Arch Gen Psychiatry 1984; 41:942–948
10. Eaton W, Kessler L (eds): Epidemiologic Field Methods in Psychiatry: The NIMH Epidemiologic Catchment Area Program. Orlando, Fla, Academic Press, 1985
11. Robins LN, Helzer JE, Cottler L, Golding E: National Institute of Mental Health Diagnostic Interview Schedule, version III, revised. St Louis, Washington University, Department of Psychiatry, 1989
12. Robins LN, Helzer JE, Croughan J, Ratcliff KS: The National Institute of Mental Health Diagnostic Interview Schedule: its history, characteristics, and validity. Arch Gen Psychiatry 1981; 38:381–389
13. Karno M, Burnam MA, Escobar J, Hough RL, Eaton WW: Development of the Spanish-language version of the National Institute of Mental Health Diagnostic Interview Schedule. Arch Gen Psychiatry 1983; 40:1183–1188
14. Burnam MA, Karno M, Hough RL, Escobar JI, Forsythe AB: The

Spanish Diagnostic Interview Schedule: reliability and comparison with clinical diagnoses. Arch Gen Psychiatry 1983; 40:1189–1196
15. Wells KB, Golding JM, Burnam MA: Psychiatric disorder and limitations in physical functioning in a sample of the Los Angeles general population. Am J Psychiatry 1988; 145:712–717
16. Wells KB, Golding JM, Burnam MA: Psychiatric disorder in a sample of the general population with and without chronic medical conditions. Am J Psychiatry 1988; 145:976–981
17. Data Collection Forms of the Hispanic HANES: Adult Sample Person Questionnaire Form PHS 6206. Washington, DC, US Department of Health and Human Services, 1982
18. Wilder CS: Health Characteristics of Persons With Chronic Activity Limitation: Data From the National Health Survey, Series 10, Number 112: Department of Health, Education and Welfare Publication HRA 77-1539. Rockville, Md, National Center for Health Statistics, 1976
19. Pearlin LI, Lieberman MA: Social sources of emotional distress. Res Community Ment Health 1979; 1:217–248
20. Golding JM: Division of household labor, strain and depressive symptoms among Mexican Americans and non-Hispanic whites. Psychol Women Q 1990; 14:103–117
21. Schluchter MD: Analysis of incomplete multivariate data using linear models with structured covariance matrices. Stat Med 1988; 7:317–324
22. Huber PJ: The behavior of maximum likelihood estimates under nonstandard conditions, in Fifth Berkeley Symposium, 1965. Berkeley, University of California Press, 1967, pp 221–233
23. Greenberg PE, Stiglin L, Finkelstein S, Berndt E: The economic burden of depression in 1990. J Clin Psychiatry 1993; 54:405–418
24. Sherbourne CD, Wells KB, Hays RD, Rogers W, Burnam MA, Judd LL: Subthreshold depression and depressive disorder: clinical characteristics of general medical and mental health specialty outpatients. Am J Psychiatry 1994; 151:1777–1784
25. Judd L: Clinical characteristics of subsyndromal symptomatic depression, in Critical Issues in the Treatment of Affective Disorders, vol 9. Edited by Langer SZ, Brunello N, Racagni G, Mendlewicz J. Basel, Switzerland, Karger (International Academy for Biomedical and Drug Research), 1994, pp 67–74

Boundaries of Major Depression: An Evaluation of DSM-IV Criteria

Kenneth S. Kendler, M.D., and Charles O. Gardner, Jr., Ph.D.

Objective: Little is known about the boundaries between major depression and milder subsyndromal depressive states. With respect to depressive symptoms, does DSM-IV "carve nature at its joints"? Method: In personally interviewed female twins from a population-based registry, the authors examined whether a range of values along three dimensions of the depressive syndrome assessed in the last year (number of symptoms listed in DSM-III-R under diagnostic criterion A for major depressive episode, level of severity or impairment required to score symptoms as present, and duration of episode) predicted future depressive episodes in the index twin and risk of major depression in the co-twin. Results: An increasing number of criterion A symptoms predicted, in a monotonic fashion, a greater risk for future depressive episodes in the index twin as well as a greater risk for major depression in the co-twin. No such consistent relationship was seen with duration of episode. For severity, a single monotonic function predicted risk in the co-twin, while index twins with severe impairment had a substantially higher risk for future episodes than did those with less severe impairment. Four or fewer criterion A symptoms, syndromes composed of symptoms involving no or minimal impairment, and episodes of less than 14 days' duration all significantly predicted both future depressive episodes in the index twin and risk of major depression in the co-twin. Conclusions: The authors found little empirical support for the DSM-IV requirements for 2 weeks' duration, five symptoms, or clinically significant impairment. Most functions appeared continuous. These results suggest that major depression—as articulated by DSM-IV—may be a diagnostic convention imposed on a continuum of depressive symptoms of varying severity and duration.

(Am J Psychiatry 1998; 155:172–177)

The depressive syndrome is one of the oldest in psychiatry, having been clearly described by the physicians of antiquity (1). Many issues have long been debated in the nosology of depression, including the relationship between "melancholic" and "neurotic/reactive" depression (2–6), the value of the primary-secondary distinction (7, 8) and "familial" subtypes (7, 9), and the diagnostic interface between depression and schizophrenia (10–12). However, less attention has been paid to the boundaries of the depressive syndrome itself. Perhaps this is because the key diagnostic question in patients with depressive symptoms in clinical settings, where most depression research has been carried out, is usually, "What is the best diagnosis?" However, in epidemiologic studies, where the range of symptoms is broader and mild cases are common, the more relevant question in individuals with depressive symptoms is often, "Is this a case of major depression?"

We evaluated two mutually exclusive hypotheses about the syndrome of major depression—as articulated in DSM-IV:

1. Is major depression a discrete syndrome with "points of rarity" at its boundaries? That is, is there a discontinuity in etiologic processes so that major depression differs qualitatively and not just quantitatively from subsyndromal conditions?

2. Is major depression a diagnostic convention imposed on a continuum of depressive symptoms of varying severity and duration?

We evaluated three key features of the syndrome of major depression: 1) number of symptoms listed under criterion A for major depressive episode (DSM-IV requires that at least five be present), 2) level of severity or impairment required for rating individual symptoms

Received Jan. 9, 1997; revision received Aug. 5, 1997; accepted Aug. 11, 1997. From the Virginia Institute for Psychiatric and Behavioral Genetics and the Department of Psychiatry and the Department of Human Genetics, Medical College of Virginia of Virginia Commonwealth University, Richmond. Address reprint requests to Dr. Kendler, P.O. Box 980126, Richmond, VA 23298-0126; kendler@hsc.vcu.edu (e-mail).

Supported by NIMH grants MH-40828, MH-49492, MH-01277, and MH-54150. The Virginia Twin Registry, established and maintained by W. Nance, M.D., Ph.D., and L. Corey, Ph.D., is supported by grant HD-26746 from the National Institute of Child Health and Human Development and grant NS-31564 from the National Institute of Neurological and Communicative Disorders and Stroke as present (DSM-IV requires either significant distress or significant impairment in functioning for the entire syndrome), and 3) duration (DSM-IV requires a minimum of 2 weeks). Our strategy was to examine, in an epidemiologic sample of female twins, individuals with depressive symptoms who reported varying numbers of symptoms, duration, and levels of severity or impairment, both above and below the DSM-IV diagnostic threshold. In these individuals, we examined how varying levels of these features predicted not only future episodes of major depression but also risk for major depression in the co-twin—two of the validating criteria most widely used for psychiatric disorders (13).

As shown in figure 1, and previously articulated by Kendell and Brockington (12), hypothesis 1 predicts a discontinuity in the relationship among symptoms, duration, and impairment and the validating criteria. For example, this hypothesis predicts a much larger difference in the risk of major depression in co-twins between individuals having four versus five of the criterion A symptoms than between those having three versus four symptoms or five versus six. By contrast, hypothesis 2 predicts that the relationship among symptoms, duration, and impairment will be relatively smooth and continuous with no apparent "breaks" at the points articulated in DSM-IV.

FIGURE 1. Two Hypothesized Relationships Between Levels of Diagnostic Criteria for Major Depression and Validating Variables[a]

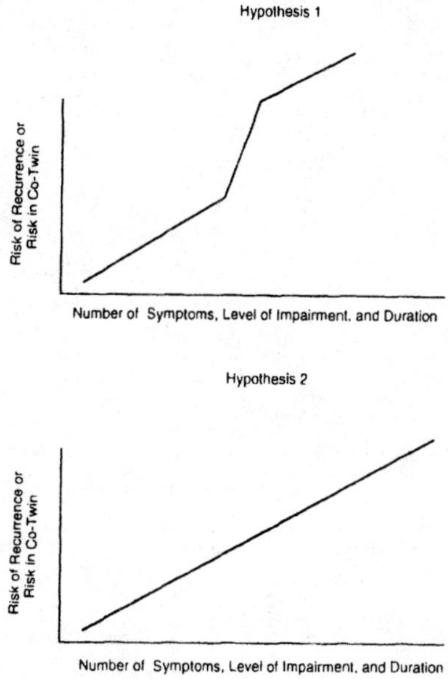

[a]With hypothesis 1, a sharp discontinuity is observed in the validating variable (risk of recurrence of major depression or risk of major depression in a co-twin) as a function of the level of the diagnostic criteria (the number of symptoms listed for criterion A in the DSM-III-R diagnosis of major depressive episode, the level of impairment required for rating a symptom as present, and the duration of episodes). Such a discontinuity may indicate a "true" diagnostic boundary in nature. By contrast, with hypothesis 2, continuity is observed between the validating variable and the diagnostic criteria. Such a pattern of results would argue that, with respect to the validators examined, the diagnostic criteria reflect a continuum of severity and not a discrete syndrome. This figure is adapted from Kendell and Brockington (12).

METHOD

Sample

The Caucasian female same-sex twins studied in this report are part of a longitudinal study of genetic and environmental risk factors for common psychiatric disorders. The twins, ascertained from the population-based Virginia Twin Registry, were eligible to participate in this study if both members of the pair had previously responded to a mailed questionnaire, to which the individual response rate was 64%. In our first series of personal interviews, we succeeded in interviewing 92% (N=2,163) of the eligible individuals. Ninety percent of the interviews were face-to-face; the rest were completed by telephone. Written informed consent was obtained before all face-to-face interviews, and personal assent was obtained for all telephone interviews. The mean age of the participating twins was 30.1 years (SD=7.6). Zygosity was determined blindly by using standard questions (14), photographs, and, when necessary, DNA testing (15).

Since the original interview, we have completed two additional series of telephone interviews, which succeeded in interviewing 2,001 (92.5%) and 1,898 (87.7%) of the originally interviewed subjects, respectively. The mean number of months between the first and third interviews was 61.3 (SD=5.1).

For these analyses, we used two subsamples: 1) individuals who completed all three personal interviews (N=1,822), in whom we attempted to predict risk for major depression at the time of either the second or third interview as a function of the characteristics of depressive syndromes reported at the first interview, and 2) members of pairs of known zygosity where both members were interviewed at least once over the first, second, and third interviews (N=2,058).

Measures

Information was collected from all respondents at each of the three interviews on the occurrence of 20 individual symptoms during the year before interview. Fourteen of these symptoms were disaggregated versions of the nine symptoms listed under criterion A for major depressive episode in DSM-III-R (p. 222). Six of the nine symptoms were each represented by a single item. Two symptoms were disaggregated into two items each: criterion A4 was divided into separate insomnia and hypersomnia items, while criterion A5 was divided into separate items assessing psychomotor agitation and retardation. Criterion A2 was disaggregated into four items: decreased appetite, increased appetite, decreased weight, and increased weight.

Symptoms were required to have a duration of at least 5 days. For every symptom reported present by the subject, the interviewer inquired as to the possibility that it was due to physical illness or medication. If in the interviewer's judgment this was the case, which occurred 17.4% of the time across all symptoms, then the symptom was considered not present.

For each symptom reported as present, we also inquired about the severity of the symptom and/or symptom-related impairment.

TABLE 1. Number of Criterion A Symptoms for DSM-III-R Major Depressive Episode as a Boundary of Major Depression in a Study of Female Twins

Number of Criterion A Symptoms	Number of Index Twins Reporting Specific Number of Symptoms at First Interview[a]	Risk of Major Depression at Second or Third Interview as a Function of Number of Criterion A Symptoms in Episode at First Interview			Number of Index Twins Reporting Specific Number of Symptoms at First, Second, or Third Interview[b]	Risk of Lifetime Major Depression in Co-Twin as a Function of Number of Criterion A Symptoms in First Episode of Index Twin		
		Odds Ratio	χ^2	p (one-tailed)		Risk Ratio	χ^2	p (one-tailed)
3	64	1.88	3.94	0.02	149	1.37	6.10	0.007
4	63	2.64	10.68	0.0005	153	1.48	9.99	0.001
5	58	3.45	17.26	0.0001	124	1.47	8.08	0.002
6	46	3.17	12.00	0.0002	119	1.85	21.80	0.0001
7	41	6.50	31.38	0.0001	99	1.94	21.85	0.0001
8 or 9	33	13.26	44.45	0.0001	72	2.55	39.58	0.0001

[a]Number of index twins who did not have a minimal depressive syndrome in the previous year at first interview was 1,517.
[b]Number of index twins who did not have a minimal depressive syndrome in previous year at first, second, or third interview was 1,447.

This was assessed in several ways. Usually, we asked how much the specific symptom (e.g., feeling of depression, tiredness/fatigue) interfered with the subject's daily life. The response options were "hardly at all," "some," "a lot," and "completely." For weight gain and loss, we asked the number of pounds lost or gained, respectively. For insomnia and hypersomnia, we asked the number of hours of lost sleep or hours spent in extra sleep, respectively. For increased or decreased appetite and for psychomotor agitation, interviewers, after probing, rated the symptom as severe, moderate, or mild. We reduced ratings of severity or impairment for each symptom into three categories—mild, moderate, and severe. For symptoms where we inquired about impairment, we converted the ratings as follows: mild=hardly at all, moderate=some, and severe=a lot or completely. For weight gain and weight loss, we defined mild, moderate, and severe as an episode-related weight change of <10 lb, 10–14 lb, and ≥15 lb, respectively. For insomnia and hypersomnia, we defined mild, moderate, and severe as an episode-related change in sleep of <2 hours, 3–4 hours, and ≥5 hours, respectively. For DSM-III-R criteria that were represented by more than one item, we took the most severe symptom-related impairment reported.

After inquiring about the individual symptoms, the interviewer asked the twin which if any of the endorsed symptoms co-occurred in the last year. For the purposes of this study, we defined a minimal depressive syndrome as consisting of at least three co-occurring depressive symptoms, regardless of level of severity or impairment—one of which had to be depressed mood or loss of interest/pleasure—and lasting at least 5 days.

To examine the impact of the number of symptoms reported, we required a minimum duration of illness of 2 weeks and, in accord with DSM-III-R, did not require any level of severity or impairment for an individual symptom to be counted as present. To examine the impact of level of severity or impairment, we required a minimum duration of 2 weeks and at least five endorsed criterion A symptoms. We then defined three hierarchically organized groups. Subjects who had five or more of the criterion A symptoms at the severe level were classified as severe. Those who had five or more criterion A symptoms at the moderate level but were not classified in the severe group were classified as moderate. Those who met five or more criteria only at the mild level (and thus did not meet criteria for either the moderate or severe group) were classified as mild. To examine the impact of duration, we required a minimum of five criterion A symptoms but no accompanying level of severity or impairment and had no requirement for a reported duration longer than 5 days.

In addition to inquiring about the history of depressive symptoms in the last year, at both the first and third interviews we inquired about the lifetime history of major depression, using a section adapted from the Structured Clinical Interview for DSM-III-R (16). We classified a twin as having a lifetime history of major depression if she reported one or more episodes meeting DSM-III-R criteria during any one of the three interviews.

Statistical Methods

Our analyses examined two potential validators of the nosologic boundaries of major depression. The first of these was risk of recurrence of DSM-III-R-defined major depression at the second and third interviews as predicted by characteristics of the depressive syndrome assessed at the first interview. These analyses were conducted by using logistic regression, operationalized by PROC LOGISTIC in SAS (17). Subgroups of twins with a depressive syndrome (e.g., those with three, four, five, or more criterion A symptoms) were compared with twins who denied a minimal depressive syndrome at the first interview.

The second validator examined was the hazard rate of lifetime major depression, defined by DSM-III-R, in the co-twin as a function of features of the first minimal depressive syndrome experienced in the first, second, or third interview. This was performed by using the Cox Proportional Hazard method, as operationalized in the PHREG procedure in SAS (17). Each group was compared with twins who denied ever experiencing even a minor depressive syndrome at all assessments. If a twin was not interviewed at all three interviews and reported no lifetime history of major depression, then her age at last interview was treated as her age.

For both the logistic and Cox analyses, we report the regression coefficient, on which tests for linearity are appropriately made, and chi-square with df=1. One-tailed p values are reported because we had a clear a priori directional hypothesis. For the logistic and Cox regression analyses, we also present, because of their ease of interpretation, the odds ratio and risk ratio, respectively.

To correct for the correlated observations in members of a twin pair, we multiplied the variance of the parameter estimate initially obtained by the following equation: ([1+r]x+y)/(x+y), where r equals the intraclass correlation in twin pairs for the dependent variable, x equals the number of complete twin pairs, and y equals the number of unpaired individuals in the analysis. This formula was algebraically derived from the formula for clustered sampling as described by Kish (18). Chi-square and p values were recalculated based on this new and larger estimate of the sampling variance.

We wished to test statistically whether the relationships between our predictor and validator variables were continuous (hypothesis 2 in figure 1) or contained a discontinuity (hypothesis 1 in figure 1). To do so, we compared the fit—measured in log likelihood units—of a series of logistic and Cox regression models, including only subjects with a minimal depressive syndrome. We first fit a "covariates only" model, where the sole predictor variable was year of birth. Next, we examined the improvement in fit obtained when a single linear function was added. This function, as depicted in figure 1 (hypothesis 2), assumes a continuous linear relationship between the predictor and validator measures and can be specified by a single parameter. Finally, we fitted a range of more complex models containing two or more parameters, which introduced discontinuities into the relationship either in the form of a second linear function or a dummy variable specifying that an individual category of the predictor variable has a

TABLE 2. Severity of Criterion A Symptoms for DSM-III-R Major Depressive Episode as a Boundary of Major Depression in a Study of Female Twins

Severity or Impairment of Criterion A Symptoms	Number of Index Twins Reporting Major Depression With Symptoms of Specific Severity or Impairment at First Interview[a]	Risk of Major Depression at Second or Third Interview as a Function of Severity of Symptoms in Episode at First Interview			Number of Index Twins Reporting Major Depression With Symptoms of Specific Severity or Impairment at First, Second, or Third Interview[b]	Risk of Lifetime Major Depression in Co-Twin as a Function of Severity of Symptoms in First Episode of Index Twin		
		Odds Ratio	χ^2	p (one-tailed)		Risk Ratio	χ^2	p (one-tailed)
Mild	37	3.97	15.07	0.0001	92	1.36	4.02	0.03
Moderate	101	3.42	28.95	0.0001	276	1.79	39.75	0.0001
Severe	40	11.64	47.99	0.0001	96	2.22	35.77	0.0001

[a]Number who did not meet DSM-III-R criteria for major depression in previous year at first interview was 1,644.
[b]Number who did not meet DSM-III-R criteria for major depression in previous year at first, second, or third interview was 1,699.

unique value. The fits of these models were compared by –2×(log likelihood), which approximates a chi-square distribution.

RESULTS

Number of Criterion A Symptoms

Compared with subjects who denied a minimal depressive syndrome during the previous year at the first interview, the future risk for an episode of DSM-III-R major depression was significantly higher for individuals with a depressive episode that included only three or four criterion A symptoms (table 1). In general, the greater the number of criterion A symptoms present, the greater the risk for a future episode of major depression. No substantial discontinuity was apparent between four and five criterion A symptoms as hypothesized by DSM-IV. However, the risk for future depressive episodes was substantially greater in subjects with seven or more than for those with six or fewer criterion A symptoms.

In modeling the relationship between the number of criterion A symptoms in subjects with a minimal depressive syndrome and the risk for future depressive episodes, we found that, compared with a covariates-only model, a marked improvement in fit was obtained by a simple model with a single linear function (χ^2=20.61, df=1, p<0.0001). No other significant improvements in fit could be found, the closest being the addition of a second linear function, which increased the slope of the regression line between six and seven criterion A symptoms (χ^2=1.60, df=1, n.s.).

Compared with subjects who denied a minimal depressive syndrome during the previous year at the first-, second-, and third interview, the risk for lifetime major depression in the co-twins was significantly greater for those twins who reported a depressive syndrome with only three or four criterion A symptoms (table 1). In general, the risk of major depression in the co-twin increased with an increasing number of criterion A symptoms. No discontinuity was seen between four and five symptoms, as hypothesized by DSM-IV, or between six and seven symptoms, as seen with the prediction of risk for future depressive episodes.

In modeling this relationship, compared with a covariates-only model, a large improvement in fit was obtained by a simple model with a single linear function (χ^2=13.94, df=1, p=0.0002). No significant improvements in fit could be found by the introduction of any discontinuities in the relationship between number of criterion A symptoms and risk for major depression in the co-twin.

Severity or Impairment

Compared with subjects who did not endorse DSM-III-R criteria for major depression in the previous year, those who met criteria for major depression only when symptoms were defined as having mild severity or impairment still had a significantly greater risk for major depression in future years (table 2). The magnitude of the increased future risk was actually less for those who met criteria when individual symptoms were required to have at least moderate severity or impairment (table 2) and substantially greater for those who met criteria when symptoms had to have severe impairment or severity to be counted present (table 2).

In modeling this relationship, compared with a covariates-only model, a significant improvement in fit was obtained by a simple model with a single linear function (χ^2=4.97, df=1, p=0.03). The addition of a second, steeper linear function between moderate and severe produced a further significant improvement in fit (χ^2=5.16, df=1, p=0.02). No other significant improvements in fit could be found.

The level of severity or impairment required for depressive symptoms predicted an increasing risk for major depression in the co-twin in what appeared to be a monotonic continuous fashion (table 2). For subjects who met criteria for major depression only when symptoms were defined as having mild severity or impairment, their co-twins had a significantly higher risk for major depression than co-twins of subjects who did not meet DSM-III-R criteria (table 2). These relative risks increased to 1.79 and 2.22, respectively, when, to be counted present, symptoms had to have moderate or severe levels of severity or impairment.

In examining a statistical model of this relationship, we found that, compared with a covariates-only model,

TABLE 3. Duration of DSM-III-R Major Depressive Episode as a Boundary of Major Depression in a Study of Female Twins

Duration of Episode (days)	Number of Index Twins Reporting Specific Duration of Episode at First Interview[a]	Risk of Lifetime Major Depression in Co-Twin as a Function of Duration of Episode at First Interview			Number of Index Twins Reporting Specific Duration of Episode at First, Second, or Third Interview[b]	Risk of Lifetime Major Depression in Co-Twin as a Function of Duration of First Episode of Index Twin		
		Odds Ratio	χ^2	p (one-tailed)		Risk Ratio	χ^2	p (one-tailed)
5–13	60	5.50	37.92	0.0001	144	1.51	10.60	0.0006
14–29	56	4.42	26.65	0.0001	154	1.58	14.79	0.0001
30–59	44	4.63	22.41	0.0001	88	1.68	11.40	0.0003
60–90	38	6.29	28.89	0.0001	84	2.64	45.66	0.0001
≥91	40	5.93	28.29	0.0001	106	1.65	13.97	0.0001

[a]Number of subjects who did not meet DSM-III-R criteria for major depression (excluding duration) in previous year at first interview was 1,584.

[b]Number of subjects who did not meet DSM-III-R criteria for major depression (excluding duration) in previous year at first, second, or third interview was 1,587.

a significant improvement in fit was obtained by a simple model with a single linear function (χ^2=5.77, df=1, p=0.02). No other significant improvements in fit could be found.

Duration

Compared with those twins who reported no major depressive episode in the last year, twins with an episode lasting 5 to 13 days had a significantly higher risk for a future episode of DSM-III-R major depression (table 3). The odds ratio for future episodes was slightly lower for those with depressive episodes lasting 14–29 or 30–59 days (table 3). A modestly greater risk for future episodes was associated with durations of greater than 60 days.

Compared with a covariates-only model, no significant improvement in fit was found with the addition of a single linear function (χ^2=0.22, df=1, n.s.), indicating no statistically significant relationship between duration and future risk for major depression. No significant improvements in fit for this model could be found.

Duration of the reported depressive episode in the index twin was an inconsistent index of the risk for major depression in the co-twin. For episodes shorter than 90 days, the risk in the co-twin increased modestly with increasing duration but decreased again with episodes of 91 or more days in length. Co-twins of subjects with a depressive episode of less than 14 days' duration had a highly significantly increased risk for major depression (table 3).

In modeling this relationship, we found that, compared with a covariates-only model, no significant improvement in fit was obtained by a model with a single linear function (χ^2=2.44, df=1, p=0.12). The only significant improvement to this was found with a model in which the twins with depressive episodes lasting for 60–90 days differed from all other categories (χ^2=8.05, df=1, p=0.005).

DISCUSSION

Our goal was to evaluate two contrasting hypotheses about the nature of the boundaries of the major depressive syndrome, illustrated in figure 1. Do DSM-IV criteria for major depression "carve nature at its joints" or is major depression a manmade concept imposed on a diagnostic continuum? We tested three fundamental features of the depressive syndrome against two key validating criteria long used in psychiatric research: occurrence of future depressive episodes and risk of major depression in a co-twin. We failed to find evidence for a discontinuity at the boundaries proposed by DSM-IV. Syndromes that met fewer than five criterion A symptoms, lasted for less than 2 weeks, or were formed of symptoms that were quite mild or produced no impairment had considerable predictive and familial validity. That is, these subsyndromes consistently predicted, at high levels of significance, the risk for subsequent DSM-III-R-defined episodes of major depression and the risk for major depression in a co-twin. We found statistical evidence for only a single discontinuity in the prediction of future depressive episodes (between those meeting symptom definitions requiring mild or moderate versus severe impairment), but this discontinuity was not in line with DSM-IV criteria, nor was it replicated in the prediction of risk of illness in the co-twin.

Nosologic Implications

We have shown that, taken one at a time, three major "gate keeping" DSM-IV criteria for major depression—symptom number, impairment, and duration—do not appear to carve nature at its joints (12). We did not perform a formal taxonomic analysis. Therefore, our results do not directly address the question of whether a discrete depressive syndrome exists in nature, as has been suggested by a number of statistical methods such as cluster analysis (19, 20), grade of membership analysis (21, 22), and latent class analysis (20, 23–25). However, our results do suggest that if a discrete depressive syndrome exists in nature, the current DSM-IV criteria that we evaluated do not perform well in detecting it.

Our results suggesting a continuity of risk between subsyndromal and syndromal major depression are not without precedent. Subsyndromal depressive symptoms have been associated with substantial social morbidity (26–28), a much greater risk for first-onset major depression (29), and a greater risk for mood disorders in first-degree relatives (30). In a recent analysis of the National Comorbidity Survey, Kessler et al. (31) examined three definitions of depression: minor (meeting two, three, or four criterion A symptoms), major (meeting five or six criterion A symptoms), and severe major (meeting seven or more criterion A symptoms). They found, across the three categories, monotonic increases for average number of episodes, average length of longest episodes, impairment, comorbidity, and parental history of psychiatric disorders.

Although the use of operationalized diagnostic criteria has resulted in substantial improvement in the reliability of psychiatric diagnoses, demonstrating their validity has been more problematic. These results suggest that our current DSM-IV diagnostic conventions for major depression, derived largely from the Washington University criteria (32) and Research Diagnostic Criteria (33), may be arbitrary and not reflective of a natural discontinuity in depressive symptoms as experienced in the general population.

Limitations

The sample studied was entirely female. Results might differ in male subjects. The history of depressive symptoms was assessed, at different points in the interview, for the last year and for lifetime. Given problems in the recall of depressive episodes (34, 35), it is possible that errors of memory might have produced a blurring of a true diagnostic boundary.

REFERENCES

1. Jackson SW: Melancholia and Depression: From Hippocratic Times to Modern Times. New Haven, Conn, Yale University Press, 1986
2. Kendell RE: The classification of depressions: a review of contemporary confusion. Br J Psychiatry 1976; 129:15–28
3. Farmer A, McGuffin P: The classification of the depressions: contemporary confusion revisited. Br J Psychiatry 1989; 155:437–443
4. Winokur G: The validity of neurotic-reactive depression: new data and reappraisal. Arch Gen Psychiatry 1985; 42:1116–1122
5. Zimmerman M, Spitzer RL: Melancholia: from DSM-III to DSM-III-R. Am J Psychiatry 1989; 146:20–28
6. Rush AJ, Weissenburger JE: Melancholic symptom features and DSM-IV. Am J Psychiatry 1994; 151:489–498
7. Andreasen NC, Winokur G: Secondary depression: familial, clinical, and research perspectives. Am J Psychiatry 1979; 136:62–66
8. Akiskal HS, Rosenthal RH, Rosenthal TL, Kashgarian M, Khani MK, Puzantian VR: Differentiation of primary affective illness from situational, symptomatic, and secondary depressions. Arch Gen Psychiatry 1979; 36:635–643
9. Winokur G: Unipolar depression: is it divisible into autonomous subtypes? Arch Gen Psychiatry 1979; 36:47–52
10. Ollerenshaw DP: The classification of the functional psychoses. Br J Psychiatry 1973; 122:517–530
11. Pope HG Jr, Lipinski JF Jr: Diagnosis in schizophrenia and manic-depressive illness: a reassessment of the specificity of "schizophrenic" symptoms in the light of current research. Arch Gen Psychiatry 1978; 35:811–828
12. Kendell RE, Brockington IF: The identification of disease entities and the relationship between schizophrenic and affective psychoses. Br J Psychiatry 1980; 137:324–331
13. Robins E, Guze SB: Establishment of diagnostic validity in psychiatric illness: its application to schizophrenia. Am J Psychiatry 1970; 126:983–987
14. Eaves LJ, Eysenck HJ, Martin NG, Jardine R, Heath AC, Feingold L, Young PA, Kendler KS: Genes, Culture and Personality: An Empirical Approach. London, Oxford University Press, 1989
15. Spence JE, Corey LA, Nance WE, Marazita ML, Kendler KS, Schieken RM: Molecular analysis of twin zygosity using VNTR DNA probes (abstract). Am J Hum Genet 1988; 43:A159
16. Spitzer RL, Williams JBW, Gibbon M: Structured Clinical Interview for DSM-III-R (SCID). New York, New York State Psychiatric Institute, Biometrics Research, 1987
17. SAS/STAT User's Guide, version 6, 4th ed, vols 1, 2. Cary, NC, SAS Institute, 1990
18. Kish L: Statistical Design for Research. New York, John Wiley & Sons, 1984
19. Paykel ES: Classification of depressed patients: a cluster analysis derived grouping. Br J Psychiatry 1971; 118:275–288
20. Grove WM, Andreasen NC, Young M, Endicott J, Keller MB, Hirschfeld RMA, Reich T: Isolation and characterization of a nuclear depressive syndrome. Psychol Med 1987; 17:471–484
21. Blazer D, Swartz M, Woodbury M, Manton KG, Hughes D, George LK: Depressive symptoms and depressive diagnoses in a community population: use of a new procedure for analysis of psychiatric classification. Arch Gen Psychiatry 1988; 45:1078–1084
22. Woodbury MA, Manton KG: Grade of membership analysis of depression-related psychiatric disorders. Sociological Methods and Res 1989; 18:126–163
23. Young MA, Scheftner WA, Klerman GL, Andreasen NC, Hirschfeld RMA: The endogenous sub-type of depression: a study of its internal construct validity. Br J Psychiatry 1986; 148:257–267
24. Eaton WW, Dryman A, Sorenson A, McCutcheon A: DSM-III major depressive disorder in the community: a latent class analysis of data from the NIMH Epidemiologic Catchment Area programme. Br J Psychiatry 1989; 155:48–54
25. Kendler KS, Eaves LJ, Walters EE, Neale MC, Heath AC, Kessler RC: The identification and validation of distinct depressive syndromes in a population-based sample of female twins. Arch Gen Psychiatry 1996; 53:391–399
26. Johnson J, Weissman MM, Klerman GL: Service utilization and social morbidity associated with depressive symptoms in the community. JAMA 1992; 267:1478–1483
27. Judd LL, Paulus MP, Wells KB, Rapaport MH: Socioeconomic burden of subsyndromal depressive symptoms and major depression in a sample of the general population. Am J Psychiatry 1996; 153:1411–1417
28. Olfson M, Broadhead WE, Weissman MM, Leon AC, Farber L, Hoven C, Kathol R: Subthreshold psychiatric symptoms in a primary care group practice. Arch Gen Psychiatry 1996; 53:880–886
29. Horwath E, Johnson J, Klerman GL, Weissman MM: Depressive symptoms as relative and attributable risk factors for first-onset major depression. Arch Gen Psychiatry 1992; 49:817–823
30. Remick RA, Sadovnick AD, Lam RW, Zis AP, Yee IML: Major depression, minor depression, and double depression: are they distinct clinical entities? Am J Med Genet Neuropsychiatr Genet 1996; 67:347–353
31. Kessler RC, Zhao S, Blazer DG, Swartz M: Prevalence, correlates, and course of minor depression and major depression in the National Comorbidity Survey. J Affect Disord 1997; 45:19–30
32. Feighner JP, Robins E, Guze SB, Woodruff RA Jr, Winokur G, Munoz R: Diagnostic criteria for use in psychiatric research. Arch Gen Psychiatry 1972; 26:57–63
33. Spitzer RL, Endicott J, Robins E: Research Diagnostic Criteria (RDC) for a Selected Group of Functional Disorders, 2nd ed. New York, New York State Psychiatric Institute, Biometrics Research, 1975
34. Bromet EJ, Dunn LO, Connell MM, Dew MA, Schulberg HC: Long-term reliability of diagnosing lifetime major depression in a community sample. Arch Gen Psychiatry 1986; 43:435–440
35. Kendler KS, Neale MC, Kessler RC, Heath AC, Eaves LJ: The lifetime history of major depression in women: reliability of diagnosis and heritability. Arch Gen Psychiatry 1993; 50:863–870

ORIGINAL ARTICLE

Prevalence of and Risk Factors for Lifetime Suicide Attempts in the National Comorbidity Survey

Ronald C. Kessler, PhD; Guilherme Borges, ScD; Ellen E. Walters, MS

Background: General population survey data are presented on the lifetime prevalence of suicide attempts as well as transition probabilities to onset of ideation, plans among ideators, and attempts among ideators either with or without a plan. Risk factors for these transitions are also studied.

Methods: Data are from part II of the National Comorbidity Survey, a nationally representative survey carried out from 1990 to 1992 in a sample of 5877 respondents aged 15 to 54 years to study prevalences and correlates of *DSM-III-R* disorders. Transitions are estimated using life-table analysis. Risk factors are examined using survival analysis.

Results: Of the respondents, 13.5% reported lifetime ideation, 3.9% a plan, and 4.6% an attempt. Cumulative probabilities were 34% for the transition from ideation to a plan, 72% from a plan to an attempt, and 26% from ideation to an unplanned attempt. About 90% of unplanned and 60% of planned first attempts occurred within 1 year of the onset of ideation. All significant risk factors (female, previously married, age less than 25 years, in a recent cohort, poorly educated, and having 1 or more of the *DSM-III-R* disorders assessed in the survey) were more strongly related to ideation than to progression from ideation to a plan or an attempt.

Conclusions: Prevention efforts should focus on planned attempts because of the rapid onset and unpredictability of unplanned attempts. More research is needed on the determinants of unplanned attempts.

Arch Gen Psychiatry. 1999;56:617-626

THIS REPORT presents nationally representative data on the prevalence and risk factors of attempted suicide in the National Comorbidity Survey (NCS).[1] The motivations are that attempted suicide is both one of the strongest risk factors for completed suicide[2-4] and an important indicator of extreme emotional distress.[5,6] Previous epidemiologic studies in the United States have estimated that between 1.1%[7] and 4.3%[8] of the population attempt suicide at some time in their life. However, no previous epidemiologic survey has investigated either trends in prevalence across cohorts or conditional risk of attempts in relation to the prior onset of ideation and plans or in relation to intercohort differences; these are a focus of the current report. This report also examines sociodemographic variables and *DSM-III-R* disorders as risk factors for attempted suicide. Previous research has documented that some demographic variables are risk factors for attempted suicide, including age,[8-10] sex (reviewed by Moscicki[11]), marital status,[12,13] education,[8,13,14] race,[13,15,16] and childbearing.[17] In addition, several studies of adults[14,18,19] and youth[9,20-23] have examined the parallel effects of demographic variables on both ideation and attempts. However, no previous study has disaggregated these effects into influences on ideation, the transition from ideation to a plan, and the transition from ideation to an attempt either in the presence or absence of a plan. As shown below, insights gleaned from this disaggregation have useful implications for targeting preventive interventions.

From the Department of Health Care Policy, Harvard Medical School, Boston, Mass (Drs Kessler and Borges and Ms Walters); and the Mexican Institute of Psychiatry, Mexico City (Dr Borges).

RESULTS

PREVALENCES

The estimated lifetime prevalences (SEs) of suicide ideation, plans, and attempts in the NCS are 13.5% (0.6), 3.9% (0.4), and 4.6% (0.4), respectively. Attempters were presented with 3 statements describing the lethality of their attempt. Of the attempters, 39.3% (3.5) endorsed the statement that they made a serious attempt, and it was only because of luck that they did not die; while 13.3% (2.1) endorsed the statement that they were serious, but knew the method was not foolproof; and the remaining 47.3% (3.9) endorsed the statement that their attempt was a cry for help, and they did not want to die.

The conditional probability of ever making a plan among lifetime ideators was

SUBJECTS AND METHODS

SAMPLE

The NCS was based on a nationally representative population survey of 8098 persons aged 15 to 54 years carried out from 1990 through 1992. Informed consent was obtained from all respondents and also from parents of minors. The response rate was 82.4%. All 8098 respondents were administered the part I interview, which averaged somewhat more than 1 hour to complete and included the assessment of *DSM-III-R* disorders. All respondents who screened positive for a lifetime prevalence of any disorder and a random subsample of other respondents were administered the part II interview. The part II interview averaged slightly more than 1 hour and consisted largely of questions about risk factors and consequences of the disorders assessed in part I. The suicidality questions were included in the part II interview. As a result, the present report is based on the 5877 respondents who participated in the part II interview. The data for these respondents were weighted to correct for differential probabilities of selection into part II as well as for differential probabilities of within-household selection and nonresponse. Comparisons of the part II NCS demographic distributions with census data show that the sample is representative of the US population on a wide range of sociodemographic variables. More details about the NCS design and data collection methods are reported elsewhere.[1,24]

MEASURES

The questions about suicide ideation, plans, and attempts are part of the life-event history section of the NCS interview. Separate questions were asked about the lifetime occurrence of suicide ideation ("Have you ever seriously thought about committing suicide?"), suicide plans ("Have you ever made a plan for committing suicide?"), and suicide attempts ("Have you ever attempted suicide?"). For each of these outcomes, information was obtained about age at first occurrence and the recency of occurrence. Lethality of intent was assessed by reading 3 statements and asking attempters to select 1 of the 3 to describe their first attempt. The first statement was "I made a serious attempt to kill myself and it was only luck that I did not succeed." The second statement was "I tried to kill myself, but I knew the method was not foolproof." The third statement was "My attempt was a cry for help; I did not want to die."

The sociodemographic variables included in the analysis are sex, marital status, cohort, educational attainment, age of youngest child, race/ethnicity, and urbanicity. Marital status was coded to differentiate the currently married, previously married (separated, divorced, widowed), and never married. Cohort was coded to differentiate respondents born in the decades 1936 to 1945, 1946 to 1955, 1956 to 1965, and 1966 to 1975. Educational attainment was coded to differentiate current students from those who had completed their schooling and, within each of these 2 categories, to differentiate those who had completed less than high school, high school, some college, or college graduation or more. Age of the respondents' youngest child was coded into 4 categories consisting of respondents who had no living child and those whose youngest child was age 1 year, between ages 2 and 10 years, and more than age 10 years. Race/ethnicity was coded to differentiate among non-Hispanic whites, non-Hispanic blacks, Hispanics, and all others (Native Americans, Asians, Pacific Islanders, and respondents who self-defined themselves as "other"). Finally, urbanicity was coded to differentiate respondents living in census-defined major metropolitan areas from those living in other census-defined urbanized areas or in census-defined nonurban areas.

DSM-III-R diagnoses were generated from a modified version of the Composite International Diagnostic Interview (CIDI),[25] a fully structured interview designed to be used by trained interviewers who are not clinicians. World Health Organization Field Trials[26] and NCS clinical reappraisal studies[27] both document good reliability and validity of most CIDI diagnoses, including mood disorders (major depression and dysthymia), anxiety disorders (panic disorder, generalized anxiety disorder, phobias, and posttraumatic stress disorder), and substance use disorders (alcohol abuse and dependence and drug abuse and dependence). However, there are 2 important exceptions involving mania[28] and nonaffective psychosis,[29] neither of which is assessed with adequate validity in the CIDI. Because of these problems, a restricted definition of mania (euphoric-grandiose subtype) and clinical diagnoses of nonaffective psychosis were used rather than the CIDI diagnoses in the analyses reported here. Conduct Disorder, Adult Antisocial Behavior, and Antisocial Personality Disorder (the conjunction of Conduct Disorder and Adult Antisocial Behavior) were assessed with the Diagnostic Interview Schedule[30] since these disorders are not included in the CIDI.

ANALYSIS PROCEDURES

All analyses were carried out using the SAS[31] software package (SAS Inc, Cary, NC). Simple cross-tabulations were used to investigate the associations among suicide ideation, plans, and attempts. Life-table methods were used to examine age-of-onset distributions. A discrete-time survival analysis with time-varying covariates[32] was used to study the risk factors of lifetime suicide ideation, plans, and attempts. The use of this method in the NCS has been described in detail previously.[33] Retrospective reports were used in the survival analyses to create the time-varying risk factors (eg, ages of changes in marital status) and to date the ages of onset of the outcome variables.

Because of the complex sample design and weighting of the NCS, SEs of the survival coefficients were estimated using the Jacknife Repeated Replications[34] simulation method implemented in an SAS macro. The Jacknife Repeated Replications estimates adjust for the clustering and weighting of cases. The survival coefficients were exponentiated and are reported below in the form of odds ratios (ORs). The 95% confidence intervals (CIs) of these coefficients are also reported and have been adjusted for design effects. Multivariate tests are based on χ^2 values computed from coefficient variance-covariance matrices that were adjusted for design effects using Jacknife Repeated Replications. When a result is specified as being significant below, it is referring to statistical significance based on 2-sided design-based tests evaluated at the .05 level.

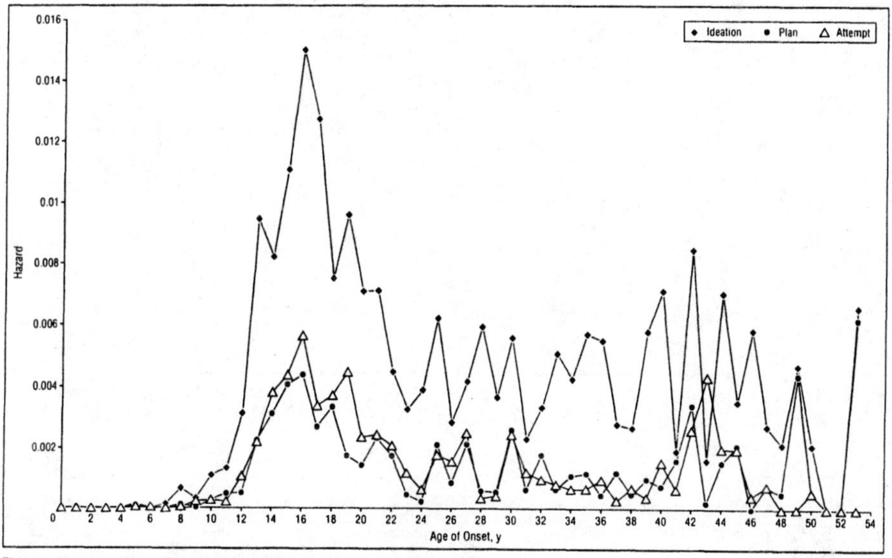

Figure 1. *Hazard functions of first onset of suicide ideation, plan, and attempt (N = 5877).*

28.9% (2.3), while the conditional probabilities of making an attempt (ignoring lethality of intent) among ideators were 57.9% (3.9) with a plan and 25.2% (1.9) without a plan. Among attempters, 46.7% (3.7) reported that they had a plan prior to making their first attempt.

ONSET DISTRIBUTIONS

Hazard curves (**Figure 1**) show that the highest risks of initial suicide ideation, plans, and attempts (ignoring lethality of intent) are in the late teens and early 20s. Age-of-onset curves (**Figure 2**) show that median ages of onset for all these outcomes are in the mid-20s. Conditional age-of-onset curves (**Figure 3**) show that progression from ideation to first onset of a plan, from a plan to first attempt, and from ideation to first attempt in the absence of a plan were all highest in the first year after onset of the earlier stage.

Two additional important results can be seen by comparing the curves for planned and unplanned attempts. One is that risk of a first attempt among ideators was substantially higher in the presence of a plan. The other is that risk of a first attempt among ideators who lack a plan was largely limited to the first year after onset of ideation. In comparison, risk of an attempt among ideators with a plan not only was very high in the year of onset of the plan, but also continued for many years afterward. In all, roughly 90% of unplanned attempts and 60% of planned attempts occurred within 1 year of the onset of ideation. Lethality of intent among attempters was not significantly related either to the presence of a plan ($\chi^2_1 = 1.0$; $P = .31$) or to speed of the attempt after onset of ideation ($\chi^2_1 = 1.2$; $P = .28$).

SOCIODEMOGRAPHIC RISK FACTORS

Risk of an attempt was significantly related to being female, being previously married, being born in a recent cohort, and having a low educational level (**Table 1**). The odds of an attempt were also lower among students than among nonstudents at the same level of educational attainment. Although non-Hispanic blacks had significantly lower odds of attempted suicide than non-Hispanic whites, the 4-category race/ethnicity variable was not significantly related to attempted suicide overall ($\chi^2_3 = 7.0$; $P = .07$).

The higher odds of an attempt among women than among men was related to 3 significant pathways, all with roughly equal ORs (1.5-1.8): higher unconditional odds of initial ideation, higher conditional odds of an attempt among ideators with a plan, and higher conditional odds of an attempt among ideators without a plan. There was no significant sex difference among ideators in the odds of making a plan. Interaction between sex and cohort in predicting attempts was also tested based on a suggestion that the sex difference might be smaller in recent cohorts.[35] No significant interaction was found ($\chi^2_3 = 5.0$; $P = .17$).

The higher odds of an attempt among previously married subjects than among currently married subjects was related to 2 of these same 3 pathways, again with roughly equal ORs (2.2): higher unconditional odds of initial ideation and higher conditional odds of an attempt among ideators with a plan. However, the second variable was not statistically significant. Unmarried ideators were not more likely than their married counterparts either to make a plan subsequent to the onset of

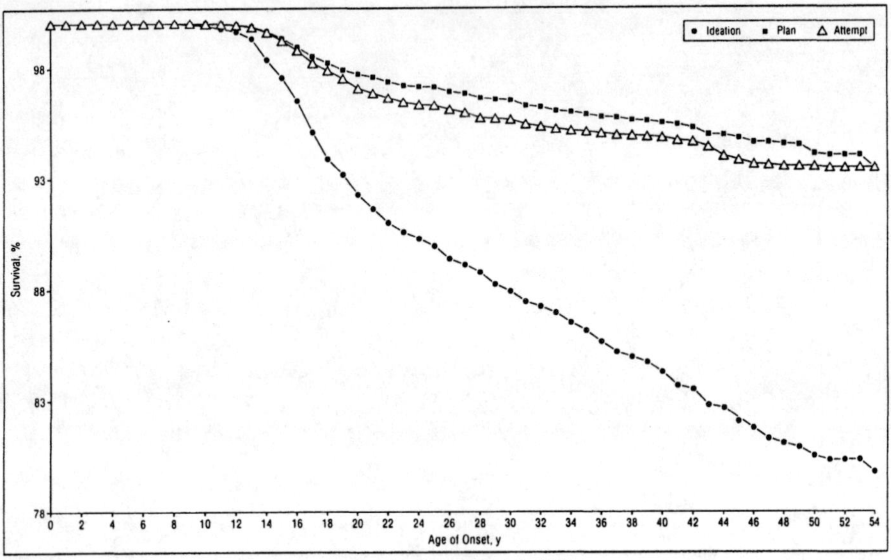

Figure 2. *Cumulative age-of-onset distribution of lifetime suicide ideation, plan, and attempt (N = 5877).*

ideation or to make an attempt in the absence of a plan. Interaction between marital status and age (coded as a dichotomy for age 18 years or younger vs age 19 years or older) was also tested based on the finding in previous research that the protective effect of marriage is less strong or even reverses at early age.[12] No significant interaction was found ($\chi^2_1 = 0.8$; $P = .39$).

The higher odds of an attempt in more recent cohorts than in earlier cohorts was related to to 3 somewhat different pathways. First, there was a significant increase across cohorts, especially strong for the most recent cohort (OR = 6.4), in the unconditional odds of ideation. Second, there was a significant but less strong increase in the conditional odds of making a plan among ideators that was very similar across all cohorts born after World War II (OR = 1.6-3.2). Third, there was a significant intercohort difference in the conditional odds of an attempt among ideators in the absence of a plan ($\chi^2_3 = 9.6$; $P = .02$). There were no significant intercohort differences in the conditional odds of an attempt among ideators in the presence of a plan ($\chi^2_3 = 3.0$; $P = .39$).

The significant negative association between education and the odds of an attempt was related to 3 pathways: a modest association with unconditional risk of ideation (OR = 1.3-2.3), a stronger association with the transition from having a plan to making an attempt (OR = 2.9-7.0), and an even stronger association with making an attempt among ideators in the absence of a plan (OR = 8.0-29.3). There was no significant association between education and the conditional odds of making a plan among ideators.

An effort was made to study the predictors of lethality of the attempt among attempters. However, the number of attempters in the NCS was too small to detect meaningful predictors with acceptable statistical power. It is of special note that neither age of first attempt ($\chi^2_4 = 3.2$; $P = .52$) nor cohort ($\chi^2_3 = 5.2$; $P = .15$) was found to be a significant predictor of lethality, although caution is needed in interpreting these negative results because of their low statistical power.

PRIOR *DSM-III-R* DISORDERS AS RISK FACTORS

Every one of the *DSM-III-R* disorders assessed in the NCS was a significant risk factor for a lifetime attempt (**Table 2**). However, the ORs for mood disorders (7.8-29.7) were substantially higher than those for any other disorders (2.1-6.5). As thoughts of death are included among the symptoms of major depression, thus creating the possibility of a confounding effect in predicting the outcomes, the analysis was also replicated with a modified definition of major depression that excluded this criterion. The OR increased from 11.0 (95% CI: 7.1-20.3) in Table 2 to 12.1 (95% CI: 9.3-15.6). Significance of variation in the effects of aggregate measures of disorders (any mood disorder, any anxiety disorder, any substance disorder, and any other disorder) as a function of both age (dichotomized at the median age of first attempt) and cohort was also tested. No significant interactions were found either with age ($\chi^2_4 = 5.8$; $P = .21$) or with cohort ($\chi^2_{12} = 14.1$; $P = .29$). In comparison, 4 significant interactions involved sex: major depression ($\chi^2_1 = 8.1$; $P = .004$), dysthymia ($\chi^2_1 = 4.5$; $P = .03$), any mood disorder ($\chi^2_1 = 6.7$; $P = .01$), and simple phobia ($\chi^2_1 = 8.5$; $P = .003$). The effect of the disorder was larger among men than among women in all 4 interactions.

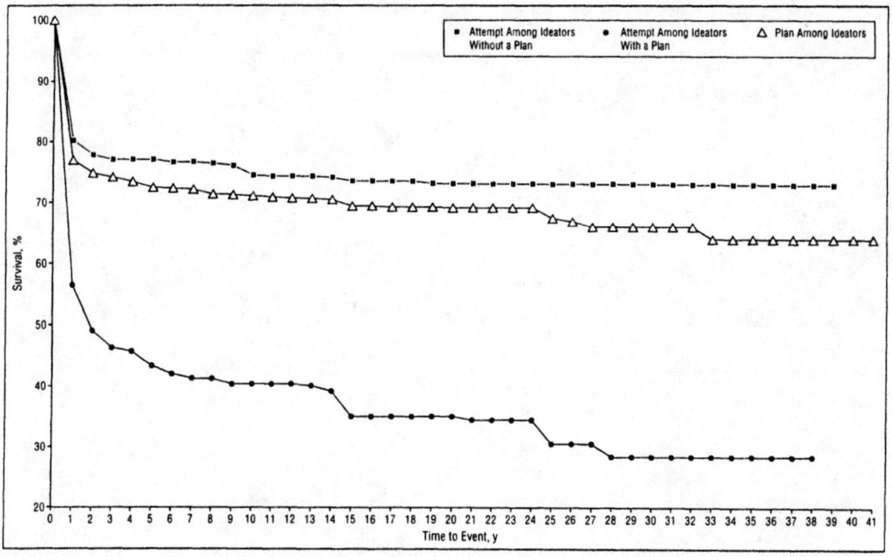

Figure 3. *Conditional, cumulative speed of onset of suicide plan among ideators (n = 230), suicide attempt among ideators without a plan (n = 145), and suicide attempt among ideators with a plan (n = 127).*

An attempt was also made to evaluate the effects of comorbidity among disorders in predicting the outcomes. As shown in the last 4 rows of Table 2, there was a significant dose-response relationship between number of prior disorders and odds of attempted suicide. Respondents with 3 or more disorders had relative odds of an attempt 19.7 times as high as respondents with no disorder. However, this result does not control for the main effects of individual disorders. When an equation was estimated that included information about each of the individual disorders as separate predictors, the incremental effect of comorbidity was found to be considerably smaller, although still statistically significant in predicting attempts, with ORs of 3.2 (95% CI: 2.0-5.2) for exactly 2 disorders and 4.1 (95% CI: 2.0-8.3) for 3 or more disorders. No significant effects of particular bivariate or multivariate comorbidity were found after controlling for number of disorders.

Three broad patterns are noteworthy in the pathways of the significant associations of prior disorders with first suicide attempts. First, there were consistently significant ORs between all of the disorders and the subsequent first onset of suicide ideation. These ORs were much higher for the mood disorders (7.7-15.5) than for any other disorders (2.2-5.3) and, within disorder, higher in predicting ideation than any other pathway for every one of the disorders. Second, the pathways associated with the conditional odds of developing a plan among ideators and of making an attempt among ideators without a plan were consistently greater than 1.0. Furthermore, ORs were roughly equal in magnitude both when compared across disorders for a particular pathway and when compared within disorders across pathways. Most of these ORs were in the range of 1.5 to 3.0. The same patterns applied to the effects of comorbidity. It is noteworthy that the much higher ORs associated with mood disorders found in other parts of the table were not found here, with the exception of strong ORs for mania with the subsequent occurrence of a plan (OR = 4.0) and an unplanned attempt (OR = 9.1). Third, the pathway associated with the conditional odds of making an attempt among ideators with a plan was generally not significant. The only exceptions were the mood disorders (OR = 1.8-3.2), panic disorder (OR = 2.0), and drug abuse (OR = 1.3).

As noted above, the sample of attempters was too small to study the predictors of lethality of the attempt with good statistical power. However, exploratory analysis shows that seriousness of attempt was positively related to total number of disorders (χ^2_{15} = 34.2; P = .003), although no particular type of disorder stands out as significantly more important than any other in the analysis of this small subsample of respondents.

COMBINING THE RISK FACTORS

Further analysis shows that the disorders considered in Table 2 partially explain the effects of the sociodemographic variables considered in Table 1. This was evaluated in a joint model to predict attempted suicide in the total sample. Results show that the significant effects of sex, cohort, and education were attenuated but remained significant when controlling for disorders. The χ^2 values for the individual predictors decreased from 34.7

Table 1. Multivariate Associations of Sociodemographic Predictors With First Onset of Attempted Suicide in the Total Sample and Disaggregated Through Pathways Involving Onset of Ideation, Plans, Impulsive Attempts, and Planned Attempts*

	Total Sample, OR (95% CI)		OR (95% CI)		
	Attempt (n = 272)	Ideation (n = 795)	Plan Among Ideators (n = 230)	Impulsive Attempt Among Ideators Without a Plan (n = 145)	Planned Attempt Among Ideators With a Plan (n = 127)
Sex					
Male	1.0	1.0	1.0	1.0	1.0
Female	2.2 (1.7-2.8)†	1.7 (1.2-2.4)†	1.2 (0.3-5.2)	1.5 (1.1-2.0)†	1.8 (1.1-2.3)†
χ^2_1/P	34.7/<.001	28.2/<.001	0.7/.41	5.9/.02	5.8/.02
Marital status					
Married	1.0	1.0	1.0	1.0	1.0
Previously married	2.6 (1.5-4.6)†	2.3 (1.7-3.0)†	1.3 (0.8-2.2)	1.1 (0.1-8.9)	2.2 (0.4-13.2)
Never married	1.2 (0.8-2.0)	1.4 (1.0-2.0)†	1.6 (0.7-3.3)	0.7 (0.4-1.3)	1.4 (0.5-4.3)
χ^2_2/P	11.7/.003	23.3/<.001	2.1/.35	1.7/.44	15.5/<.001
Cohort (year of birth)					
1966-1975	6.0 (3.9-9.2)†	6.4 (5.0-8.3)†	3.2 (1.8-5.4)†	1.0 (0.3-3.1)	1.4 (0.4-5.5)
1956-1965	2.2 (1.3-3.5)†	2.2 (1.6-3.0)†	2.2 (1.2-3.8)†	0.9 (0.6-1.4)	1.6 (0.1-21.6)
1946-1955	1.7 (0.9-3.1)	2.0 (1.4-2.7)†	1.6 (1.0-2.6)†	0.5 (0.2-1.2)	1.6 (0.3-9.8)
1936-1945	1.0	1.0	1.0	1.0	1.0
χ^2_3/P	92.0/<.001	352.0/<.001	16.6/<.001	9.6/.02	3.0/.39
Education status/y					
Student/<12	6.2 (2.3-16.7)†	2.3 (1.0-5.3)†	0.5 (0.2-1.7)	8.5 (0.8-92.3)	2.9 (0.6-14.3)
Student/12+	3.2 (1.4-7.2)†	1.4 (0.8-2.4)	0.9 (0.1-6.4)	8.0 (0.5-121.7)	5.3 (1.4-20.2)†
Nonstudent/<12	10.6 (5.2-21.3)†	2.1 (0.3-13.6)	0.9 (0.3-3.0)	29.3 (2.4-354.5)†	7.0 (1.6-29.9)†
Nonstudent/12	4.8 (2.4-10.0)†	1.6 (1.1-2.4)†	0.9 (0.4-1.9)	14.4 (1.3-158.5)†	3.5 (0.7-16.9)
Nonstudent/13-15	4.0 (1.8-8.6)†	1.3 (0.7-2.2)	1.0 (0.5-1.9)	8.1 (0.7-95.5)	6.9 (2.3-20.7)†
Nonstudent/16+	1.0	1.0	1.0	1.0	1.0
χ^2_5/P	56.7/<.001	18.7/.002	1.7/.89	50.0/<.001	17.4/.004
Age of youngest child, y					
None	1.0	1.0	1.0	1.0	1.0
1	0.8 (0.2-4.1)	1.2 (0.7-2.1)	0.8 (0.3-1.9)	0.8 (0.0-14.3)	0.5 (0.1-2.1)
2-10	1.2 (0.4-3.9)	1.3 (0.9-2.0)	0.8 (0.5-1.5)	0.8 (0.4-2.0)	1.1 (0.4-3.1)
≥11	1.9 (0.7-4.7)	1.7 (1.0-2.9)†	0.9 (0.2-4.3)	0.6 (0.2-1.7)	1.5 (0.0-79.8)
χ^2_3/P	2.2/.54	3.9/.27	0.5/.93	0.3/.96	3.0/.38
Race/ethnicity					
Non-Hispanic white	1.0	1.0	1.0	1.0	1.0
Non-Hispanic black	0.6 (0.4-0.9)†	0.7 (0.4-1.2)	0.7 (0.3-1.8)	0.8 (0.5-1.4)	1.0 (0.6-1.8)
Hispanic	1.2 (0.7-1.9)	0.9 (0.6-1.4)	1.2 (0.7-2.1)	1.7 (0.9-3.5)	1.0 (0.5-2.1)
Other	1.0 (0.5-2.3)	0.9 (0.5-1.4)	0.5 (0.1-1.9)	2.4 (1.0-5.6)	0.4 (0.0-3.5)
χ^2_3/P	7.0/.07	5.9/.12	4.0/.26	7.4/.06	2.4/.49
Urbanicity					
Metropolitan	1.2 (0.7-2.1)	1.2 (0.9-1.6)	1.2 (0.7-2.1)	1.0 (0.6-1.6)	1.0 (0.6-1.6)
Other urban	0.9 (0.2-3.4)	0.9 (0.7-1.2)	1.2 (0.7-2.0)	0.8 (0.5-1.4)	0.9 (0.5-1.7)
Rural	1.0	1.0	1.0	1.0	1.0
χ^2_2/P	3.5/.17	6.4/.04	0.8/.66	0.7/.71	.05/.77
Total model					
χ^2_{21}/P	823.0/<.001	837.5/<.001	27.8/.09	73.2/<.001	50.0/<.001

*Odds ratios (ORs) were obtained by exponentiating coefficients from discrete-time survival models. The 95% confidence intervals (CIs) were obtained using the method of Jacknife Repeated Replications to adjust for clustering and weighting of data. A single model was estimated for each of the 5 outcomes that included all the predictors and controls for person-year. Wald χ^2 values were obtained from design-based variance-covariance coefficient matrices that adjust for clustering and weighting of the data.

†$P<.05$ by 2-sided test.

to 22.7 ($P<.001$) for sex, from 92.0 to 33.6 ($P<.001$) for cohort, and from 56.7 to 29.4 ($P<.001$) for education. In comparison, the significant effect of marital status and near-significant effect of race/ethnicity in Table 1 are largely explained by mental disorders, with the χ^2 values changing from 11.7 to 4.6 ($P=.10$) for marital status and from 7.0 to 1.5 ($P=.22$) for race/ethnicity.

Survival analysis for all possible subsets was used to develop a parsimonious risk factor equation for first attempts based on the results of these multivariate models. The final equation included terms for age 15 to 24 years, female, most recent cohort, nonstudents with 12 or fewer years of education, any mood disorder, nonaffective psychosis, posttraumatic stress disorder, any substance disorder, and antisocial personality disorder. There was a dramatic dose-response relationship between number of risk factors and relative odds of first suicide attempt (**Table 3**). Inspection of the disaggregated coefficients in Table 3 shows, similar to Table 2, that the highest ORs were associated with the unconditional odds of onset of initial suicide ideation and the lowest ORs were associated with the conditional odds of a first attempt among ideators with a plan.

Table 2. Multivariate Associations of National Comorbidity Survey/*DSM-III-R* Disorders With Subsequent First Onset of Attempted Suicide in the Total Sample and Disaggregated Through Pathways Involving Onset of Ideation, Plans, Impulsive Attempts, and Planned Attempts*

	Total Sample, OR (95% CI)		OR (95% CI)		
	Attempt (n = 272)	Ideation (n = 795)	Plan Among Ideators (n = 230)	Impulsive Attempt Among Ideators Without a Plan (n = 145)	Planned Attempt Among Ideators With a Plan (n = 127)
Mood disorders					
Major depressive episode	11.0 (7.1-20.3)†	9.6 (7.5-12.3)†	1.7 (1.1-2.5)†	1.9 (1.3-2.9)†	2.1 (1.2-3.7)†
Dysthymia	7.8 (4.6-13.5)†	7.7 (5.9-10.1)†	1.9 (1.4-2.8)†	1.5 (0.9-2.5)	1.8 (1.1-2.9)†
Mania	29.7 (11.7-75.1)†	15.5 (8.9-26.8)†	4.0 (1.4-11.7)†	9.1 (1.7-50.3)†	3.2 (1.1-9.0)†
Any mood disorder	12.9 (7.8-21.3)†	10.7 (8.4-13.5)†	1.9 (1.3-2.8)†	1.7 (1.2-2.6)†	2.0 (1.2-3.4)†
Anxiety disorders					
Generalized anxiety disorder	5.6 (2.8-11.1)†	4.2 (3.1-5.9)†	2.6 (1.3-5.0)†	2.5 (1.2-5.5)†	1.1 (0.4-2.8)
Agoraphobia	2.8 (1.6-5.1)†	2.9 (2.2-3.9)†	1.5 (0.8-2.7)	1.1 (0.7-1.9)	1.2 (0.7-1.9)
Simple phobia	3.1 (1.8-5.3)†	2.9 (2.3-3.6)†	1.5 (1.1-2.2)†	1.2 (0.8-1.7)	1.3 (0.6-2.1)
Social phobia	2.1 (1.3-3.6)†	2.2 (1.7-2.9)†	1.5 (1.0-2.4)†	1.1 (0.9-1.4)	0.9 (0.6-1.3)
Panic disorder	5.6 (2.9-10.7)†	3.9 (2.8-5.3)†	1.6 (0.8-3.2)	2.0 (1.1-3.5)†	2.0 (1.0-4.0)†
Posttraumatic stress disorder	6.0 (3.4-10.7)†	5.1 (3.9-6.8)†	2.4 (1.7-3.3)†	1.7 (1.1-2.7)†	1.0 (0.6-1.6)
Any anxiety	3.2 (2.0-5.2)†	2.8 (2.2-3.5)†	1.7 (1.1-2.5)†	1.3 (1.0-1.7)†	1.0 (0.7-1.5)
Substance disorders					
Alcohol abuse	4.8 (2.8-8.1)†	3.4 (2.7-4.3)†	1.6 (1.1-2.4)†	1.5 (0.9-2.3)	1.5 (0.9-2.6)
Alcohol dependence	6.5 (3.6-11.5)†	4.6 (3.5-6.1)†	1.9 (1.3-2.9)†	1.4 (0.8-2.5)	1.8 (0.9-3.7)
Drug abuse	5.9 (3.4-10.2)†	4.9 (3.8-6.1)†	1.6 (1.1-2.3)†	1.5 (1.0-2.4)†	1.3 (1.0-1.9)†
Drug dependence	5.8 (3.3-10.1)†	5.3 (4.1-6.9)†	1.5 (1.0-2.3)†	1.4 (0.8-2.3)	1.3 (0.8-2.1)
Any substance disorder	5.8 (3.5-9.7)†	3.9 (3.1-4.9)†	1.8 (1.3-2.6)†	1.8 (1.3-2.7)†	1.4 (0.9-1.9)
Other disorders					
Conduct disorder	4.2 (2.5-6.9)†	3.2 (2.6-3.9)†	2.1 (1.5-2.9)†	1.6 (1.0-2.5)†	1.2 (0.8-1.8)
Adult antisocial behavior	5.7 (3.1-10.3)†	4.2 (3.2-5.6)†	2.1 (1.2-3.6)†	2.9 (1.5-5.5)†	0.7 (0.4-1.4)
Antisocial personality disorder	5.7 (2.9-11.2)†	4.6 (3.2-6.5)†	2.2 (1.2-4.0)†	1.8 (0.8-4.2)	1.1 (0.5-2.2)
Nonaffective psychosis	5.7 (2.6-12.4)†	4.2 (2.7-6.7)†	2.4 (1.0-6.1)†	2.8 (0.9-8.8)	0.8 (0.2-3.7)
No. of total disorders					
Any	6.7 (4.1-11.0)†	5.7 (4.4-7.3)†	1.4 (0.9-2.3)	1.7 (1.1-2.5)†	1.0 (0.6-1.7)
1	3.8 (2.1-6.9)†	3.4 (2.7-4.3)†	1.2 (0.7-2.1)	1.6 (1.0-2.6)†	0.5 (0.2-1.0)
2	6.1 (4.1-9.2)†	6.1 (4.5-8.3)†	1.0 (0.2-5.3)	1.4 (0.8-2.6)	1.0 (0.5-2.1)
≥3	19.7 (13.2-29.3)†	14.3 (11.4-18.1)†	2.4 (0.9-6.4)	2.3 (1.4-3.7)†	1.1 (0.6-2.1)

**Odds ratios (ORs) were obtained by exponentiating coefficients from discrete-time survival models. Disorders were defined without diagnostic hierarchy rules. The 95% confidence intervals (CIs) were obtained using the method of Jacknife Repeated Replications to adjust for clustering and weighting of data. Each column in this table presents the results of 22 models. Each model controls for person-year and the sociodemographic variables in Table 1. In addition, each model contains (a) exactly 1 of the 17 individual disorders, (b) exactly 1 of the 3 summary measures (any mood, any anxiety, any substance), (c) a single dichotomous measure that distinguishes between respondents with any disorders and those with no disorders, or (d) the set of summary measures of number of disorders (exactly 1, exactly 2, and 3 or more).*

†P<.05 by 2-sided test.

Inspection of the distribution of the summary risk factor count in the sample of person-years used in the survival analysis (**Table 4**) shows that the extremely high OR of a suicide attempt associated with having 5 or more risk factors accounts for only 7.0% of the people who made a lifetime attempt. This is because only a tiny fraction of the population (0.4%) had this large number of risk factors. People with 3 or more risk factors, who made up 9.2% of the population, accounted for 55.1% of all people who made a lifetime suicide attempt.

COMMENT

The results reported here are limited by the fact that the NCS is a cross-sectional survey in which information about lifetime suicide behaviors is based on retrospective reports. Because of this limitation, prevalences are likely to be lower bound estimates. The estimated effects of cohort and other risk factors could be caused, at least in part, by systematic differences in accuracy of recall related to these risk factors.[36] Furthermore, no reliability or validity data were obtained on the measures of ideation, plans, attempts, or lethality. Finally, the ability to study the distribution and predictors of lethality is constrained by the fact that the sample excluded people who completed suicide. This selection bias might account for the failure to find a significant positive association between age of first attempt and lethality of intent, an association that has been found when both attempters who died and those who survived have been considered in the same analysis.[37]

Within the context of these limitations, the 4.6% estimated lifetime prevalence of attempted suicide is above the high end of the range of estimates reported in previous US general population surveys.[15] Also, the 13.5% estimated prevalence of suicide ideation is at the high end of the range of previous estimates.[19,38,39] However, the question wording to assess ideation varied in important ways in earlier surveys,[40] sometimes asking about "thoughts" of suicide,[19] "serious" thoughts,[39] and "serious thoughts

Table 3. Multivariate Associations of the Summary Risk Score With Subsequent First Onset of Attempted Suicide in the Total Sample and Disaggregated Through Pathways Involving Onset of Ideation, Plans, Impulsive Attempts, and Planned Attempts*

	Total Sample, OR (95% CI)		OR (95% CI)		
Risk Factors	Attempt (n = 272)	Ideation (n = 795)	Plan Among Ideators (n = 230)	Impulsive Attempt Among Ideators Without a Plan (n = 145)	Planned Attempt Among Ideators With a Plan (n = 127)
None	1.0	1.0	1.0	1.0	1.0
1	6.1 (1.3-27.7)†	2.9 (2.0-4.3)†	2.3 (0.4-14.0)	2.5 (0.3-22.6)	1.5 (0.0-108.3)
2	21.4 (4.8-95.9)†	8.3 (5.6-12.4)†	2.0 (0.4-10.2)	5.4 (0.6-50.8)	1.5 (0.0-113.0)
3	124.7 (27.4-568.9)†	32.2 (21.0-49.4)†	4.6 (0.9-24.2)	10.8 (1.1-107.2)†	2.3 (0.0-171.5)
4	213.3 (47.7-953.9)†	61.7 (39.8-95.6)†	6.6 (1.3-32.9)†	7.0 (0.6-81.7)	3.8 (0.1-278.8)
≥5	477.0 (90.5-2512.7)†	115.2 (64.4-206.2)†	10.8 (1.9-61.5)†	26.8 (0.2-4445.9)	2.3 (0.0-192.1)
χ^2_5/P	312.9/<.001	736.8/<.001	51.1/<.001	54.3/<.001	6.4/.27

Odds ratios (ORs) were obtained by exponentiating coefficients from discrete-time survival models. The 95% confidence intervals (CIs) were obtained using the method of Jacknife Repeated Replications to adjust for clustering and weighting of data. The summary risk score is a count of the following risk factors: age 15 to 24 years, female, most recent cohort, nonstudent with 12 or fewer years of education, any mood disorder, nonaffective psychosis, posttraumatic stress disorder, any substance use disorder (alcohol or drug abuse or dependence), and antisocial personality disorder. A single model was estimated for each of the 5 outcomes, including separate dummy predictor variables for each level of risk. The subsample of respondents with none of the risk factors is the contrast category.

†*P*<.05 by 2-sided test.

Table 4. Distribution of the Summary Risk Score in the Total Sample, Conditional Per-Annum Probability of First Attempt, and the Distribution of Lifetime Attempts

Risk Factors	Distribution, % (SE)	Per-Annum Conditional Probability of First Attempt, % (SE)*	Lifetime Attempt, % (SE)*
None	21.8 (0.9)	0.0 (0.0)	1.7 (1.0)
1	42.2 (0.9)	0.1 (0.0)	16.8 (2.5)
2	26.8 (0.9)	0.2 (0.0)	26.3 (3.7)
3	6.7 (0.3)	1.0 (0.0)	32.3 (3.2)
4	2.1 (0.2)	1.6 (0.3)	15.8 (2.0)
≥5	0.4 (0.1)	3.6 (1.0)	7.0 (1.8)

By level of risk score.

or plans,"[38] making it difficult to make direct comparisons with the NCS findings.

There is no basis for comparing the 3.9% estimate of lifetime plans obtained in the NCS, as, to our knowledge, no previous population surveys assessed plans separate from thoughts. The finding that risk of an attempt was significantly higher among ideators with than without a plan is consistent with previous studies of period prevalence.[9,41] The finding that having a plan was unrelated to lethality of intent among attempters is inconsistent with the finding in one previous study that planned suicide attempts were generally more serious than unplanned attempts.[42]

Although, to our knowledge, no previous general population surveys estimated the age-of-onset distribution of attempted suicide, related research carried out with students confirms the NCS finding that risk begins to rise during the teenage years.[10] This is also consistent with the finding in cross-sectional surveys of adults that period prevalence of attempted suicide is inversely related to age,[8] and in longitudinal research that period prevalence decreases as a cohort moves into adulthood.[9] The NCS finding of rapid transition from first onset of suicide ideation and plans to attempts cannot be compared with previous research, as no other population surveys have examined this issue.

The risk factors considered here were examined in a survival framework to study the predictors of first attempts. Previous research has generally studied cross-sectional associations between current measures of risk factors and lifetime measures of attempts. This difference in methods could lead to discrepancies in results. Therefore, it is striking that most of the NCS risk factor results are consistent with those found in previous research. These include the higher lifetime prevalence of attempted suicide among women than among men,[11] the higher prevalence among previously married people,[13] and the inverse association with education,[8] although the education association was stronger in the NCS than in other recent studies.[13,14] The significantly lower odds of an attempt among non-Hispanic blacks than among whites is consistent with the trend in previous studies (reviewed by Moscicki[15]), although some studies did not find a race difference.[13,16] The analysis fails to replicate the finding of a decrease in the sex difference over recent cohorts[35] or the finding that the protective effect of being married is reversed among very young people.[12]

The NCS provides the first nationally representative general population data on intercohort difference in lifetime suicide attempts. This finding is consistent with independent evidence that could not be explained by a methodological artifact, including increasing prevalences of completed suicide in the United States[43] and elsewhere[44] in recent cohorts and increasing prevalences of attempted suicide among young people in clinical settings.[45-47] To our knowledge, there is no previous research to compare with the findings reported here of insignificant effects of urbanicity or age of youngest child. The finding that a substantial part of this cohort effect is explained by controlling for disorders means that increasing prevalences of mental disorders in recent cohorts account for most but not all of the cohort effect in suicide attempts.

The strong associations of *DSM-III-R* disorders with subsequent attempted suicide and the dose-response relationship between the number of these disorders and attempts are consistent with other cross-sectional[8,19,48] and longitudinal[9,13,18] community epidemiologic surveys. The finding that mood disorders are stronger predictors than other mental or substance use disorders is also consistent with earlier studies. The NCS results do not confirm the findings in some earlier studies, however, of especially strong effects of substance use disorders,[49] antisocial personality disorder,[14] or panic disorder.[19] Stronger associations might have been obtained if the analysis had examined the effects of critical symptoms, such as hopelessness, rather than exclusively focusing on diagnoses.

THE FINDING THAT comorbidity is a significant predictor of suicide attempts over and above the effects of individual disorders is consistent with many recent studies among both children[50,51] and adults.[52-54] While some of these earlier reports suggest a special role of particular types of comorbidity, none of them controlled rigorously for both specific individual disorders and global patterns of comorbidity (ie, number of disorders). When such controls were introduced, no special effects of comorbidity involving particular disorders were found. Total number of disorders, rather than the types of disorders involved in the comorbidity, were found to be the strongest predictors of suicide attempts.

The finding that comorbidity is a significant predictor of lethality is also important and is an exception to the more general failure to document significant predictors of lethality of intent among attempters in the NCS. This failure is inconsistent with findings from previous studies that have documented several significant predictors of lethality, including having a plan and late age of first attempt, that were found not to be significant in the NCS.[31,33,37,55] As noted above, the low statistical power to study lethality of intent in the NCS, coupled with the fact that suicide completers were excluded from the analysis, might account for the failure to replicate these previous findings regarding significant predictors of lethality.

The findings that rapid-onset attempts account for more than 90% of unplanned first attempts and approximately two thirds of planned first attempts are in need of replication in both clinical samples and general population samples before they can be accepted. If confirmed, the finding that the vast majority of unplanned first attempts occur shortly after the onset of suicide ideation means that efforts to intervene after the onset of ideation to prevent a first unplanned attempt would be impractical unless a patient presented for treatment within a year of first onset of ideation. In cases in which this occurs, the obvious implications are that the clinician should search for modifiable risk factors (eg, depression) and should engage in especially aggressive treatment over the high-risk period of the first year.[56,57] As noted by Brent,[55] it is also important to make sure patients at risk of impulsive attempts do not have access to medications that can be used to make a suicide attempt, as risk of unplanned attempts may be increased by easy access to such agents.

The only potentially realistic high-risk population prevention efforts aimed at first suicide attempts after the first year of ideation would deal with planned attempts. The retrospective NCS results suggest that approximately one half of the people in the general population with a history of a suicide plan who do not make an attempt during their first year of ideation make an attempt at some later date. The combination of high conditional risk and a long risk period in a fairly small proportion of the population (about 2% of the population in recent cohorts) makes it likely that focused interventions in this subgroup would be cost-effective.

The risk factors considered in this report are more directly related to first attempts among ideators with a plan than to unplanned attempts. This can be seen most clearly in Table 3, where the OR comparing the highest- and lowest-risk groups is 2.3 for predicting a first attempt among ideators with a plan compared with between 10.8 and 115.2 for the other pathways in the table. Clearly, if effective interventions to prevent first attempts among ideators with a plan are to be developed, they will need to go beyond the standard set of risk factors considered in the current report and elsewhere in the literature to gain insights into possible intervention targets in this high-risk segment of the population.

Accepted for publication March 30, 1999.

This study was supported by grants R01 MH46376, R01 MH49098, and R01 MH52861 from the National Institute of Mental Health, Bethesda, Md, with supplemental support by grant MH46376 from the National Institute on Drug Abuse, Bethesda, and grant 90135190 from the William T. Grant Foundation, New York, NY (Dr Kessler). Preparation of this report was also supported by Research Scientist Award K05 MH00507 from the National Institutes of Health, Bethesda (Dr Kessler), and by a joint fellowship from NIDA/INVEST (National Institute on Drug Abuse International Visiting Scientists and Technical Exchange Program) and CONACYT (Consejo Nacional de Ciencia y Tecnología), Mexico City, Mexico (Dr Borges).

Collaborating National Comorbidity Survey sites and investigators are The Addiction Research Foundation, Toronto, Ontario (Robin Room, PhD); Duke University Medical Center, Durham, NC (Dan Blazer, MD, PhD, Marvin Swartz, MD); Harvard Medical School, Boston, Mass (Richard Frank, PhD, Ronald Kessler, PhD); Johns Hopkins University, Baltimore, Md (James Anthony, PhD, William Eaton, PhD, Philip Leaf, PhD); the Max Planck Institute of Psychiatry Clinical Institute, Munich, Germany (Hans-Ulrich Wittchen, PhD); the Medical College of Virginia, Richmond (Kenneth Kendler, MD); the University of Miami, Miami, Fla (R. Jay Turner, PhD); the University of Michigan, Ann Arbor (Lloyd Johnston, PhD, Roderick Little, PhD); New York University, New York (Patrick Shrout, PhD); State University of New York, Stony Brook (Evelyn Bromet, PhD); and Washington University School of Medicine, St Louis, Mo (Linda Cottler, PhD, Andrew Heath, DPhil).

A complete list of all National Comorbidity Survey publications, along with abstracts, study documentation, interview schedules, and the raw National Comorbidity Survey public use data files, can be obtained directly from the National Comorbidity Survey home page: http://www.hcp.med.harvard.edu/ncs.

Corresponding author: Ronald C. Kessler, PhD, Department of Health Care Policy, Harvard Medical School, 180 Longwood Ave, Boston, MA 02115-5899 (e-mail: Kessler@hcp.med.harvard.edu).

REFERENCES

1. Kessler RC, McGonagle KA, Zhao S, Nelson CB, Hughes M, Eshleman S, Wittchen HU, Kendler KS. Lifetime and 12-month prevalence of *DSM-III-R* psychiatric disorders in the United States: results from the National Comorbidity Survey. *Arch Gen Psychiatry.* 1994;51:8-19.
2. Brent DA, Perper JA. Research in adolescent suicide: implication for training, service delivery and public policy. *Suicide Life Threat Behav.* 1995;25:222-230.
3. Nordstrom P, Samuelsson M, Asberg M. Survival analysis of suicide risk after attempted suicide. *Acta Psychiatr Scand.* 1995;91:336-340.
4. Johnsson-Fridell E, Ojehagen A, Traskman-Bendz L. A 5-year follow-up study of suicide attempts. *Acta Psychiatr Scand.* 1996;93:151-157.
5. Moscicki EK. Epidemiology of suicidal behavior. *Suicide Life Threat Behav.* 1995; 25:22-35.
6. Lewinsohn PM, Clark GN, Seeley JR, Rohde P. Major depression in community adolescents: age at onset, episode duration, and time to recurrence. *J Am Acad Child Adolesc Psychiatry.* 1994;33:809-818.
7. Paykel ES, Myers JK, Lindenthal JJ, Tanner J. Suicidal feelings in the general population: a prevalence study. *Br J Psychiatry.* 1974;124:460-469.
8. Moscicki EK, O'Carroll P, Rae DS, Locke BZ, Roy A, Regier DA. Suicide attempts in the Epidemiologic Catchment Area Study. *Yale J Biol Med.* 1988;61:259-268.
9. Lewinsohn PM, Rohde P, Seeley JR. Adolescent suicidal ideation and attempts: prevalence, risk factors, and clinical implications. *Clin Psychol Sci Pract.* 1996; 3:25-46.
10. Bolger N, Downey G, Walker E, Steininger P. The onset of suicidal ideation in childhood and adolescence. *J Youth Adolesc.* 1989;18:175-190.
11. Moscicki EK. Gender differences in completed and attempted suicides. *Ann Epidemiol.* 1994;4:152-158.
12. Kreitman N. Suicide, age and marital status. *Psychol Med.* 1988;18:121-128.
13. Petronis KR, Samuels JF, Moscicki EK, Anthony JC. An epidemiologic investigation of potential risk factors for suicide attempts. *Soc Psychiatry Psychiatr Epidemiol.* 1990;25:193-199.
14. Sorenson SB, Golding JM. Suicide ideation and attempts in Hispanics and non-Hispanic whites: demographic and psychiatric disorder issues. *Suicide Life Threat Behav.* 1988;18:205-218.
15. Moscicki EK. Identification of suicide risk factors using epidemiologic studies. *Psychiatr Clin North Am.* 1997;20:499-518.
16. Roberts RE, Chen YR, Roberts CR. Ethnocultural differences in prevalence of adolescent suicidal behaviors. *Suicide Life Threat Behav.* 1997;27:208-217.
17. Appelby L, Turnbull G. Parasuicide in the first postnatal year. *Psychol Med.* 1995; 25:1087-1090.
18. Juon HS, Ensminger ME. Childhood, adolescent, and young adult predictors of suicidal behaviors: a prospective study of African Americans. *J Child Psychol Psychiatry.* 1997;38:533-563.
19. Weissman MM, Gerald LK, Markowitz JS, Ouellette R. Suicidal ideation and suicide attempts in panic disorder and attacks. *N Engl J Med.* 1989;321:1209-1214.
20. Brent DA, Kalas R, Edelbrock C, Costello AJ, Dulcan MK, Conover N. Psychopathology and its relationship to suicidal ideation in childhood and adolescence. *J Am Acad Child Psychiatry.* 1986;25:666-673.
21. Reinherz HZ, Giaconia RM, Silverman AB, Friedman A, Pakiz B, Frost AK, Cohen E. Early psychosocial risks for adolescent suicidal ideation and attempts. *J Am Acad Child Adolesc Psychiatry.* 1995;34:599-611.
22. Gould MS, King R, Greenwald S, Fisher P, Schwabstone M, Kramer R, Flisher AJ, Goodman S, Canino G, Shaffer D. Psychopathology associated with suicidal ideation and attempts among children and adolescents. *J Am Acad Child Adolesc Psychiatry.* 1998;37:915-923.
23. Goldston DB, Daniel SS, Reboussin BA, Reboussin DM, Kelley AE, Frazier RH. Psychiatric diagnoses of previous suicide attempters, first-time attempters, and repeat attempters on an adolescent inpatient psychiatry unit. *J Am Acad Child Adolesc Psychiatry.* 1998;37:924-932.
24. Kessler RC, Little RJA, Groves RM. Advances in strategies for minimizing and adjusting for survey nonresponse. *Epidemiol Rev.* 1995;17:192-204.
25. World Health Organization. *Composite International Diagnostic Interview (CIDI), Version 1.0.* Geneva, Switzerland: World Health Organization; 1990.
26. Wittchen H-U. Reliability and validity studies of the WHO Composite International Diagnostic Interview (CIDI): a critical review. *J Psychiatr Res.* 1994;28: 57-84.
27. Kessler RC, Wittchen H-U, Abelson JM, McGonagle KA, Schwartz N, Kendler KS, Knäuper B, Zhao S. Methodological studies of the Composite International Diagnostic Interview (CIDI) in the U.S. National Comorbidity Survey. *Int J Meth Psychiatr Res.* 1998;7:33-55.
28. Kessler RC, Rubinow DR, Holmes C, Abelson JM, Zhao S. The epidemiology of *DSM-III-R* bipolar I disorder in a general population survey. *Psychol Med.* 1997; 27:1079-1089.
29. Kendler KS, Gallagher TJ, Abelson JM, Kessler RC. Lifetime prevalence, demographic risk factors, and diagnostic validity of nonaffective psychosis as assessed in a US community sample: the National Comorbidity Survey. *Arch Gen Psychiatry.* 1996;53:1022-1031.
30. Robins LN, Wing J, Wittchen HU, Helzer JE, Babor TF, Burke J, Farmer A, Jablenski A, Pickens R, Regier DA, Sartorious N, Towle LH. The Composite International Diagnostic Interview: an epidemiologic instrument suitable for use in conjunction with different diagnostic systems and in different cultures. *Arch Gen Psychiatry.* 1988;45:1069-1077.
31. SAS Inc. *STAT User's Guide, Version 6.* Cary, NC: SAS Institute; 1990.
32. Efron B. Logistic regression, survival analysis, and the Kaplan-Meier curve. *J Am Sociol Assoc.* 1988;83:414-425.
33. Kessler RC, Sonnega A, Bromet E, Hughes M, Nelson CB. Posttraumatic stress disorder in the National Comorbidity Survey. *Arch Gen Psychiatry.* 1995;52: 1048-1060.
34. Kish L, Frankel MR. Balanced repeated replications for standard errors. *J Am Stat Assoc.* 1970;65:1071-1094.
35. Kessler RC, McRae JA. Trends in the relationship between sex and attempted suicide. *J Health Soc Behav.* 1983;24:98-110.
36. Giuffra LA, Risch N. Diminished recall and the cohort effect of major depression: a simulation study. *Psychol Med.* 1994;24:375-383.
37. Safer DJ. Adolescent/adult differences in suicidal behavior and outcome. *Ann Clin Psychiatry.* 1997;9:61-66.
38. Ramsay R, Bagley C. The prevalence of suicidal behaviors, attitudes and associated social experiences in an urban population. *Suicide Life Threat Behav.* 1985; 15:151-167.
39. Schwab JJ, Warheit GJ, Holzer CE. Suicidal ideation and behavior in a general population. *Dis Nerv Syst.* 1972;33:745-748.
40. O'Carroll P, Berman AL, Maris RW, Moscicki EK, Tanney BL, Silverman MM. Beyond the Tower of Babel: a nomenclature for suicidology. *Suicide Life Threat Behav.* 1996;26:237-252.
41. Garrison CZ, McKeown RE, Valois RF, Vincent ML. Aggression, substance use, and suicidal behaviors in high school students. *Am J Public Health.* 1993;83: 179-184.
42. Brown LK, Overholser JC, Spirito A, Fritz GK. The correlates of planning in adolescent suicide attempts. *J Am Acad Child Adolesc Psychiatry.* 1991;30:95-99.
43. Kachur SP, Potter LB, James SP, Powell KE. *Suicide in the United States, 1980-1992.* Atlanta, Ga: National Center for Injury Prevention and Control, Centers for Disease Control and Prevention; 1995. Violence Surveillance Summary Series, No. 1.
44. Diekstra CZ, Gulbinat W. The epidemiology of suicidal behavior: a review of three continents. *World Health Stat Q.* 1993;46:52-68.
45. Hawton K, Fagg J. Deliberate self-poisoning and self-injury in adolescents: a study of characteristics and trends in Oxford, 1976-89. *Br J Psychiatry.* 1992;161:816-823.
46. McEvedy CJ. Trends in self-poisoning: admissions to a central London hospital, 1991-1994. *J R Soc Med.* 1997;90:496-498.
47. Bille-Brahe U. The role of sex and age in suicidal behavior. *Acta Psychiatr Scand.* 1993;371(suppl):21-27.
48. Beautrais AL, Joyce PR, Mulder RT, Fergusson DM, Deavoll BJ, Nightingale SK. Prevalence and comorbidity of mental disorders in persons making serious suicide attempts: a case-control study. *Am J Psychiatry.* 1996;153:1009-1014.
49. Adams DM, Overholser JC. Suicidal behavior and history of substance abuse. *Am J Drug Alcohol Abuse.* 1992;18:343-354.
50. Wonderlich U, Bronisch T, Wittchen H-U. Comorbidity patterns in adolescents and young adults with suicide attempts. *Eur Arch Psychiatry Clin Neurosci.* 1998; 248:87-95.
51. Lewinsohn PM, Rohde P, Seeley JR. Adolescent psychopathology, III: the clinical consequences of comorbidity. *J Am Acad Child Adolesc Psychiatry.* 1995; 34:510-519.
52. Suominen K, Henriksson M, Suokas J, Isometsä E, Ostamo A, Lönnqvist J. Mental disorders and comorbidity in attempted suicide. *Acta Psychiatr Scand.* 1996; 94:234-240.
53. Rudd MD, Dahm PF, Rajab MH. Diagnostic comorbidity in persons with suicidal ideation and behavior. *Am J Psychiatry.* 1993;150:928-934.
54. Bronisch T, Wittchen H-U. Suicidal ideation and suicide attempts: comorbidity with depression, anxiety disorders, and substance abuse disorder. *Eur Arch Psychiatry Clin Neurosci.* 1994;244:93-98.
55. Brent DA. Correlates of the medical lethality of suicide attempts in children and adolescents. *J Am Acad Child Adolesc Psychiatry.* 1987;26:87-91.
56. van der Sande R, Buskens E, Allart E, van der Graaf Y, van Engeland H. Psychosocial intervention following suicide attempt: a systematic review of treatment interventions. *Acta Psychiatr Scand.* 1997;96:43-50.
57. Power K, Davies C, Swanson V, Gordon D, Carter H. Case-control study of GP attendance rates by suicide cases with or without a psychiatric history. *Br J Gen Pract.* 1997;47:211-215.

ORIGINAL ARTICLE

A 40-Year Perspective on the Prevalence of Depression

The Stirling County Study

Jane M. Murphy, PhD; Nan M. Laird, PhD; Richard R. Monson, MD, DSc; Arthur M. Sobol, MA; Alexander H. Leighton, MD

Background: According to epidemiologic studies that use recall of lifetime episodes, the prevalence of depression is increasing. This report from the Stirling County Study compares rates of current depression among representative samples of adults from a population in Atlantic Canada.

Methods: Sample sizes were 1003, 1201, and 1396 in 1952, 1970, and 1992, respectively. The depression component of the study's method, the DPAX (DP for depression and AX for anxiety), was employed. The original procedure (DPAX-1) was applied in all years. A revision (DPAX-2) was used in 1970 and 1992. The Diagnostic Interview Schedule (DIS) was also used in 1992.

Results: With the DPAX-1, the overall prevalence of current depression was steady at 5% over the 2 early samples but declined in 1992 because of vernacular changes referring to dysphoria. The DPAX-2 gave a stable overall prevalence of 5% in the 2 recent samples, but indicated that women and younger people were at greater risk in 1992 than in 1970. The DIS, like the DPAX-2, found a current 1992 rate of 5% for major depressive episodes combined with dysthymia. Recalled lifetime rates using the DIS showed the same profile interpreted in other studies as suggesting an increase in depression over time.

Conclusions: Three samples over a 40-year period showed a stable current prevalence of depression using the DPAX methods that was comparable in 1992 with the current rates using the DIS. This casts doubt on the interpretation that depression is generally increasing. Within the overall steady rate observed in this study, historical change was a matter of redistribution by sex and age, with a higher rate among younger women being of recent origin.

Arch Gen Psychiatry. 2000;57:209-215

The Epidemiologic Catchment Area (ECA) program, the National Comorbidity Survey, the Edmonton Psychiatric Epidemiology Study in Canada, and the Lundby Study in Sweden suggest that rates of depression are increasing.[1-9] These studies used methods that ask subjects to recall episodes of depression and have been criticized for the fact that such memories may be unreliable.[10-13]

See also pages 217, 223, 227, and 230

This report takes a different approach, in that we focus on what subjects said about their current moods, symptoms, and impairment when interviewed as members of representative samples from the same general population at 3 points (1952, 1970, and 1992), thus providing a population perspective that makes long-term recall unnecessary. As in an earlier report that dealt with 1952 and 1970, we use the study's traditional methods for diagnosing disorders.[14-16] We added the Diagnostic Interview Schedule (DIS) of the ECA for the 1992 survey so that comparisons could be drawn with other studies.[17]

The research site, given the pseudonym *Stirling County* and located in Canada on the eastern side of the Gulf of Maine, was selected for its socioeconomic and cultural diversity.[18-20] The population numbered 19 989 in the early 1950s and 21 255 in the 1990s. As a region, it has experienced the social trends that characterize North America generally. These include the social advances of a rising standard of living, improved health care delivery, and increased educational opportunities. The changing times have also brought disadvantages, such as racial tension and increases in crime, including illegal drug use; loosening of family ties; and weakening of religious values. The economic picture has fluctuated, rising to a

From the Departments of Psychiatry, Harvard Medical School (Dr Murphy) and Massachusetts General Hospital (Dr Murphy and Mr Sobol); the Departments of Epidemiology (Drs Murphy and Monson) and Biostatistics (Dr Laird), Harvard School of Public Health, Boston, Mass; and the Departments of Psychiatry and of Community Health and Epidemiology, Dalhousie University, Halifax, Nova Scotia (Dr Leighton).

PARTICIPANTS AND METHODS

SAMPLING

The sampling procedures for 1952 and 1970 have been described previously.[14,19,21] The following points are relevant to the sample of 1992: (1) Research maps and the census were updated and continued to provide the means for selecting and locating subjects. (2) The 1952 sample was a selection of heads of households, while the samples of 1970 and 1992 were selections of all adults 18 years and older, among whom heads of households were designated. (3) Communities of special interest because of socioeconomic and cultural contrasts were consistently oversampled using identical procedures. (4) For the remaining communities, the 1952 sample used variable sampling rates, the 1970 sample was based on selecting every ninth name from the census, and the 1992 sample used computer techniques to make a random selection from the census.

We have found that being a head of household was not related to the prevalence of depression and thus this report draws on all subjects with complete information (**Table 1**). Subjects gave informed consent to be interviewed. After the first survey, follow-up interviewing of subjects from earlier samples was coordinated with interviewing new subjects.[22-29] Because of this, interviewing for the second and third samples took longer than interviewing for the first sample. For the 1970 sample, interviewing extended from the summer of 1969 through 1971, and for the recent sample, from 1992 through 1995. Therefore, current point prevalence should be interpreted as referring to the disorders present at the time of interview.

INTERVIEW METHODS AND DEFINITIONS OF DEPRESSION

Two methods of data gathering and analysis employed herein were developed within the Stirling County Study and have been described elsewhere.[15,16] They are named for the diagnostic focus on depression and anxiety (DPAX [DP for depression and AX for anxiety]), with the second (DPAX-2) being a revision of the first (DPAX-1) and with depression being separately analyzed in this report.

The original interview schedule used in the Stirling County Study contained only one question about dysphoria (using the word *spirits* to represent mood) and only one about functional impairment. According to psychometric principles, the greater the number of questions asked on a given theme, the greater the reliability.[30] Thus, for the 1970 phase, several questions were added and they have been maintained in the subsequent issues of the schedule. By the 1990s, positive responses to the question about spirits had declined, while the proportion who responded positively to other questions about dysphoria ("feeling low and hopeless" and "wondering if anything is worthwhile anymore") increased. This suggested that phrases such as *poor spirits* or *low spirits*, like *melancholy*, were waning as familiar ways of talking about depressed mood. Thus, the DPAX-2 was prepared to make use of the new questions.

These methods employ a concept of depression that approximates the one used in the *DSM-III* and *DSM-IV*.[31-33] Both the original and revised versions follow an algorithm that takes into account "essential features," "associated symptoms," "impairment," and "duration."

For essential features, the DPAX-1 requires a response of *sometimes* or *rarely* to the question "Do you feel in good spirits?" responses that we will describe by the term *poor spirits*. The DPAX-2 requires a positive response to at least 1 of 3 questions (poor spirits, low and hopeless, or wondering if things are worthwhile).

For associated symptoms, the DPAX-2 needs positive evidence in each of the 3 clusters of symptoms concerning disturbances of appetite, sleep, and energy, but the DPAX-1 allows only 2 clusters to be represented if the subject is frequently in poor spirits. It is in the area of associated symptoms that both versions of the DPAX are limited in congruence to criteria spelled out in *DSM-III* and *DSM-IV*.

period of prosperity in the 1980s followed by a recent downturn. The primary industries have declined, large numbers of women have entered the labor force, the service and information industries have grown, and urbanism has increased through the media and travel.

RESULTS

ESTIMATES OF CURRENT DEPRESSION FOR THREE SAMPLES

The overall prevalence of depression according to the DPAX-1 remained stable at 5.3% in 1952 and 1970 but decreased significantly to 2.9% in 1992 (**Table 2**). The rates for women were somewhat higher than those for men in each year but the differences were not significant. Age was significantly related to the rates of depression in 1952 and 1970 but not in 1992. However, the patterns of association with age were not consistent over time or by sex.

The DPAX-2 indicated that the rate of depression was 5.3% in 1970 and 5.7% in 1992. In 1970, the prevalence of depression in men and women was not significantly different. In 1992, the rate for women was significantly higher than that for men. Age was significantly related to depression in 1970 but not in 1992.

The DIS results for 1992 indicated that the 1-month rate for MDE was 2.6%, while the rate for dysthymia without MDE was 2.9%; when these rates were combined, the current prevalence of acute and chronic depression was 5.5%. Women had a significantly higher prevalence of the combined disorders than men, but age was not significantly associated with the rate.

AGREEMENT AND DISAGREEMENT BETWEEN THE DPAX-1 AND THE DPAX-2

To explore reasons why the 2 DPAX methods gave different rates in 1992 in contrast to the similarity of rates in 1970, we compared the results as they applied to individual cases. Agreement was better in 1970 than 1992 (**Figure 1**). To meet the criteria for essential features in the DPAX-2, at least 1 of 3 indicators of dysphoria was

For functional impairment, both DPAX methods are similar to the model provided in *DSM-IV*, in which the following criterion was added: "The symptoms cause clinically significant distress or impairment in social, occupational, or other important areas of functioning."[32(p327)] The DPAX-1 requires a positive response to its one question about "going easy on work," while the DPAX-2 involves a larger array of questions. Two of them are general and deal with not being able to "get going" and not being "healthy enough to do things," while the others are linked specifically with depression and concern hospitalization and interference with work, family, and social activities.

Where duration is concerned, the DPAX-2 estimates the time of occurrence and the duration of the episode using supplemental questions, which are asked if positive evidence has been given about the essential features. These questions concern when the symptoms started, whether they still bother the subject, and, if not, when they stopped being bothersome. For the DPAX-1, time of occurrence is based on the period of going easy on work. Both algorithms require a minimum duration of 1 month, but the actual durations have been found to be longer. The average duration of essential symptoms found by the DPAX-2 varied between 10 and 11 years in 1970 and 1992; the average duration of impairment found by the DPAX-1 was about 8 years in each of the 3 surveys. This information does not mean that all aspects of essential features, associated symptoms, and impairment occurred together throughout these durations. Nevertheless, a sizable proportion of the DPAX depressive disorders seemed to be chronic.

The complete module for depression from the DIS, as used in the ECA, was added to the Stirling interview protocol for the 1990s.[17] The purpose was to compare the DPAX findings with those of the ECA and other DIS studies that use *DSM-III* criteria, especially the other main North American investigation, the Edmonton Psychiatric Epidemiology Study.[6,34,35] Major depressive episode (MDE) and dysthymia were used in combination for comparison with the DPAX, since the latter involves both acute and chronic disorders. One-month and lifetime rates of MDE were computed. One-month rates include episodes in existence at the time of interview or within the month preceding the interview. Lifetime rates include all episodes recalled as occurring at any time during the subject's life up to and including the time of interview. We followed the convention of the ECA in considering dysthymia to be a current disorder.[36]

STATISTICAL METHODS

The dependent variable for this study is the current prevalence of depression. Three explanatory variables are used: year of study, sex, and age. The main statistical procedure employed was hierarchical modeling, using a form of logistic regression known as log-linear analysis.[37-39] For analysis focused on between-year comparisons, year of study was investigated first in terms of a model that assessed its association with current depression controlling for age and sex, then by models that assessed the 2-way interactions of year of study with sex and age. The levels of significance were based on maximum likelihood χ^2 statistics with appropriate degrees of freedom. To facilitate comparison with other investigations, within-year analysis was also carried out. Each of the 3 years was assessed individually for the associations of sex and age with current depression.

To adjust for variable sampling rates, we divided the county into 3 districts (2 for the oversampled and contrasting communities and 1 for the remainder of the county). The rates were standardized by the direct method to the pooled adult populations of the county for 1952, 1970, and 1992.[40] The age profile of the population of Stirling County changed in ways similar to that for North America generally because of the increase of births after World War II. Since our goal was a comparison of rates over the years of study, we standardized the rates to the pooled population rather than choosing one year as opposed to another.

Table 1. Data Completeness, Age, and Sex for the 3 Samples

	Year of Sample Selection					
	1952		1970		1992	
No. selected	1098		1369		1618	
Complete interviews, No. (%)	1003 (91)		1201 (88)		1396 (86)	
	Female	Male	Female	Male	Female	Male
Age, No. (%)						
<45 y	281 (51.3)	192 (42.1)	271 (44.9)	242 (40.5)	333 (43.9)	280 (43.9)
45-64 y	175 (32.0)	168 (36.8)	221 (36.6)	234 (39.2)	249 (32.9)	230 (36.0)
≥65 y	91 (16.6)	96 (21.0)	112 (18.5)	121 (20.2)	176 (23.2)	128 (20.0)
Total*	**547** (100)	**456** (100)	**604** (100)	**597** (100)	**758** (100)	**638** (100)

**In some columns, percentages do not add to 100% because of rounding.*

needed, including poor spirits. In the DPAX-1, poor spirits was the sole and necessary indicator of dysphoria. Therefore, if a subject fulfilled the criteria for essential features in the DPAX-1, that person automatically fulfilled the criteria in the DPAX-2. The obverse was not true; therefore, a main reason for disagreement was that a subject could exhibit dysphoria according to the DPAX-2 but not according to the DPAX-1 (**Table 3**).

Another contribution to disagreement was that only one question was available for disability in the

Table 2. Standardized Current Prevalence Rates of Depression Identified by 3 Methods in 1952, 1970, and 1992*

	Prevalence (SE) of Depression (per 100)											
	1952 (n = 1003)				1970 (n = 1201)				1992 (n = 1396)			
	Age, y				Age, y				Age, y			
Method	<45	45-64	≥65	Total	<45	45-64	≥65	Total	<45	45-64	≥65	Total
DPAX-1†												
Female	4.5 (1.2)	6.1 (1.9)	11.0 (3.3)	6.4 (1.1)	3.9 (1.2)	6.7 (1.8)	7.7 (2.6)	5.6 (1.0)	4.4 (1.2)	3.3 (1.2)	2.2 (1.1)	3.6 (0.7)
Male	2.3 (1.1)	7.0 (2.0)	4.4 (2.1)	4.1 (0.9)	3.1 (1.1)	10.0 (2.0)	1.9 (1.3)	5.0 (0.9)	1.8 (0.9)	2.1 (1.0)	3.8 (1.7)	2.3 (0.6)
Total	3.4 (0.8)	6.6 (1.4)	7.9 (2.0)	5.3 (0.7)	3.5 (0.8)	8.4 (1.3)	5.0 (1.5)	5.3 (0.6)	3.1 (0.7)	2.7 (0.8)	3.0 (1.0)	2.9 (0.5)
DPAX-2‡												
Female					3.3 (1.1)	8.1 (1.9)	8.9 (2.7)	5.9 (1.0)	8.2 (1.6)	6.6 (1.6)	5.7 (1.7)	7.1 (1.0)
Male					2.8 (1.1)	9.3 (2.0)	1.9 (1.3)	4.6 (0.8)	3.2 (1.1)	4.7 (1.4)	6.2 (2.1)	4.2 (0.8)
Total					3.0 (0.8)	8.7 (1.4)	5.6 (1.6)	5.3 (0.6)	5.6 (1.0)	5.6 (1.1)	5.9 (1.3)	5.7 (0.6)
DIS§												
Female									9.3 (1.7)	7.6 (1.8)	4.8 (1.7)	7.8 (1.0)
Male									3.7 (1.2)	2.9 (1.1)	2.6 (1.5)	3.2 (0.7)
Total									6.4 (1.0)	5.2 (1.0)	3.8 (1.1)	5.5 (0.6)

**DPAX-1 and DPAX-2 indicate the original and revised methods of the Stirling County Study method for diagnosing depression (DP) and anxiety (AX); DIS, Diagnostic Interview Schedule. The DPAX rates are point prevalence rates for depression, and the DIS rates combine major depressive episode (1-month prevalence) and dysthymia.*

†Between-year comparisons for DPAX-1 indicated that the year of study was not significant for 1952 vs 1970 but was significant for 1970 vs 1992 (χ^2_1 = 8.95; P = .003). There were no significant interactions. Within-year comparisons indicated that sex was not significant for any year but age was significant in 1952 (χ^2_2 = 7.08; P = .03) and also in 1970 (χ^2_2 = 8.11; P = .02) but not in 1992.

‡Between-year comparisons for DPAX-2 indicated that the year of study was not significant. Sex did not interact significantly with year of study but age did (χ^2_2 = 7.96; P = .02). Within-year comparisons indicated that age was significant in 1970 (χ^2_2 = 13.33; P<.001) but not in 1992, while sex was not significant in 1970 but was significant in 1992 (χ^2_1 = 5.95; P = .02).

§Within-year comparisons for DIS indicated that sex was significant (χ^2_1 = 10.16; P = .001) but age was not.

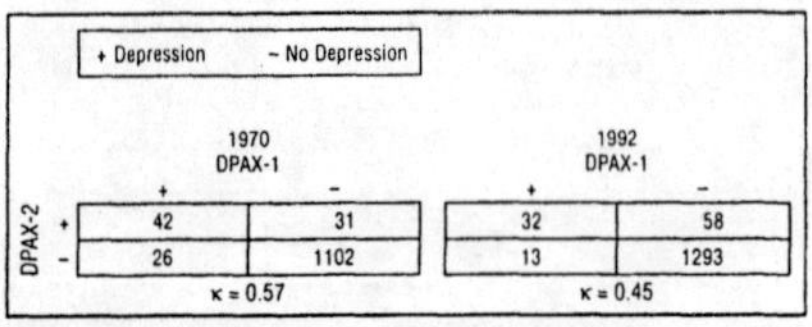

Figure 1. *Levels of agreement between the DPAX-1 and the DPAX-2 in 1970 and 1992. Numbers are numbers of subjects. DPAX-1 and DPAX-2 (DP for depression and AX for anxiety) indicate the original and revised methods for diagnosing depression.*

DPAX-1, while the DPAX-2 has multiple indicators of disability. These 2 types of disagreements could be expected to lead to higher prevalence according to the DPAX-2, because it offered more options to describe mood and impairment. However, another type of disagreement constrained such a tendency—the DPAX-2 had more stringent criteria for associated symptoms than the DPAX-1.

The 2 DPAX methods produced similar prevalence rates in 1970 because positive responses about poor spirits had not yet declined seriously and because the number of subjects who did not meet the DPAX-1 criteria for poor spirits was about equal to the number who did not meet the DPAX-2 criteria for associated symptoms. The reason the 2 methods agree less well in 1992 relates primarily to the decreased use of poor spirits and secondarily to declining use of the concept of going easy on work as an indicator of impairment.

This comparison of the 2 DPAX methods suggests that the 1992 results based on the DPAX-1 are probably

Table 3. Numbers of Discordant Cases in Categories of Disagreement Using the DPAX-1 and DPAX-2*

	1970		1992	
Analytic Components	DPAX-1+ DPAX-2−	DPAX-2+ DPAX-1−	DPAX-1+ DPAX-2−	DPAX-2+ DPAX-1−
Essential features	0	19	0	34
Both impairment and associated symptoms	7	0	2	1
Associated symptoms only	12	7	9	9
Impairment only	3	2	0	9
Time of occurrence	4	3	2	5
Total	**26**	**31**	**13**	**58**

**DPAX-1 and DPAX-2 indicate the original and revised methods of the Stirling County Study methods for diagnosing depression (DP) and anxiety (AX). Plus sign indicates positive for depression; minus sign, negative for depression.*

related to changing vernacular usage rather than to changing rates.

COMPARISON WITH OTHER DIS STUDIES FOR MDE

Comparisons based on using the DIS in 3 North American studies (ECA, Edmonton, and Stirling County) can be made for MDE as a separate disorder rather than in combination with dysthymia, as in the rest of this report.[2,6,34-36,41] Overall lifetime rates for MDE varied across the studies only from 6.3% to 8.6%, and 1-month rates from 2.2% to 2.6% (**Table 4**). In all comparisons, the rates for women were about 2 times higher than those

Table 4. Lifetime and 1-Month Prevalence Rates of Major Depressive Episode (MDE) Based on the Diagnostic Interview Schedule in 3 North American Studies

	Prevalence of MDE (per 100)					
	Epidemiologic Catchment Area (ECA) Study 1980-1984* (n = 18571)		Edmonton Epidemiologic Study 1983-1986† (n = 3258)		Stirling County Study 1992-1995 (n = 1396)	
	Lifetime	1-Month	Lifetime	1-Month	Lifetime	1-Month
Overall	6.3	2.2	8.6	2.3	7.9	2.6
Sex						
Female	8.7	2.9	11.4	2.9	11.5	3.6
Male	3.6	1.6	5.9	1.7	4.4	1.5
Female-male ratio	2.4/1	1/8	1/9	1/7	2/6	2/4
Age, y						
<45	7.7	2.8	8.8	2.3	9.4	3.7
45-64	4.8	2.2	10.1	3.0	8.2	1.9
≥65	1.9	1.0	4.1	0.7	4.1	0.9
<45-to-≥65 ratio	4/0	2/8	2/1	3/3	2/3	4/1

*For the ECA study, the lifetime rates for MDE are shown in the study by Weissman et al[41] and the 1-month rates in the study by Regier et al.[36] To show the rates for 3 age groups, the public-use tape containing the ECA data was used with the recommended weights. The published data by age for the lifetime rates are, for 18 to 29 years, 6.7%; for 30 to 44 years, 9.5%; for 45 to 64 years, 5.0%; and for 65 years or older, 2.0%. The published data by age for the 1-month rates are, for 18 to 24 years, 2.2%; for 25 to 44 years, 3.0%; for 45 to 64 years, 2.0%; and for 65 years or older, 0.7%.

†For the Edmonton study, the lifetime rates for MDE are shown in the study by Bland et al[34] and the overall 1-month rates in the study by Bland et al.[35] The adjustment to show 3 age groups was provided by the Edmonton research group.

for men. From both the lifetime and 1-month perspectives, younger people had higher prevalence than older people. In the Stirling County and Edmonton studies, the rates for the 2 younger age categories were more uniform than in the ECA study. However, the ratios comparing subjects younger than 45 years with those 65 years or older exhibit 2-fold to 4-fold differences.

TIME, SEX, AND AGE

Based on the evidence that the DPAX-1 findings for 1992 were influenced by vernacular changes, the most appropriate time comparisons from this study involve the DPAX-1 for 1952 and the DPAX-2 for 1970 and 1992, the latter being selected for the last 2 samples because its coverage of impairment is more congruent with the intent of the disability criterion of *DSM-IV* and because its requirement for 3 associated symptoms is a closer approximation of the 4 needed according to both *DSM-III* and *DSM-IV*.[31,32] Using this selection of findings, it seemed worthwhile to compare current prevalence using a single threshold for age (<45 years vs ≥45 years). This threshold was chosen because the ECA findings of higher prevalence among those younger than 45 years have drawn considerable attention and influenced the design of the National Comorbidity Survey in terms of its focus on younger persons.[2,4,41] Under these circumstances, the DPAX rates of depression in the 2 early samples were quite similar for women and men, and prevalence increased with age for both women and men (**Figure 2**). In 1992, the DPAX and DIS rates for women were similar and different from those in the earlier years. Both methods emphasized that the highest prevalence of depression was among younger women. The rates for younger men were similar across time and across method. The DPAX and DIS rates for older men differed, however, in that the

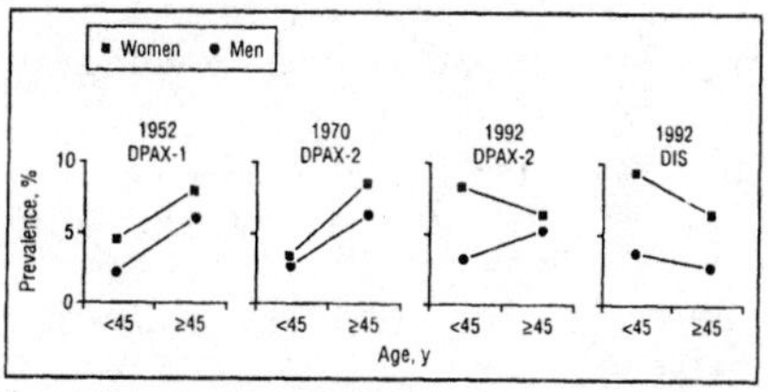

Figure 2. *Current prevalence of depression by sex and age using the DPAX-1 for 1952, the DPAX-2 for 1970 and 1992, and the DIS for 1992. DPAX-1 and DPAX-2 (DP for depression and AX for anxiety) indicate the original and revised methods for diagnosing depression; DIS, Diagnostic Interview Schedule.*

DPAX showed the prevalence of depression rising with age, while it declined somewhat according to the DIS.

COMMENT

The conclusion we draw from this longitudinal analysis is that the current prevalence of depression in Stirling County remained steady at about 5% among successive samples of adults over the period from 1952 to 1992 and that these depressions tended to be chronic. At the end point of the study, the current prevalence of acute and chronic depression based on the DIS method was also about 5%.

At the same time, this study illustrates the problems posed for time-trend analysis by changes in the language people use to describe their moods and by the evolution of diagnostic criteria. There are 3 ways in which time can influence prevalence: show an increase, show a decrease, or maintain a stable rate. Each of these possibilities was, to some extent, evident. The DPAX-1 indicated a decrease by 1992, the DPAX-2 indicated stable prevalence, and the use of recalled lifetime evidence based on the DIS gave information of the same type that in other studies has been interpreted as showing an increase.

Our analysis of the DPAX-1 results indicated that the decrease in prevalence was influenced by changes in the vernacular and should therefore be discounted as showing a real decrease in prevalence. Where diagnostic standards are concerned, the methods used throughout this study share with contemporary approaches the concept that a diagnosis involves essential features, associated symptoms, duration, and impairment. At the level of several of the specific criteria, however, the DPAX and DIS methods differ, pointing to a dilemma for analyzing time trends. Use of the specific criteria of *DSM-III*, as with the DIS, depends on reconstructing the past by asking people to recall their psychiatric histories; such recollections may involve inaccuracies. On the other hand, data that do not require long-term memory, as in the use of current DPAX depression in samples dating back to 1952, cannot take into account all of the specific criteria that became standardized in *DSM-III*.

A question can be raised as to whether there is any common ground between the findings about a steady current prevalence of depression and findings that indicate increasing lifetime rates of depression. A stable current prevalence rate is not necessarily incompatible with increasing lifetime rates. If most of the disorders registered in the lifetime rates were short-lived, either because of their nature or because of effective treatment, their increase would have only small influence on current prevalence. Thus, at least theoretically, rising lifetime rates of acute depression and steady prevalence of chronic depression can occur together.

Increasingly, it is recognized that depression is an etiologically complex disorder that often runs a recurrent or chronic course.[22,29,42-44] In reporting the Stirling County findings comparing 1952 and 1970, we suggested that stable prevalence is more realistic than marked change for a type of disorder that exhibits such features.[14] It seems unlikely, for example, that genetic and social circumstances would combine in a coordinated way during the same period to foster a pronounced increase or decrease. If changes were found to occur in a circumscribed historical period, it is likely that they would reflect social influences, but even where social experiences are concerned, there are cross-currents of advantages and disadvantages in a population at large that may give protection for some and have noxious effects for others. Thus, small changes in the distribution of depression may be more credible than wide fluctuations.

In considering these possibilities, the generalizability of the information from this study is an important issue. If the environment of the study area is unique and homogeneous, the findings would not have as much general relevance as if the region were typical of many others. Like most rural areas, this one has not grown much in population size, the way cities have, but its population is heterogeneous and its history has been molded by the same forces commonly observed throughout North America. In terms of psychiatric features, the DIS information from Stirling County in the present decade indicates that the prevalence of MDE is similar to what has been found elsewhere. This raises the possibility that other places might have appeared similar to Stirling County if the DPAX methods had been used. The population studies of similar vintage, such as the Lundby and Midtown Manhattan investigations, did not use structured diagnostic methods, thus making comparison problematic.[8,45,46] Many of the other earlier studies used short inventories of symptoms with cases identified by a cutoff point rather than diagnostically oriented interviews.[47-51]

While the methods used in this study (the DPAX and the DIS) show advances over the use of symptom inventories, both have limitations. It has been suggested that when the available methods for tracing trends are imperfect, it is useful to "pursue multiple pathways and look for agreements across them" (L. E. Robins, PhD, letter, March 3, 1998). Since 1980 most studies have employed either the DIS or the Composite International Diagnostic Interview (CIDI).[52] The findings have been consistent in regard to 2 points. One is that the prevalence of MDE is about twice as high among women as men, and the other is that both lifetime and recent prevalence rates are higher among younger than older persons.[1-7,34-36,41,53-57] The results from the 1952 and 1970 samples in Stirling County were not congruent with these DIS and CIDI results. After 1970, however, the DPAX methods indicated that, within an overall stable rate, women were about twice as likely to report depression as men and that the burden of prevalence was moving toward younger women. In these terms, then, the DIS and DPAX methods provide mutual corroboration, although the DPAX findings point to the fact that the associations seen with consistency in DIS and CIDI studies may be of fairly recent origin.

This study suggests that interpretations about a general increase in depression should be tempered or modified in favor of a redistribution of prevalence by sex and age. The higher prevalence of depression among women younger than 45 years in the recent survey in Stirling County is especially worthy of attention. This change refers to a specific time span and a specific segment of the population. Therefore, it may be possible to develop testable hypotheses for investigation that would throw light on the origins of change, especially as these refer to the portion of prevalence that may be under the influence of social and historical circumstances.

Accepted for publication April 29, 1999.

This work was supported by grant MH39576 from the National Institute of Mental Health, Rockville, Md (Dr Murphy).

A preliminary version of this article was presented at grand rounds, Department of Psychiatry, Dalhousie University Faculty of Medicine, April 15, 1998, Halifax, Nova Scotia.

We thank Patricia Merritt, Barbara Burns, and Ellen Krystofik for field management and data processing; Ellen Krystofik and Barbara Burns for manuscript preparation; and Stephen C. Newman, MD, and Roger C. Bland, MB, for providing the lifetime and 1-month rates from the Edmonton study in the age categories used in this article.

Reprints: Jane M. Murphy, PhD, Department of Psychiatry, Room 9155, Massachusetts General Hospital, 149 13th St, Charlestown, MA 02129-2000 (e-mail: murphy@a1.mgh.harvard.edu).

REFERENCES

1. Klerman GL, Weissman MM. Increasing rates of depression. *JAMA.* 1989;261: 2229-2235.
2. Robins LN, Regier DA, eds. *Psychiatric Disorders in America: The Epidemiologic Catchment Area Study:* New York, NY: Free Press; 1991.
3. Cross-National Collaborative Group. The changing rate of major depression: cross-national comparisons. *JAMA.* 1992;268:3098-3105.
4. Kessler RC, McGonagle KA, Zhao S, Nelson CB, Hughes M, Eshleman S, Wittchen HU, Kendler KS. Lifetime and 12-month prevalence of *DSM-III-R* psychiatric disorders in the United States: results from the National Comorbidity Survey. *Arch Gen Psychiatry.* 1994;51:8-19.
5. Kessler RC, McGonagle KA, Nelson CB, Hughes M, Swartz M, Blazer DG. Sex and depression in the National Comorbidity Survey, II: cohort effects. *J Affect Disord.* 1994;30:15-26.
6. Bland RC, Newman SC, Orn H, eds. Epidemiology of psychiatric disorders in Edmonton. *Acta Psychiatr Scand Suppl.* 1988;338:1-80.
7. Bland RC. Epidemiology of affective disorders: a review. *Can J Psychiatry.* 1997; 42:367-377.
8. Hagnell O, Lanke J, Rorsman B, Öjesjö L. Are we entering an age of melancholy? depressive illnesses in a prospective epidemiological study over 25 years: the Lundby Study, Sweden. *Psychol Med.* 1982;12:279-289.
9. Grof P. The age of misery: affective disorders on the rise. *Can J Psychiatry.* 1997; 42:361-362.
10. Parker G. Are the lifetime prevalence estimates in the ECA study accurate? *Psychol Med.* 1987;17:275-282.
11. Giuffra LA, Risch N. Diminished recall and the cohort effect of major depression: a simulation study. *Psychol Med.* 1994;24:375-383.
12. Simon GE, VonKorff M, Ustun TB, Gater R, Gureje O, Sartorius N. Is the lifetime risk of depression actually increasing? *J Clin Epidemiol.* 1995;48:1109-1118.
13. Angst J. Epidemiology of depression. *Psychopharmacology.* 1992;106(suppl): S71-S74.
14. Murphy JM, Sobol AM, Neff RK, Olivier DC, Leighton AH. Stability of prevalence: depression and anxiety disorders. *Arch Gen Psychiatry.* 1984;41:990-997.
15. Murphy JM, Neff RK, Sobol AM, Rice JX, Olivier DC. Computer diagnosis of depression and anxiety: the Stirling County Study. *Psychol Med.* 1985;15:99-112.
16. Murphy JM, Monson RR, Laird NM, Sobol AM, Leighton AH. Identifying depression and anxiety in a forty-year epidemiologic investigation: the Stirling County Study. *Int J Methods Psychiatr Res.* 1998;7:89-109.
17. Robins LN, Helzer JE, Croughan J, Ratcliff KS. National Institute of Mental Health Diagnostic Interview Schedule: its history, characteristics, and validity. *Arch Gen Psychiatry.* 1981;38:381-389.
18. Leighton AH. *My Name Is Legion: The Stirling County Study of Psychiatric Disorder and Sociocultural Environment.* Vol 1. New York, NY: Basic Books Inc; 1959.
19. Hughes CC, Tremblay MA, Rapoport RN, Leighton AH. *People of Cove and Woodlot: The Stirling County Study of Psychiatric Disorder and Sociocultural Environment.* Vol 2. New York, NY: Basic Books Inc; 1960.
20. Leighton DC, Harding JS, Macklin DB, Macmillan AM, Leighton AH. *The Character of Danger: The Stirling County Study of Psychiatric Disorder and Sociocultural Environment.* Vol 3. New York, NY: Basic Books Inc; 1963.
21. Murphy JM. The Stirling County Study: then and now. *Int Rev Psychiatry.* 1994; 6:329-348.
22. Murphy JM, Olivier DC, Sobol AM, Monson RR, Leighton AH. Diagnosis and outcome: depression and anxiety in a general population. *Psychol Med.* 1986;16: 117-126.
23. Murphy JM, Monson RR, Olivier DC, Sobol AM, Leighton AH. Affective disorders and mortality: a general population study. *Arch Gen Psychiatry.* 1987;44: 473-480.
24. Murphy JM, Olivier DC, Monson RR, Sobol AM, Leighton AH. Incidence of depression and anxiety: the Stirling County Study. *Am J Public Health.* 1988;78: 534-540.
25. Murphy JM, Sobol AM, Olivier DC, Monson RR, Leighton AH, Pratt LA. Prodromes of depression and anxiety: the Stirling County Study. *Br J Psychiatry.* 1989;155:490-495.
26. Murphy JM. Diagnostic comorbidity and symptom co-occurrence: the Stirling County Study. In: Maser JD, Cloninger CR, eds. *Comorbidity of Mood and Anxiety Disorders.* Washington, DC: American Psychiatric Press; 1990:153-176.
27. Murphy JM, Olivier DC, Monson RR, Sobol AM, Federman EB, Leighton AH. Depression and anxiety in relation to social status: a prospective epidemiologic study. *Arch Gen Psychiatry.* 1991;48:223-229.
28. Murphy JM, Monson RR, Olivier DC, Zahner GE, Sobol AM, Leighton AH. Relations over time between psychiatric and somatic disorders: the Stirling County Study. *Am J Epidemiol.* 1992;136:95-105.
29. Murphy JM. What happens to depressed men? *Harv Rev Psychiatry.* 1995;3: 47-49.
30. Nunnally JC. *Psychometric Theory.* New York, NY: McGraw-Hill Book Co; 1978.
31. American Psychiatric Association. *Diagnostic and Statistical Manual of Mental Disorders, Third Edition.* Washington, DC: American Psychiatric Association; 1980.
32. American Psychiatric Association. *Diagnostic and Statistical Manual of Mental Disorders, Fourth Edition.* Washington, DC: American Psychiatric Association; 1994.
33. Murphy JM. Continuities in community-based psychiatric epidemiology. *Arch Gen Psychiatry.* 1980;37:1215-1223.
34. Bland RC, Orn H, Newman SC. Lifetime prevalence of psychiatric disorders in Edmonton. *Acta Psychiatr Scand Suppl.* 1988;338:24-32.
35. Bland RC, Newman SC, Orn H. Period prevalence of psychiatric disorders in Edmonton. *Acta Psychiatr Scand Suppl.* 1988;338:33-42.
36. Regier DA, Boyd JH, Burke JD Jr, Rae DS, Myers JK, Kramer M, Robins LN, George LK, Karno M, Locke BZ. One-month prevalence of mental disorders in the United States: based on five Epidemiologic Catchment Area sites. *Arch Gen Psychiatry.* 1988;45:977-986.
37. Everitt BS. *The Analysis of Contingency Tables.* London, England: Chapman & Hall Ltd; 1977.
38. Laird N, Olivier D. Covariance analysis of censored survival data using log-linear analysis techniques. *J Am Stat Assoc.* 1981;76:231-240.
39. Bishop YMM, Fienberg SE, Holland PW. *Discrete Multivariate Analysis: Theory and Practice.* Cambridge, Mass: MIT Press; 1975.
40. Anderson A, Auguier A, Hauck WW, Oakes D, Vandaele W, Weisberg HI. *Statistical Methods for Comparative Studies.* New York, NY: John Wiley & Sons Inc; 1980.
41. Weissman MM, Bruce ML, Leaf PJ, Florio LP, Holzer C. Affective disorders. In: Robins LN, Regier DA, eds. *Psychiatric Disorders in America: The Epidemiologic Catchment Area Study.* New York, NY: Free Press; 1991:53-80.
42. Klerman GL. Depression and related disorders of mood (affective disorders). In: Nicholi AM, ed. *The New Harvard Guide to Psychiatry.* Cambridge, Mass: Harvard University Press; 1988:309-336.
43. Sargeant JK, Bruce ML, Florio LP, Weissman MM. Factors associated with 1-year outcome of major depression in the community. *Arch Gen Psychiatry.* 1990;47: 519-526.
44. Judd LL. The clinical course of unipolar major depressive disorders. *Arch Gen Psychiatry.* 1997;54:989-991.
45. Srole L, Langner TS, Michael ST, Opler MK, Rennie TA. *Mental Health in the Metropolis: The Midtown Manhattan Study.* New York, NY: McGraw-Hill Book Co; 1962.
46. Srole L, Fischer AK. The Midtown Manhattan Longitudinal Study vs 'The Mental Paradise Lost' doctrine: a controversy joined. *Arch Gen Psychiatry.* 1980;37: 209-221.
47. Comstock GW, Helsing KJ. Symptoms of depression in two communities. *Psychol Med.* 1976;6:551-563.
48. Finlay-Jones RA, Burvill PW. The prevalence of minor psychiatric morbidity in the community. *Psychol Med.* 1977;7:475-489.
49. Link B, Dohrenwend BP. Formulation of hypotheses about the true prevalence of demoralization in the United States. In: Dohrenwend BP, Dohrenwend BS, Gould MS, Link B, Neugebauer R, Wunsch-Hitzig R, eds. *Mental Illness in the United States: Epidemiologic Estimates.* New York, NY: Praeger Publishers; 1980:114-132.
50. Phillips DL. The 'true prevalence' of mental illness in a New England state. *Community Ment Health J.* 1966;2:35-40.
51. Schwab JJ, Bell RA, Warheit GJ, Schwab RB. *Social Order and Mental Health: The Florida Health Study.* New York, NY: Brunner/Mazel Publishers; 1979.
52. Robins LN, Wing J, Wittchen HU, Helzer JE, Babor TF, Burke J, Farmer A, Jablenski A, Pickens R, Regier DA, Sartorius N, Towle LH. The Composite International Diagnostic Interview: an epidemiologic instrument suitable for use in conjunction with different diagnostic systems and in different cultures. *Arch Gen Psychiatry.* 1988;45:1069-1077.
53. Canino GJ, Bird HR, Shrout PE, Rubio-Stipec M, Bravo M, Martinez R, Sesman M, Guevara LM. The prevalence of specific psychiatric disorders in Puerto Rico. *Arch Gen Psychiatry.* 1987;44:727-735.
54. Wells JE, Bushnell JA, Hornblow AR, Joyce PR, Oakley-Browne MA. Christchurch Psychiatric Epidemiology Study, part I: methodology and lifetime prevalence for specific psychiatric disorders. *Aust N Z J Psychiatry.* 1989;23:315-326.
55. Offord DR, Boyle MH, Campbell D, Goering P, Lin E, Wong M, Racine YA. One-year prevalence of psychiatric disorder in Ontarians 15 to 64 years of age. *Can J Psychiatry.* 1996;41:559-563.
56. Kessler RC, McGonagle KA, Swartz M, Blazer DG, Nelson CB. Sex and depression in the National Comorbidity Survey, I: lifetime prevalence, chronicity and recurrence. *J Affect Disord.* 1993;29:85-96.
57. Weissman MM, Bland R, Joyce PR, Newman S, Wells JE, Wittchen HU. Sex differences in rates of depression: cross-national perspectives. *J Affect Disord.* 1993; 29:77-84.

ORIGINAL ARTICLE

Depressive Symptomatology and Incident Cognitive Decline in an Elderly Community Sample

Shari S. Bassuk, ScD; Lisa F. Berkman, PhD; David Wypij, PhD

Background: It is not known whether depression is a cause or consequence of progressive cognitive decline. We assessed the relationship between depressive symptoms and subsequent cognitive decline in the community-dwelling elderly population.

Methods: Data were from a population-based cohort study that enrolled 2812 noninstitutionalized elderly residents of New Haven, Conn, and followed them with in-home visits in 1982, 1985, 1988, and 1994. Cognitive function was assessed with the Short Portable Mental Status Questionnaire (SPMSQ). Response to the SPMSQ was scored as high, medium, and low, and cognitive decline was defined as a transition to a lower category. Depressive symptoms were measured with the Center for Epidemiological Studies Depression Scale.

Results: An elevated level of depressive symptoms was associated with an increased risk of incident cognitive decline among medium SPMSQ performers (3-year odds ratio [OR], 1.72; 95% confidence interval [CI], 1.04-2.82, $P=.03$; 6-year OR, 2.40; 95% CI, 1.33-4.34; $P=.004$; 12-year OR, 1.65; 95% CI, 0.62-4.38; $P=.31$) but not among high performers (3-year OR, 0.93; 95% CI, 0.62-1.39; $P=.71$; 6-year OR, 1.03; 95% CI, 0.67-1.58; $P=.90$; 12-year OR, 1.26; 95% CI, 0.59-2.71; $P=.55$), after adjustment for age, sex, race, education, income, housing type, functional disability, cardiovascular profile, and alcohol use.

Conclusions: Depressive symptoms, particularly dysphoric mood, presage future cognitive losses among elderly persons with moderate cognitive impairments. However, the data do not provide support for the hypothesis that depressive symptoms are associated with the onset or rate of cognitive decline among cognitively intact elderly persons.

Arch Gen Psychiatry. 1998;55:1073-1081

It is not known whether depression, particularly at subclinical levels, contributes to the onset or course of cognitive decline in old age or instead is a consequence of cognitive impairment. Epidemiologic studies have been primarily limited to cross-sectional investigations that are consistent in showing a positive correlation between depressive symptoms and poorer cognitive performance in putatively nondemented individuals,[1-3] as well as between depressive symptoms and severe cognitive deficits indicative of dementia in population-based samples,[4-7] but reveal little about the causal direction of this association.

See also page 1082

Dementia, defined as chronic and substantial decline in 2 or more areas of cognitive function sufficient to interfere significantly with work, social activities, and interpersonal relationships, affects an estimated 15% of the United States population older than 65 years.[8] Clinical and neuropathologic studies suggest that Alzheimer disease (AD) accounts for at least 50% of dementia cases.[9] Caring for dementia patients imposes enormous psychosocial and economic burdens on family and other caregivers.[10] In the United States, the total societal cost of caring for all persons first diagnosed with AD in 1991 alone has been estimated at $67.3 billion.[11] Aside from age and genetic factors,[12] there are few established risk factors for AD.[9]

Case-control investigations of depression and cognitive function have focused on AD patients. A pooled reanalysis of studies conducted before 1990 suggests that a history of medically treated depression occurring at least 1 year prior to AD

From the Departments of Epidemiology (Drs Bassuk and Berkman), Health and Social Behavior (Dr Berkman), and Biostatistics (Dr Wypij), Harvard School of Public Health, Boston, Mass.

SUBJECTS AND METHODS

RESPONDENTS

The study population was drawn from the New Haven, Conn, site of the Established Populations for Epidemiologic Studies of the Elderly (EPESE) project, described in detail elsewhere.[18] The New Haven cohort is a multistage probability sample of 2812 noninstitutionalized persons 65 years and older living in New Haven in 1982. Samples were drawn from 3 housing strata: public housing for elderly persons (age- and income-restricted), private housing for elderly persons (age-restricted), and community housing. All eligible men were sampled; women were randomly subsampled to achieve roughly equal representation of both sexes. The response rate at baseline was 82%. Trained lay examiners interviewed the cohort in their homes in 1982, 1985, 1988, and 1994 and by telephone in intervening years.

MEASURES

Cognitive Function

Cognitive performance was measured during in-home interviews with the 10-item Short Portable Mental Status Questionnaire[19] (SPMSQ). (The original item "What is the name of this place?" was changed to "What is your address?" as this seemed more appropriate for community-dwelling residents.) Correct answers receive 1 point; possible scores range from 0 to 10. If 4 or more items were refused or missing, the SPMSQ was not scored. Otherwise, refusals were scored as incorrect, and scores on missing items were imputed by assigning the mean of nonmissing items. For some analyses, we trichotomized scores into 3 categories: high (9-10), medium (7-8), and low (0-6).

Depressive Symptomatology

The Center for Epidemiological Studies Depression Scale[20] (CES-D), a self-report measure of current depressive symptomatology, was administered during in-home interviews. Possible scores range from 0 to 60; higher scores indicate more severe symptoms. The conventional cutpoint of 16 was used to classify respondents as "depressed" or "nondepressed." For some analyses, depressed respondents were further subdivided into cases of "severe" (CES-D score ≥26) vs "mild/moderate" (16≤ CES-D score ≤25) depression based on tertiles of the CES-D distribution. An alternative scoring approach employed a diagnostic algorithm[21] designed to capture the presence of dysphoria (low mood), considered the essential feature of clinical depression.[22]

Covariates

The following self-reported variables were viewed as potential confounders because of their associations with depressive symptoms or cognitive function among New Haven[23] or other community-dwelling elders,[4,16] or because of their status as established risk factors for vascular dementia,[24] the most common cause of progressive cognitive decline in elderly persons after AD[25]: age (coded as a continuous covariate); sex; race (white or nonwhite); education (≥12 or <12 years); yearly income (<$5000, ≥$5000, or missing); housing; functional disability (defined as requiring assistance with 1 or more activities of daily living[26] [walking across a room, dressing, eating, bed-to-chair transferring, bathing, using toilet]); cardiovascular profile (low- or high-risk, where high-risk is defined as a history of physician-diagnosed stroke, diabetes, myocardial infarction, or a measured sitting blood pressure of at least 160/95 mm Hg); and cigarette and alcohol consumption.

diagnosis is associated with an elevated risk of dementia in persons 70 years and older.[13] However, a recent case-control study that paid closer attention to the temporal ordering between depression and dementia found that treated depression occurring more than 1 year prior to earliest AD symptoms did not predict AD onset.[14] Two recently published cohort studies of depression and subsequent cognitive impairment also yield discrepant results. Devanand et al[15] report that depressed mood was strongly predictive of incident AD among 478 individuals identified through a New York City dementia registry and followed from 1 to 5 years. In contrast, Dufouil et al[16] found that depressive symptoms were not associated with cognitive deterioration during a 3-year period in a community-based sample of 1600 elderly French persons.

Given the inconclusive evidence, additional population-based longitudinal investigations are needed. We determined whether an elevated level of depressive symptomatology is predictive of an increased incidence of cognitive impairment or a faster rate of cognitive decline in a cohort of community-dwelling elderly persons. Clarifying the temporal relationship between depressive states and cognitive dysfunction may be helpful in elucidating the etiology of these conditions. Furthermore, given the failure of many primary care physicians to recognize or treat depression in elderly patients,[17] a positive finding would suggest the need to incorporate depression screening into medical practice to identify individuals at high risk for cognitive decline and should stimulate investigation of the efficacy of various treatments for depression in slowing the rate of progressive cognitive impairment.

RESULTS

In 1982, 2754 (98%) of the 2812 respondents had valid SPMSQ scores (**Table 1**). At the 3-year assessment, 2030 respondents (87% of those alive) completed the SPMSQ. After 6 years, 1447 respondents (80% of those alive) were retested, and 756 (73% of those alive) had valid SPMSQ scores at the 12-year assessment.

At baseline, 2412 individuals had high or medium scores on the SPMSQ and were therefore at risk of cognitive decline (**Table 2**). The 342 low-scoring respondents were significantly more likely to be older, female, nonwhite, poor, disabled, less educated, live in public housing, abstain from alcohol, and have an elevated CES-D score than were higher scorers. Compared with nondepressed respondents, depressed individuals had a greater odds of low cognitive performance at baseline (age-

ANALYSES

Outcomes of interest are (1) onset of cognitive impairment and (2) course of cognitive change during the study period.

Depression and Onset of Cognitive Impairment

Cognitive decline was defined as a transition to a lower SPMSQ category (high to medium or low, or medium to low) during a given interval. Respondents with low SPMSQ scores at the beginning of an interval were excluded from consideration during that period.

Incidence of cognitive decline by initial depression status and SPMSQ category was estimated during intervals of 3 lengths: 1982 to 1985 and 1985 to 1988 (3 years); 1982 to 1988 and 1988 to 1994 (6 years); and 1982 to 1994 (12 years). Polytomous logistic regression was used to estimate the relative risk of cognitive decline or death in depressed vs nondepressed respondents, controlling for potential confounders. The 3 outcomes—maintenance of cognitive function, cognitive decline, and death—were treated as unordered categorical variables. Preliminary analyses showed that the magnitude of the depression effect was comparable for the two 3-year intervals, as were results from the two 6-year intervals. Thus, data from intervals of equal length were combined to achieve maximal power.

Sociodemographic covariates were included in multivariate models. To maximize efficiency, health-related covariates were retained only if the covariate was a significant predictor ($P<.05$) of decline in multivariate modeling or if its inclusion changed the magnitude of the depression coefficient by at least 10%. Accordingly, only smoking status was not included in final models. Values of time-varying covariates were updated at the start of each interval; when missing data occurred, values from the previous interval were substituted.

Depression and Mean Cognitive Performance Over Time

Multiple linear regression was used to estimate mean SPMSQ scores at the end of an interval as a function of depression status at the start of an interval, controlling for initial cognitive performance and confounders. The hypothesis that depression is associated with a more rapid rate of decline was tested by inclusion of interaction terms between initial depression status and indicator variables for length of time elapsed. If any covariate exhibited significant interactions with time, then these interactions were included before introducing the depression × time terms. High or medium SPMSQ scorers with at least 1 subsequent test contributed data to reported analyses. Restricting analyses to respondents with 4 valid SPMSQ scores yielded little change in parameter estimates.

To eliminate the possibility that observed associations between elevated CES-D scores and cognitive performance were due solely to poor physical health without underlying psychological disorder, we also estimated the effect of dysphoric mood alone on cognitive decline. To address dose-response issues, we examined whether severity of a depressive episode and consistency of depression history would affect the likelihood of decline. In separate logistic models, we examined the depression-decline association in younger vs older respondents to determine if the relationship was stronger at older ages, as suggested by case-control data.[13] In addition, because the cognitive manifestation of AD may be accentuated in the presence of vascular disease,[27] data were stratified by cardiovascular profile.

Computing was done using the statistical package SUDAAN, version 7.0.[28] The estimating equations approach[29] was used to adjust standard errors for the clustering due to the sampling scheme and repeated measurements. Estimates were weighted to reflect differential sampling, coverage, and response rates within housing and sex strata.

adjusted odds ratio [OR], 1.75; 95% confidence interval [CI], 1.19-2.57; $P=.005$), although the association was somewhat attenuated when the above covariates were controlled (OR, 1.37; 95% CI, 0.92-2.05; $P=.12$).

Among all at-risk respondents, those with elevated CES-D scores were more likely to decline cognitively in any given interval than were those with lower scores, though the increase in risk was statistically significant only for the 6-year interval (**Table 3**). On closer examination, the association between depression and subsequent decline seemed to be confined to respondents whose SPMSQ scores at the start of an interval were in the medium rather than high category. The significant association between depression and decline persisted in medium scorers after adjustment for potential confounders (**Table 4**). Depressed respondents were also more likely than nondepressed respondents to die than to maintain cognitive function, particularly during longer intervals.

To examine whether observed effects were related specifically to depressed mood rather than the cumulative number of symptoms, we performed the multivariate analyses with dysphoria as the predictor of interest. Among medium scorers, dysphoria was more strongly associated with cognitive decline than was an elevated total CES-D score. Compared with nondysphoric persons, medium scorers with depressed mood had 1.76 times the odds of declining by the 3-year assessment (95% CI, 0.93-3.36; $P=.08$); such odds jumped to 2.57 by 6 years (95% CI, 1.30-5.08; $P=.007$), and to 2.91 by 12 years (95% CI, 1.00-8.42; $P=.05$). Among high scorers, there was no association between dysphoria and decline (3-year OR, 0.71; 95% CI, 0.44-1.15; $P=.16$; 6-year OR, 0.89; 95% CI, 0.52-1.51; $P=.66$; 12-year OR, 0.74; 95% CI, 0.30-1.80; $P=.50$).

To address the possibility that trichotomous classification of SPMSQ scores might have obscured small shifts in cognitive performance over time and to determine whether depression is associated with the rate of cognitive change, we also treated the SPMSQ as a continuous outcome variable in linear regression modeling. Initially depressed respondents turned in poorer cognitive performances at follow-up than did nondepressed respondents, though between-group differences were greatly attenuated after adjustment for covariates (**Table 5**). Consistent with the hypothesis that depression is associated with a more rapid rate of decline, the magnitude of the comparative deficit of the depressed group steadily increased with length of follow-up (from 0.15 to 0.20 to 0.44 SPMSQ points). However, depression × time interactions were not statistically significant. Stratification by initial SPMSQ performance again reveals that the detrimental effect of de-

Table 1. Unweighted Distribution of Follow-up Status and Cognitive Performance on the Short Portable Mental Status Questionnaire (SPMSQ)

	No. (%)			
	Baseline, 1982	3-Y Follow-up, 1985	6-Y Follow-up, 1988	12-Y Follow-up, 1994
Valid SPMSQ	2754 (97.9)	2030 (72.2)	1447 (51.5)	756 (26.9)
Partial/proxy interview	58 (2.1)	136 (4.8)	224 (8.0)	186 (6.6)
Not interviewed	0 (0.0)	156 (5.5)	146 (5.2)	95 (3.4)
Deceased	0 (0.0)	490 (17.4)	995 (35.4)	1775 (63.1)
Total	**2812 (100.0)**	**2812 (100.0)**	**2812 (100.0)**	**2812 (100.0)**
Among those with valid SPMSQ				
SPMSQ category				
High	1643 (59.7)	1219 (60.0)	794 (54.9)	365 (48.3)
Medium	769 (27.9)	512 (25.2)	432 (29.9)	198 (26.2)
Low	342 (12.4)	299 (14.7)	221 (15.3)	193 (25.5)
Total	**2754 (100.0)**	**2030 (100.0)**	**1447 (100.0)**	**756 (100.0)**
Among high/medium scorers at baseline				
Mean ± SD SPMSQ score	8.92 ± 1.00	8.57 ± 1.70	8.33 ± 1.80	7.73 ± 2.40
Decline from baseline, %*	NA	24.8	29.1	37.6

**Weighted percentages. NA indicates not applicable.*

pression was observed exclusively among medium scorers. After adjustment for confounders, the main-effects estimate for depression among medium scorers was −0.44 points (95% CI, −0.78 to −0.09; $P=.01$); among high scorers, the corresponding estimate was −0.06 points (95% CI, −0.31 to 0.19; $P=.64$).

Severity of depressive symptoms did not exhibit a consistent relationship to the probability of cognitive decline across the 3 follow-ups. At the 3- and 6-year assessments, after adjustment for confounders, mildly to moderately depressed persons were at increased risk of decline compared with the nondepressed persons (3-year OR, 1.34; 95% CI, 0.95-1.89; $P=.09$; 6-year OR, 1.50; 95% CI, 1.04-2.16; $P=.03$), but severely depressed persons were not (3-year OR, 0.67; 95% CI, 0.39-1.16; $P=.15$; 6-year OR, 0.95; 95% CI, 0.43-2.13; $P=.91$). Conversely, by 12 years, the excess risk was confined to the severely depressed subgroup (OR, 3.32; 95% CI, 0.94-11.69; $P=.06$); mild/moderate depression was not associated with decline (OR, 1.02; 95% CI, 0.48-2.15; $P=.97$). These trends were far more pronounced among medium performers (data not shown).

Contrary to expectation, the depression–cognitive decline association was not stronger in respondents who exhibited a consistent history of depression (ie, who had high CES-D scores at 2 or more points prior to the interval during which cognitive change was assessed) as compared with those with only 1 prior elevated CES-D score (**Table 6**). Indeed, among medium performers, recent-onset depression (depression occurring at the start of an interval but not earlier) appeared to be as or more predictive of subsequent decline as a consistent history of depression. Furthermore, an isolated depressive episode occurring 3 to 6 years prior to the start of a given interval had less prognostic significance than recent-onset depression.

Stratified multivariate analyses of younger (65-74 years) and older (≥75 years) subgroups provide some support for the hypothesis that depression is a better predictor of cognitive decline in the older old, but only for medium SPMSQ scorers. While depression was associated with an equivalent increase in risk after 3 years in both older (multivariate OR, 1.83; 95% CI, 0.92-3.61; $P=.08$) and younger medium scorers (OR, 1.80; 95% CI, 0.87-3.73; $P=.11$), the 6- and 12-year ORs jumped to 3.33 (95% CI, 1.51-7.34; $P=.003$) and 1.92 (95% CI, 0.37-10.10; $P=.44$), respectively, in the older subgroup but fell to 1.33 (95% CI, 0.55-3.19; $P=.53$) and 1.14 (95% CI, 0.31-4.16; $P=.84$) in the younger. However, depression × age interactions were not statistically significant.

Stratification by cardiovascular profile reveals that the association between depression and cognitive decline was stronger among persons with high-risk profiles, but again only for medium SPMSQ scorers and only at longer intervals. Among medium scorers with high-risk cardiovascular profiles, the relative odds of decline associated with depression were 1.70 (95% CI, 0.78-3.70; $P=.18$) at 3 years, 3.19 (95% CI, 1.21-8.35; $P=.02$) at 6 years, and 6.42 (95% CI, 1.06-38.80; $P=.04$) at 12 years. Among medium scorers with a low-risk profile, the corresponding estimates were 1.67 (95% CI, 0.86-3.26; $P=.13$) at 3 years, 2.29 (95% CI, 1.08-4.85; $P=.03$) at 6 years, and 0.90 (95% CI, 0.27-3.02; $P=.86$) at 12 years. The depression × cardiovascular profile interaction was significant ($P=.03$) in the 12-year analysis.

The clinical relevance of a medium SPMSQ score is ambiguous without knowledge of premorbid performance.[19] Some respondents (eg, the less educated) would probably have "tested medium" throughout adulthood; their scores may not reflect incident impairment. For others, medium scores represent decline from higher levels of functioning. To examine more closely the relationship between depression and decline among medium scorers, we subdivided respondents with medium scores in 1985 or 1988 according to their baseline (1982) SPMSQ category. Among medium scorers who had previously performed at a higher level, the association between depression and subsequent decline was striking. That is, among persons with medium scores in 1985 but high scores in 1982, depres-

Table 2. Baseline Characteristics of 2412 Respondents at Risk of Cognitive Decline*

Characteristic	No. (%)†
Age, y	
65-74	1412 (61.5)
75-84	813 (31.7)
>85	187 (6.8)
Sex	
Male	1026 (37.2)
Female	1386 (62.8)
Education, y	
<12	1546 (59.6)
≥12	827 (39.1)
Yearly income, $	
0 to <5000	803 (26.9)
5000 to <15 000	1119 (48.0)
≥15 000	223 (13.4)
Race	
White	1937 (83.3)
Nonwhite (90% black)	475 (16.7)
Housing	
Public	584 (8.1)
Private	748 (14.1)
Community	1080 (77.8)
Physical disability	
Yes	285 (9.8)
No	2127 (90.2)
Cardiovascular profile	
High risk	799 (31.0)
Low risk	1613 (69.0)
Current smoker	
Yes	512 (19.9)
No	1898 (80.0)
Drink alcohol in past month	
Yes	1258 (55.0)
No	1152 (44.9)
CES-D‡ score	
≥16	372 (15.4)
<16	2009 (83.4)
Dysphoria	
Yes	248 (10.2)
No	2129 (88.3)

*Unweighted sample sizes are given. Percentages are from the weighted data.

†Total number for each covariate may sum to less than 2412 (and percentages may sum to less than 100%) because of missing values.

‡Center for Epidemiological Studies Depression Scale.[20]

sion in 1985 predicted decline during 1985 to 1988 (3-year OR, 4.91; 95% CI, 1.64-14.64; $P=.004$); similarly, among persons with medium scores in 1988 but high scores in 1982, depression in 1988 predicted decline during 1988 to 1994 (6-year OR, 5.48; 95% CI, 1.47-20.43; $P=.01$). On the other hand, among medium scorers whose performance history did not indicate a prior drop in cognitive function (ie, who had also scored medium at baseline), such depression had little prognostic significance with respect to future decline (3-year OR, 1.08; 95% CI, 0.28-4.20; $P=.92$; 6-year OR, 1.87; 95% CI, 0.35-10.16; $P=.47$).

COMMENT

Depressive symptoms, particularly dysphoric mood, were strongly predictive of subsequent decline among respondents with medium SPMSQ scores. However, this association was most marked in those medium scorers who had already experienced a decrement in cognitive performance (ie, who had transitioned from a baseline high to a medium SPMSQ category). Our interpretation is that the depression did not clearly precede, and may in fact have been a reaction to, eroding cognitive capacities. Supporting this interpretation is the finding that, in medium performers, recent-onset depression was more strongly associated with subsequent decline than a distal or even multiple past depressive episodes. Moreover, an elevated CES-D score was not associated with decline in cognitive function among respondents with the best initial SPMSQ scores. Overall, the data do not provide convincing support for the hypothesis that depression is a risk factor for cognitive decline or that it plays an etiologic role in the development of AD.

Our study has many strengths, most notably a prospective design with multiple direct assessments of depressive symptomatology and cognitive status, a large population-based inception cohort, and minimal loss to follow-up even after 12 years. These features allowed us to examine in more detail issues raised by earlier studies, including the role of initial cognitive status, the dose-response gradient (ie, severity and consistency of depressive symptoms), and potential dependence of the depression–cognitive decline relationship on age and cardiovascular profile.

Case-control investigations suggest that medically treated depression is a risk factor for AD,[13] but methodologic limitations preclude a rigorous assessment of depression's hypothesized etiologic role. Exposure information was often obtained by family report, raising the possibility of recall bias. The timing of depression in relation to onset (as opposed to clinical diagnosis) of dementia is unclear. The question of whether untreated or undiagnosed depression is associated with incipient dementia has generally not been addressed. If individuals with depression secondary to underlying dementia are more likely to seek treatment than those with depression occurring in the absence of nascent dementia, a likely scenario,[30] then the depression-AD association would be inflated in such studies.

Longitudinal data on depression as a risk factor for dementia have been gathered primarily in small clinical samples of depressed patients already evincing pronounced cognitive deficits.[31] However, 2 well-designed cohort studies have examined the issue. Devanand et al[15] found that depressed mood was associated with a significant 2-fold risk of incident dementia, as diagnosed by standardized neuropsychological tests and evidence of impaired function. Excluding persons with moderate cognitive impairment at baseline did not attenuate the association; however, the relative risk that would have been observed had mildly impaired individuals, who comprised a disproportionate percentage of the sample, also been excluded was not reported. This study did not rule out depression as a prodromal feature of subclinical dementia. Dufouil et al[16] reported no relationship between elevated CES-D scores and subsequent cognitive deterioration, defined as a drop of 5 or more points on the Mini-Mental State Examination.[32] Unfortunately, the authors chose a conservative cutpoint (score ≥23) for clas-

Table 3. Depressive Symptomatology and Incidence of Cognitive Decline as Measured by a Transition to Lower Category on the Short Portable Mental Status Questionnaire (SPMSQ) Among Respondents Surviving to End of Designated Interval*

	CES-D† Score ≥16		CES-D Score <16				
SPMSQ Category at Start of Interval	No.	% Decline	No.	% Decline	Odds Ratio‡	95% Confidence Interval	*P*
3-y follow-up (1982-1985, 1985-1988)							
High or medium	433	26.6	2620	25.0	1.28	0.94-1.75	.12
High	247	29.6	1936	27.3	1.08	0.73-1.60	.70
Medium	186	27.3	684	17.4	1.77	1.10-2.84	.02
6-y follow-up (1982-1988, 1988-1994)							
High or medium	264	37.3	1697	29.8	1.55	1.11-2.15	.01
High	151	36.0	1248	32.3	1.23	0.82-1.86	.32
Medium	113	39.4	449	21.5	2.35	1.34-4.11	.003
12-y follow-up (1982-1994)							
High or medium	87	46.9	618	36.4	1.54	0.86-2.76	.15
High	59	49.6	468	37.7	1.55	0.78-3.11	.21
Medium	28	42.0	150	31.7	1.51	0.55-4.16	.42

*Unweighted sample sizes are given. Percentages and odds ratios are estimated from the weighted data.
†CES-D indicates Center for Epidemiological Studies Depression Scale.[20]
‡Odds ratios are adjusted for age and SPMSQ category at start of interval.

Table 4. Adjusted Odds Ratios for Cognitive Decline or Death (vs Maintenance of Cognitive Function) According to Depression Status at Start of Interval (CES-D Score ≥16 vs CES-D Score <16)*

		Decline vs Maintain Function			Death vs Maintain Function		
SPMSQ Category at Start of Interval	No.	Odds Ratio†	95% Confidence Interval	*P*	Odds Ratio†	95% Confidence Interval	*P*
3-y follow-up (1982-1985, 1985-1988)							
High or medium							
Depressed	554	1.10	0.81-1.51	.54	1.13	0.81-1.58	.46
Nondepressed	3167						
High only							
Depressed	307	0.93	0.62-1.39	.71	1.32	0.85-2.05	.22
Nondepressed	2291						
Medium only							
Depressed	247	1.72	1.04-2.82	.03	1.02	0.64-1.61	.94
Nondepressed	876						
6-y follow-up (1982-1988, 1988-1994)							
High or medium							
Depressed	495	1.32	0.95-1.85	.10	1.61	1.18-2.20	.003
Nondepressed	2662						
High only							
Depressed	268	1.03	0.67-1.58	.90	1.61	1.06-2.44	.03
Nondepressed	1859						
Medium only							
Depressed	227	2.40	1.33-4.34	.004	1.70	1.08-2.67	.02
Nondepressed	803						
12-y follow-up (1982-1994)							
High or medium							
Depressed	341	1.40	0.76-2.56	.28	1.47	0.91-2.37	.11
Nondepressed	1799						
High only							
Depressed	196	1.26	0.59-2.71	.55	1.30	0.69-2.46	.41
Nondepressed	1261						
Medium only							
Depressed	145	1.65	0.62-4.38	.31	1.70	0.82-3.52	.15
Nondepressed	538						

*Unweighted sample sizes are given. Odds ratios are estimated from the weighted data. CES-D indicates Center for Epidemiological Studies Depression Scale.[20]
†Odds ratios are adjusted for age, Short Portable Mental Status Questionaire (SPMSQ) category at start of interval, sex, race, education, income, housing type, functional disability, cardiovascular profile, and alcohol use.

Table 5. Effect of Depression (CES-D* Score ≥16) on Predicted Short Portable Mental Status Questionnaire (SPMSQ) Score Over Time Among Respondents With High or Medium SPMSQ Score at Start of Interval (Weighted Data)

	Adjusted for Age and Initial SPMSQ Category			Multivariate Model†		
	β	95% Confidence Interval	P	β	95% Confidence Interval	P
Interaction model						
Predicted difference in SPMSQ scores between subjects depressed and subjects not depressed at start of interval						
After 3 y	-.29	-0.52 to -0.06	.01	-.15	-0.37 to 0.07	.17
After 6 y	-.35	-0.65 to -0.06	.02	-.20	-0.49 to 0.09	.18
After 12 y	-.58	-1.26 to 0.10	.10	-.44	-1.09 to 0.22	.19
Predicted difference in effect of depressed mood at start of interval on SPMSQ score over time (depression × time interaction)						
After 6 vs 3 y	-.06	-0.35 to 0.23	.69	-.05	-0.34 to 0.24	.75
After 12 vs 3 y	-.28	-0.96 to 0.39	.41	-.29	-0.94 to 0.37	.39
Main effects only model						
Predicted difference in SPMSQ score between subjects depressed and subjects not depressed at start of interval, averaged over all follow-up times	-.35	-0.57 to -0.12	.002	-.20	-0.42 to 0.01	.06

*CES-D indicates Center for Epidemiological Studies Depression Scale.[20]

†Adjusted for age, initial SPMSQ category, sex, race, education, income, housing type, functional disability, cardiovascular profile, alcohol use, age × time, and education × time interactions.

sifying female respondents as depressed; if milder depressive episodes predict decline, as suggested by our and others' findings,[13,15] then grouping individuals with mild symptoms and those with no symptoms into one unexposed category would dilute the observed association.

One possible explanation for the apparent discrepancy between our results and those of Devanand et al is that we used an epidemiologic screening instrument rather than clinical assessment to ascertain cognitive status. The limitations of using brief screeners to detect mild cognitive dysfunction are well known.[33] While the SPMSQ has good stability in the ostensible absence of true cognitive change,[19] its responsiveness to small changes in cognition over time is unclear. Nevertheless, using the SPMSQ, we detected strong relationships between other known risk factors (eg, age, lack of education) and cognitive decline (data not shown, but see White et al[34]), suggesting that a major nondifferential misclassification of cognitive change did not occur. Furthermore, we followed up the cohort for 12 years; because the median time from AD onset to death is 8 to 10 years,[35] many incident cases would have presumably progressed to moderate or severe dementia and thus been detected with high probability. The SPMSQ's validity as a measure of cognitive impairment has been assessed in a subsample of respondents at another EPESE site.[36] Participants received a detailed medical examination to determine the presence and severity of impairment. When the middle SPMSQ and mild impairment categories were excluded, the SPMSQ's sensitivity in identifying moderate or severe impairment was 85% and the specificity was 96%.[37]

Although the SPMSQ seems to capture the presence of at least moderate cognitive dysfunction, it provides no indication of the underlying medical condition responsible for such impairment. However, AD and vascular dementia account for the majority of irreversible pathologic cognitive decline in elderly populations.[24] Among medium performers, we found that the relationship between depression and decline was stronger in the presence of a high-risk cardiovascular profile. A history of hypertension has been linked to the development of AD as well as vascular dementia,[38] and cerebrovascular disease may potentiate the clinical expression of pathologic features of AD.[27] Moreover, depression increases the risk of other adverse outcomes (reoccurrence or death) in myocardial infarction[39] and stroke[40] patients. Given these findings, the observed interaction between depression and cardiovascular profile is not surprising. That we failed to detect any association between depressive symptoms and decline among those high SPMSQ performers at greatest risk for the outcome—either because of their cardiovascular history or advanced age—supports the conclusion that depression is not a risk factor for dementia among elderly respondents with no apparent cognitive impairment at baseline.

While the CES-D may be useful in quantifying the severity of depressive states, it does not yield clinical diagnoses, such as major depression, dysthymia, or transient grief reactions. When we employed a diagnostic rather than the traditional approach to scoring the CES-D, the association between depressive symptoms and cognitive decline was enhanced. That this occurred only among medium SPMSQ scorers, however, implies that lack of diagnostic specificity is not a compelling explanation for the negative findings among their higher-scoring counterparts. Furthermore, we observed no noticeable increase in risk of decline among high-scoring respondents with a consistent as opposed to a sporadic history of depressive symptoms. However, additional prospective investigations using comprehensive clinical assessments of both mood and dementing disorders are necessary to determine whether there are stronger relationships between specific clinical syndromes than might be surmised from our findings.

Table 6. Adjusted Odds Ratios for Cognitive Decline (vs Maintenance of Cognitive Function) on the Short Portable Mental Status Questionnaire (SPMSQ) According to Consistency of Depression History*

SPMSQ Category at Start of Interval	CES-D† Score ≥ 16 in Year(s)	Depression History	No.	Odds Ratio‡	95% Confidence Interval	P
3-y follow-up (1985-1988)						
High or medium	1982 and 1985	Consistent	66	0.98	0.45-2.13	.96
	1982 only	Sporadic, past	92	1.74	0.97-3.11	.06
	1985 only	Sporadic, recent	91	1.52	0.84-2.75	.16
	No year	None	965	1.00	...	
High only	1982 and 1985	Consistent	39	0.59	0.23-1.52	.28
	1982 only	Sporadic, past	66	1.85	0.95-3.63	.07
	1985 only	Sporadic, recent	48	1.19	0.57-2.50	.64
	No year	None	736	1.00	...	
Medium only	1982 and 1985	Consistent	27	3.00	0.86-10.51	.09
	1982 only	Sporadic, past	26	2.49	0.64-9.67	.19
	1985 only	Sporadic, recent	43	3.65	1.12-11.87	.03
	No year	None	229	1.00	...	
6-y follow-up (1988-1994)						
High or medium	1982/1985§ and 1988	Consistent	35	1.54	0.54-4.36	.42
	1982/1985 only	Sporadic, past	70	0.95	0.46-1.94	.88
	1988 only	Sporadic, recent	49	1.28	0.61-2.70	.51
	No year	None	462	1.00	...	
High only	1982/1985 and 1988	Consistent	19	1.23	0.25-6.02	.80
	1982/1985 only	Sporadic, past	51	0.88	0.41-1.90	.74
	1988 only	Sporadic, recent	24	0.72	0.25-2.11	.55
	No year	None	321	1.00	...	
Medium only	1982/1985 and 1988	Consistent	16	2.34	0.64-8.54	.20
	1982/1985 only	Sporadic, past	19	1.01	0.18-5.78	.99
	1988 only	Sporadic, recent	25	3.00	0.90-9.97	.07
	No year	None	141	1.00	...	

*Unweighted sample sizes are given. Odds ratios are estimated from the weighted data.
†CES-D indicates Center for Epidemiological Studies Depression Scale.[20]
‡Odds ratios are adjusted for age, SPMSQ category of start of interval, sex, race, education, income, housing type, functional disability, cardiovascular profile, and alcohol use. Results of logistic regression (deaths not included) were used.
§1982/1985 indicates at least 1 CES-D score of 16 or higher in 1982 or 1985.

The occurrence of missing data due to mortality and nonresponse is an inherent feature of longitudinal studies of elderly populations. In our sample, both depressive symptoms and lower cognitive scores at baseline were significantly associated with death; among survivors, lower cognitive performance was also associated with subsequent missing SPMSQ scores. If depression was a stronger predictor of (unobserved) decline among respondents who died or refused reinterview than among those who were retested, our estimates will be biased downward. Several procedures were used to evaluate the effect of the potential bias. When decline and death were combined into 1 category, or, alternatively, when respondents with partial or proxy interview at follow-up were assumed to have declined cognitively, the pattern of results remained essentially unchanged from that of Table 4.

The prevalence of depression among AD patients is markedly higher than in the general elderly population,[31] although it is unclear whether dementia predisposes to depression more than other illnesses.[41] Both psychosocial and physiologic explanations could account for this relationship. Depression could develop in reaction to the realization of one's failing capacities or could arise as a result of neuroanatomic damage in the brain.[42] For example, degenerative changes in the locus ceruleus are observed more frequently in AD patients with depression than in their nondepressed counterparts,[43-45] a finding consistent with the catecholaminergic deficit hypothesis of depression.[46] We regard these as important areas for further examination.

In conclusion, the data from this population-based longitudinal study do not indicate that depressive symptoms are associated with the onset or rate of cognitive decline among cognitively intact community-dwelling elderly persons. On the other hand, the results do show that dysphoric mood strongly presages future cognitive losses among elderly persons with questionable cognitive status, ie, who may already be evincing some difficulties. Although the depression may be a consequence rather than cause of progressive decline, these data may be of use in forecasting the service needs and designing interventions for aged persons with mild or moderate cognitive deficits. Targeted depression screening of this subgroup may be warranted. However, while treatment for depression has other documented benefits for elderly persons with[47] and without[48] cognitive impairment, our findings should restrain expectations that such treatment will delay the onset of dementia or prevent future cognitive decline.

Accepted for publication September 23, 1997.

This research was supported by grant T32-MH17119 (National Research Service Award to Dr Bassuk) from the National Institute of Mental Health, Rockville, Md, and by grants R01-AG11042, N01-AG02105, and N01-AG12102 from the National Institute on Aging, Bethesda, Md.

Reprints: Lisa F. Berkman, PhD, Department of Health and Social Behavior, Harvard School of Public Health, 677 Huntington Ave, Boston, MA 02115.

REFERENCES

1. Rabbitt P, Donlan C, McInnes L, Watson P, Bent N. Unique and interactive effects of depression, age, socioeconomic advantage, and gender on cognitive performance of normal healthy older people. *Psychol Aging.* 1995;10:307-313.
2. LaRue A, Swan GE, Carmelli D. Cognition and depression in a cohort of aging men: results from the Western Collaborative Group Study. *Psychol Aging.* 1995;10:30-33.
3. Jones KJ, Albert MS, Duffy FH, Hyde MR, Naeser M, Aldwin C. Modeling age using cognitive, psychosocial, and physiologic variables: the Boston Normative Aging Study. *Exp Aging Res.* 1991;17:227-242.
4. Scherr PA, Albert MS, Funkenstein HH, Cook NR, Hennekens CH, Branch LG, White LR, Taylor JO, Evans DA. Correlates of cognitive function in an elderly community population. *Am J Epidemiol.* 1988;128:1084-1101.
5. O'Connor DW, Pollitt PA, Roth M. Coexisting depression and dementia in a community survey of the elderly. *Int Psychogeriatr.* 1990;2:45-53.
6. Fuhrer R, Antonucci RC, Gagnon M, Dartigues JF, Barberger-Gateau P, Alperovitch A. Depressive symptomatology and cognitive functioning: an epidemiological survey in an elderly community sample in France. *Psychol Med.* 1992;22:159-217.
7. Forsell Y, Jorm AF, Winblad B. Association of age, sex, cognitive dysfunction, and disability with major depressive symptoms in an elderly sample. *Am J Psychiatry.* 1994;151:1600-1604.
8. Larson EB, Kukull WA, Katzman RL. Cognitive impairment: dementia and Alzheimer's disease. *Annu Rev Public Health.* 1992;13:431-449.
9. Breteler MMB, Claus JJ, van Duijn CM, Launer LJ, Hofman A. Epidemiology of Alzheimer's disease. *Epidemiol Rev.* 1992;14:59-81.
10. George LK, Gwyther LP. Caregiver well-being: a multidimensional examination of family caregivers of demented adults. *Gerontologist.* 1986;26:253-259.
11. Ernst RL, Hay JW. The US economic and social costs of Alzheimer's disease revisited. *Am J Public Health.* 1994;84:1261-1264.
12. Plassman BL, Breitner JCS. The genetics of dementia in late life. *Psychiatr Clin North Am.* 1997;20:59-76.
13. Jorm AF, van Duijn CM, Chandra V, Fratiglioni L, Graves AB, Heyman A, Kokmen E, Kondo K, Mortimer JA, Rocca WA, Shalat SL, Soininen H, Hofman A. Psychiatric history and related exposures as risk factors for Alzheimer's disease: a collaborative re-analysis of case-control studies. *Int J Epidemiol.* 1991;20(suppl):43-47.
14. Speck CE, Kukull WA, Brenner DE, Bowen JD, McCormick WC, Teri L, Pfanschmidt ML, Thompson JD, Larson EB. History of depression as a risk factor for Alzheimer's disease. *Epidemiology.* 1995;6:366-369.
15. Devanand DP, Sano M, Tang MX, Taylor S, Gurland BJ, Wilder D, Stern Y, Mayeux R. Depressed mood and the incidence of Alzheimer's disease in the elderly living in the community. *Arch Gen Psychiatry.* 1996;53:175-182.
16. Dufouil C, Fuhrer R, Dartigues JF, Alperovitch A. Longitudinal analysis of the association between depressive symptomatology and cognitive deterioration. *Am J Epidemiol.* 1996;144:634-641.
17. Woolley DC. Geriatric psychiatry in primary care. *Psychiatr Clin North Am.* 1997;20:241-260.
18. Cornoni-Huntley J, Ostfeld AM, Taylor JO, Wallace RB, Blazer D, Berkman LF, Evans DA, Kohout FJ, Lemke JH, Scherr PA, Korper SP. Established Populations for Epidemiologic Studies of the Elderly: study design and methodology. *Aging Clin Exp Res.* 1993;5:27-37.
19. Pfeiffer E. A short portable mental status questionnaire for the assessment of organic brain deficit in elderly patients. *J Am Geriatr Soc.* 1975;23:433-441.
20. Radloff LS. The CES-D scale: a self-report depression scale for research in the general population. *Appl Psychol Meas.* 1977;1:385-401.
21. Schoenbach VJ, Kaplan BH, Grimson RC, Wagner EH. Use of a symptom scale to study the prevalence of a depressive syndrome in young adolescents. *Am J Epidemiol.* 1982;116:791-800.
22. American Psychiatric Association. *Diagnostic and Statistical Manual of Mental Disorders, Fourth Edition.* Washington, DC: American Psychiatric Association; 1994.
23. Berkman LF, Berkman CS, Kasl S, Freeman DH, Leo L, Ostfeld AM, Cornoni-Huntley J, Brody JA. Depressive symptoms in relation to physical health and functioning in the elderly. *Am J Epidemiol.* 1986;124:372-388.
24. Hebert R, Brayne C. Epidemiology of vascular dementia. *Neuroepidemiology.* 1995;14:240-257.
25. Skoog I. Risk factors for vascular dementia: a review. *Dementia.* 1994;5:127-144.
26. Katz S, Downs TD, Cash HR, Grotz RC. Progress in the development of an index of ADL. *Gerontologist.* 1970;10:20-30.
27. Snowdon DA, Grenier LH, Mortimer JA, Riley KP, Grenier PA, Markesbery WR. Brain infarction and the clinical expression of Alzheimer's disease. *JAMA.* 1997;277:813-817.
28. Shah BV, Barnwell BG, Bieler GS. *SUDAAN User's Manual, Version 7.0.* Research Triangle Park, NC: Research Triangle Institute; 1996.
29. Zeger SL, Liang KY, Albert PS. Models for longitudinal data: a generalized estimating equation approach. *Biometrics.* 1988;44:1049-1060.
30. Henderson AS. Co-occurence of affective and cognitive symptoms: the epidemiological evidence. *Dementia.* 1990;1:119-123.
31. Teri L, Wagner A. Alzheimer's disease and depression. *J Consult Clin Psychol.* 1992;60:379-391.
32. Folstein MF, Folstein SE, McHugh PR. "Mini-Mental State": a practical method for grading the cognitive state of patients for the clinician. *J Psychiatr Res.* 1975;12:189-198.
33. Colsher PL, Wallace RB. Epidemiologic considerations in studies of cognitive function in the elderly: methodology and nondementing acquired dysfunction. *Epidemiol Rev.* 1991;13:1-27.
34. White L, Katzman R, Losonczy K, Salive M, Wallace R, Berkman L, Taylor J, Fillenbaum G, Havlik R. Association of education with incidence of cognitive impairment in three established populations for the epidemiologic studies of the elderly. *J Clin Epidemiol.* 1994;47:363-374.
35. Walsh JS, Welch HG, Larson EB. Survival of outpatients with Alzheimer-type dementia. *Ann Intern Med.* 1990;113:429-434.
36. Albert MS, Smith LA, Scherr PA, Taylor JO, Evans DA, Funkenstein HH. Use of brief cognitive tests to identify individuals in the community with clinically diagnosed Alzheimer's disease. *Int J Neurosci.* 1991;57:167-178.
37. Field TS. Risk factors for change in the ability to perform basic activities of daily living among the elderly [dissertation]. Boston, Mass: Boston University School of Public Health; 1993.
38. Skoog I, Lernfelt B, Landahl S, Palmertz B, Andreasson L, Nilsson L, Persson G, Oden A, Svanborg A. 15-year longitudinal study of blood pressure and dementia. *Lancet.* 1996;347:1141-1145.
39. Carney RM, Freedland KE, Rich MW, Jaffe AS. Depression as a risk factor for cardiac events in established coronary heart disease: a review of possible mechanisms. *Ann Behav Med.* 1995;17:142-149.
40. Morris PLP, Robinson RG, Andrzejewksi P, Samuels J, Price TR. Association of depression with 10-year poststroke mortality. *Am J Psychiatry.* 1993;150:124-129.
41. Alexopoulos GS, Abrams RC. Depression in Alzheimer's disease. *Psychiatr Clin North Am.* 1991;14:327-340.
42. Liston EH, Jarvik LF, Gerson S. Depression in Alzheimer's disease: an overview of adrenergic and cholingeric mechanisms. *Compr Psychiatry.* 1987;28:444-457.
43. Zweig RM, Ross CA, Hedreen JC, Steele C, Cardillo JE, Whitehouse PJ, Folstein MF, Price DL. The neuropathology of aminergic nuclei in Alzheimer's disease. *Ann Neurol.* 1988;24:233-242.
44. Zubenko GS, Moossy J. Major depression in primary dementia: clinical and neuropathologic correlates. *Arch Neurol.* 1988;45:1182-1186.
45. Forstl H, Burns A, Luthert P, Cairns N, Lantos P, Levy R. Clinical and neuropathological correlates of depression in Alzheimer's disease. *Psychol Med.* 1992;22:877-884.
46. Schildkraut JJ. The catecholamine hypothesis of affective disorders: a review of supporting evidence. *Am J Psychiatry.* 1965;122:483-497.
47. American Psychiatric Association. Practice guideline for the treatment of patients with Alzheimer's disease and other dementias of late life. *Am J Psychiatry.* 1997;154(suppl):1-33.
48. Blazer DG. Depression in the elderly: myths and misconceptions. *Psychiatr Clin North Am.* 1997;20:111-119.

Lost Human Capital From Early-Onset Chronic Depression

Ernst R. Berndt, Ph.D.

Lorrin M. Koran, M.D.

Stan N. Finkelstein, M.D.

Alan J. Gelenberg, M.D.

Susan G. Kornstein, M.D.

Ivan M. Miller, Ph.D.

Michael E. Thase, M.D.

George A. Trapp, M.D.

Martin B. Keller, M.D.

Objective: Chronic depression starts at an early age for many individuals and could affect their accumulation of "human capital" (i.e., education, higher amounts of which can broaden occupational choice and increase earnings potential). The authors examined the impact, by gender, of early- (before age 22) versus late-onset major depressive disorder on educational attainment. They also determined whether the efficacy and sustainability of antidepressant treatments and psychosocial outcomes vary by age at onset and quantified the impact of early- versus late-onset, as well as never-occurring, major depressive disorder on expected lifetime earnings.

Method: The authors used logistic and multivariate regression methods to analyze data from a three-phase, multicenter, double-blind, randomized trial that compared sertraline and imipramine treatment of 531 patients with chronic depression aged 30 years and older. These data were integrated with U.S. Census Bureau data on 1995 earnings by age, educational attainment, and gender.

Results: Early-onset major depressive disorder adversely affected the educational attainment of women but not of men. No significant difference in treatment responsiveness by age at onset was observed after 12 weeks of acute treatment or, for subjects rated as having responded, after 76 weeks of maintenance treatment. A randomly selected 21-year-old woman with early-onset major depressive disorder in 1995 could expect future annual earnings that were 12%–18% lower than those of a randomly selected 21-year-old woman whose onset of major depressive disorder occurred after age 21 or not at all.

Conclusions: Early-onset major depressive disorder causes substantial human capital loss, particularly for women. Detection and effective treatment of early-onset major depressive disorder may have substantial economic benefits.

(Am J Psychiatry 2000; 157:940–947)

Many young adults pursue further education after high school graduation. By foregoing current income and incurring the tuition costs of higher education, these individuals invest in their futures. This foregone income and higher education cost may be considered a form of human capital investment and accumulation. Payoffs from these human capital investments include increases in expected subsequent productivity and earnings (1).

The ability of young adults to successfully accumulate human capital depends in part on their health status during the years in which most post-high-school education typically occurs, i.e., ages 18–30. Illnesses with an early age at onset that substantially reduce physical, social, or cognitive functioning are particularly burdensome. The costs of such disorders include not only direct and indirect medical costs but also costs associated with reduced functioning and impaired ability to accumulate human capital. Detection and effective treatment of such early-onset disorders could reduce these costs.

This study examines the impact of early-onset major depressive disorder. About 15.7% of the U.S. population is estimated to have experienced an episode of major depressive disorder between the ages of 15 and 24, with a higher incidence seen in young women than in young men (20.8% versus 11.0%) (2). Depression produces similar or greater functional impairments than many other episodic and chronic medical illnesses (3–9). Depression is frequently underdiagnosed and inadequately treated (9–18). Guideline-consistent treatments for episodic depression produce success rates of 60%–70% for those patients who complete a trial (18–20). Moreover, antidepressants have been shown to be effective in the prophylaxis of recurrent mood disorders (21, 22).

This study reports the impact of early- (before age 22) versus late-onset—as well as never-occurring—major depression on human capital accumulation. Four issues are addressed: 1) Does early-onset major depressive disorder reduce educational attainment more than late-onset major depressive disorder? 2) Do human capital impairments associated with early-onset major depressive disorder vary by gender? 3) Do the efficacy and sustainability of antidepressant treatments for chronic depression and the psychosocial outcomes vary by initial age at onset? 4) Among individuals in the United States in 1995 who were 21 years of age, what are the differences in future lifetime expected mean earnings, by gender, attributable to lost human capital for those who experienced early-onset major depressive disorder versus those in whom it occurred later or not at all?

Method

The data for this study were derived from two sources: 1) a clinical trial that involved 635 chronically depressed outpatients; and 2) the Current Population Survey, which was conducted by the U.S. Bureau of the Census in March 1996.

Clinical Trial Data

A 12-site, double-blind, randomized, parallel-group trial compared the efficacy of sertraline and imipramine in the acute and maintenance treatment of 635 outpatients, aged 21–65 years, with DSM-III-R-defined chronic major or double depression (23, 24). After complete description of the study to subjects, written informed consent was obtained. The trial consisted of a 12-week acute phase (with a 12-week crossover phase for patients who did not respond), a 16-week continuation phase, and a 76-week maintenance phase (23). All patients entering the trial had a 24-item Hamilton Depression Rating Scale total score of ≥18 after a 1-week, single-blind placebo washout.

Patients excluded from the study were those with DSM-III-R-defined diagnoses of organic mental syndrome; current or lifetime bipolar disorder or cyclothymia; schizophrenia or other psychotic disorder; obsessive-compulsive disorder; antisocial, schizotypal, or severe borderline personality disorder; a principal diagnosis of panic disorder, generalized anxiety disorder, or post-traumatic stress disorder within the past 6 months; anorexia or bulimia nervosa within the past year; or drug or alcohol abuse or dependence within the past 6 months. The protocol criteria excluded individuals who required concomitant therapy with any psychotropic drug (except chloral hydrate or temazepam, used sparingly for sleep disorders) and patients who had failed a previous adequate trial of sertraline or imipramine. Because the intent of the trial was to examine the efficacy of antidepressant medications, psychotherapy was prohibited during the study unless it had been initiated at least 3 months before randomization.

After a complete medical/psychiatric history and physical examination, subjects entered a 1-week, single-blind washout phase and then were randomly assigned to treatment with either sertraline or imipramine in a 2:1 ratio. Assessments of various demographic and socioeconomic characteristics, including educational attainment, were made at baseline. A number of medical and psychosocial measures were collected at various points during the trial (23). Age at onset of major depressive disorder was determined by the Structured Clinical Interview for DSM-III-R (25), which was conducted by a certified rater.

Patients' response to treatment at various trial milestone points was measured by using the 24-item Hamilton depression scale (administered by investigating physicians or certified trained raters) and the Clinical Global Impression (CGI) improvement and severity measures (always administered by a physician). A satisfactory therapeutic response was defined as an improvement of at least 50% from baseline Hamilton depression scale score, a CGI improvement rating of 1 or 2 (very much or much improved), a total Hamilton depression scale score of ≤15, and a final CGI severity rating of ≤3 (no more than mildly ill). Patients not meeting this definition of therapeutic response were classified as nonresponders.

Various instruments and subscales were employed to measure psychosocial functioning and to compare scores of clinical trial subjects with those from "normal populations," which were based on community studies (26). We used data from the Medical Outcomes Study Health Status Questionnaire and the Medical Outcomes Study 36-item Short-Form Health Survey (27, 28).

The 635 patients in the clinical trial were stratified into two age groups: those less than age 30 (N=104) and those age 30 or older (N=531) at baseline. The age 30 cutoff was selected to ensure that all subjects had ample opportunity for post-high-school human capital accumulation. Comparisons of categorical variable means were based on Cochran-Mantel-Haenszel chi-square tests, while comparisons of continuous variable means used analysis of variance (ANOVA) F tests. To test whether the onset groups scored below community norms on the various domains of the Short-Form Health Survey instrument, one-tailed ANOVA F tests were performed. Various binary measures of behavioral and educational attainment were used as dependent variables in logistic regressions. Explanatory variables included patient's current age, age squared, as well as binary variables for gender, onset of major depressive disorder (early versus late), and the interaction between gender and age at onset. Statistical inference in the logistic regressions was based on Wald chi-square tests, and statistical inference in the linear regressions was based on t tests.

U.S. Census Data

The U.S. Census Bureau's Current Population Survey provides data on the demographic structure and earnings of the population (29). We used data for calendar year 1995, taken from a publicly available CD-ROM, for 83,007 individuals between ages 19 and 70, with nonnegative potential work experience (defined as age minus years of schooling minus 6). We defined an individual as having been in the labor force if 1995 total annual earnings from employment or self-employment were greater than $260 (average $5 per week).

The 0/1 binary variable for labor force participation is specified as the dependent variable in logistic regressions, estimated separately by gender. Conditional on the individual being in the labor force, annual employment earnings are related to the socioeconomic variables; the natural logarithm of annual earnings is the dependent variable in least squares regressions (30). Once estimated, these labor force participation and earnings equations provide the basis for a quantitative evaluation of changes in expected annual earnings (the product of the predicted probability of labor force participation=1 times predicted earnings conditional on labor force participation=1) associated with reductions in educational attainment (human capital accumulation), controlling for other socioeconomic characteristics. The software used for both logistic and ordinary least squares estimation was Stata, version 5.0 (Stata Corp., College Station, Tex.).

The 1995 U.S. Census Bureau's Current Population Survey data on educational attainment histories of recent cohorts of individuals (between ages 25 and 40 in 1995) were then used to construct educational attainment transition probability matrices, by gender, for the entire U.S. population, which indicated the proportion of individuals who completed successively higher levels of education.

Integration of Clinical Trial and U.S. Census Data

To assess the differential probabilities of educational attainment attributable to age of initial onset of major depressive disorder, the clinical trial data was integrated with U.S. Census Bureau's Current Population Survey population data. Results from the logistic regressions that related educational attainment of trial subjects to initial age of major depressive disorder onset were used to compute odds ratios for attainment of successively higher levels of education for the U.S. population, separately by age at onset and gender (31). When statistically different from even, these differential odds ratios were applied to the educational attainment transition probabilities for the U.S. male and female

TABLE 1. Demographic and Clinical Characteristics of 531 Patients Aged 30 and Over With Major Depressive Disorder of Either Early or Late Onset[a]

Characteristic	Early Onset (N=226)		Late-Onset (N=305)		Analysis	
	N	%	N	%	Cochran-Mantel-Haenszel χ^2 (df=1)	p
Female	148	65.5	177	58.0	3.03	0.08
White	209	92.5	278	91.1	0.30	0.58
Never married	166	73.5	253	83.0	6.92	0.009
History of alcohol abuse	80	35.4	70	23.0	10.12	0.001
History of drug abuse	54	23.9	36	11.8	13.64	0.001
Highest education level					1.36[b]	0.51
Partial college	95	42.0	104	34.1		
College graduation	55	24.3	66	21.6		
Graduate training	30	13.3	63	20.7		
Employed or in labor force	159	70.4	210	68.9	0.16	0.69
Current depression type					1.16[c]	0.28
Chronic major	99	43.8	148	48.5		
Double depression	127	56.2	157	51.5		
Early-onset dysthymia	104	46.0	87	28.5	17.22	0.001

[a] Early onset=before age 22; late onset=at age 22 or later. [b] df=3. [c] df=2.

TABLE 2. Impact of Major Depressive Disorder on Marital Status, Substance Abuse History, and Educational Attainment for 531 Patients Aged 30 and Over, by Age at Onset and Gender[a]

Variable	Number of Observations	Early Versus Late Onset: Women Odds Ratio	p^b	Early Versus Late Onset: Men Odds Ratio	p^b	Men Versus Women: Late Onset Odds Ratio	p^b	Men Versus Women: Early Onset Odds Ratio	p^b
Never married	530	0.89	0.69	2.31	0.03	0.84	0.62	2.19	0.02
History of alcohol abuse	530	2.45	0.002	1.22	0.50	3.78	<0.001	1.89	0.04
History of drug abuse	530	2.67	0.005	1.48	0.27	2.61	0.009	1.45	0.27
Attended some college	528	1.25	0.41	1.11	0.77	1.39	0.23	1.24	0.55
Completed college degree	409	0.57	0.04	1.14	0.69	0.94	0.83	1.89	0.05
Some postgraduate schooling	212	0.50	0.09	0.94	0.89	0.95	0.90	1.79	0.22

[a] Early onset=before age 22; late onset=at age 22 or later.
[b] Determined by Wald chi-square test (df=1), where value represents the significance of the observed odds ratio's difference from unity. Current age and current age squared were added as control variables.

populations, based on recent cohorts (ages 25–40 in 1995) in the U.S. Census Bureau's Current Population Survey data set. Through early-onset major depressive disorder prevalence estimates from the National Comorbidity Survey (15% lifetime prevalence for women by age 21, 8% for men) (2), synthetic education transition probability matrices were constructed for populations who at age 21 had experienced early-onset major depressive disorder, and for those who will have experienced depression after age 21 or will never experience major depressive disorder.

The expected annual future lifetime earnings of the early-onset population at age 21 in 1995 was then computed as a weighted average of expected income by educational attainment, where weights reflected the proportions of those with early-onset major depressive disorder who achieved successively higher levels of post-high-school education. A similar calculation was made for the population at age 21 in 1995 who would be expected to develop major depressive disorder after age 21 or never.

Results

Clinical Trial: Pretreatment Patient Characteristics

Of the 635 trial subjects, 531 were age 30 and over at baseline. Among this subgroup, the 226 patients (42.6%) with early-onset major depressive disorder differed in a number of important ways from the 305 patients (57.4%) with late-onset major depressive disorder. As shown in Table 1, subjects with early onset of major depressive disorder were more likely to be female, to have never married, and to have had a history of alcohol or drug abuse. The early-onset patients were also significantly younger than those patients with late-onset major depressive disorder (mean=41.3 years [SD=7.6] versus 45.7 years [SD=8.4], respectively) (F=6.26, df=1, 529, p<0.001). There was no significant difference between early- and late-onset subjects in employment status, educational attainment, or current type of depression, and the two groups were similar in terms of baseline severity of depression as measured by their Hamilton depression scale scores (mean=24.8 [SD=5.3] and 24.8 [SD=5.6], respectively) (F=0.07, df=1, 529, p=0.95). Almost half (46.0%) of the patients with early-onset major depressive disorder also had a history of early-onset dysthymia, whereas early-onset dysthymia occurred in only 28.5% of the patients with late-onset major depressive disorder.

Levels of educational attainment, whether the patient ever married, and histories of alcohol or drug abuse depended in part on age. To account for possible age confounds, and to permit identification of gender-specific impacts, multivariate logistic regressions were performed. Results of these logistic regressions, expressed in the form of odds ratios, are given in Table 2.

The impact of early-onset major depressive disorder on whether the patient had never married varied by gender. The likelihood of women with early-onset depression never having married was not significantly different from

TABLE 3. Attrition, Response, and Change in Depression Scores During Pharmacotherapy for 531 Patients Aged 30 and Over With Major Depressive Disorder of Either Early or Late Onset[a]

Phase and Comparison	Subject Attrition (N=531)		Treatment Response (N=403)		Change in Hamilton Depression Rating Scale Score (N=403)	
	Odds Ratio	p[b]	Odds Ratio	p[b]	Odds Ratio	p[c]
Acute phase (12 weeks)						
Early versus late onset						
Women	0.88	0.65	1.07	0.85	–0.25	0.77
Men	1.58	0.17	0.95	0.89	1.16	0.29
Men versus women						
Late onset	0.86	0.59	1.00	0.99	–0.85	0.32
Early onset	1.54	0.18	0.88	0.76	0.56	0.61
Subsequent phases[d]						
Early versus late onset						
Women	1.65	0.22	1.55	0.30	–0.52	0.61
Men	1.48	0.39	0.74	0.68	–0.83	0.56
Men versus women						
Late onset	1.78	0.16	3.27	0.02	–1.30	0.22
Early onset	1.60	0.29	1.57	0.49	–1.61	0.24
Placebo versus active medication	0.79	0.49	0.29	<0.001	4.08	<0.001

[a] Early onset=before age 22; late onset=at age 22 or later.
[b] Determined through logistic regression on the basis of Wald chi-square tests (df=1). Value represents the significance of the odds ratio's difference from unity.
[c] Determined through linear regression on the basis of t tests, df=396 (acute phase) and df=208 (continuation phase). Value represents the significance of the parameter's difference from zero (no change).
[d] Odds ratio reflects likelihood of event during continuation and maintenance phases for subject attrition (N=285) and change in Hamilton score (N=216). For treatment response, odds ratio reflects likelihood of maintaining response during maintenance phase (N=208).

that of women whose onset was later. However, men with early-onset depression were more than twice as likely to have never married than were men whose depressive onset occurred later. While men and women with late-onset major depressive disorder did not differ from each other, men with early-onset depression were more than twice as likely to have never married than were women with early-onset depression. For men, the impact of early-onset major depressive disorder was most apparent on this simple index of intimate relationships.

Impacts of early-onset major depressive disorder on substance abuse also varied by gender. Women with early-onset major depressive disorder were much more likely than those with late-onset depression to have a history of alcohol or drug abuse. Age at onset did not significantly affect the risk of having a history of alcohol or drug abuse for men. The propensity for men to have a history of alcohol or drug abuse was generally larger than that for women. However, although men with late-onset major depressive disorder had an almost fourfold greater risk of alcohol abuse history than women with late-onset depression, the male-female relative risk dropped by about half when both genders had early-onset major depressive disorder.

Although the likelihood of having attended college was unaffected by age at onset, for those who attended college, early-onset major depressive disorder negatively affected the probability of graduating, particularly for women. Women with early-onset major depressive disorder were about half as likely to obtain a college degree as their older-onset counterparts. Further, within the early-onset group, men were almost twice as likely as women to graduate. This large negative impact of early-onset major depressive disorder for women appeared to continue beyond college into graduate studies, as women with early-onset major depressive disorder were half as likely as those with late-onset depression to seek postgraduate training. For men, however, the likelihood of attempting a postgraduate degree was unaffected by age at onset.

In terms of the six domains of psychological functioning measured at baseline by the Short-Form Health Survey, subjects with early- and late-onset major depressive disorder scored significantly lower than the "normal" population in each of the domains (results not shown, one-tailed ANOVA, df=1, 529, all F>20 and p<0.001). Between the early- and late-onset patients, scores were significantly different only for the domains of physical functioning (two-tailed ANOVA, F=6.60, df=1, 529, p=0.01) and work/daily activities—physical (two-tailed ANOVA, F=4.93, df=1, 529, p=0.03), with the late-onset patients having scores on both that indicated greater impairment. Further details are available upon request from the corresponding author (L.M.K.).

Clinical Trial: Treatment Response

Symptomatic treatment responsiveness was independent of age at onset, both in terms of subject attrition during phases of the trial and treatment responsiveness for those who completed a trial phase (Table 3). The likelihood of dropping out during the acute phase, or of dropping out during the continuation or maintenance phase, was not significantly affected by age of major depressive disorder onset or gender; no odds ratio significantly differed from unity. For patients who completed the acute phase, the probability of achieving a satisfactory acute-phase therapeutic response was independent of age at onset. Among the acute-phase responders, age of major de-

TABLE 4. Highest Level of Education Attained by All Women in the U.S. Population and by Female Patients Aged 30 and Over With Either Early-Onset or Late-Onset/Never Occurring Major Depressive Disorder[a]

	Percent of Women[b]		
Highest Level of Education Attained	U.S. Population	With Early-Onset Major Depressive Disorder	With Late-Onset/Never-Occurring Major Depressive Disorder
High school diploma	36.83	36.83	36.83
Some college	33.87	45.32	31.85
College degree	22.71	15.76	23.71
Master's degree or equivalent[c]	4.95	1.89	5.56
Ph.D. or equivalent[c]	1.64	0.29	2.05

[a] Early onset=before age 22; late onset=at age 22 or later.

[b] Percentages for the U.S. population were taken from the U.S. Census Bureau's Current Population Survey (29). Percentages for early- versus late-onset educational attainment were calculated from odds ratios presented in Table 2. The assumed lifetime prevalence of early-onset depression for women is 15% (2). The calculations assume that early-onset major depressive disorder did not affect the probability of obtaining a high school diploma and that subsequent education attainment probabilities at age 21 are the same for women for whom the onset of major depressive disorder occurs after age 21 or not at all.

[c] The clinical trial did not assess specific postgraduate educational attainment. Percentages are calculated on the basis of the U.S. population data and the corresponding relative odds ratios from Table 2 for "some postgraduate schooling," with the master's degree percentages also including those who pursued but did not complete a doctoral degree program.

FIGURE 1. Expected Mean Annual Earnings for Women With Early-Onset Major Depressive Disorder Versus Those of Women With Late-Onset/Never-Occurring Major Depressive Disorder[a]

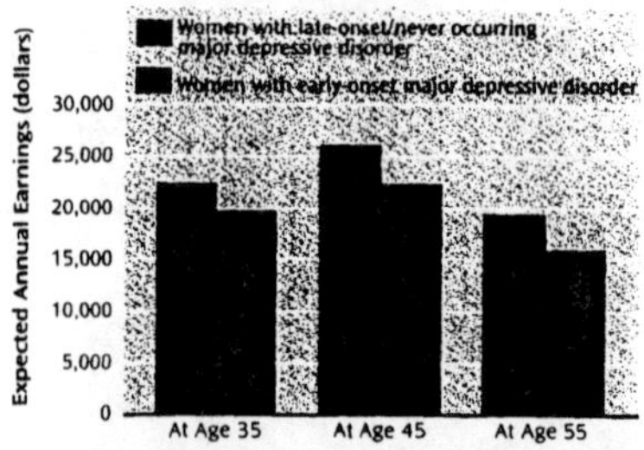

[a] Early onset=before age 22; late onset=at age 22 or later. Bars represent the average earnings a 21-year-old woman in 1995 could expect to receive in the future depending on the presence and age at onset of major depressive disorder.

pressive disorder onset did not affect the likelihood of maintaining the therapeutic response during the maintenance phase of the trial, although among the subjects with late-onset major depressive disorder, the likelihood was significantly greater for men than for women. The likelihood of patients randomly assigned to receive placebo maintaining a therapeutic response during this trial phase was only one-quarter that of patients randomly assigned to receive sertraline.

Least squares regression estimates, where the dependent variable is the change in Hamilton depression scale score since the beginning of that trial phase (negative implies improvement), and with beginning-phase Hamilton depression scale score as an additional regressor, indicate that the amount of change in Hamilton depression scale score was unaffected by gender or age of major depressive disorder onset. However, during the maintenance phase, being randomly assigned to receive placebo in place of sertraline resulted in a mean 4-point worsening in score on the Hamilton depression scale.

The Short-Form Health Survey results (not shown) suggest that therapeutic responders returned to levels of psychosocial functioning generally comparable to community norms, regardless of major depressive disorder age at onset. In four of the six domains (general health, pain, work/daily activities—physical, and interpersonal functioning), therapeutic responders after the 12-week acute phase were insignificantly different from normal community populations (one-tailed ANOVA, $df=1, 529$, all $F\leq1.17$ and $p\geq0.14$). In the physical functioning domain, late-onset subjects had slightly but significantly lower scores than the community subjects (one-tailed ANOVA, $df=1, 529$, $F=6.40$, $p=0.006$). In the work/daily activities—emotional domain, both early and late-onset subjects had slightly but significantly lower scores than the community subjects (one-tailed ANOVA, $df=1, 529$, $F=3.25$ and $F=3.23$, $p=0.04$ for both). In each of the six domains, however, the mean scores of the early- and late-onset patients were not significantly different from each other (two-tailed ANOVA, $df=1, 529$, all $F\leq2.96$ and $p\geq0.09$). Further details are available upon request from the corresponding author.

Education and Earnings Impacts of Lost Human Capital

The impact of early-onset depression on future earnings arise in our framework because of associated reductions in educational attainment. Trial data indicated that for men, early-onset major depressive disorder did not affect subsequent educational attainment. For women, however, the likelihood of completing a college degree for those attending college was only 57% as high for those with early- versus late-onset major depressive disorder, and for college degree recipients, the odds for pursuing postgraduate training were only 50% as high.

As seen in the final two columns of Table 4, in relation to the female U.S. population in 1995, early-onset major depressive disorder resulted in considerable reductions in highest educational attainment, i.e., in lost human capital. More women with early- than late-onset major depressive disorder attended college but did not complete a college degree program, which resulted in a smaller proportion of early-onset women having a college degree as their highest level of educational attainment.

To assess the earnings impact of reductions in human capital accumulation associated with early-onset major depressive disorder for women, we related 1995 earnings of U.S. women ages 19–70 to levels of educational attainment. Although not shown here, consistent with other labor market studies (30), we found that annual earnings are greater and peak at older ages with successive increases in educational attainment.

When these age at onset, educational attainment, and income data are combined, they reveal significant declines in expected future annual earnings for women experiencing early-onset versus late-onset/never-occurring major depressive disorder. As shown in Figure 1, expected annual earnings at age 35 for two women 21 years of age in 1995 would be $22,461 for the woman with late-onset/never-occurring major depressive disorder but only $19,795 ($2,666, or 11.9% less) for the woman with early-onset major depressive disorder. At age 45, the expected annual earnings gap widens to $26,071 versus $22,341 ($3,730, or 14.3% less), respectively, and at age 55 expected annual earnings are $19,415 versus $15,937 ($3,478, or 17.9% less). We emphasize that these are annual decrements. Were they to be summed over a lifetime in the workforce, these decrements would be more substantial. Thus, early-onset major depressive disorder has considerable consequences for the expected earnings of women.

Discussion

The clinical trial data provide strong empirical support for the hypothesis that early-onset major depressive disorder adversely affects the final educational attainment of young women. Early-onset major depressive disorder does not exhibit a significant effect on the educational attainment of young men. The negative educational attainment effect for women constitutes one form of lost human capital from early-onset major depressive disorder; the expected future earnings of these women with early-onset major depressive disorder are decreased by about 12%–18% relative to women whose onset occurred after age 21 or not at all. While employment rates for patients with early- and late-onset major depressive disorder were similar, the reduced educational attainment of women with early-onset major depressive disorder results in lower expected income.

A second important finding is that both the symptomatic relief and the psychosocial improvement that follow acute-phase and longer-term antidepressant treatment were independent of age of depression onset. As reported elsewhere (24), 60% of the chronically depressed patients who completed the acute phase of this trial were classified as therapeutic responders. The odds of a patient completing the various phases of this trial were independent of age of major depressive disorder onset. Moreover, the psychosocial functioning of therapeutic responders, as measured by various domains of the Short-Form Health Survey, was comparable to community norms regardless of age of major depressive disorder onset.

Together, these findings lead us to conclude that early-onset major depressive disorder causes substantial human capital loss. Early detection and appropriate antidepressant treatment of major depressive disorder among the young could have substantial economic benefits, particularly for women (32).

We have confined our analysis to the economic implications resulting from reduced educational attainment associated with early-onset major depressive disorder. Our analysis does not take into account whether the amount and quality of learning achieved at each education level are affected by early-onset major depressive disorder, as well as any earnings implications of these possible impacts. This study did not assess related effects of early-onset major depressive disorder on human capital formation involving marital status or drug and alcohol abuse, each of which was significantly affected by early-onset major depressive disorder. Moreover, our analysis of the burden of early-onset major depressive disorder did not encompass important noneconomic factors, such as the patients' satisfaction and quality of life and that of their families and friends.

Because college graduation is more likely to occur by age 22 than age 21, we defined early-onset major depressive disorder as occurring before age 22. Although not reported here, our principal findings are essentially unaffected when early onset is defined as occurring up to age 18 or to age 21 (the DSM-IV definition), rather than to age 22. These findings are robust to other modifications, such as 1) when the older subgroup is categorized as those over age 35, or over age 40, rather than using the age-30 demarcation; 2) when the lifetime prevalence of major depressive disorder for 21-year-old women is 10% or 20%, rather than 15%; or 3) when labor force participation is defined as occurring when annual earnings are several multiples of $260. Moreover, the educational attainment results for women with early- versus late-onset major depressive disorder are unaffected when drug and/or alcohol abuse histories are added as explanatory variables to the logistic regressions.

Our results amplify earlier reported gender differences in dysthymia and chronic major and double depression and buttress the findings of others relating to early-onset chronic depression and comorbidity with selected personality disorders (32–36). There is some evidence that early-onset major depressive disorder is associated with a greater degree of comorbidity than early-onset dysthymia and may represent a more serious form of the disorder (33, 34). The clinical trial data indicated that unlike early-onset major depressive disorder, early-onset dysthymia did not have statistically significant impacts on patients' marital, substance abuse, or education attainment histories, either when considered by itself or in combination with early-onset major depressive disorder. Whether early-onset dysthymia and major depressive disorder have different impacts on human capital accumulation merits further research.

Several additional caveats should be noted. First, the trial included only subjects with chronic depression. We could not assess whether a single episode of early-onset major depressive disorder with no subsequent relapse or recurrence would have a significant impact on human capital formation. The risks of recurrence and relapse from initial and subsequent episodes of major depressive disorder have been shown, however, to be considerable (37–40). Second, our clinical trial data may understate the impact of chronic depression. Specifically, prospective patients with profound comorbid illnesses or treatment resistance to multiple therapies were not included in the trials. Third, we cannot ascertain whether patients with early-onset major depressive disorder would have responded equally if they had been appropriately treated years earlier at the initial onset of major depressive disorder. However, selective serotonin reuptake inhibitor response rates of young major depressive disorder patients have been shown to be equivalent to those of older subjects (41).

Our results extend available knowledge concerning the impact of undifferentiated recent psychiatric disorders on labor market outcomes (42). Further research into these relationships can provide important inputs into policy discussions on the cost effectiveness of medical care expenditures.

Received Feb. 9, 1999; revisions received July 7, Sept. 9, and Nov. 29, 1999; accepted Dec. 27, 1999. From the Massachusetts Institute of Technology, Cambridge; Stanford University, Stanford, Calif.; the University of Arizona, Tucson; Virginia Commonwealth University, Richmond; Brown University, Providence, R.I.; University of Pittsburgh, Pittsburgh; the University of Texas Southwestern Medical Center at Dallas; and the VA Medical Center, Dallas. Address reprint requests to Dr. Koran, OCD Clinic Room 2363, 401 Quarry Rd., Stanford, CA 94305.

This study was supported by Pfizer Inc.

The authors thank Howard Birnbaum, Paul E. Greenberg, Amy Grudzinski, James M. Russell, and Jason Verner for their assistance with this study.

References

1. Becker GS: Human Capital: A Theoretical and Empirical Analysis, With Special Reference to Education. New York, National Bureau of Economic Research, 1964
2. Kessler RC, McGonagle KA, Swartz M, Blazer DG, Nelson CB: Sex and depression in the National Comorbidity Survey, I: lifetime prevalence, chronicity and recurrence. J Affect Disord 1993; 29:85–96
3. Broadbent WE, Blazer DG, George LK, Tse CK: Depression, disability days, and days lost from work in a prospective epidemiologic survey. JAMA 1990; 264:2524–2528
4. Conti DJ, Burton WN: The economic impact of depression in a workplace. J Occup Med 1994; 36:983–988
5. Greenberg PE, Kessler RC, Nels TL, Finkelstein SN, Berndt ER: Depression in the workplace: an economic perspective, in Selective Serotonin Reuptake Inhibitors: Advances in Basic Research and Clinical Practice, 2nd ed. Edited by Feighner JP, Boyers WF. Chichester, UK, John Wiley & Sons, 1996, pp 321–358
6. Wells KB, Stewart AL, Hays RD, Burnam MA, Rogers WH, Daniels M, Berry S, Greenfield S, Ware JE Jr: The functioning and well-being of depressed patients. JAMA 1989; 262:914–919
7. Klerman GL: Depressive disorders: further evidence for increased medical morbidity and impairment of social functioning. Arch Gen Psychiatry 1989; 46:856–858
8. Hays RD, Wells KB, Sherbourne CD, Rogers WH, Spritzer K: Functioning and well-being outcomes of patients with depression compared with chronic general medical illness. Arch Gen Psychiatry 1995; 52:11–19
9. Wells KB, Sturm R, Sherbourne CD, Meredith LS: Caring for Depression. Cambridge, Mass, Harvard University Press, 1996
10. Wells KB, Hays RD, Burnham MA, Rogers WH, Greenfield S, Ware JE Jr: Detection of depressive disorder for patients receiving prepaid or fee for service practices; results from the Medical Outcomes Study. JAMA 1989; 262:925–930
11. Katon W, Von Korff M, Lin EHB, Bush T, Ormel J: Adequacy and duration of antidepressant treatment in primary care. Med Care 1992; 30:67–76
12. Keller MB, Klerman GL, Lavori PW, Fawcett JA, Coryell WA, Endicott J: Treatment received by depressed patients. JAMA 1982; 248:1848–1855
13. Keller MB, Lavori PW, Klerman GL, Andreasen NC, Endicott J, Coryell W, Fawcett J, Rice JP, Hirschfeld RM: Low levels and lack of predictors of somatotherapy and psychotherapy received by depressed patients. Arch Gen Psychiatry 1986; 43:458–466
14. Keller MB: Undertreatment of major depression. Psychopharmacol Bull 1988; 24:75–80
15. Kocsis JH, Frances AJ, Voss C, Mann JJ, Mason BJ, Sweeney J: Imipramine treatment for chronic depression. Arch Gen Psychiatry 1988; 45:253–257
16. Keller MB, Harrison WM, Fawcett JA, Gelenberg AJ, Hirschfeld RMA, Klein D, Kocsis JH, McCullough JP, Rush AJ, Schatzberg AF, Thase ME: Treatment of chronic depression with sertraline or imipramine: preliminary blinded response rates and high rates of undertreatment in the community. Psychopharmacol Bull 1995; 31:205–212
17. Perez-Stable EJ, Miranda J, Munoz RF, Ying YW: Depression in medical outpatients: underrecognition and misdiagnosis. Arch Intern Med 1990; 150:1083–1088
18. Regier DA, Hirschfeld RMA, Goodwin FK, Burke JD Jr, Lazar JB, Judd LL: The NIMH Depression Awareness, Recognition and Treatment Program: structure, aims, and scientific basis. Am J Psychiatry 1988; 145:1351–1357
19. Baldessarini RJ: Current status of antidepressants: clinical pharmacology and therapy. J Clin Psychiatry 1985; 50:117–126
20. American Psychiatric Association: Practice Guideline for Major Depressive Disorder in Adults. Am J Psychiatry 1993; 150(April suppl)
21. Kupfer DJ, Frank E, Perel JM, Cornes C, Mallinger AC, Thase ME, McEachran AB, Grochocinski VJ: Five year outcomes for maintenance therapies in recurrent depression. Arch Gen Psychiatry 1992; 49:769–773
22. Keller MB, Kocsis JH, Thase ME, Gelenberg AJ, Rush AJ, Koran LM, Schatzberg AF, Russell JM, Hirschfeld RMA, Klein DN, McCullough JP, Fawcett JA, Kornstein SM, LaVange L, Harrison WM: Maintenance phase efficacy of sertraline for chronic depression, a randomized controlled trial. JAMA 1998; 280:1665–1672
23. Rush AJ, Koran LM, Keller MB, Markowitz JC, Harrison WM, Miceli RJ, Fawcett JA, Gelenberg AJ, Hirschfeld RMA, Klein DN, Kocsis JH, McCullough JP, Schatzberg AF, Thase ME: The treatment of chronic depression, part 1: study design and rationale for evaluating the comparative efficacy of sertraline and imipramine as acute crossover, continuation, and maintenance phase therapies. J Clin Psychiatry 1998; 59:589–597

24. Keller MB, Gelenberg AJ, Hirschfeld RMA, Rush AJ, Thase ME, Kocsis JH, Markowitz JC, Fawcett JA, Koran LM, Klein DN, Russell JM, Kornstein SG, McCullough JP, Davis SM, Harrison WM: The treatment of chronic depression, part 2: a double-blind, randomized trial of sertraline and imipramine. J Clin Psychiatry 1998; 59:598–607
25. Spitzer RL, Williams JBW, Gibbon M, First MB: The Structured Clinical Interview for DSM-III-R (SCID), I: history, rationale, and description. Arch Gen Psychiatry 1992; 49:624–629
26. Miller IW, Keitner GI, Schatzberg AF, Klein DN, Thase ME, Rush AJ, Markowitz JC, Schlager D, Kornstein SG, Davis SM, Harrison WM, Keller MB: The treatment of chronic depression, part 3: psychosocial functioning before and after treatment with sertraline or imipramine. J Clin Psychiatry 1998; 59:608–617
27. Tarlov AR, Ware JE Jr, Greenfield S, Nelson EC, Perrin E, Zubkoff M: Medical Outcomes Study: an application of methods for evaluating the results of medical care. JAMA 1989; 262:907–913
28. Ware JE Jr, Sherbourne CD: The MOS 36-Item Short-Form Health Survey (SF-36), I: conceptual framework and item selection. Med Care 1992; 30:473–483
29. US Bureau of the Census: Current Population Survey: Current Population Reports, Series P-20 and P-60. Washington DC: US Government Printing Office, March 1997
30. Berndt ER: Analyzing determinants of wages and measuring wage discrimination: dummy variables in regression models, in The Practice of Econometrics: Classic and Contemporary. Edited by Berndt ER. Reading, Mass, Addison-Wesley, 1991, pp 150–223
31. Kocsis JH, Frances AJ, Voss C, Mason BJ, Mann JJ, Sweeney J: Imipramine and social-vocational adjustment in chronic depression. Am J Psychiatry 1988; 145:997–999
32. Kornstein SG, Schatzberg AF, Thase ME, Yonkers KA, McCullough JP, Keitner GI, Gelenberg AJ, Ryan CE, Hess AL, Harrison WM, Davis SM, Keller MB: Gender differences in chronic major and double depression. J Affect Disord (in press)
33. Fava M, Alpert JE, Borus JS, Nierenberg AA, Pava JA, Rosenbaum JF: Patterns of personality disorder comorbidity in early-onset versus late-onset major depression. Am J Psychiatry 1996; 153:1308–1312
34. Kash KL, Klein DN: The relationship between age at onset and comorbidity in psychiatric disorders. J Nerv Ment Dis 1996; 184:703–707
35. Rohde P, Lewinsohn PM, Seeley JR: Comorbidity of unipolar depression, II: comorbidity with other mental disorders in adolescents and adults. J Abnorm Psychol 1991; 100:214–222
36. Klein DN, Schatzberg AF, McCullough JP, Keller MB, Dowling F, Goodman D, Howland RH, Markowitz JC, Smith C, Miceli RJ, Harrison WM: The early versus late distinction in dysthymic disorder: comparison on demographic and clinical variables, family history, and treatment response in outpatients with superimposed major depressive episodes. J Affect Disord 1999; 52:187–196
37. Keller MB, Shapiro RW, Lavori PW, Wolfe N: Recovery in major depressive disorder. Arch Gen Psychiatry 1982; 39:905–910
38. Keller MB, Lavori PW, Endicott J, Coryell W, Klerman GL: "Double depression": two-year follow-up. Am J Psychiatry 1983; 140:689–694
39. Keller MB, Klerman GL, Lavori PW, Coryell WA, Endicott J, Taylor J: Long-term outcome of episodes of major depression. JAMA 1984; 252:788–792
40. Keller MB, Lavori PW, Rice JB, Coryell W, Hirschfeld RMA: The persistent risk of chronicity in recurrent episodes of nonbipolar major depressive disorder: a prospective follow-up. Am J Psychiatry 1986; 143:24–28
41. Emslie GJ, Rush AJ, Weinberg WA, Kowatch RA, Hughes CW, Carmody T, Rintelman J: A double-blind, randomized, placebo-controlled trial of fluoxetine in children and adolescents with depression. Arch Gen Psychiatry 1997; 54:1031–1037
42. Ettner SL, Frank RG, Kessler RC: The impact of psychiatric disorders on labor market outcomes. Ind Labor Relat Rev 1997, 51. 64–81

Annu. Rev. Psychol. 1997. 48:191–214

THE EFFECTS OF STRESSFUL LIFE EVENTS ON DEPRESSION

Ronald C. Kessler

Department of Health Care Policy, Harvard Medical School, Boston, Massachusetts 02115

KEY WORDS: life events, stress

ABSTRACT

This chapter reviews recent research on the relationship between stressful life experiences and depression. A distinction is made between aggregate studies of overall stress effects and focused studies of particular events and difficulties. A distinction is also made between effects of life stress on first onset of depression and on the subsequent course of depression. Although the available evidence suggests that acute stressful life events can lead to the recurrence of episodes of major depression, a series of methodological problems compromise our ability to make clear causal inferences about the effects of life events on first onset of major depression or about the effects of chronic stress on either onset or recurrence of depression. The main problems of this sort are discussed, and recommendations made for ways of addressing these problems in future studies.

CONTENT

INTRODUCTION

Despite ample theories of psychopathology and many associated empirical studies, it is uncertain whether stressful life events promote psychiatric disorders. This chapter reviews contemporary theorizing and research about mental health in the context of stress. Although I focus on major depression, the most commonly investigated outcome, effects of stress on other psychiatric disorders are also considered (e.g. Blazer et al 1987, Dohrenwend et al 1995, Falsetti et al 1995, Kessler et al 1995).

The fundamental question—Does stress cause depression?—can only be evaluated rigorously in an experiment. Two different experimental literatures have developed to address this question. One addresses the effects of stress on what appear to be episodes of depression in animals (Soumi 1991a,b), and one addresses the effects of experimentally manipulated presumed mediating or modifying variables in field experiments of people facing serious stressors (Mrazek & Haggerty 1994). Both paradigms are limited in the evidence they provide about the effects of stress on major depression. It is unclear whether the results of animal studies generalize to human beings. Intervention experiments, which provide more direct evidence about major stress effects on human beings, are limited in that they manipulate stress mediators or modifiers rather than stress itself. In such work, the range within which stress effects can be changed is evaluated rather than the magnitude of these effects.

Because of these limitations, most evidence for a depressogenic effect of stressful life events comes from nonexperimental research. Inferences about the effects of stress in nonexperimental research are based on attempts to approximate the conditions of experimental random exposure by some combination of matching and use of control variables. Several methodological problems exist in most of these studies that make it difficult to estimate the effects of life events on depression and make it even more difficult to address complex questions about the importance of refining life event measures, distinguishing the effects of life events on onset and course of depression, and investigating stress-modifying effects. The review discusses these questions in sections. Each section begins with a review of the literature and then discusses theoretical and methodological problems. Sections end with suggestions to resolve these problems and advance the substantive research agenda.

ESTIMATING THE SHORT-TERM EFFECTS OF STRESS ON DEPRESSION

Aggregate Life Event Studies

The most common study estimating the effects of life events on depression focuses on short-term effects, typically a recall period of no more than one year. These studies compare scores on aggregated stressful life event scales between persons who did and did not report the recent onset of an episode of major depression. Community surveys (e.g. Brown & Harris 1978) and case-control studies of depressed patients and matched nondepressed controls (Dohrenwend et al 1995) have been used to make these comparisons. The comparisons have generally been, of necessity, retrospective in the sense that information about stress exposure was gathered after onset of depression. Retrospective life event assessment is the norm even in prospective studies, where information about intercurrent events and depressive episodes between waves of data collection is collected in the later wave (e.g. Lewinsohn et al 1988).

Many such studies have been conducted in the past two decades (Bidzinska 1984, Billings et al 1983, Brown et al 1987, Hammen et al 1985, Holahan & Moos 1991, Kendler et al 1995a, Lloyd 1980, Patrick et al 1978, Paykel 1979, Shrout et al 1989, Williamson et al 1995) and mainly show the following: 1. There is a consistently documented association between exposure to stressful life events and subsequent onset of episodes of major depression. 2. However, the magnitude of this association varies across studies depending on how life events are measured, with associations generally stronger when "contextual" measures are used rather than simple life event checklists. 3. There is consistent evidence for a dose-response relationship between stressful events and depression, with severe events more strongly associated with depression than nonsevere events. 4. Stressful life events are highly prevalent in these studies. Although the majority of depressed people report the occurrence of a stressful event shortly before the onset of their depression, only a minority of those people exposed to such events become depressed.

Two main methodological problems compromise our ability to make causal inferences about stress effects from these studies. First, most of the studies failed to consider that accuracy in reporting life events is associated with depression. These studies failed to adjust for the bias introduced by this possibility. For example, many studies failed to confirm whether events occurred before depression. Because depression can cause some events (Hammen 1991) and because people with a history of depression have more events than others even when not in episodes of depression (Kessler & Magee 1993), there may be a bias toward finding specious associations between life events and depression. A number of researchers have found, consistent with this concern, that the relationship between "dependent" events and depression is stronger than the relationship between "independent" events and depression (Williamson et al 1995), where a dependent event was defined as one that could plausibly be a consequence of the respondent's own actions (e.g. being fired from a job) while an independent event could not be defined so (e.g. losing a job due to a plant closing).

The fact that independent events were generally significant predictors of depression in those studies that distinguished independent and dependent events has been considered evidence that life events do cause depression (e.g. Brown & Harris 1978). However, another type of confounding could have led to the association between independent events and depression. Retrospective reports about event exposure might have been biased in these studies by differential recall accuracy or differential willingness to disclose and discuss stressful experiences among currently (at the time of interview) depressed versus nondepressed respondents in such a way that created the appearance that life events cause depression. Consistent with this possibility, experimental research has shown that induction of depressed mood can lead to a significant increase in reports of past stressful events (Cohen et al 1988). Furthermore, recent research with twins has documented a significant heritable component in reports about the occurrence of both independent and dependent life events, which could be due to a stable difference in reporting styles that is associated with liability to depression (Kendler et al 1993).

The problems of accuracy of life event reporting and dating can be partially overcome by obtaining independent reports about life events from informants or archival records. However, this is seldom practiced, and even when it is, these procedures can only provide a partial solution because it is impossible to find informants for all study respondents, many important events will not be known to informants even when they exist, informants will not be perfectly accurate even when they are aware of all relevant events, and archival records exist for only a small fraction of all relevant events.

A second methodological problem compromising our ability to make causal inferences about stress effects involves the logic of causal analysis used in nonexperimental studies of aggregate stress effects. As noted above, these studies interpret the associations between life events and depression as indicating a causal effect of the former on the latter. The assumption implicit in this interpretation is that exposure to life events occurs randomly with respect to other causes of depression. However, this assumption is generally incorrect. Some researchers have attempted to adjust for this problem statistically by introducing controls for confounding variables in multivariate causal models. The recent statistical literature shows quite clearly, though, that efforts of this sort are doomed to failure in the absence of highly unrealistic assumptions about completeness of controls and linearity-additivity of multivariate influences (Holland 1986, Sobel 1990).

It is important to emphasize in this regard that misspecification can invalidate the control variable approach even when confounding variables are correctly measured. The most obvious example involves the case where the researcher assumes that confounding variables have additive effects. Given what we know about stress-modifying effects, it is almost certain that this is not the case in most applications. Common causes of event exposure and depression, such as a genetic liability or various aspects of personality or access to supportive social relationships, are likely to modify the impact of stressful life events on depression and lead to a biased estimate of the magnitude of this impact in the absence of a correct specification of interactions between the events and the controls.

Focused Studies of Individual Events

Because of the methodological problems enumerated above, the studies cited above cannot be interpreted as providing unequivocal support for the view that aggregated stressful life events cause depression. However, other studies do provide support. Such studies exploit the fact that the relationship between a stressful life event and a health outcome can be interpreted as if it were based on an experiment when exposure to the event occurred for reasons that are random with respect to the outcome. There are cases where this situation occurs, but these are almost entirely limited to single events such as job loss due to economic conditions, exposure to an unanticipated natural disaster, or involvement in a fatal automobile accident where the other driver was at fault. These "natural experiments," each focusing on a single fairly common event such as job loss (e.g. Dew et al 1987), widowhood (e.g. Umberson et al 1992), and divorce (e.g. Aseltine & Kessler 1993), provide the strongest evidence about the effects of stressful life events on depression. This evidence is especially strong when the sample of people exposed to these events is obtained from archival data so that there is no risk of selective recall bias. All these studies show that serious stressful events are associated with a substantial increase in depressive episodes.

A New Emphasis on Chronic Stress

Although early research on life stress and depression was almost exclusively concerned with life events, the past decade has seen a new interest in chronic stress. This interest draws on a long-standing epidemiological research tradition that has studied the health-damaging effects of chronic work stress (e.g. House & Cottington 1986, Karasak & Theorell 1990, Kasl 1978) and a growing body of literature on the relationship between chronic marital difficulties and depression (e.g. Beach et al 1990, Gotlib & McCabe 1990). We know from these studies that chronic role-related stresses are significantly associated with chronically depressed mood (Mirowsky & Ross 1989, Pearlin 1989). We also know from the handful of life event studies that have included assessments of them that chronic stresses are often associated with an exacerbation of the effects of life events on episodes of major depression, especially when the life domains affected by the events are the same as the domains affected by the chronic stresses (Brown et al 1987, McGonagle & Kessler 1990).

Recent research has also begun to focus on chronic stresses as mediators of the effects of life events on depression. These studies suggest that enduring stressful sequelae of stressful events account for most of the effects of life events on major depression. For example, the adverse effects of unemployment on depression are partly mediated by resultant financial stresses (Kessler et al 1987), while the relationship between loss of spouse and depression is partly mediated by social isolation (Umberson et al 1992). As discussed below, an exciting opportunity for increasing our understanding of the processes linking life events to depression involves the disaggregation of life event effects through these mediating chronic stresses.

Future Directions

AGGREGATE LIFE EVENT STUDIES It is important for researchers to grapple more seriously with the complex methodological problems involved in conducting naturalistic studies of aggregate stress effects in community samples. Focused studies of individual randomly occurring events are limited because few life events occur for reasons that are entirely random with respect to the outcome of interest. This means that reliance on those few opportunities where natural experiments present themselves or the somewhat larger set of opportunities where design enhancements can be used to develop the functional equivalents of natural experiments (Kessler et al 1996b), while providing clear documentation that life events lead to depression, provide no insights into the dynamics of the much more common situations in which potentially dependent events occur before the onset of depression. Yet we need to study these complex situations because they are most commonly associated with depression. It is a challenge for future research to develop procedures to do this. These procedures will presumably require innovations in research design and analysis (Kessler et al 1996b).

FOCUSED STUDIES OF INDIVIDUAL EVENTS In addition, life events researchers need to begin working more seriously with studies of individual events to better understand causal relationships. Many focused studies already exist on the stress and coping processes associated with such important stressors as unemployment (Feather 1990), bypass surgery (Kulik & Mahler 1993), and rape (Von et al 1991). However, the vast majority of these studies are by clinicians interested in treatment effects rather than life event effects. As a result, the studies generally lack control groups and usually focus on people in treatment rather than on representative community samples of those who have been exposed to the event under investigation. Consequently, it is impossible to draw any inferences about stress effects (Burgess & Holstrom 1979). Despite such limitations, the results from these studies provide a rich source of information about the meanings of stressful events in the lives of the people who experience them, the coping challenges these events elicit, and the resources and vulnerabilities associated with successful and unsuccessful coping efforts. These results could be invaluable to future researchers who attempt to apply the logic of nonexperimental causal analysis to new investigations of the effects of these events on depression. Such studies should include prospective designs and use carefully constructed control groups in an effort to estimate the magnitude of life event effects, the pathways through which these effects operate, and the modifying factors that lead these events to vary in their effects across respondents.

CHRONIC STRESS STUDIES The methodological issues are a good deal more complex in research on the relationship between chronic stress and chronic depression. The possibility that chronic role-related stress is an important determinant of chronic depression is certainly consistent with the observation that people who have chronic major depression or dysthymia often report ongoing problems in one or more of their central life roles. However, a major problem in interpreting this fact is that both the chronic role-related stresses and the chronic depression by definition have occurred for so long that deciding unambiguously which came first is difficult. No serious efforts address this problem of causal order. The researcher, however, may focus on stresses that can be assumed to have occurred randomly with respect to other risk factors of depression and to be inescapable, in which case matched comparison can be used to make causal inferences about long-term stress effects. A good example is the matched comparison of the parents of children having cancer, diabetes, or some other serious childhood physical disorder with the parents of healthy children. Disorders of this sort are quite common and occur, in most cases, for reasons that are unrelated to other risk factors for parental psychiatric disorder (Pless 1994). The small amount of research shows that these childhood physical disorders have significant psychiatric effects on the family (Jessop et al 1988, Krosnick 1970).

The more usual case, however, is one in which nonrandom exposure to the chronic stress cannot be ruled out, as in studies of the relationship between chronic marital difficulties and chronic depression. Frequently an added complication is systematic selection out of exposure (e.g. differential likelihood of seeking a less stressful job based on individual differences in the depressogenic effects of job stress). Standard longitudinal data collection methods have limited potential for studying chronic stress situations because these situations, by their very nature, are quite stable. These problems make it much more difficult to assess the long-term effects of chronic stress on chronic depression than the short-term effects of life events on episodic depression. Nevertheless, there are some opportunities for making provisional assessments of this sort when exposure is nonrandom. For example, prospective research can be carried out to investigate role entry (e.g. the first few years of marriage or of employment) in an effort to study selection processes into and out of stressful situations in light of the prior existence of both depression and risk factors for depression (Orbuch et al 1993, Veroff et al 1993). Another opportunity for making provisional assessment of causal effects is to focus on microprocesses of chronic stress effects using daily diaries or other fine-grained time-series methods (Csikszentmihalyi & Larson 1987, Eckenrode & Bolger 1995).

REFINING LIFE EVENT MEASURES

Checklists versus Contextual Measures

As noted above, there is considerable variation in the estimated effects of life events, depending on whether scores are based on checklists or contextual measures. The intellectual origin of the checklist approach is usually traced to Adolf Meyer's use of a "life chart" to summarize information provided by patients at intake (Lief 1948), the subsequent use of the life chart method by Wolff and his colleagues (1950) to study the relationship between life change and illness onset, and the eventual refinement of this method by Holmes & Rahe (1967) in the Social Readjustment Rating Scale (SRRS). The SRRS was a checklist of 43 stressful experiences generated on the basis of clinical research to characterize the events that most often occurred to patients before seeking treatment. Separate life change unit (LCU) weights were generated by a panel of raters for each event in the SRRS and used to construct a summary LCU score from this checklist.

The publication of the SRRS led to an enormous amount of research on the relationship between life events and various types of illness onset, with over 1000 papers using the SRRS published in the first decade after its development (Holmes 1979). Subsequent research with mental health outcomes (typically screening scales of nonspecific psychological distress) led to refinements and proliferation of life event checklists (Turner & Wheaton 1995). Refinements included the following: 1. At least three of the events in the SRRS were thought by many critics to be better conceptualized as early symptoms of illness (change in sleeping habits, change in eating habits, sexual difficulties) than life events. Subsequent checklists eliminated these events. 2. Many of the events in the SRRS were actually vaguely defined categories of events (e.g. business readjustment, change in financial state). Subsequent checklists replaced these with a longer set of more concretely defined events within each of these categories. 3. The SRRS was a fairly short checklist that omitted a great many stressful events (e.g. rape, criminal victimization, witnessing a traumatic event). Subsequent checklists added these events and sometimes customized event lists to special populations (e.g. Kessler et al 1992).

In addition, methodological studies of the SRRS and the various checklists based on it were carried out. The main results of these studies were as follows: 1. Negative events are much more powerful predictors of mental health outcomes than positive events (Zautra & Reich 1983), which led to the conclusion that life change is not the central dimension linking stressful life events to psychological disorder and that the LCU weighting approach in the SRRS leads to an underestimation of life event effects. 2. Within the set of fairly serious events typically included in life event checklists like the SRRS, the use of differential weights does not markedly increase the association between negative life event scales and measures of psychological distress (Zimmerman 1983). 3. However, distinctions along a number of other dimensions (e.g. amount of loss, amount of threat, degree of controllability of consequences of the event) do lead to substantial increases in the association between negative life event scales and measures of distress (Thoits 1983).

A key feature of the checklist approach is that all life events of a given type are treated as equivalent. Death of a spouse, for example, was assigned a 100 point LCU score on the SRRS irrespective of the suddenness of the death, the quality of the marriage, or any circumstances surrounding the death that might have made it more stressful (e.g. the death occurred in an automobile accident in which the respondent was driving) or less stressful (e.g. the death occurred peacefully after the spouse had spent many years suffering from a degenerative illness). There is clear evidence from focused studies of individual events that the strength of the relationship between life events and depression increases substantially when these sorts of distinctions are made. Based on this observation, a number of researchers have attempted to modify the checklist approach in such a way as to consider these distinctions.

Two strategies have been used to make these adjustments. One is to allow each respondent to assign a subjective weight to his or her own events (Sarason et al 1978). The other is to use objective information about the person and his life situation to construct an independent judgment of how stressful the event would be for a typical person in that same situation. The first of these strategies has been rejected as confounding measurement of the event with emotional reaction to the event (Turner & Wheaton 1995, Zimmerman 1983) and has consequently been abandoned. The second strategy has evolved into what has been termed the "contextual" approach to rating life events.

The intellectual origins of the contextual approach can be traced to the work of Brown & Harris (1978), who developed a method of using a rating panel to assign scores on a variety of dimensions to stressful life events. According to this rating scheme, the death of a neighbor would be rated as more severe than otherwise if the respondent who reported it was a rural elderly person who lived alone and was a housebound invalid whose main source of social contact was the weekly visit of the neighbor for lunch. To obtain adequate contextual information for rating events, the Brown & Harris method requires intensive personal interviews and qualitative probes to specify precisely the characteristics of the events believed to be relevant to contextual ratings. Detailed probing is also used to establish the timing of the event in relation to the onset of the depression. Precise dating is also used to identify the aspects of the event that are thought to affect depression onset.

Methodological studies suggest that such intensive interviewing is much more effective than the comparatively mechanical procedures used in the administration of checklists in avoiding misdating of events (McQuaid et al 1992), communicating to the respondent the importance of accurate recall (Cannell et al 1981), and facilitating the use of memory aids to improve recall of events and accurate dating of event occurrence (e.g. calendars, visual representations, reminders of personally salient events reported previously in the interview). Such aids have been shown to significantly improve accuracy of life event reports (Sobell et al 1990). Furthermore, the use of contextual ratings has been shown to substantially reduce the response errors in checklist measures due to individual differences, such as checking off the occurrence of a "serious physical illness" that, in fact, was only a cold, or otherwise giving reports that are inconsistent with the implied severity thresholds in the checklist events (Kessler & Wethington 1991, Raphael et al 1991).

There are two practical problems with the contextual rating approach to life events measurement. The first is that great care is needed to make sure information about the occurrence of depression after the event does not contaminate the ratings of context, possibly by highlighting to the interviewer an aspect of the respondent's life situation that would not have been known were it not for the fact that the respondent became depressed. Concerns have been raised that some users of the Brown & Harris method are not sufficiently attentive to this possibility, which can result in confounding of stress ratings with outcomes (Bebbington 1986). The second practical problem is that the intensive interviews used to make contextual life event ratings are very labor intensive. Interviewers must be highly trained. Interviews can take as much as five hours to complete. A complicated rating scheme typically requiring several additional hours to complete is needed to review interview audiotapes. Weekly panel meetings sometimes last an entire day to review these ratings (Brown

1989). Several attempts have been made to evaluate whether a short-cut can be devised to approximate the Brown & Harris method (Cooke 1985, Dohrenwend et al 1993, Kessler & Wethington 1991, Miller & Salter 1984). The most promising of these is a structured version of the method, still being pilot tested, that appears to generate information similar to the original in a shorter interview period and with fewer demands for complex postprocessing (Wethington et al 1995).

There is also a conceptual problem with the contextual rating method. As described below, life events researchers are greatly interested in stress-modifying factors: aspects of the personal and situational environments of people exposed to stressful events that are associated with variation in the impact of these events on their probability of becoming depressed. The contextual rating method subverts this investigation by absorbing information about stress modifiers into the ratings of life event severity. Indeed, the information used by the Brown & Harris ratings panel can be seen as hypotheses concerning stress modifiers that never have a chance to be investigated because they are assumed in rating event severity. A clearly preferable approach would be to subject these hypotheses to empirical test. The difficulty of doing so until now, though, has been that studies of the sort using the Brown & Harris method have all had quite small sample sizes due to the labor-intensive nature of the method. This has meant that the number of subjects has been too small to test specific hypotheses about the modifying effects of particular aspects of context.

Unpacking Events in Focused Studies of Individual Events

The confounding of measures of life event severity with stress modifiers can work in the opposite way as well, by suggesting that there are individual differences in emotional reactivity to an event when, in fact, the event is not the same for all people who experience it. A good illustration is found in research on the relationship between widowhood and depression, which consistently shows that death of a spouse is more strongly associated with depression among men than women (Stroebe & Stroebe 1983). Does this mean that men are less capable of coping with emotional losses than women? Or, alternatively, is widowhood a different stress for men than women? One way to distinguish these two possibilities is to carry out focused studies in which the researcher attempts to disaggregate widowhood in such a way as to unpack its stress components and study how these components explain the effect of the event on depression.

Several recent studies of this sort have been carried out, each focused on a single major event such as divorce (Aseltine & Kessler 1993), unemployment (Turner et al 1991), and widowhood (Umberson et al 1992). The basic approach in each study has been to start with a conceptual model of the dimensions that lead to the effects of the event on depression and then measure these dimensions longitudinally in a sample of people who were exposed to the event and in an appropriate comparison sample of people not exposed to it. Standard multivariate procedures have then been used to study the mediating effects of the stress dimensions on the overall relationship between the event and depression. Umberson et al (1992), for example, examined how much the observed gender difference in the impact of widowhood on depression in a national sample was due to male-female differences in the impact of widowhood on stress dimensions versus differences in the impact of these dimensions on depression. The analysis documented that the greater depressogenic effect of widowhood on men than women is, at least in part, because the death of a spouse leads to a number of secondary stresses for men that do not exist for women. For example, death of a spouse leads to a significant decrease in contact and emotional closeness between the surviving parent and adult children among widowed men but not widowed women.

A consistent result in these studies has been that most of the association between some stressful events and depression is due to a mediating effect on role-related stresses. Caution is needed in interpreting this result, however, in light of the fact that only one of the three studies (Aseltine & Kessler 1993) was truly prospective (i.e. assessed both depression and the mediators before the onset of the stressful event) and none of them controlled for other possible confounding effects. Future work on unpacking life event effects needs to be based on prospective designs that use carefully matched control groups and use intensive interview methods and contextual ratings to define the intervening chronic stress dimensions.

DISTINGUISHING THE EFFECTS OF STRESS ON ONSET AND COURSE ON DEPRESSION

The Effects of Traumatic Stress on Lifetime Depression

The results discussed so far have focused on the short-term effects of recent stressful life events on episodes of depression. Another area of stress research is concerned with the long-term effects of previous stresses (usually either childhood or lifetime traumatic stresses) on lifetime depression. The only programmatic research of this sort we know of is that of Kessler & Magee (1993, 1994a), who analyzed lifetime retrospective data on the relationship between childhood adversities and lifetime depression in a nationally representative general population sample of adults. They concluded that most severe childhood adversities have significant effects on early-onset depression (defined as an onset before age 20) but not on later-onset depression, which indicates that there is some risk period for the impact of childhood adversities beyond which they lose their depressogenic effects. Subsequent work by the same investigators in two other large-scale community surveys yielded similar results (Kessler et al 1996a).

This investigation has the potential to yield important information about life course variations in the effects of traumatic events. By studying differential effects as a function of time since occurrence of the event, it might be possible to document variation in both initial impact and in the length of the risk period associated with the event. We would expect these effects to vary depending on the event and the age of exposure. An investigation of the association between childhood parental loss and clinical depression, for example, would probably look for fairly rapid onset of the disorder after the traumatic event, while an investigation of the association between childhood sexual abuse and lifetime depression might be interested in the possibility of more long-term delayed reactions. By investigating the possibility of variation in the long-term effects of traumas as a function of the respondent's age at occurrence, in comparison, the researcher can investigate the hypothesis that some traumas have their most powerful health-damaging effects during certain critical developmental phases of the life course.

The Long-Term Effects of Traumatic Stress on Current Depression

Related research considers the long-term effects of traumatic stress on current adult depression. A number of studies have been carried out in both psychiatric patient samples and general population samples. These studies have all been based on retrospective data and comparative analyses of persons who are depressed with those who are not. The studies consistently find that depressed adults report the occurrence of more childhood adversities such as separation from a parent, family turmoil, parental psychopathology, and physical/sexual abuse than those who are not depressed (e.g. Birtchnell et al 1988, Brown & Anderson 1991, Bryer et al 1987, Earls et al 1988, Faravelli et al 1986, Fendrich et al 1990, Holmes & Robins 1988, McLeod 1991, Rutter 1989, Tennant 1988, West & Prinz 1987, Stein et al 1988, Yama et al 1993).

The use of long-term retrospective recall to assess these relationships raises concerns about confounding based on selective recall as a function of current depression even though there is evidence that fairly objective adversities such as parental death or divorce are recalled with good reliability (Brewin et al 1993). It is important, in light of these concerns, that researchers who work with retrospective data maximize accuracy of assessment, perhaps by using follow-back designs based on archival records or relying on evaluation of the effects of self-reports about fairly objective and major childhood stressors. In addition, it is important that methodological research be conducted to refine methods of collecting retrospective data to improve the accuracy of respondent reports (Kessler et al 1997).

Disaggregating Long-Term Stress Effects on Onset and Course

History of depression might explain, either in whole or in part, the relationship between childhood adversities and current depression. The plausibility of this hypothesis is supported by research showing that many forms of childhood adversity are associated with increased risk of depression in adolescence and early adulthood (Fleming & Offord 1990, Goodyear 1990) and that early-onset depression is associated with high recurrence risk (Lewinsohn et al 1988). Recent research, in fact, suggests that there is specificity in the continuation of depression between childhood and adulthood (Harrington et al 1990). Because of this observation, it is important for research on the long-term effects of childhood adversities on current depression to control for history and distinguish effects on first onset, recurrence, and speed of episode recovery.

Analyses of this type could shed light on the pathways involved in the long-term effects of early adversities. What little is known about these pathways suggests that childhood adversities are associated with difficulties in making successful role transitions into early adulthood, which in turn are associated with depression during the adult years (McLeod 1991, Quinton et al 1984). Childhood adversities have also been linked to intrapsychic factors that predict adult depression, such as helplessness, low self-esteem, and interpersonal dependency (Brown et al 1987). However, an important limitation in this research is that prior history of depression has not been considered a potential confounding variable. This makes it much more difficult to interpret the true effects of other mediating variables than it would be otherwise.

A good illustration of this problem is provided by Parker & Hadzi-Pavlovic's (1984) investigation of women whose mothers died during the women's childhoods. Retrospective reports about lack of care from fathers and stepmothers after the death of the mothers were significantly associated with high adult scores on screening scales of both state depression and trait depression. These associations were attenuated among respondents with supportive spouses, which led the authors to conclude that success in forming intimate relationships "largely corrected any diathesis to greater depression created by uncaring parenting." However, this conclusion ignores the alternative hypothesis that lack of success in forming a supportive marriage and current depression were both due to a history of depression that began after the death of the mother but before marriage. If this is true, there might be no causal effect of success in forming a supportive marriage on subsequent depression even though there is a significant association between these two variables.

As noted above, Kessler and his associates (Kessler & Magee 1993, 1994b; Kessler et al 1996a) examined these issues and found that a wide variety of retrospectively reported childhood adversities are associated with lifetime onset of depression before age 20 and that few of these adversities continue to be associated with later risk of either first onset or episode recurrence. Their studies have not examined the relationships between childhood adversities and speed of episode recovery. Replications and extensions of these studies are needed in more focused samples.

Controlling History in Studying the Determinants of Episode Onset

An understanding of history of depression could be important in evaluating the short-term effects of stressful life events on episode onset. The literature on sex differences in depression provides an interesting illustration of this situation. Point prevalence of depression is much higher among women than men (Blazer et al 1994, Weissman et al 1988). However, there is no sex difference in recurrence of depression (Coryell et al 1991), nor in speed of episode recovery of depression (Kessler et al 1993), which means that the higher rate of current depression typically found among women is presumably due to a relationship between sex and lifetime depression (Eaton et al 1989, Weissman et al 1988). We know that the average age of onset of depression for both men and women is in the early twenties (Sorenson et al 1991). However, the sex difference in prevalence of depression is more pronounced in mid-life because the density of recurrent episodes of depression is greatest in this period of the life cycle. This mid-life bulge in the sex difference in depression has been considered by many commentators as evidence that chronic life stresses associated with sex roles explain the sex difference in depression (e.g. Ensel 1982). However, a consideration of sex differences in first onset and in recurrence shows that the mid-life increase in the sex difference is largely because of a sex difference in lifetime onset of depression that occurs by the early twenties. The implications of this observation for current ideas about the relationship between the chronic stresses associated with adult sex roles and depression are profound.

An informative illustration of the importance of controlling for depression history in studying the short-term effects of stressful life events comes from reanalysis of date collected in the Epidemiologic Catchment Area (ECA) study, a major five-site collaborative study of the epidemiology of adult psychiatric disorders (Robins & Regier 1991). Data from the ECA public-use file shows that 91% of the respondents who reported an episode of depression in the 12 months before the baseline ECA interview had a previous history of depression. An obvious question is whether prior depression should be considered a predictor in studies of the short-term effects of stressful life events on episodes of depression. It is clear that such a variable would be a powerful predictor of subsequent episode onset. In the ECA data, history of depression had an odds-ratio close to 40.0 in predicting an episode onset in the 12 months before the baseline ECA interview, an association that dwarfs the effects of any other risk factor in the literature on depression.

Much evidence is consistent with the possibility that history might be an important predictor of current stress, in which case failure to control history could lead to serious bias in estimation of short-term stress effects. History of depression, for example, is thought to influence interpersonal style in ways that provoke other people to act toward depressed people in ways that are nonsupportive and that could lead to increased exposure to interpersonal loss events (Coyne 1976, Monroe & Steiner 1986). This possibility implies that a risk-factor analysis that includes history of depression as a control variable might find that social support and interpersonal loss are less powerful predictors of episode onset than an analysis that failed to control for history.

There is only one published report that investigated this possibility empirically. Kessler & Magee (1994b) introduced a control for history of depression into a risk-factor model for episode onset of recent depression and found that a number of previously significant predictors became insignificant. As discussed below, they also found that history significantly modified the relationships between most other risk factors, which suggests that future work on risk factors for depressive episodes needs to look separately at the predictors of onset and recurrence. As a practical matter, given that the vast majority of episode onsets in adulthood are recurrences, this injunction implies that studies of the relationship between stressful life events and depression in adult samples should explicitly recognize that they are, in effect, studying recurrence of depression. Therefore, the appropriate comparison group is the subsample of respondents with a lifetime history of depression who have not had a recent recurrence and where controls or matching should be used to adjust for variation in age of onset and course of depression before the onset of events as well as for the possibility of selection into dependent events on the basis of prior course of the disorder.

Stress Effects on Speed of Episode Recovery

A number of studies have examined the relationship between stressful life experiences that occurred before the onset of depressive episodes and speed of recovery of these episodes. Most were carried out in patient samples (Brugha et al 1990, Huxley et al 1979, Karp et al 1993, Keller et al 1986, Krantz & Moos 1988, Mann et al 1981, Monroe et al 1992, Parker et al 1988, Weissman et al 1978), although a few were carried out in community samples (Beiser 1976, McLeod et al 1992, Sargeant et al 1990). In these studies, stressful life events and chronic difficulties were generally found to predict slow speed of recovery. A smaller number of studies examined the relationship between intercurrent life events and speed of episode recovery (Brown & Moran 1994, Brown et al 1995, Tennant 1988). These studies found that events arising in the midst of a depressive episode impede recovery if they exacerbate the stressful situations that triggered the episode (e.g. foreclosure in the wake of a job loss). However, events that reverse or resolve an earlier stress are associated with more rapid recovery (e.g. reemployment after a job loss). An especially interesting result is that otherwise negative events can sometimes lead to episode recovery either because they resolve an ongoing difficulty (e.g. separation from an abusive spouse) or because they put the event that triggered the episode into perspective (e.g. a near-death experience in an automobile accident leading to the realization that a recent job loss was not really life-shattering).

STRESS-MODIFYING EFFECTS

Substantive Modifiers

I have focused until now on investigations that document the existence of aggregate effects of stress on depression. However, contemporary research on stress and depression typically accepts this association as a given and focuses more on the consistent finding that the majority of people exposed to all but the most extreme stressful life experiences do not become depressed. An attempt is made to explain this finding and, more generally, individual differences in stress reactivity by searching for characteristics of the individual or the environment in which the individual is embedded that modify stress effects. These modifying factors are sometimes referred to as stress-buffering factors, vulnerability factors, or stress-diathesis factors.

It is beyond the scope of this review to provide an overview of the enormous literature that has accumulated over the past decade to study this diverse array of modifying factors. Instead, see reviews by Gotlib & Hammen (1992), Mrazek & Haggerty (1994), and Taylor & Aspinwall (1996). Several factors have been repeatedly shown to predict an attenuation of the relationship between subsequent events and episode onset of depression, including access to social support, various aspects of personality, appraisal processes, intellectual capabilities such as cognitive flexibility and effective problem-solving skills, interpersonal skills such as social competence and communication ability, and various coping strategies.

History of Depression as a Modifier

There is a problem with interpreting these substantive results in causal terms because virtually none of the studies distinguished modifiers of the stress-depression relationship for first onset of depression from the modifiers of the stress-depression relationship for recurrence of depression, nor did they control for the possible confounding effect of history of depression. As noted above, Kessler & Magee (1994b) found that a number of previously significant stress-modifying factors became statistically insignificant, and the effects of others were substantially attenuated, when they controlled for history of depression and considered that history operates as a stress modifier. Failure to introduce similar controls seriously compromises our ability to draw any inferences from the larger literature on stress-modifying factors in depression.

It is important to reemphasize two earlier points in making this criticism of the literature on stress-modifying effects. First, recurrent major depression can profoundly affect most of the individual-level and environmental factors that have been studied in the modifier literature. Consistent with this observation, Kessler & Magee (1994b) found strong relationships between retrospective reports of a lifetime history of depression and current scores on most of the variables that are normally considered to be stress modifiers in their nationally representative survey. Second, history of depression is itself a stress modifier. That is, the relationship between stressful life events and first onset of depression in the subsample of adult respondents who report no prior history of depression is much weaker than the relationship between stressful life events and recurrence of depression in the subsample of adult respondents who report having a prior history (Kessler & Magee 1994b). The conjunction of these two observations implies that many of the variables currently thought to be stress modifiers will appear to have modifying effects even if they do not. This will occur because they are related to history of depression.

Number of Prior Episodes of Depression as a Modifier

In addition to the distinction between people who have and have not previously been depressed, recent research has shown that number of episodes in the subsample of people with a history is also significantly related to stress reactivity. Post et al (1986) were the first to report this phenomenon and noted that even though stressful life events often precipitate early episodes of depression, as the number of episodes increases "the illness appears to evolve with its own rhythmicity and spontaneity, independent of life events." A subsequent review of epidemiologic studies supported this clinical observation (Post 1992), which led Post to postulate that "sensitization to stressors and episode sensitization occur and become encoded at the level of gene expression" in such a way that responsivity to stress is permanently altered.

Genetic Predisposition as a Modifier

A related line of research has examined the possibility that genetic factors influence stress reactivity. The plausibility of this possibility is suggested by a variety of twin and adoption studies that document genetic influences on major depression (Kendler et al 1992, Tsaung & Farone 1990). However, these genetic effects could occur either independent of environmental stress effects or in interaction with stress by affecting emotional vulnerability to the effects of stress. A recent study by Kendler et al (1995a) in a general population sample of adult female twins investigated this issue by using information on zygosity and co-twin history of depression to define a gradient of genetic vulnerability to depression. The results showed that genetic liability is associated with a threefold increase in the stress-depression relationship.

It is also important to recognize that genetic influences can account for what appears to be an effect of a substantive stress-modifying variable. Kessler et al (1992) found in a study of the stress-buffering effect of social support on the relationship between life events and depression that it was not support itself but the genetically determined component of social support that became more strongly associated with depression in the presence of stressful life events. Future research on stress modifiers should use genetically informative designs, such as twin or adoption studies, to investigate related possibilities in more detail.

OVERVIEW

The evidence reviewed above clearly shows that inventories of stressful events predict subsequent depression. A smaller number of controlled comparative studies of people exposed to single major life events provide strong evidence that at least part of this association is due to events causing depression. It is also clear from other studies that this relationship can be reciprocal and that depression can elicit or exacerbate certain stressful events and difficulties.

In addition, much evidence from prospective studies shows that the association between stressful life events and depression varies considerably depending on prior characteristics of the people exposed to the events and the environments in which these people are embedded. However, this evidence cannot be interpreted unequivocally as demonstrating that these factors are stress modifiers. The reason for this is that unmeasured variables such as prior history of depression or genetic vulnerability could be confounding factors that explain the associations between the presumed stress modifiers and depression.

The results of experimental interventions aimed at preventing depression among people exposed to particular life events offer great promise for reducing this uncertainty about stress modifiers. A number of such interventions have been shown to reduce the depressogenic effects of certain otherwise stressful events by manipulating either stress modifiers and/or the secondary stresses created by the events (Bloom et al 1985, Heaney 1992, Price et al 1992), which shows that some aspects of the stress process can be modified. However, it has not been possible to use this information to make informed judgments about the significance of individual stress modifiers.

There are two reasons for this. First, all the interventions had multiple components. Further nonexperimental process evaluation of their outcome results would consequently be needed to make informed judgments about the effects of separate intervention components. Second, none of these interventions included carefully matched control groups of people who were not exposed to the events, which made it impossible to distinguish stress-modifying effects from the effects of presumed modifiers operating in exactly the same way among people who were not exposed to the events used to define the intervention subjects.

It is unclear why there has not been more collaboration between interventionists and nonexperimental stress researchers. It is conceivable that disciplinary differences in orientation are involved. Preventive interventions are typically carried out by clinical or community psychologists, while naturalistic stress studies are typically conducted by personality/social psychologists, epidemiologists, and sociologists. Future advances in our understanding of the relationship between life events and depression, in my view, will require a collaboration between both perspectives.

The above review has repeatedly implied why such a collaboration would be useful to naturalistic researchers but has also emphasized that these researchers must work harder at approximating the conditions of experiments to clarify the meanings of their results. One unique way of doing this is to work with interventionists to construct control groups of people who were not exposed to the events under investigation and to use the manipulation of intervention exposure with parallel measurement in the control group to facilitate analysis of stress-modifying effects. It is also important to recognize, though, that there is another side of the exchange: Nonexperimental studies are equally important for intervention specialists. Such studies are needed to select intervention targets and to interpret the pathways involved in the effects of successful interventions. Once reliable data on pathways are obtained, nonexperimental studies should search for factors that might effectively block these pathways. This kind of iterative cross-fertilization is our best hope for advancing research on stressful events and depression in the future.

Literature Cited

Aseltine RH Jr, Kessler RC. 1993. Marital disruption and depression in a community sample. *J. Health Soc. Behav.* 34:237–51

Beach SRH, Sandeen EE, O'Leary KD. 1990. *Depression in Marriage: A Model for Etiology and Treatment.* New York: Guilford

Bebbington P. 1986. Establishing causal links: recent controversies. In *Life Events and Psychiatric Disorder: Controversial Issues*, ed. H Katchnig, pp. 188–200. Cambridge: Cambridge Univ. Press

Beiser M. 1976. Personal and social factors associated with the remission of psychiatric symptoms. *Arch. Gen. Psychiatry* 33:941–45

Bidzinska E. 1984. Stress factors in affective diseases. *Br. J. Psychiatry* 144:161–66

Billings A, Cronkite R, Moos R. 1983. Social-environmental factors in unipolar depression: comparisons of depressed patients and nondepressed controls. *J. Abnorm. Psychol.* 93:119–33

Birtchnell J, Evans C, Kennard J. 1988. Life history factors associated with neurotic symptomatology in a rural community sample of 40–49 year old women. *J. Affect. Disord.* 3:271–85

Blazer D, Hughes D, George LK. 1987. Stressful life events and the onset of a generalized anxiety syndrome. *Am. J. Psychiatry* 144:1178–83

Blazer DG, Kessler RC, McGonagle KA, Swartz MS. 1994. The prevalence and distribution of major depression in a national community sample: the National Comor-

bidity Survey. *Am. J. Psychiatry* 151: 979–86
Bloom BL, Hodges WF, Kerns MB, McFadden SC. 1985. A preventive intervention program for the newly separated. *Am. J. Orthopsychiatry* 55:9–26
Brewin CR, Andrews B, Gotlib IH. 1993. Psychopathology and early experience: a reappraisal of retrospective reports. *Psychol. Bull.* 113:82–98
Brown GR, Anderson B. 1991. Psychiatric morbidity in adult inpatients with childhood histories of sexual and physical abuse. *Am. J. Psychiatry* 148:55–61
Brown GW. 1989. Life events and measurement. In *Life Events and Illness*, ed. GW Brown, TO Harris, pp. 3–45. New York: Guilford
Brown GW, Bifulco A, Harris TO. 1987. Life events, vulnerability and onset of depression: some refinements. *Br. J. Psychiatry* 150:30–42
Brown GW, Harris TO. 1978. *Social Origins of Depression: A Study of Psychiatric Disorder in Women.* New York: Free Press
Brown GW, Harris TO, Hepworth C. 1995. Loss, humiliation and entrapment among women developing depression: a patient and nonpatient comparison. *Psychol. Med.* 25:7–21
Brown GW, Moran P. 1994. Clinical and psychosocial origins of chronic depressive episodes. I. A community survey. *Br. J. Psychiatry* 165:447–56
Brugha TS, Bebbington PE, MacCarthy B, Sturt S, Wykes T, Potter J. 1990. Gender, social support and recovery from depressive disorders: a prospective clinical study. *Psychol. Med.* 20:147–56
Bryer JB, Nelson BA, Miller JB, Krol PA. 1987. Childhood sexual and physical abuse as factors in adult psychiatric illness. *Am. J. Psychol.* 144:1426–30
Burgess AW, Holmstrom LL. 1979. Adaptive strategies and recovery from rape. *Am. J. Psychol.* 136:1278–82
Cannell CF, Miller PV, Oksenberg L. 1981. Research on interviewing techniques. In *Sociological Methodology* 1981, ed. S Leinlandt, pp. 389–437. San Francisco: Jossey-Bass
Cohen LH, Towbes LC, Flocco R. 1988. Effects of induced mood on self-reported life events and perceived and received social support. *J. Pers. Soc. Psychol.* 55:669–74
Cooke DJ. 1985. The reliability of a brief life event interview. *J. Psychosom. Res.* 29: 361–65
Coryell W, Endicott J, Keller MB. 1991. Predictors of relapse into major depressive disorder in a nonclinical population. *Am. J. Psychol.* 148:1353–58
Coyne JC. 1976. Depression and the response of others. *J. Abnorm. Psychol.* 85:186–93
Csikszentmihalyi M, Larson R. 1987. Validity and reliability of experience sampling method. *J. Nerv. Ment. Dis.* 175:526–36
Dew MA, Bromet EH, Schulberg HC. 1987. A comparative analysis of two community stressors' long-term mental health effects. *Am. J. Community Psychol.* 15:167–84
Dohrenwend BP, Raphael KG, Schwartz S, Stueve A, Skoldol A. 1993. The structured event probe and narrative rating method for measuring stressful life events. See Mazure 1995, pp. 174–99
Dohrenwend BP, Shrout PE, Link BG, Skodol AE, Stueve A. 1995. Life events and other possible psychosocial risk factors for episodes of schizophrenia and major depression: a case-control study. See Mazure 1995, pp. 43–66
Earls F, Reich W, Jung KG, Cloninger CR. 1988. Psychopathology in children of alcoholic and antisocial parents. *Alcohol Clin. Exp. Res.* 12:481–87
Eaton WW, Kramer M, Anthony JC, Dryman A, Shapiro S, Locke BZ. 1989. The incidence of specific DIS/DSM-III mental disorders: data from the NIMH epidemiologic catchment area program. *Acta Psychiatr. Scand.* 79:163–78
Eckenrode J, Bolger N. 1995. Daily and within-day event measurement. See Cohen et al 1995, pp. 80–101
Ensel WM. 1982. The role of age in the relationship of gender and marital status to depression. *J. Nerv. Ment. Dis.* 170:536–43
Falsetti SA, Resnick HS, Dansky BS, Lydiard RB, Kilpatrick DG. 1995. The relationship of stress to panic disorder: cause or effect? See Mazure 1995, pp. 111–48
Faravelli C, Sacchetti E, Ambonetti A, Conte G, Pallanti S, Vita A. 1986. Early life events and affective disorder revisited. *Br. J. Psychiatry* 148:288–95
Feather NT. 1990. *The Psychological Impact of Unemployment.* New York: Springer-Verlag
Fendrich M, Warner V, Weissman MM. 1990. Family risk factors, parental depression, and psychopathology in offspring. *Dev. Psychol.* 26:40–50
Fleming JE, Offord DR. 1990. Epidemiology of childhood depressive disorders: a critical review. *J. Am. Acad. Child Adolesc. Psychiatry* 29:571–80
Goodyear IM. 1990. Family relationships, life events and childhood psychopathology. *J. Child Psychol. Psychiatry* 31:161–92
Gotlib IH, Hammen C. 1992. *Psychological Aspects of Depression: Toward a Cognitive-Interpersonal Integration.* New York: Wiley
Gotlib IH, McCabe SB. 1990. Marriage and

psychopathology. In *The Psychology of Marriage: Basic Issues and Applications*, ed. F Fincham, T Bradbury, pp. 226–55. New York: Guilford

Hammen C. 1991. The generation of stress in the course of unipolar depression. *J. Abnorm. Psychol.* 100:555–61

Hammen C, Marks T, Mayol A, Deayo R. 1985. Depressive self-schemas, life stress, and vulnerability to depression. *J. Abnorm. Psychol.* 94:308–19

Harrington R, Fudge H, Rutter M, Pickles A, Hill J. 1990. Adult outcomes of childhood and adolescent depression. *Arch. Gen. Psychiatry* 47:465–73

Heaney CA. 1992. Enhancing social support at the workplace: assessing the effects of the Caregiver Support Program. *Health Ed. Q.* 18:477–94

Holahan C, Moos R. 1991. Life stressors, personal and social resources, and depression: a 4-year structural model. *J. Abnorm. Psychol.* 100:31–38

Holland PW. 1986. Statistics and causal inference (with discussion). *J. Am. Stat. Assoc.* 81:945–70

Holmes SJ, Robins LN. 1988. The role of parental disciplinary practices in the development of depression and alcoholism. *Psychiatry* 51:24–36

Holmes TH. 1979. Development and application of a quantitative measure of life change magnitude. In *Stress and Mental Disorder*, ed. JE Barrett, RM Rose, GL Klerman, pp. 37–54. New York: Raven

Holmes TH, Rahe RH. 1967. The social adjustment rating scale. *J. Psychosom. Res.* 11: 213–18

House JS, Cottington E. 1986. Health and the workplace. In *Applications of Social Science to Clinical Medicine and Health Policy*, ed. LH Aiken, D Mechanic, pp. 382–415. New Brunswick, NJ: Rutgers Univ. Press

Huxley PJ, Goldberg DP, Maguire GP, Kincey VA. 1979. The prediction of the course of minor psychiatric disorders. *Br. J. Psychiatry* 135:535–43

Jessop DJ, Riessman CK, Stein RE. 1988. Chronic childhood illness and maternal mental health. *J. Dev. Behav. Pediatr.* 9: 147–56

Karasek RA, Theorell T. 1990. *Healthy Work*. New York. Basic Books

Karp JF, Frank E, Anderson B, George CG, Reynolds CF, et al. 1993. Time to remission in late-life depression: analysis of effects of demographic, treatment, and life-events measures. *Depression* 1:250–56

Kasl SV. 1978. Epidemiological contributions to the study of work stress. In *Stress at Work*, ed. C Cooper, R Payne, pp. 3–48. New York: Wiley

Keller MB, Lavori PW, Rice J, Coryell W, Hirschfeld RWA. 1986. The persistent risk of chronicity in recurrent episodes of nonbipolar major depressive disorder: a prospective follow-up. *Am. J. Psychiatry* 143: 24–28

Kendler KS, Kessler RC, Walters EE, MacLean C, Neale MC, et al. 1995a. Stressful life events, genetic liability, and onset of an episode of major depression in women. *Am. J. Psychiatry* 152:833–42

Kendler KS, Neale MC, Kessler RC, Heath AC, Eaves LJ. 1992. A population-based twin study of major depression in women: the impact of varying definitions of illness. *Arch. Gen. Psychiatry* 49:257–66

Kendler KS, Neale MC, Kessler RC, Heath AC, Eaves LJ. 1993. A twin study of recent life events and difficulties. *Arch. Gen. Psychiatry* 50:789–96

Kendler KS, Walters EE, Neale MC, Kessler RC, Heath AC, Eaves LJ. 1995b. The structure of the genetic and environmental risk factors for six major psychiatric disorders in women. *Arch. Gen. Psychiatry* 52: 374–83

Kessler RC, Gillis-Light J, Magee WJ, Kendler KS, Eaves LJ. 1996a. Childhood adversity and adult psychopathology. In *Trajectories and Turning Points: Stress and Adversity Over the Life Course*, ed. IH Gotlib, B Wheaton. New York: Cambridge Univ. Press. In press

Kessler RC, Kendler KS, Heath A, Neale MC, Eaves LJ. 1992. Social support, depressed mood, and adjustment to stress: a genetic epidemiologic investigation. *J. Pers. Soc. Psychol.* 62:257–72

Kessler RC, Magee WJ. 1993. Childhood adversities and adult depression: basic patterns of association in a U.S. National Survey. *Psychol. Med.* 23:679–90

Kessler RC, Magee WJ. 1994a. Childhood family violence and adult recurrent depression. *J. Health Soc. Behav.* 35:13–27

Kessler RC, Magee WJ. 1994b. The disaggregation of vulnerability to depression as a function of the determinants of onset and recurrence. In *Stress and Mental Health: Contemporary Issues and Prospects for the Future*, ed. WR Avison, IH Gotlib, pp. 239–58. New York: Plenum

Kessler RC, Magee WJ, Nelson CB. 1996b. Analysis of psychosocial stress. In *Psychosocial Stress: Perspective on Structure, Theory, Life Course and Methods*, ed. H Kaplan, pp. 333–66. Academic

Kessler RC, McGonagle KA, Swartz M, Blazer DG, Nelson CB. 1993. Sex and depression in the National Comorbidity Survey I. Lifetime prevalence, chronicity, and recurrence. *J. Affect. Disord.* 29:85–96

Kessler RC, Mroczek DK, Belli RF. 1997. Retrospective adult assessment of childhood psychopathology. In *Assessment in Child Psychopathology*, ed. D Shaffer, J Richeters. New York: Guilford. In press

Kessler RC, Sonnega A, Bromet E, Hughes M, Nelson CB. 1995. Posttraumatic stress disorder in the National Comorbidity Survey. *Arch. Gen. Psychiatry* 52:1048–60

Kessler RC, Turner JB, House JS. 1987. Intervening processes in the relationship between unemployment and health. *Psychol. Med.* 17:949–61

Kessler RC, Wethington E. 1991. The reliability of life event reports in a community survey. *Psychol. Med.* 21:723–38

Krantz SE, Moos RH. 1988. Risk factors at intake predict nonremission among depressed patients. *J. Consult. Clin. Psychol.* 56:863–69

Krosnick A. 1970. Psychiatric aspects of diabetes. In *Diabetes Mellitus: Theory and Practice*, ed. M Ellenberg, H Rifkin, pp. 920–33. New York: McGraw-Hill

Kulik JA, Mahler HIM. 1993. Emotional support as a moderator of adjustment and compliance after coronary artery bypass surgery: a longitudinal study. *J. Behav. Med.* 16:45–64

Lewinsohn PM, Hoberman HM, Rosenbaum M. 1988. A prospective study of risk factors for unipolar depression. *J. Abnorm. Psychol.* 97:251–64

Lief A. 1948. *The Commonsense Psychiatry of Dr. Adolf Meyer*. New York: McGraw-Hill

Lloyd C. 1980. Life events and depressive disorders reviewed. II. Events as precipitating factors. *Arch. Gen. Psychiatry* 37:541–48

Mann AH, Jenkins R, Belsey E. 1981. The twelve-month outcome of patients with neurotic illness in general practice. *Psychol. Med.* 11:535–50

Mazure C, ed. 1995. *Does Stress Cause Psychiatric Illness?* Washington, DC: Am. Psychiatr. Press

McGonagle KA, Kessler RC. 1990. Chronic stress, acute stress, and depressive symptoms. *Am. J. Community Psychol.* 18:681–705

McLeod JD. 1991. Childhood parental loss and adult depression. *J. Health Soc. Behav.* 35: 205–20

McLeod JD, Kessler RC, Landis KR. 1992. Speed of recovery from major depressive episodes in a community sample of married men and women. *J. Abnorm. Psychol.* 101: 277–86

McQuaid J, Monroe SM, Roberts JR, Johnson SL, Garamoni GL, et al. 1992. Toward the standardization of life stress assessment: definitional discrepancies and inconsistencies in method. *Stress Med.* 8:47–56

Miller P, Salter DP. 1984. Is there a short-cut? An investigation into the life event interview. *Acta Psychiatr. Scand.* 70:417–27

Mirowsky J, Ross C. 1989. *Social Causes of Psychological Distress*. New York: Aldine de Gruyter

Monroe SM, Kupfer DJ, Frank E. 1992. Life stress and treatment outcome of recurrent depression. I. Response during index episode. *J Consult. Clin. Psychol.* 60:718–24

Monroe SM, Steiner SC. 1986. Social support and psychopathology: interrelations with preexisting disorder, stress, and personality. *J. Abnorm. Psychol.* 95:29–39

Mrazek PB, Haggerty RJ. 1994. *Reducing Risks for Mental Disorders: Frontiers for Preventive Intervention Research*. Washington, DC: Natl. Acad. Press

Orbuch TL, Veroff J, Holmberg D. 1993. Becoming a married couple: the emergence of meaning in the first years of marriage. *J. Marriage Fam.* 55:815–26

Parker G, Bliguault I, Manicavasagar V. 1988. Neurotic depression: delineation of symptom profiles and their relation to outcome. *Br. J. Psychiatry* 152:15–23

Parker G, Hadzi-Pavlovic D. 1984. Modification of levels of depression in mother-bereaved women by parental and marital relationships. *Psychol. Med.* 14:125–35

Patrick V, Dunner D, Fieve R. 1978. Life events and primary affective illness. *Acta Psychiatr. Scand.* 58:48–55

Paykel E. 1979. Recent life events in the development of the depressive disorders. In *The Psychobiology of the Depressive Disorders: Implications for the Effects of Stress*, ed. R Depue, pp. 245–62. New York: Academic

Pearlin LI. 1989. The sociological study of stress. *J. Health Soc. Behav.* 30:241–56

Pless IB. 1994. *The Epidemiology of Childhood Disorders*. New York: Oxford Univ. Press

Post RM. 1992. Transduction of psychosocial stress into the neurobiology of recurrent affective disorder. *Am. J. Psychiatry* 149: 999–1010

Post RM, Rubinow DR, Ballenger JC. 1986. Conditioning and sensitisation in the longitudinal course of affective illness. *Br. J. Psychiatry* 149:191–201

Price RH, Van Ryn N, Vinokur A. 1992. Impact of a preventive job search intervention on the likelihood of depression among the unemployed. *J. Health Soc. Behav.* 33: 158–67

Quinton D, Rutter M, Liddle C. 1984. Institutional rearing, parenting, difficulties and marital support. *Psychol. Med.* 14:107–24

Raphael KG, Cloitre N, Dohrenwend BP. 1991. Problems with recall and misclassification with checklist methods of measuring stressful life events. *Health Psychol.* 10: 62–74

Robins LN, Regier DA. 1991. *Psychiatric Disorders in America: The Epidemiologic Catchment Area Study*. New York: Free Press

Rutter M. 1989. Pathways from childhood to adult life. *J. Child Psychol. Psychiatry* 30: 23–51

Sarason IG, Johnson JH, Siegel JM. 1978. Assessing the impact of life change: development of the Life Experiences Survey. *J. Consult. Clin. Psychol.* 46:32–46

Sargeant JK, Bruce ML, Florio LP, Weissman MM. 1990. Factors associated with 1-year outcome of major depression in the community. *Arch. Gen. Psychiatry* 47:519–26

Shrout PE, Link B, Dohrenwend B, Skodol AE. 1989. Characterizing life events as risk factors for depression: the role of fateful loss events. *J. Abnorm. Psychol.* 98:460–67

Sobel ME. 1990. Effect analysis of causation in linear structural equation models. *Psychometrika* 55:495–515

Sobell LG, Toneatto T, Sobell MB, Schuller R, Maxwell M. 1990. A procedure for reducing error in reports of life events. *J. Psychosom. Res.* 2:163–70

Sorenson SB, Rutter CM, Aneshensel CS. 1991. Depression in the community: an investigation into age of onset. *J. Consult. Clin. Psychol.* 59:541–46

Soumi SJ. 1991a. Adolescent depression and depressive symptoms: insights from longitudinal studies with rhesus monkeys. *J. Youth Adolesc.* 20:272–87

Soumi SJ. 1991b. Primate separation models of affective disorders. In *Neurobiology of Learning, Emotion and Affect*, ed. J Madden IV, pp. 195–214. New York: Raven

Stein JA, Golding JM, Siegel JM, Burnam MA, Sorenson SB. 1988. Long-term psychological sequelae of child sexual abuse: the Los Angeles Epidemiologic Catchment Areas Study. In *Lasting Effects of Child Sexual Abuse*, ed. GE Wyatt, GJ Powell, pp. 135–54. Newbury Park, CA: Sage

Stroebe MS, Stroebe W. 1983. Who suffers most? Sex differences in health risks of the widowed. *Psychol. Bull.* 93:279–301

Taylor SE, Aspinwall LG. 1996. Mediating and moderating processes in psychosocial stress: appraisal, coping, resistance, and vulnerability. In *Psychosocial Stress, Perspective on Structure, Theory, Life-Course, and Methods*, ed. H Kaplan, pp. 71–110. San Diego: Academic

Tennant C. 1988. Parental loss in childhood: its effect in adult life. *Arch. Gen. Psychiatry* 45:1045–50

Thoits PA. 1983. Dimensions of life events that influence psychological distress: an evaluation and synthesis of the literature. In *Psychosocial Stress: Trends in Theory and Research*, ed. HB Kaplan, pp. 33–103. New York: Academic

Tsaung MT, Farone SV. 1990. *The Genetics of Mood Disorders*. Baltimore: Johns Hopkins Univ. Press

Turner JB, Kessler RC, House JS. 1991. Factors facilitating adjustment to unemployment: implications for intervention. *Am. J. Community Psychol.* 19:521–42

Turner RJ, Wheaton B. 1995. Checklist Measurement of Stressful Life Events. See Cohen et al 1995, pp. 29–53

Umberson D, Wortman CB, Kessler RC. 1992. Widowhood and depression: explaining long-term gender differences in vulnerability. *J. Health Soc. Behav.* 33:10–24

Veroff J, Douvan E, Hatchett S. 1993. Marital interaction and marital quality in the first year of marriage. In *Advances in Personal Relationships*, ed. W Jones, D Pearlman, 4:103–37. Greenwich, CT: JAI

Von JM, Kilpatrick DG, Burgess AW, Hartman CR. 1991. Rape and sexual assault, In *Violence in America: A Public Health Approach*, ed. ML Rosenberg, MA Finley, pp. 95–122. New York: Oxford Univ. Press

Weissman MM, Leaf PJ, Tischler GL, Blazer DG, Karno M, et al. 1988. Affective disorders in five United States communities. *Psychol. Med.* 18:141–53

Weissman MM, Prusoff BA, Klerman GL. 1978. Personality and the prediction of long-term outcome of depression. *Am. J. Psychiatry* 135:797–800

West MO, Prinz RJ. 1987. Parental alcoholism and childhood psychopathology. *Psychol. Bull.* 102:204–18

Wethington E, Brown GW, Kessler RC. 1995. Interview measurement of stressful life events. See Cohen et al 1995, pp. 59–79

Williamson DE, Birmaher B, Anderson BP, Al-Shabbout M, Ryan ND. 1995. Stressful life events in depressed adolescents: the role of dependent events during the depressive episode. *J. Acad. Child Adolesc. Psychiatry* 34:591–98

Wolff HG, Wolf S, Hare CC. 1950. *Life Stress and Bodily Disease*. Baltimore: Williams & Wilkins

Yama MF, Tovey SL, Fogas BS. 1993. Childhood family environment and sexual abuse as predictors of anxiety and depression in adult women. *Am. J. Orthopsychiatry* 63: 136–41

Zautra AJ, Reich JW. 1983. Life events and perceptions of life quality: developments in a two-factor approach. *J. Community Psychol.* 1:121–32

Zimmerman M. 1983. Methodological issues in the assessment of life events: a review of issues and research. *Clin. Psychol. Rev.* 3: 339–70

Natural Course of Adolescent Major Depressive Disorder in a Community Sample: Predictors of Recurrence in Young Adults

Peter M. Lewinsohn, Ph.D.

Paul Rohde, Ph.D.

John R. Seeley, M.S.

Daniel N. Klein, Ph.D.

Ian H. Gotlib, Ph.D.

Objective: The primary purpose was to identify factors related to the recurrence of major depressive disorder during young adulthood (19–23 years of age) in a community sample of formerly depressed adolescents.

Method: A total of 274 participants with adolescent-onset major depressive disorder were assessed twice during adolescence and again after their 24th birthday. Lifetime psychiatric information was obtained from their first-degree relatives. Adolescent predictor variables included demographic characteristics, psychosocial variables, characteristics of adolescent major depressive disorder, comorbidity, family history of major depressive disorder and nonmood disorder, and antisocial and borderline personality disorder symptoms.

Results: Low levels of excessive emotional reliance, a single episode of major depressive disorder in adolescence, low proportion of family members with recurrent major depressive disorder, low levels of antisocial and borderline personality disorder symptoms, and a positive attributional style (males only) independently predicted which formerly depressed adolescents would remain free of future psychopathology. Female gender, multiple major depressive disorder episodes in adolescence, higher proportion of family members with recurrent major depressive disorder, elevated borderline personality disorder symptoms, and conflict with parents (females only) independently predicted recurrent major depressive disorder. Comorbid anxiety and substance use disorders in adolescence and elevated antisocial personality disorder symptoms independently distinguished adolescents who developed recurrent major depressive disorder comorbid with nonmood disorder from those who developed pure major depressive disorder.

Conclusions: Formerly depressed adolescents with the risk factors identified in this study are at elevated risk for recurrence of major depressive disorder during young adulthood and therefore warrant continued monitoring and preventive or prophylactic treatment.

(Am J Psychiatry 2000; 157:1584–1591)

It is now well documented that major depressive disorder is one of the most common mental disorders in adolescence (e.g., references 1–3). Given the high prevalence of major depressive disorder in adolescence, examining the natural course of episodes in this age group is clearly important. In a previous study (4), we found that individuals who had experienced an episode of major depressive disorder by age 19 were at significantly elevated risk for future major depressive disorder, compared to participants with adolescent-onset nonmood disorders and adolescents with no disorder. In these three groups, rates of major depressive disorder over the 5-year period from age 19 through 23 were 45.0%, 28.2%, and 18.5%, respectively. In addition, compared to no-disorder comparison subjects, formerly depressed adolescents had significantly higher rates of nonmood disorder in the follow-up period (33.2% versus 19.5%). The primary purpose of the study reported here was to identify the factors in formerly depressed adolescents that predict major depressive disorder recurrence in young adulthood.

To our knowledge, only six studies have examined predictors of recurrence of major depressive disorder in depressed children or adolescents. Five studies examined patient groups (5–9), and one examined the offspring (6–23 years of age) of adults treated for depression (10). The results of these studies are inconsistent, perhaps because of the generally small size of the study groups and the considerable variation in participants' ages, duration of the follow-up periods, treatment settings, and assessment methods.

The framework that guides our research is based on an integrative, multifactorial model (11), in which depression is conceptualized as the end result of environmentally initiated changes in behavior, affect, and cognitions. The model distinguishes between antecedents, which occur before the onset of the depression, and consequences, which are observable during and after an episode of depression and which may influence the risk of recurrence. Antecedents examined in the study reported here included having lived in a stressful environment during adolescence (e.g., a nonintact household, a high level of conflict with parents, stressful life events). The model also recognizes individual differences (vulnerabilities and protective factors) that increase or decrease the impact of the antecedent events and moderate the impact of the consequences of depression on recurrence. Vulnerabilities examined in this study included psychopathology among family members, female gender (which has often been shown to be a risk factor), elevated level of depression symptoms, depressotypic cognitions, and excessive emotional reliance. Protective factors included self-rated social competence and positive coping skills. The model, like most other current theories of the etiology of depression, does not distinguish between first onset and recurrent episodes of depression, even though the results of other studies (12–14) have suggested that these two types of episodes may be predicted by different variables.

Consistent with the expectation that having experienced an episode of depression creates vulnerabilities that effect recurrence, clinical aspects of the episode of major depressive disorder in adolescence (e.g., early onset, longer duration, recurrence during adolescence, greater severity, treatment utilization, and suicide attempts) were hypothesized to be associated with recurrence. Comorbid adolescent psychopathology was also hypothesized to be a vulnerability for recurrence. Last, traits measuring selected young adult personality disorders (i.e., antisocial and borderline personality disorders) were posited to reflect stable characteristics of the person that constitute vulnerabilities for recurrence.

This study focuses on individuals who experienced and recovered from an episode of major depressive disorder during adolescence, which we defined as before age 19. On the basis of their psychiatric outcome between age 19 and 23, individuals were assigned to four mutually exclusive groups: 1) those with no further disorder, 2) those with a recurrent episode of major depressive disorder but no comorbid mental disorder, 3) those with a recurrent episode of major depressive disorder that was accompanied by a nonmood disorder, and 4) those with no recurrence of major depressive disorder but who experienced a nonmood disorder.

This design allowed us to address three questions. First, what factors predict staying well (group 1 versus groups 2, 3, and 4). Second, what factors predict major depressive disorder recurrence (groups 1 and 4 versus groups 2 and 3). Third, what factors predict pure (i.e., noncomorbid) major depressive disorder versus major depressive disorder with a co-occurring nonmood disorder (group 2 versus group 3).

Method

Participants

Probands. Participants were a subset of individuals from the Oregon Adolescent Depression Project. Participants were originally randomly selected from nine senior high schools in western Oregon. A total of 1,709 adolescents (ages 14–18; mean age at initial assessment=16.6 years, SD=1.2) completed the initial assessment (time 1), which consisted of an interview and questionnaires, between 1987 and 1989. Approximately 1 year later (time 2), 1,507 participants (88.2%) participated in a reassessment that used the same interview questions and questionnaires (mean interval between time 1 and time 2=13.8 months, SD=2.3) (additional details are provided elsewhere [2]).

As probands from the Oregon Adolescent Depression Project reached their 24th birthday, participants with a history of major depressive disorder at time 2 (N=360), those with a history of nonmood disorder at time 2 (N=284), and a subset of those with no history of mental disorder at time 2 (N=457) were invited to participate in a time 3 interview. The no-disorder comparison group was representative of the entire group of participants with no mental disorder at time 2 (N=863) in age and gender within age; all participants with nonwhite ethnicity were invited to participate in the time 3 assessment.

Of the 1,101 young adults selected for time 3 interview, 940 participated (85.4%). Of those participants, 57.2% were female, 89.0% were white, 34.1% were married, 96.8% had graduated from high school, and 31.4% had a bachelor's degree or a higher educational level. Their average age at time 3 was 24.2 years (SD=0.6). Women were more likely than men to complete the time 3 assessments (88.9% versus 81.0%) (χ^2=13.55, df=1, N=1,101, p<0.001). Differences in time 3 participation as a function of other demographic characteristics or time 2 diagnostic status were nonsignificant.

A total of 315 time 3 participants had experienced an episode of major depressive disorder before age 19. Forty-one of these participants were deselected to better clarify the predictors of major depressive disorder recurrence between age 19–23: 22 were experiencing the major depressive disorder episode at the time of their 19th birthday, three met criteria for bipolar disorder after age 19, three met criteria for dysthymia but not major depressive disorder after age 19, and 13 met criteria for adjustment disorder with depressed mood but not for major depressive disorder after age 19. Thus, the reference group for the present study consisted of 274 participants who had experienced and recovered from an episode of major depressive disorder by age 19.

Family members. Lifetime psychiatric information was obtained from the first-degree relatives over the age of 13 (biological parents, full siblings) of the Oregon Adolescent Depression Project participants in the time 3 assessment. To supplement the direct interviews, informant psychiatric data were collected from probands or another first-degree relative. Our goal was to collect diagnostic data from two sources for each family member. Diagnostic information was available for the relatives of 234 of the 274 probands with a history of major depressive disorder during adolescence (85.4%). Of the 761 first-degree relatives for whom diagnostic information was collected, direct interviews were obtained for 442 (58.1%); data for 145 (19.1%) of the family members were based on a single source.

After a thorough description of the study, written informed consent was obtained from Oregon Adolescent Depression Project probands (and their guardians, if applicable) and from the family members.

Diagnostic Interviews

Oregon Adolescent Depression Project probands. Participants were interviewed at time 1 with a version of the Schedule for Affective Disorders and Schizophrenia for School-Age Children (K-SADS) that combined features of the epidemiologic version (15) and the present episode version and included additional items to derive DSM-III-R diagnoses. At time 2 and time 3, participants were interviewed with the Longitudinal Interval Follow-Up Evaluation (16), which elicited detailed information about the course of psychiatric symptoms and disorders since the previous interview. Time 3 interviews were conducted by telephone, and time 3 diagnoses were made by using DSM-IV criteria.

Most diagnostic interviewers had an advanced degree in clinical or counseling psychology or social work, and all were extensively trained before data collection. Interrater reliability for lifetime diagnoses in a randomly selected subsample at time 1 (N=233) was moderate to excellent: kappa=0.86 for major depressive disorder, and kappa=0.76–0.89 for nonmood disorder categories. For a randomly selected subsample at time 3 (N=178), interrater reliability was excellent for the primary categories of major depressive disorder (kappa=0.87) and nonmood disorder (kappa=0.82).

Family members. Parents and siblings were interviewed with either the Structured Clinical Interview for DSM-III-R, Nonpatient Version (SCID-NP) (17) or the K-SADS employed in the time 1 proband assessment, modified for collection of DSM-IV criteria. Family history data were collected by using the revised Family Informant Schedule and Criteria (18), which is based on the Family History Research Diagnostic Criteria (19), modified for DSM-IV criteria. Using all available data, the project's four senior diagnosticians (P.R., D.N.K., P.M.L., and Nicholas Allen), who were blind to proband diagnoses, derived best-estimate diagnoses (20) for relatives.

Outcome Variable: Psychopathology in Early Adulthood

The primary outcome variable used in this study was the development of another episode of major depressive disorder during early adulthood. The 274 formerly depressed participants were categorized into four groups: 1) no disorder, consisting of 87 participants (31.8%) who experienced neither major depressive disorder nor a nonmood disorder from age 19 through 23; 2) major depressive disorder, consisting of 58 participants (21.2%) who had a recurrence of major depressive disorder by age 24 but no nonmood disorder during the 19–23 age period; 3) major depressive disorder plus nonmood disorder, consisting of 67 participants (24.5%) who had a recurrence of major depressive disorder and experienced a nonmood disorder during the 19–23 age period; and 4) nonmood disorder, consisting of 62 participants (22.6%) who experienced a nonmood disorder but did not have a recurrence of major depressive disorder during the 19–23 age period. Of the 129 participants with a nonmood disorder during the 19–23 age period, 99 (76.7%) had a diagnosis of substance use disorder, 44 (34.1%) anxiety disorder, three (2.3%) oppositional defiant disorder, three (2.3%) conduct disorder, two (1.6%) eating disorder, one (0.8%) schizophreniform disorder, and one (0.8%) somatoform disorder. The majority of these nonmood disorder episodes (58.1%) were new disorders that began after age 19 (i.e., did not represent the continuation of a nonmood disorder that began before age 19 and persisted into the 19–23 age period). Twenty-two of the 274 participants (8.0%) were experiencing a current major depressive disorder episode at the time 1 assessment; differences in diagnostic outcome as a function of time 1 current major depressive disorder status were nonsignificant (χ^2=3.39, df=3, N=274, n.s.).

Predictor Variables

Demographic characteristics. Four dichotomous time 1 variables were included: 1) gender; 2) family intactness (living with versus not living with both biological parents); 3) highest parental education within the household (bachelor's degree versus less than a bachelor's degree), which was included as a proxy measure of socioeconomic status; and 4) ethnicity (white or nonwhite).

Psychosocial variables. An extensive battery of psychosocial measures was administered at time 1 to all participants. All measures had been previously shown to possess very good psychometric properties (21, 22)). Variables were standardized and scored such that higher values reflected more problematic functioning.

Current depression was assessed by using the 20-item National Institute of Mental Health Center for Epidemiologic Studies Depression Scale (CES-D Scale) (23) (alpha=0.89; time 1–time 2 r=0.61) (df=1505, p<0.001 for all correlations). Negative cognitions were assessed with 27 items on self-reinforcement, likelihood of future positive events, dysfunctional attitudes, and perceived control over one's life (alpha=0.81; time 1–time 2 r=0.61). Attributional style was assessed with the 48-item Kastan Attributional Style Questionnaire for Children (N. Kaslow, R.L. Tanenbaum, M.E.P. Seligman, unpublished 1978 questionnaire) (alpha=0.63; time 1–time 2 r=0.55). Self-esteem was assessed with nine items on physical appearance and general self-esteem (alpha=0.81; time 1–time 2 r=0.62). Excessive emotional reliance was assessed with 10 items on the extent to which the individual desires excessive support and approval from others and is interpersonally sensitive (alpha=0.83; time 1–time 2 r=0.54). Self-rated social competence was assessed with 12 items (alpha=0.85; time 1–time 2 r=0.64). Coping skills were assessed with 17 items (alpha=0.76, time 1–time 2 r=0.55). Social support from friends was assessed with 13 items (alpha=0.81, time 1–time 2 r=0.60). Social support from family was assessed with 22 items (alpha=0.86, time 1–time 2 r=0.64). Conflict with parents was assessed with the 45-item Issues Checklist scale (24) (alpha=0.81; time 1–time 2 r=0.51). Daily hassles were assessed with 20 items from the Unpleasant Events Schedule (25) (alpha=0.79; time 1–time 2 r=0.55). Major life events were assessed by using questions about 11 negative life events involving self or significant other (parent, sibling, other relative, close friend) during the past year (alpha=0.78; time 1–time 2 r=0.52). Academic problems were assessed with nine items from the questionnaire and the time 1 K-SADS interview (e.g., lifetime occurrence of school expulsion or suspension, truancy, repeating a grade in school, most recent grade point average). Physical illness at time 1 was assessed by using 90 items on physical symptoms, number of sick days, and physician visits during the past year. Cigarette use was assessed in the time 1 K-SADS interview with a question about whether the participant had been a daily cigarette smoker.

Adolescent major depressive disorder. The following six characteristics of adolescent major depressive disorder were included in the analysis: 1) age at onset of first major depressive disorder episode before age 13 years (N=47 of 274, 17.2%) versus at age 13 or older, 2) duration of the first major depressive disorder episode of 2–8 weeks (N=136 of 274, 49.6%) versus 9 or more weeks, 3) single major depressive disorder episode before age 19 (N=207 of 274, N=75.5%) versus two or more episodes, 4) severity of the worst episode indicated by the presence of five to seven DSM-IV symptoms (N=175 of 274, 63.9%) versus eight or nine symptoms, 5) treatment utilization (outpatient or inpatient treatment or medications) for major depressive disorder during adolescence (N=58 of 274, 21.2%) versus no treatment, and 6) history of a suicide attempt during adolescence (N=62 of 274, 22.6%) versus no attempt.

Psychiatric comorbidity during adolescence. Four categories of comorbid psychiatric disorders occurring before age 19 were examined: 1) dysthymia (N=20 of 274, 7.3%), 2) anxiety disorders (N=74 of 274, 27.0%), 3) substance use disorder (N=80 of 274, 29.2%), and 4) conduct disorder/oppositional defiant disorder (N=35 of 274, 12.7%). For the 143 participants with nonmood comorbidity during adolescence, the major depressive disorder episode was categorized as either primary (N=42, 29.4%) or secondary (N=101, 70.6%) on the basis of the age at onset of the two disorders; primary major depressive disorder could not be determined for eight participants due to simultaneous onset with the nonmood disorder.

Family history of psychopathology. Three variables were included as indications of the degree of psychopathology in the family: 1) the proportion of first-degree relatives (parents and siblings) with major depressive disorder, 2) the proportion of relatives with recurrent major depressive disorder, and 3) the proportion of relatives with nonmood disorder.

Personality disorders. The two most frequent and relevant DSM-IV personality disorders (antisocial and borderline) were assessed by using relevant portions of the Personality Disorder Examination (26). Personality Disorder Examination dimensional scores (i.e., summation of partial and full symptom criteria) were used in the analyses. The interrater reliability of the Personality Disorder Examination dimensional scores was excellent (intraclass correlation coefficients>0.80).

Statistical Analyses

To address the three primary questions posed in this study (What are the predictors of staying well, of major depressive disorder recurrence, and of pure depression?), three multiple logistic regression analyses were conducted with each potential predictor variable. The first multiple logistic regression analysis compared the no-disorder control group to the remaining three outcome groups (i.e., major depressive disorder, major depressive disorder plus nonmood disorder, and nonmood disorder). The second multiple logistic regression analysis identified the predictors of major depressive disorder recurrence by comparing participants who experienced major depressive disorder (i.e., the groups with major depressive disorder and with major depressive disorder plus nonmood disorder) with those who did not (i.e., the groups with no disorder and with nonmood disorder). The third multiple logistic regression analysis compared predictors of pure major depressive disorder versus comorbid major depressive disorder plus nonmood disorder. To test for possible moderating effects of gender, gender was entered in the model in a second block within each multiple logistic regression analysis, and the predictor-by-gender interaction term was entered in the third block. By using variables that emerged as significant univariate predictors of the specific contrast, three summary multiple logistic regression models with the likelihood ratio backward selection procedure were conducted to identify unique predictors (i.e., variables that remained significant when controlling for other variables in the model).

The strength of the associations is illustrated by the odds ratio with 95% confidence interval (CI). For the examined contrasts and for interactions with gender, with alpha set to 0.05, statistical power was sufficient (>0.80) to detect medium effect sizes or larger (Cohen's w>0.30). Although numerous tests were performed, thereby inflating the type I error rate, statistical significance was based on $p<0.05$ to identify predictors of potential clinical relevance.

Results

Univariate Predictors

Adolescent predictor variables with one or more significant contrasts are shown in Table 1. The first four columns of Table 1 illustrate the percentage or mean value of the variable in the four diagnostic outcome groups. The last six columns of Table 1 present odds ratios and CIs for the three contrasts.

Gender interactions. Two variables interacted significantly with gender. Although nonsignificant as a main effect, attributional style had a significant interaction with gender in the first contrast, predicting staying well (χ^2=4.83, df=1, N=274, $p<0.05$). When the results were examined separately by gender, positive attributional style predicted no-disorder status between age 19 and 23 for male participants (odds ratio=2.21, 95% CI=1.20–4.09) but not female participants (odds ratio=1.06, 95% CI=0.79–1.42). In the second contrast, conflict with parents had a significant gender interaction in predicting recurrent major depressive disorder (χ^2=5.47, df=1, N=274, $p<0.05$), having a significant effect for female participants (odds ratio=1.38, 95% CI=1.01–1.87) but not for male participants (odds ratio=0.71, 95% CI=0.43–1.16).

Multivariate Predictors

To examine whether the variables distinguishing the outcome groups remained significant when controlling for the effects of the other variables, summary multiple logistic regression analyses using the likelihood ratio backward selection procedure were conducted for each of the three contrasts. The variables with unique and independent main effects retained in the final model for each contrast are indicated in Table 1.

Of the variables predicting which formerly depressed adolescents remained free of future psychopathology, low levels of excessive emotional reliance, a single (as opposed to multiple) major depressive disorder episode in adolescence, a low proportion of family members with recurrent major depressive disorder, low rates of antisocial and borderline personality disorder symptoms, and the interaction of attributional style and gender were retained in the first contrast. The solution correctly classified 78.0% of the participants (sensitivity=77.4%).

In the second contrast, female gender, multiple major depressive disorder episodes in adolescence, a higher proportion of family members with recurrent major depressive disorder, elevated rates of borderline personality disorder symptoms, and the interaction of conflict with parents and gender were retained as predictive of recurrent major depressive disorder in young adulthood. The solution correctly classified 72.0% of participants (sensitivity=72.6%). Although female gender was retained as an independent predictor of recurrent major depressive disorder, examining the gender composition of the four outcome groups indicated that gender differences between no-disorder, major depressive disorder, and major depressive disorder plus nonmood disorder groups were not statistically significant, suggesting that formerly depressed young men made up a significantly higher proportion of the pure nonmood disorder group.

In the third contrast, comorbid anxiety disorder and substance use disorder in adolescence and elevated levels of

TABLE 1. Characteristics of Subjects With a History of Major Depressive Disorder in Adolescence by Diagnostic Outcome at Age 19–23 Years and Comparisons of Diagnostic Outcome Groups

	Diagnostic Outcome at Age 19–23 Years				Planned Contrasts					
					Group 1 Versus Groups 2–4		Groups 1 and 4 Versus Groups 2 and 3		Group 2 Versus Group 3	
Characteristic in Adolescence	1. No Disorder (N=87)	2. Major Depressive Disorder (N=58)	3. Major Depressive Disorder Plus Nonmood Disorder (N=67)	4. Nonmood Disorder (N=62)	Odds Ratio	95% CI	Odds Ratio	95% CI	Odds Ratio	95% CI
Female gender (%)	71.3	86.2	73.1	50.0	0.92	0.53–1.61	2.29*[a]	1.33–3.95	0.44	0.17–1.09
Psychosocial variables[b]										
Emotional reliance (mean z score)	–0.21	0.01	0.27	0.00	1.38*[a]	1.06–1.79	1.31*	1.03–1.67	1.29	0.91–1.84
Conflict with parents (mean z score)	–0.21	0.05	0.10	0.14	1.38*	1.05–1.81	1.15	0.91–1.47	1.07	0.73–1.56
Daily hassles (mean z score)	–0.19	0.12	0.11	0.03	1.34*	1.02–1.75	1.24	0.97–1.57	0.98	0.70–1.39
Academic problems (mean z score)	–0.20	–0.31	0.23	0.33	1.36*	1.04–1.77	0.96	0.75–1.22	1.80*	1.21–2.67
Cigarette use (%)	23.0	19.0	43.3	33.9	1.62	0.90–2.91	1.24	0.74–2.09	3.26*	1.44–7.37
Characteristics of depressive episodes										
Duration of first episode ≥9 weeks (%)	40.2	58.6	55.4	50.8	1.81*	1.08–3.03	1.64*	1.01–2.66	0.88	0.43–1.79
≥2 episodes (%)	11.5	36.2	27.7	24.6	3.20*[a]	1.54–6.65	2.30*[a]	1.29–4.05	0.67	0.31–1.45
Severity of worst episode consisted of eight or nine symptoms of DSM-III-R major depressive disorder (%)	23.0	44.8	38.5	40.0	2.33*	1.30–4.15	1.65	1.00–2.74	0.77	0.37–1.58
Suicide attempt (%)	14.9	20.7	31.3	25.8	2.02*	1.03–3.96	1.48	0.84–2.62	1.75	0.77–3.97
Comorbidity										
Anxiety disorder (%)	21.8	13.8	40.3	32.3	1.49	0.82–2.71	1.09	0.64–1.87	4.22*[a]	1.73–10.29
Substance use disorder (%)	14.9	10.3	49.3	45.2	3.18*	1.64–6.15	1.19	0.71–2.01	8.41*[a]	3.18–22.22
Conduct disorder/ oppositional defiant disorder (%)	6.9	5.2	20.9	19.4	2.48	0.99–6.21	1.15	0.56–2.33	4.84*	1.32–17.82
Primary major depressive disorder in subjects with nonmood comorbidity (%)	28.6	45.5	18.0	34.9	0.95	0.38–2.37	1.34	0.65–2.75	3.80*	1.26–11.48
Family history of psychopathology (mean proportion of first-degree relatives with disorder)										
Major depressive disorder	0.27	0.33	0.44	0.28	2.65*	1.02–6.92	3.59*	1.50–8.63	2.90	0.87–9.66
Recurrent major depressive disorder	0.11	0.23	0.27	0.14	7.42*[a]	1.89–29.11	9.46*[a]	2.92–30.61	1.64	0.43–6.25
Nonmood disorder	0.45	0.46	0.59	0.51	2.00	0.85–4.69	1.70	0.77–3.75	3.77*	1.13–12.55
Axis II psychopathology[c]										
Borderline (mean score out of a possible 18)	0.20	0.98	2.25	0.70	2.73*[a]	1.73–4.31	1.80*[a]	1.42–2.28	1.34*	1.09–1.65
Antisocial (mean score out of a possible 44)	0.87	1.00	4.11	3.89	1.41*[a]	1.20–1.67	1.04	0.97–1.11	1.51*[a]	1.22–1.86

[a] Variable was a unique and independent predictor in the summary multiple logistic regression.
[b] Measured with an extensive battery of psychosocial measures (21, 22).
[c] Measured with the relevant sections of the Personality Disorder Examination (27).
*$p<0.05$.

borderline personality disorder symptoms were retained as unique measures distinguishing adolescents who developed recurrent major depressive disorder comorbid with nonmood disorder from those who developed pure major depressive disorder in early adulthood. The solution correctly classified 77.2% of participants (sensitivity=80.0%).

Discussion

Formerly depressed adolescents who developed psychiatric problems during young adulthood were characterized during adolescence by more severe depressive episodes (e.g., longer episode duration, multiple episodes, greater number of symptoms, history of suicide attempts); by elevated stress, conflict, and interpersonal dependency; and, for males only, by a negative attributional style. These individuals also had an elevated rate of substance use disorder during adolescence, and, as young adults, they showed traits associated with borderline and antisocial personality disorder. In addition, their parents and siblings were more likely to have experienced both single-episode and recurrent major depressive disorder. Variables that independently contributed to the prediction of psychopathology in young adulthood included emotional reliance, multiple depressive episodes, a family history of recurrent major depressive disorder, borderline and antisocial personality disorder symptoms, and attributional style (for males). Excessive emotional reliance is a component of the broader construct of interpersonal dependency (27), which has been implicated theoretically in the etiology of depression, especially in the psychoanalytic literature (e.g., references 28, 29). We previously reported that excessive emotional reliance predicted depression onset in adolescents (22) and that emotional reliance remained elevated after major depressive disorder recovery (30). The results reported here indicate that emotional reliance is also predictive of the recurrence of psychopathology, particularly of major depressive disorder, underscoring both the centrality of emotional reliance to depression theory and its potential explanatory breadth to other disorders.

Variables that specifically predicted major depressive disorder recurrence included multiple depressive episodes in adolescence, a family history of recurrent major depressive disorder, borderline personality disorder symptoms, and, for females only, increased conflict with parents. Gender was retained in the multivariate solution, but this finding appeared to be due to the greater likelihood that formerly depressed male adolescents would develop pure nonmood disorders in young adulthood. These findings suggest that clinical characteristics, both of the proband and of the first-degree relatives, are among the strongest predictors of major depressive disorder recurrence.

There was no evidence that adolescent comorbidity acted as a risk factor for pure major depressive disorder in young adulthood. The presence of nonmood disorders in adolescence predicted nonmood disorders in young adulthood, generally comorbid with recurrent major depressive disorder. Contrary to previous research (e.g., references 7, 10), comorbid dysthymia in the present study failed to predict major depressive disorder recurrence. Unlike previous research on the impact of double depression (i.e., major depressive disorder superimposed on a preexisting dysthymia), adolescent major depressive disorder and dysthymia in the present study occurred largely at different periods. Additional research is needed to disentangle whether concurrent comorbidity of major depressive disorder and dysthymia specifically confers a risk for major depressive disorder recurrence.

Familial psychopathology was a significant predictor in all three contrasts. Most significantly, the proportion of family members with recurrent major depressive disorder predicted major depressive disorder recurrence in the offspring, with and without a nonmood disorder. These findings are consistent with previous research indicating that the presence of major depressive disorder in family members significantly increases the likelihood of major depressive disorder recurrence in adults (e.g., references 31–34). The results reported here extend previous research by indicating that recurrent depression breeds true from parent to offspring.

Both elevated antisocial and borderline personality disorder symptoms were significant in multiple contrasts. Several adult studies have suggested strong comorbidity between depression and borderline personality disorder symptoms (e.g., references 35–38) and a small number of studies of adult patients have shown that axis II pathology, especially cluster B disorders (i.e., antisocial, borderline, narcissistic, histrionic), increases the likelihood of depression recurrence in treated adult patients (e.g., references 39–41). Our findings on axis II psychopathology need to be qualified in two respects. First, rates of personality disorders were low, so elevated dimensional scores were generally in the subthreshold range. Second, the data on axis II psychopathology were obtained at time 3. Therefore, the direction of these associations cannot be determined, although previous research supports the hypothesis that adolescent depression precedes the onset of personality disorder symptoms (42).

The majority of psychosocial variables assessed during adolescence were not found to predict recurrence of psychopathology, including negative cognitions, self-esteem, social skills, coping, life events, social support, and elevated depression symptoms (as measured by the CES-D Scale). The most plausible explanation for these nonsignificant findings is that their prognostic impact in previous studies was time limited. Thus, the extent to which a variable's predictive ability diminishes as a function of time needs to be explored in future research. A second explanation is that the assessment of these variables in the design of the study reported here may have occurred before, during, or after the adolescent major depressive disorder episode.

A depressotypic attributional style predicted future psychopathology in formerly depressed young men. There is a large literature, conducted primarily with adults, examining the role of depressotypic cognitions in predicting recurrence. The findings of these studies are mixed, with some investigations reporting significant results (e.g., reference 43) and others reporting nonsignificant effects (e.g., reference 41). Important issues that need to be addressed in future research concern whether depressotypic cognitions are measured at intake or at the end of treatment, whether results obtained with adults are replicated in samples of adolescents and children, and whether the cognitions specifically predict depression.

A number of limitations of the present study should be acknowledged. Given the absence of previous research in this area, a stringent correction for type I error was not applied, and the results need to be considered preliminary pending independent replication. Second, although a relatively large number of predictors were examined, some potentially important categories of predictors (e.g., biological measures, childhood physical and sexual abuse) were not represented. Third, although our sample was community based, which reduced a number of selection biases, the sample selection may also limit the applicability of our findings to clinical practice. Offsetting these limitations were several noteworthy strengths of this study, including the large sample size, prospective design, rigorous diagnostic interviews, and assessment of a broad array of predictors, including direct interview data on family history of psychopathology. Overall, the findings support arguments by Warner et al. (10), Ilardi et al. (41), and Goodyer et al. (44) that the predictors of depression onset, duration (persistence), and recurrence may differ in important ways.

The clinical implications of this study are straightforward. Clinicians are routinely faced with decisions about what to do with youngsters with a history of major depressive disorder. We previously demonstrated that all individuals with a history of major depressive disorder during adolescence are at very high risk for major depressive disorder recurrence and for other psychiatric disorders during young adulthood (4). In the study reported here, roughly one-fourth of formerly depressed adolescents experienced subsequent pure major depressive disorder, one-fourth experienced comorbid major depressive disorder, and one-fourth remained free from depression recurrence but experienced a nonmood disorder. Earlier and better identification of the most salient risk factors is the first step in avoiding a protracted course of disorder. Depressed female adolescents (especially those who experience high conflict with parents), adolescents with multiple major depressive disorder episodes, and adolescents with a family history of recurrent depression are at particularly high risk for depression recurrence and should be closely monitored or receive continued prophylactic treatment. The association between recurrent depression and borderline personality disorder features indicates that individuals with recurrent depression may warrant additional treatment focused on emerging axis II psychopathology.

Received June 14, 1999; revisions received Jan. 27 and Apr. 28, 2000; accepted May 12, 2000. From the Oregon Research Institute; the Department of Psychology, State University of New York, Stony Brook; and the Department of Psychology, Stanford University, Stanford, Calif. Address reprint requests to Dr. Lewinsohn, Oregon Research Institute, 1715 Franklin Blvd., Eugene, OR 97403-1983.

This research was supported in part by NIMH grants MH-40501, MH-50522, and MH-52858.

References

1. Fleming JE, Offord DR: Epidemiology of childhood depressive disorders: a critical review. J Am Acad Child Adolesc Psychiatry 1990; 29:571–580
2. Lewinsohn PM, Hops H, Roberts RE, Seeley JR, Andrews JA: Adolescent psychopathology, I: prevalence and incidence of depression and other DSM-III-R disorders in high school students. J Abnorm Psychol 1993; 102:133–144
3. Reinherz HZ, Giaconia RM, Lefkowitz ES, Pakiz B, Frost AK: Prevalence of psychiatric disorders in a community population of older adolescents. J Am Acad Child Adolesc Psychiatry 1993; 32:369–377
4. Lewinsohn PM, Rohde P, Klein DN, Seeley JR: Natural course of adolescent major depressive disorder, I: continuity into young adulthood. J Am Acad Child Adolesc Psychiatry 1999; 38:56–63
5. Emslie GJ, Rush AJ, Weinberg WA, Gullion CM, Rintelmann J, Hughes CW: Recurrence of major depressive disorder in hospitalized children and adolescents. J Am Acad Child Adolesc Psychiatry 1997; 36:785–792
6. Harrington RC, Fudge H, Rutter M, Pickles A, Hill J: Adult outcomes of childhood and adolescent depression, I: psychiatric status. Arch Gen Psychiatry 1990; 47:465–473
7. Kovacs M, Feinberg TL, Crouse-Novack MA, Paulauskas SL, Finkelstein R: Depressive disorders in childhood, I: a longitudinal prospective study of characteristics and recovery. Arch Gen Psychiatry 1984; 41:229–237
8. McCauley E, Myers K, Mitchell J, Calderon R, Schloredt K, Trader R: Depression in young people: initial presentation and clinical course. J Am Acad Child Adolesc Psychiatry 1993; 32:714–722
9. Rao U, Ryan ND, Birmaher B, Dahl RE, Williamson DE, Kaufman J, Rao R, Nelson B: Unipolar depression in adolescents: clinical outcome in adulthood. J Am Acad Child Psychiatry 1995; 34:566–578
10. Warner V, Weissman MM, Fendrich M, Wickramaratne P, Moreau D: The course of major depression in the offspring of depressed parents: incidence, recurrence, and recovery. Arch Gen Psychiatry 1992; 49:795–801
11. Lewinsohn PM, Hoberman H, Teri L, Hautzinger M: An integrative theory of depression, in Theoretical Issues in Behavior Therapy. Edited by Reiss S, Basin R. San Diego, Academic Press, 1985, pp 331–359
12. Post RM, Weiss SB, Leverich GS: Recurrent affective disorder: roots in developmental neurobiology and illness progression based on changes in gene expression. Dev Psychopathol 1994; 6:781–813
13. Monroe SM, Rohde P, Seeley JR, Lewinsohn PM: Life events and depression in adolescence: relationship loss as a prospective risk factor for first onset of major depressive disorder. J Abnorm Psychol 1999; 108:606–614
14. Lewinsohn PM, Allen NB, Seeley JR, Gotlib IH: First onset versus recurrence of depression: differential processes of psychosocial risk. J Abnorm Psychol 1999; 108:483–489
15. Orvaschel H, Puig-Antich J, Chambers WJ, Tabrizi MA, Johnson R: Retrospective assessment of prepubertal major depression with the Kiddie-SADS-E. J Am Acad Child Psychiatry 1982; 21:392–397

16. Keller MB, Lavori PW, Friedman B, Nielsen E, Endicott J, McDonald-Scott P, Andreasen NC: The Longitudinal Interval Follow-Up Evaluation: a comprehensive method for assessing outcome in prospective longitudinal studies. Arch Gen Psychiatry 1987; 44:540–548
17. Spitzer RL, Williams JBW, Gibbon M, First MB: The Structured Clinical Interview for DSM-III-R (SCID), I: history, rationale, and description. Arch Gen Psychiatry 1992; 49:624–629
18. Mannuzza S, Fyer AJ: Family Informant Schedule and Criteria (FISC), July 1990 revision. New York, New York State Psychiatric Institute, Anxiety Disorders Clinic, 1990
19. Endicott J, Andreasen N, Spitzer RL: Family History Research Diagnostic Criteria, 3rd ed. New York, New York State Psychiatric Institute, Biometrics Research, 1978
20. Leckman JF, Sholomskas D, Thompson D, Belanger A, Weissman MM: Best estimate of lifetime psychiatric diagnosis: a methodological study. Arch Gen Psychiatry 1982; 39:879–883
21. Andrews JA, Lewinsohn PM, Hops H, Roberts RE: Psychometric properties of scales for the measurement of psychosocial variables associated with depression in adolescence. Psychol Rep 1993; 73:1019–1046
22. Lewinsohn PM, Roberts RE, Seeley JR, Rohde P, Gotlib IH, Hops H: Adolescent psychopathology, II: psychosocial risk factors for depression. J Abnorm Psychol 1994; 103:302–315
23. Radloff LS: The CES-D Scale: a self-report depression scale for research in the general population. J Applied Psychol Measurement 1977; 1:385–401
24. Robin AL, Weiss JG: Criterion-related validity of behavioral and self-report measures of problem-solving communication skills in distressed and nondistressed parent-adolescent dyads. Behavioral Assessment 1980; 2:339–352
25. Lewinsohn PM, Mermelstein RM, Alexander C, MacPhillamy DJ: The Unpleasant Events Schedule: a scale for the measurement of aversive events. J Clin Psychol 1985; 41:483–498
26. Loranger AW, Susman VL, Oldham JM, Russakoff M: The Personality Disorder Examination (PDE) Manual. Yonkers, NY, DV Communications, 1988
27. Hirschfeld RMA, Klerman GL, Lavori P, Keller MB, Griffith P, Coryell W: Premorbid personality assessments of first onset of major depression. Arch Gen Psychiatry 1989; 46:345–350
28. Blatt S, Quinlan D, Chevron E, McDonald C, Zuroff D: Dependency and self-criticism: psychological dimensions of depression. J Consult Clin Psychol 1982; 50:113–124
29. Hirschfeld RMA, Klerman GL, Chodoff P, Korchin S, Barrett J: Dependency–self-esteem–clinical depression. J Am Acad Psychoanal 1976; 4:373–388
30. Rohde P, Lewinsohn PM, Seeley JR: Are adolescents changed by an episode of major depression? J Am Acad Child Adolesc Psychiatry 1994; 33:1289–1298
31. Bland RC, Newman SC, Orn H: Recurrent and nonrecurrent depression: a family study. Arch Gen Psychiatry 1986; 43:1085–1089
32. Gonzales LR, Lewinsohn PM, Clarke GN: Longitudinal follow-up of unipolar depressives: an investigation of predictors of relapse. J Consult Clin Psychol 1985; 53:461–469
33. Merikangas KR, Wicki W, Angst J: Heterogeneity of depression: classification of depressive subtypes of longitudinal course. Br J Psychiatry 1994; 164:342–348
34. Weissman MM, Gammon GD, John K, Merikangas KR, Warner V, Prusoff BA, Sholomskas D: Children of depressed parents: increased psychopathology and early onset of major depression. Arch Gen Psychiatry 1987; 44:847–853
35. Farmer R, Nelson-Gray RO: Personality disorders and depression: hypothetical relations, empirical findings, and methodological considerations. Clin Psychol Rev 1990; 10:453–475
36. Akiskal HS, Hirschfeld RMA, Yerevanian BI: The relationship of personality to affective disorders. Arch Gen Psychiatry 1983; 40:801–810
37. Oldham JM, Skodol AE, Kellman HD, Hyler SE, Doidge N, Rosnick L, Gallagher PE: Comorbidity of axis I and axis II disorders. Am J Psychiatry 1995; 152:571–578
38. Skodol AE, Stout RL, McGlashan TH, Grilo CM, Gunderson JG, Shea MT, Morey LC, Zanarini MC, Dyck IR, Oldham JM: The co-occurrence of mood and personality disorders: a report from the Collaborative Longitudinal Personality Disorders Study (CLPS). Depress Anxiety 1999; 10:175–182
39. Peselow ED, Fieve RR, DiFiglia C: Personality traits and response to desipramine. J Affect Disord 1992; 24:209–216
40. Pfohl B, Coryell W, Zimmerman M, Stangl D: Prognostic validity of self-report and interview measures of personality disorder in depressed inpatients. J Clin Psychiatry 1987; 48:468–472
41. Ilardi SS, Craighead WE, Evans DD: Modeling relapse in unipolar depression: the effects of dysfunctional cognitions and personality disorders. J Consult Clin Psychol 1997; 65:381–391
42. Cohen P: Childhood risks for young adult symptoms of personality disorder: method and substance. Multivariate Behavioral Res 1996; 31:121–148
43. Simons AD, Murphy GE, Levine JL, Wetzel RD: Cognitive therapy and pharmacotherapy for depression: sustained improvement over one year. Arch Gen Psychiatry 1986; 43:43–48
44. Goodyer IM, Herbert J, Secher SM, Pearson J: Short-term outcome of major depression, I: comorbidity and severity at presentation as predictors of persistent disorder. J Am Acad Child Adolesc Psychiatry 1997; 36:179–187

Recurrence After Recovery From Major Depressive Disorder During 15 Years of Observational Follow-Up

Timothy I. Mueller, M.D., Andrew C. Leon, Ph.D., Martin B. Keller, M.D., David A. Solomon, M.D., Jean Endicott, Ph.D., William Coryell, M.D., Meredith Warshaw, M.S.S., M.A., and Jack D. Maser, Ph.D.

Objective: The recurrence of an affective disorder in people who initially recover from major depressive disorder was characterized by using the unique longitudinal prospective follow-up data from the National Institute of Mental Health Collaborative Program on the Psychobiology of Depression—Clinical Studies. **Method:** Up to 15 years of prospective follow-up data on the course of major depressive disorder were available for 380 subjects who recovered from an index episode of major depressive disorder and for 105 subjects who subsequently remained well for at least 5 years after recovery. Baseline demographic and clinical characteristics were examined as predictors of recurrence of an affective disorder. The authors also examined naturalistically applied antidepressant therapy. **Results:** A cumulative proportion of 85% (Kaplan-Meier estimate) of the 380 recovered subjects experienced a recurrence, as did 58% (Kaplan-Meier estimate) of those who remained well for at least 5 years. Female sex, a longer depressive episode before intake, more prior episodes, and never marrying were significant predictors of a recurrence. None of these or any other characteristic persisted as a predictor of recurrence in subjects who recovered and were subsequently well for at least 5 years. Subjects reported receiving low levels of antidepressant treatment during the index episode, which further decreased in amount and extent during the well interval. **Conclusions:** Few baseline demographic or clinical characteristics predict who will or will not experience a recurrence of an affective disorder after recovery from an index episode of major depressive disorder, even in persons with lengthy well intervals. Naturalistically applied levels of antidepressant treatment are well below those shown effective in maintenance pharmacotherapy studies.

(Am J Psychiatry 1999; 156:1000–1006)

"Single episodes are extremely rare if the period of observation is significantly extended."

—Angst et al. (1)

For the majority of people with major depressive disorder, recurrence after recovery is the rule. Although resolution of the signs and symptoms of depression is the major goal of treatment, the maintenance of that state of well-being is one of the current challenges for the mental health field. Both naturalistic and treatment studies of major depression have highlighted the high rate of recurrence after recovery (2–6). A greater number of prior episodes of major depression is the strongest baseline predictor of the duration of the well interval; the greater the number of prior episodes, the more rapid the recurrence (4–6). Other factors that predict a more rapid recurrence are secondary subtype of depression (6) and the persistence of subsyndromal symptoms (L.L. Judd et al., 1998 unpublished paper). The literature is inconsistent regarding the effect of age on recurrence risk. Lower age has been

Presented in part at the 149th annual meeting of the American Psychiatric Association, New York, May 4–9, 1996. Received June 12, 1998; revision received Oct. 21, 1998; accepted Nov. 17, 1998.
From the NIMH Collaborative Program on the Psychobiology of Depression—Clinical Studies; and the Department of Psychiatry and Human Behavior, Brown University School of Medicine. Address reprint requests to Dr. Mueller, Department of Psychiatry and Human Behavior, Brown University School of Medicine, c/o Butler Hospital, 345 Blackstone Blvd., Providence, RI 02906; Timothy_Mueller@brown.edu (e-mail).
This manuscript has been reviewed by the Publication Committee of the Collaborative Depression Study and has its endorsement.

The authors thank Rita Misek for manuscript preparation.

positively associated with greater risk in some studies of clinical samples (4, 7) and a nonclinical sample (8) and negatively associated with greater risk in other clinical samples (6).

The National Institute of Mental Health Collaborative Program on the Psychobiology of Depression—Clinical Studies is a prospective naturalistic study of a cohort of people who sought treatment for an affective disorder at one of five university medical centers between 1978 and 1981. This cohort has been followed since intake with attention to course and outcome of their mental disorders. We have reported (9) on the 10-year course of the index episode of major depressive disorder, focusing on the subjects who remained ill for 5 years of prospective follow-up. Over the 10 years of follow-up, 401 (93% by Kaplan-Meier estimate) out of 431 subjects eventually recovered. In the 35 subjects who were continuously ill for 5 years, 13 (38% by Kaplan-Meier estimate) subsequently recovered in the next 5 years.

The current report complements the description of 10 years of observation of the first cycle of major depressive disorder by describing the well interval following recovery from the intake episode, on the basis of 15 years of follow-up data, which have recently become available. In addition to the subjects who recovered at some point in the 15 years, we focus on the subgroup of subjects who recovered from the index episode of depression and subsequently remained well for at least 5 years. We chose 5 years to parallel the time frame used in the prior work (9). In this report we specifically address the following questions: 1) What proportion of subjects with major depressive disorder develop another episode of affective disorder? 2) Do subject age, number of prior episodes, and presence of secondary major depression persist as significant baseline predictors of recurrence? 3) What clinical or demographic features distinguish the group of subjects who recovered and then stayed well for at least 5 years after recovery? 4) Do subjects continue to experience recurrences after 5 years of recovery? and 5) What was the level of antidepressant treatment in the groups who stayed well for at least 5 years after recovery?

METHOD

Between the years 1978 and 1981, 955 patients who sought psychiatric treatment for a mood disorder at one of five U.S. medical centers (in Boston, Chicago, Iowa City, New York, and St. Louis) were entered into a prospective, naturalistic follow-up study. This report extends to 15 years of follow-up previous analyses on the 431 subjects with only major depressive disorder at intake who had no prior history of mania, hypomania, schizoaffective disorder, chronic intermittent depressive disorder, or minor depression of at least 2 years' duration at intake. After complete description of the study to the subjects, written informed consent was obtained. We have distinguished two nested groups. The first consists of the 380 subjects who recovered from the index episode at some time while still in active follow-up during the 15 years of observational follow-up. From them come the second group of 105, a subset who recovered from the index episode and subsequently remained well for at least 5 years.

Assessments

The details of the assessment procedures are described elsewhere (6, 9). Briefly, all subjects were assessed at intake with the Schedule for Affective Disorders and Schizophrenia (SADS) (10), and this information was used with medical records to make diagnoses according to the Research Diagnostic Criteria (RDC) (11). The subjects were interviewed every 6 months for the first 5 years and every year thereafter by means of the Longitudinal Interval Follow-Up Evaluation (12). This follow-up instrument measures the level of psychopathology for each RDC major affective disorder on a 6-point scale called the "psychiatric status rating" (9). A score of 1 denotes no symptoms of the disorders, and a score of 6 denotes fulfillment of the full diagnostic criteria with psychosis or severe impairment. For these 431 subjects with major depression, recovery was considered to begin with the first of 8 consecutive weeks of no or minimal symptoms (psychiatric status rating of 1 or 2). Until recovery occurred, a subject remained in an episode of major depressive disorder, with psychiatric status ratings of 1–6. The continuous string of psychiatric status ratings for major depressive disorder lasting up to 780 weeks was the source of data for the analyses of the course of illness.

Predictors of Course

We examined demographic and clinical characteristics determined at intake as predictors of the subsequent course of major depressive disorder. In addition, we used the extracted score on the Hamilton Depression Rating Scale (10) and the score on the Global Assessment Scale (GAS) from data collected at the 5-year point to reflect the "current" status for the subgroup of subjects who remained well for at least 5 years.

Treatment

Antidepressant treatment was coded weekly by using a 5-point composite antidepressant scale, which quantifies all antidepressant somatotherapy, including ECT and pharmacotherapy (9). A score of 0 means that no antidepressant somatic treatment was provided for that week. A score of 1 represents a daily dose of 1–99 mg of imipramine or its equivalent. A score of 2 represents a daily dose of 100–199 mg of imipramine or equivalent, 3 represents 200–299 mg of imipramine equivalent, and 4 represents 300 mg or more of imipramine equivalent. The study protocol did not influence the treatment provided by the patient's physician.

Statistical Methods

The outcome of interest in these analyses was recurrence of an affective disorder. The data were censored either by loss to follow-up or end of the assessment period. Survival analysis was used to analyze time until recurrence during the follow-up. The Kaplan-Meier product limit was used to estimate the cumulative probability of recurrence (13). Analyses were conducted for the entire group of 380 subjects with major depressive disorder at baseline who experienced a recovery and for the 105 subjects who subsequently remained well for at least 5 years after recovery from the index episode and for whom additional follow-up data were available.

For predictor analyses and to account for length of follow-up, clinical and demographic variables were entered into a Cox regression to evaluate the strength of their associations with recurrence after other variables in the model were controlled for. A two-tailed alpha of 0.05 was considered statistically significant. For analyses of treatment, the t test and Fisher's exact test were used. To account for multiple univariate tests, a two-tailed alpha of 0.01 was used to determine level of statistical significance.

RESULTS

The results are organized to reflect the two groups that are the focus of this study: the complete cohort who recovered within 15 years (N=380) and the subset

TABLE 1. Relation of Clinical and Demographic Features to Recurrence Over 15 Years for 380 Subjects Who Recovered From an Index Episode of Major Depressive Disorder

Characteristic	No Recurrence (N=101)		Recurrence (N=279)		Adjusted Odds Ratio	95% CI	Wald χ^2 (df=1)	p
	Mean	*SD*	*Mean*	*SD*				
Age at intake (years)	39.6	14.2	37.7	14.7	1.00	0.99–1.01	0.18	0.67
Duration of depressive episode before intake (weeks) (odds ratio calculated per year)	50	85	68	108	1.11	1.05–1.18	12.59	0.0004
Hamilton depression score before intake[a]	19.4	7.3	20.3	7.1	1.01	0.99–1.03	0.80	0.37
GAS score before intake[a]	42.3	10.8	40.4	11.0	1.00	0.99–1.01	0.00	0.97
	N	*%*	*N*	*%*				
Female gender	52	51	178	64	1.43	1.10–1.86	7.20	0.007
Number of episodes of major depressive disorder before intake					1.18	1.06–1.31	9.51	0.002
0	48	48	93	33				
1	26	26	64	23				
2	10	10	40	14				
≥3	17	17	82	29				
Primary major depressive disorder at intake	60	59	164	59	0.80	0.62–1.03	2.91	0.09
Psychotic subtype at intake	7	7	29	10	1.17	0.77–1.79	0.53	0.47
Marital status at intake								
Married	58	57	133	48	1.00			
Divorced, separated, or widowed	24	24	56	20	1.01	0.73–1.40	0.00	0.96
Never married	19	19	90	32	1.55	1.14–2.10	7.83	0.005

[a] Owing to missing data, N=95 and N=271, respectively.

FIGURE 1. Time to Recurrence of Affective Disorder for 380 Subjects Who Recovered From an Index Episode of Major Depressive Disorder

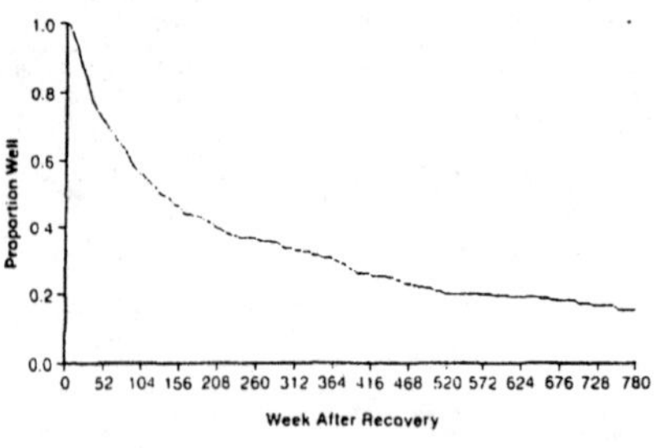

of this group who subsequently remained well for at least 5 years (N=105).

Complete Cohort

Of the 380 subjects in this study group, 279 were followed until a recurrence, 66 remained well and were followed until "lost to follow-up," and 35 remained well and were followed to the 15-year point. In the survival analyses that follow, these last two groups are classified as censored. Table 1 summarizes the demographic and clinical features for the group who recovered and did not have a recurrence (N=101) and for those who recovered and eventually did experience a recurrence (N=279); it also presents the results of a Cox regression model that examined each variable as a predictor of recurrence. Women were 43% more likely to experience a recurrence. Those who had never married were 55% more likely to experience a recurrence than those in the other two categories of marital status. Longer duration of depressive episode before intake was associated with a higher risk, such that each additional year was associated with an 11% greater likelihood of recurrence. Similarly, each additional episode of major depression before intake was associated with an 18% increase in the risk of recurrence.

Figure 1 presents the survival curve for the 380 subjects. Subjects began their well intervals at different calendar dates and thus have different lengths of follow-up, from 28 weeks to 15 full years (780 weeks total). The median time to recurrence (length of the well interval) was 132 weeks, and the cumulative proportion (Kaplan-Meier) of recurrence at 15 years was 85%. The mean time to recurrence in the total group of subjects (including censored subjects) was 145 weeks (SD=160). Some of the 279 subjects with major depressive disorder at intake who had a recurrence received a different diagnosis during the recurrence: nine (3%) developed schizoaffective disorder (depressed, manic, or mixed); 17 (6%) developed mania; and 36 (13%) developed hypomania. For 78% (N=217), however, the recurrence was major depressive disorder.

To assess the level of naturalistic somatic antidepressant treatment, we determined the proportion of weeks during the episode of illness that any such treatment was received, the mean scores on the composite antidepressant scale during those weeks of treatment, and the proportion of subjects who received no antidepressant treatment. During their in-

TABLE 2. Relation of Clinical and Demographic Features to Recurrence Over 15 Years for 105 Subjects Who Remained Well for at Least 5 Years After Recovery From an Index Episode of Major Depressive Disorder

Characteristic	No Recurrence (N=53)		Recurrence (N=52)		Adjusted Odds Ratio	95% CI	Wald χ^2 (df=1)	p
	Mean	*SD*	*Mean*	*SD*				
Age at intake (years)	39.5	12.8	38.5	15.8	1.01	0.98–1.03	0.40	0.52
Duration of depressive episode before intake (weeks) (odds ratio calculated per year)	56	103	42	50	0.97	0.73–1.29	0.05	0.82
Hamilton depression score before intake[a]	18.1	7.0	20.8	7.7	1.00	0.95–1.05	0.01	0.92
GAS score before intake	43.1	11.7	37.8	13.3	0.99	0.96–1.01	0.87	0.35
Hamilton depression score at 5 years[b]	4.1	3.8	4.8	3.9	1.08	0.97–1.19	1.96	0.16
GAS score at 5 years	77.0	9.7	72.7	11.8	0.99	0.96–1.03	0.11	0.74
	N	*%*	*N*	*%*				
Female gender	26	49	32	62	1.16	0.62–2.16	0.22	0.64
Number of episodes of major depressive disorder before intake					1.15	0.88–1.50	1.05	0.31
0	24	45	18	35				
1	13	25	11	21				
2	6	11	10	19				
≥3	10	19	13	25				
Primary major depressive disorder at intake	33	62	33	63	0.69	0.37–1.30	1.33	0.25
Marital status at intake								
Married	32	60	28	54	1.00			
Divorced, separated, or widowed	13	25	7	13	1.04	0.42–2.60	0.01	0.93
Never married	8	15	17	33	1.92	0.92–4.02	3.04	0.08

[a] Owing to missing data, N=51 and N=52, respectively.
[b] Owing to missing data, N=42 and N=49, respectively.

dex episode of major depressive disorder, the group with a recurrence (N=279) and the group without a recurrence (N=101) received antidepressant treatment for similar percentages of the weeks during follow-up (mean=68%, SD=36%, versus mean=70%, SD=40%, respectively) (t=0.40, df=378, p=0.69). These groups also received similar levels of antidepressant treatment, as represented by the score on the composite antidepressant scale (mean=1.70, SD=1.08, versus mean=1.64, SD=1.08) (t=–0.45, df=378, p=0.66). In addition, 11% of the group with a recurrence (30 of 279) versus 16% of the group with no recurrence (16 of 101) received no antidepressant treatment during the index episode of major depressive disorder (χ^2=1.81, df=1, p=0.18).

Subjects Who Remained Well for at Least 5 Years

In this subsample of 105 subjects, 52 were followed until a recurrence, 18 remained well and were followed until "lost to follow-up," and 35 remained well and were followed to the 15-year point. In the survival analyses that follow, these last two groups are classified as censored. Table 2 presents the demographic and clinical information for the 105 subjects who experienced a well interval of 5 years or longer and were followed for up to 10 additional years (15 years total). Many of these subjects remained well; however, 52 (58% Kaplan-Meier estimate) experienced a recurrence of an affective disorder during the subsequent prospective follow-up period. The subjects who did not experience a recurrence were followed for a mean of 676 weeks (SD=165), whereas those who did experience a recurrence were followed for 722 weeks (SD=116). Scores on the GAS and Hamilton depression scale at 5 years indicated a relatively high level of functioning and few depressive symptoms. The variables in table 2 were entered into a Cox regression model. None of these clinical or demographic variables predicted time to recurrence.

FIGURE 2. Time to Recurrence of Affective Disorder for 105 Subjects Who Remained Well for at Least 5 Years After Recovery From an Index Episode of Major Depressive Disorder

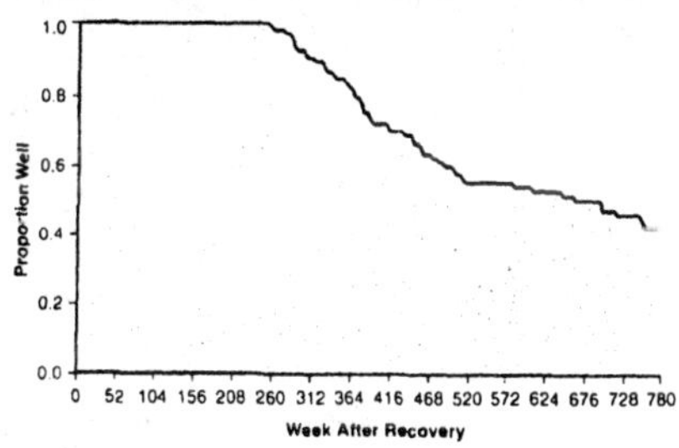

Figure 2 illustrates the survival curve for this subgroup of subjects. The median time to recurrence was 394 weeks, or 134 weeks beyond the requisite 260 weeks of recovery. Most of those who experienced a recurrence of an affective disorder after 5 years of wellness (N=52) developed only major depressive disorder (N=47, 90%). However, five (10%) developed hypomania; none developed schizoaffective disorder or mania. The pattern of recurrence of major affective disor-

TABLE 3. Relation of Recurrence Over 15 Years to Antidepressant Treatment Received During the Well Interval for 105 Subjects Who Remained Well for at Least 5 Years After Recovery From an Index Episode of Major Depressive Disorder

	No Recurrence (N=53)				Recurrence (N=52)				Analysis		
Period and Measure	N	%	Mean	SD	N	%	Mean	SD	t	df	p
Year 1 of well interval											
Subjects who received no antidepressant treatment	17	32			21	40					0.42[a]
Percentage of weeks in which antidepressant treatment was received	66	37					80	26	−1.68	65	0.10
Score on composite antidepressant scale for subjects receiving antidepressant treatment[b]			1.54	0.99			1.86	0.91	−1.39	65	0.17
Year 2 of well interval											
Subjects who received no antidepressant treatment	35	66			30	58					0.43[a]
Percentage of weeks in which antidepressant treatment was received	91	22					66	38	2.47	38	0.02
Score on composite antidepressant scale for subjects receiving antidepressant treatment[b]			1.99	0.95			1.37	1.10	1.89	38	0.07
Years 3–5 of well interval											
Subjects who received no antidepressant treatment	32	60			37	71					0.31[a]
Percentage of weeks in which antidepressant treatment was received	70	40					62	41	0.54	34	0.59
Score on composite antidepressant scale for subjects receiving antidepressant treatment[b]			1.49	1.09			1.34	0.95	0.43	34	0.67

[a] Fisher's exact test.
[b] A score of 1 represents 1–99 mg/day of imipramine or equivalent; 4 represents ≥300 mg/day of imipramine or equivalent.

der in this subgroup is similar to the overall pattern in the larger group of 279 subjects described earlier who recovered from the index episode and subsequently had a recurrence. Recurrence of major depressive disorder is the predominant pattern.

The antidepressant treatment for the group of subjects who stayed well for at least 5 years was examined. For the index episode of major depression we determined the proportion of weeks in which any antidepressant treatment was received, the mean level of antidepressant treatment in those weeks, and the proportion of subjects who received no antidepressant treatment. In addition, for all of these subjects we determined the same data at years 1, 2, and 3–5 of the well interval to gain a view of naturalistically applied "maintenance antidepressant treatment," and for the subjects with a recurrence we determined the antidepressant treatment during the 4 weeks just before recurrence. Those remaining well received antidepressant treatment for a mean of 63% (SD=44%) of the index episode of major depressive disorder, compared to 65% (SD=40%) for those who experienced a recurrence, and those who did and did not remain well had treatment levels corresponding to mean scores on the composite antidepressant scale of 1.48 (SD=1.15) and 1.59 (SD=1.15). Neither of these small differences was statistically significant. In addition, during the index episode, 21% of the well group (11 of 53) and 19% of the group who experienced a recurrence (10 of 52) received no antidepressant treatment (χ^2=0.04, df=1, p=0.85).

After recovery from the index episode, the subjects continued to receive antidepressant somatic therapy. Table 3 summarizes the antidepressant treatment received during the first 5 years of the well interval. Using a conservatively set alpha of 0.01 for statistical significance, we found no differences between those who did and did not have a recurrence in the proportion of weeks in which any antidepressant treatment was received, the mean score on the composite antidepressant scale for those who did receive treatment, or the proportion who received none. For the group who experienced a recurrence (N=52), we examined the level of antidepressant treatment during the month just before recurrence. The mean scores on the composite antidepressant scale for this time period were distributed as follows: score=0 (no treatment), N=40 (77%); score ≥1, N=12 (23%), score ≥2, N=8 (15%); score ≥3, N=1 (2%); score ≥4, N=0.

DISCUSSION

It may be that recurrence after recovery from major depressive disorder is not inevitable. These results extend our knowledge through careful prospective observation. It appears that some people with major depression do not develop another episode with observational periods of up to 15 years. What baseline characteristics distinguish these people from those who do have recurrences?

In the entire group of 380 subjects who recovered, a greater likelihood of recurrence of an affective disorder was associated with being female, having more prior episodes, never marrying, and having a longer duration of depression before intake. Age and primary versus secondary depressive episode did not distinguish the two groups in this long-term study, a finding contrary to the findings of reports from the collaborative depression study based on briefer follow-up periods (6). None of the other clinical or demographic characteristics assessed at baseline distinguished the two groups. Recent work by our group (unpublished 1998 paper), which broadens the strictly syndromal view of major depressive disorder to include subsyndromal symptoms, illustrates that the persistence of subsyndromal symptoms in subjects who would classically be categorized as recovered predicts a threefold shorter time to recurrence than that seen in subjects who achieve a fully asymptomatic state (68 versus 231 weeks). In fact, this prospectively observed clinical characteristic appears to be a stronger predictor of recurrence than the aforementioned baseline measures.

The presence of psychotic features was not a significant predictor in this sample. Coryell and colleagues (14) demonstrated that the presence of psychotic features in subjects with depression in the collaborative depression study predicted greater psychosocial impairment, longer illness episodes, and shorter times to first and second recurrences. We did not find this to be the case in this group. The important distinction is that the current group was more restrictive and did not include any subjects with schizoaffective disorder, whereas the group in the study by Coryell et al. did.

A meaningful minority of subjects developed mania as the manifestation of their recurrent affective disorder. The rate of 6.1% for the larger group (N=380) is comparable to the 5.2% in the collaborative depression study (15), which was based on 10 years of follow-up data. As reviewed in the report on that study, previous investigators using widely differing methods and patient populations report a rate of switching from unipolar to bipolar depression that ranges from 0% to 37.5%, with a median of 9.7%. The longitudinal design of this study lends strength to our finding, which indicates a slight increase from 10 years of follow-up to the currently reported 15 years.

The gender difference in diagnosed major depressive disorder is well known. Most but not all studies reveal a 2:1 (female to male) ratio in prevalence and an earlier onset of depression and more recurrence for women than for men (16). The greater risk of recurrence for women is not universally reported; in fact, in studies using retrospectively collected data and sophisticated methods of analysis, no gender effect was apparent (17, 18). Earlier reports from the collaborative depression study on probands and family members (6, 8), including work on only subjects with a first episode of major depressive disorder (19), revealed no gender difference in time to recurrence. However, another analysis of data from the collaborative depression study, based on longer follow-up times, showed a gender difference among a group with heterogeneous numbers of episodes (20). That analysis indicates that a longer follow-up is needed to demonstrate a gender effect on recurrence. This effect disappears when the group is restricted to subjects with 5 years of recovery, suggesting that this subgroup "behaves" like the first-episode group in regard to the effect of gender on recurrence.

The second subject group in our study represents a unique collection of people. To our knowledge, this is the first report of a group of people with major depressive disorder who recovered from an episode of illness, subsequently remained well for 5 years, and were prospectively followed for up to 10 additional years. Our earlier work (8) demonstrated that although 67% (Kaplan-Meier estimate) recover from major depressive disorder within the first year, with a median time to recovery of 16 weeks (Kaplan-Meier), a small but meaningful fraction of people continue to recover for up to the 10-year follow-up point. The persistently well subjects (N=105) reported here recovered fairly promptly after intake (median time to recovery=13.27 weeks), and 80% were well at 1 year of follow-up. Even with the lengthy well interval, 58% (Kaplan-Meier estimate) subsequently experienced a recurrence. None of the baseline demographic and clinical characteristics that predicted recurrence in the larger group persisted as significant in this well group.

Our analysis of the antidepressant treatment received by the entire group of 380 subjects who recovered provides some insights into naturalistically applied treatments as prospectively observed over 15 years. The subjects who did and did not have a recurrence received similar amounts of antidepressant treatment during the index episode, and they received treatment for similar proportions of the index episode. Insofar as treatment is a reflection of clinical characteristics of the depression, the comparability of the treatment received lends further support to the clinical similarity of the index episodes of depression for the two groups.

The smaller group of 105 subjects who experienced at least 5 years of recovery provide another view of naturalistically applied treatments. As the well interval progressed, the proportion of weeks that any antidepressant treatment was received and the mean level of that treatment did not differ to a statistically significant degree between the group who did not experience a recurrence and the group who did. In addition, the proportion of subjects receiving no antidepressant treatment increased from around 35% to 65% over the 5 years.

Furthermore, of the subjects who eventually experienced a recurrence, 77% were receiving no antidepressant treatment during the month just before the recurrence. In the remaining 23% who did receive treatment, the modal level of treatment was between antidepressant scale scores of 2 and 3, or between 100 and 199 mg of imipramine equivalents per day. It appears that whether ill or well, this cohort of affectively ill subjects received roughly equivalent and rather low levels of somatic antidepressant therapy during the lengthy well interval, and the majority of subjects received no antidepressant therapy just before recurrence. Whether or not the recurrence rate would be reduced if the level of antidepressant treatment were greater cannot be determined by these data. Our data on nonsomatic therapies, such as psychotherapy or family therapy, are not systematic or comprehensive enough for us to comment on their application in this group.

Being female, having a longer episode of illness before seeking treatment, never being married, and having more prior episodes are characteristics that may suggest to the treating clinician that a patient will have a recurrence after recovering from major depressive disorder. From the data we are reporting it was discouraging to find so little information with which to predict which subjects are still at risk for recurrence even after half a decade of recovery. Unfortunately, in this study group we found that people continue to experience recurrences even after long periods of wellness. The paucity of predictors and the persistent possibility of recurrence should guide clinicians and patients to be ever vigilant for a recurrence of depression and the pernicious subsyndromal symptoms of depression (our 1998 unpublished paper). This somewhat discouraging admonition is tempered by our report (9) that some people can recover after even extremely long and seemingly interminable episodes of major depressive disorder and by others' findings (2) that suggest that effective application of long-term antidepressant pharmacotherapy may maintain a state of well being.

ACKNOWLEDGMENTS

The NIMH Collaborative Program on the Psychobiology of Depression—Clinical Studies was conducted with the participation of the following investigators: M.B. Keller, M.D. (chairperson, Providence, R.I.); W. Coryell, M.D. (co-chairperson, Iowa City); J.D. Maser, Ph.D. (Washington, D.C.); T.I. Mueller, M.D., M.T. Shea, Ph.D. (Providence, R.I.); J. Haley (Iowa City); J. Endicott, Ph.D., A.C. Leon, Ph.D., J. Loth, M.S.W. (New York); and J. Rice, Ph.D., T. Reich, M.D. (St. Louis). Other contributors include H.S. Akiskal, M.D., N.C. Andreasen, M.D., Ph.D., P.J. Clayton, M.D., J. Croughan, M.D., R.M.A. Hirschfeld, M.D., M.M. Katz, Ph.D., P.W. Lavori, Ph.D., R.L. Spitzer, M.D., and M.A. Young, Ph.D. Deceased: G.L. Klerman, M.D., E. Robins, M.D., R.W. Shapiro, M.D., and G. Winokur, M.D.

REFERENCES

1. Angst J, Baastrup P, Grof P, Hippius H, Poldinger W, Weis P: The course of monopolar depression and bipolar psychoses. Psychiatr Neurol Neurochir 1973; 76:489–500
2. Frank E, Kupfer DJ, Peral JM, Cornes C, Jarrett DB, Mallinger AG, Thase ME, McEachran AB, Grochocinski VJ: Three-year outcomes for maintenance therapies in recurrent depression. Arch Gen Psychiatry 1990; 47:1093–1099
3. Roy-Byrne P, Post RM, Uhde TW, Porcu T, Davis D: The longitudinal course of recurrent affective illness: life chart data from research patients at the NIMH. Acta Psychiatr Scand Suppl 1985: 71:3–34
4. Gonzales LR, Lewinsohn PM, Clarke GN: Longitudinal follow-up of unipolar depressives: an investigation of predictors of relapse. J Consult Clin Psychol 1985; 53:461–469
5. Maj M, Veltro F, Pirozzi R, Lobrace S, Magliano L: Pattern of recurrence of illness after recovery from an episode of major depression: a prospective study. Am J Psychiatry 1992; 149: 795–800
6. Keller MB, Lavori PW, Lewis CE, Klerman GL: Predictors of relapse in major depressive disorder. JAMA 1983; 250:3299–3304
7. Giles DE, Jarrett RB, Biggs MM, Guzick DS, Rush AJ: Clinical predictors of recurrence in depression. Am J Psychiatry 1989; 146:764–767
8. Coryell W, Endicott J, Keller MB: Predictors of relapse into major depressive disorder in a nonclinical population. Am J Psychiatry 1991: 148:1353–1358
9. Mueller TI, Keller MB, Leon AC, Solomon DA, Shea MT, Coryell W, Endicott J: Recovery after five years of unremitted major depressive disorder. Arch Gen Psychiatry 1996; 53: 794–799
10. Endicott J, Spitzer RL: A diagnostic interview: the Schedule for Affective Disorders and Schizophrenia. Arch Gen Psychiatry 1978; 35:837–844
11. Spitzer RL, Endicott J, Robins E: Research Diagnostic Criteria: rationale and reliability. Arch Gen Psychiatry 1978; 35: 773–782
12. Keller MB, Lavori PW, Friedman B, Nielsen E, Endicott J, McDonald-Scott P, Andreasen NC: The Longitudinal Interval Follow-Up Evaluation: a comprehensive method for assessing outcome in prospective longitudinal studies. Arch Gen Psychiatry 1987; 44:540–548
13. Kaplan EL, Meier P: Nonparametric estimation from incomplete observations. J Am Stat Assoc 1958; 53:457–481
14. Coryell W, Leon A, Winokur G, Endicott J, Keller M, Akiskal H, Solomon D: Importance of psychotic features to long-term course in major depressive disorder. Am J Psychiatry 1996; 153:483–489
15. Coryell W, Endicott J, Maser JD, Keller MB, Leon AC, Akiskal HS: Long-term stability of polarity distinctions in the affective disorders. Am J Psychiatry 1995; 152:385–390
16. Pajer K: New strategies in the treatment of depression in women. J Clin Psychiatry 1995; 56(Feb suppl):30–37
17. Kessler RC, McGonagle KA, Swartz M, Blazer DG, Nelson CB: Sex and depression in the National Comorbidity Survey, I: lifetime prevalence, chronicity and recurrence. J Affect Disord 1993; 29:85–96
18. Kessing LV: Recurrence in affective disorder, II: effect of age and gender. Br J Psychiatry 1998; 172:29–34
19. Simpson HB, Nee JC, Endicott J: First-episode major depression: few sex differences in course. Arch Gen Psychiatry 1997; 54:633–639
20. Winokur G, Coryell W, Keller M, Endicott J, Akiskal H: A prospective follow-up of patients with bipolar and primary unipolar affective disorder. Arch Gen Psychiatry 1993; 50:457–465

ORIGINAL INVESTIGATION

Association Between Depression and Mortality in Older Adults

The Cardiovascular Health Study

Richard Schulz, PhD; Scott R. Beach, PhD; Diane G. Ives, MPH; Lynn M. Martire, PhD; Abraham A. Ariyo, MD, MPH; Willem J. Kop, PhD

Background: Studies of the association between depressive symptoms and mortality in elderly populations have yielded contradictory findings. To address these discrepancies, we test this association using the most extensive array of sociodemographic and physical health control variables ever studied, to our knowledge, in a large population-based sample of elderly individuals.

Objective: To examine the relation between baseline depressive symptoms and 6-year all-cause mortality in older persons, systematically controlling for sociodemographic factors, clinical disease, subclinical disease, and health risk factors.

Methods: A total of 5201 men and women aged 65 years and older from 4 US communities participated in the study. Depressive symptoms and 4 categories of covariates were assessed at baseline. The primary outcome measure was 6-year mortality.

Results: Of the 5201 participants, 984 (18.9%) died within 6 years. High baseline depressive symptoms were associated with a higher mortality rate (23.9%) than low baseline depression scores (17.7%) (unadjusted relative risk [RR], 1.41; 95% confidence interval [CI], 1.22-1.63). Depression was also an independent predictor of mortality when controlling for sociodemographic factors (RR, 1.43; 95% CI, 1.23-1.66), prevalent clinical disease (RR, 1.25; 95% CI, 1.07-1.45), subclinical disease indicators (RR, 1.35; 95% CI, 1.15-1.58), or biological or behavioral risk factors (RR, 1.42; 95% CI, 1.22-1.65). When the best predictors from all 4 classes of variables were included as covariates, high depressive symptoms remained an independent predictor of mortality (RR, 1.24; 95% CI, 1.06-1.46).

Conclusions: High levels of depressive symptoms are an independent risk factor for mortality in community-residing older adults. Motivational depletion may be a key underlying mechanism for the depression-mortality effect.

Arch Intern Med. 2000;160:1761-1768

From the Department of Psychiatry (Drs Schulz and Martire), the University Center for Social and Urban Research (Drs Schulz, Beach, and Martire), and the Department of Epidemiology, Graduate School of Public Health (Ms Ives), University of Pittsburgh, Pittsburgh, Pa; the Department of Cardiology, University of California, Davis Medical Center, Sacramento (Dr Ariyo); and the Department of Medical and Clinical Psychology, Uniformed Services University of the Health Sciences, and the Division of Cardiology, Georgetown University Medical Center, Washington, DC (Dr Kop).

THE LINK between depression and mortality in older persons continues to be a hotly debated issue,[1,2] with some investigators[3-11] demonstrating that depression is an independent risk factor for mortality and others[12-18] failing to find this association. Although researchers may argue about the reasons for these inconsistent findings (measures of depression used, sample used, the length of the observation period for ascertaining mortality, and choice of covariates), individuals in both camps would agree that a fair test of the depression-mortality hypothesis requires that known demographic and physical health status predictors of mortality be controlled. Moreover, the better and more extensive the health controls used in a study, the more conclusive would be a finding linking depression to mortality.

The Cardiovascular Health Study (CHS), a large population-based study of older persons, affords a unique opportunity to test the association between depression and mortality because of the extensive array of sociodemographic, objective clinical disease, subclinical disease, and health risk factor variables available as covariates. The association between more than 70 predictor variables

For editorial comment see page 1731

and 5-year mortality for this sample was recently reported by Fried and colleagues.[19] While Fried and colleagues used an exploratory approach, relying on stepwise Cox proportional hazards regression procedures to determine the best predictors of mortality, we use a more theoretical, hypothesis-based approach in this article. We extend the work of Fried and colleagues by testing specific multivariate models linking depression to 6-year mortality in this sample. Five distinct mod-

PARTICIPANTS AND METHODS

STUDY POPULATION

The sample used for this study was from the CHS, a prospective, observational study designed to determine the risk factors for and consequences of cardiovascular disease in older adults. Beginning in 1989, a total of 5201 men and women aged 65 years or older were recruited in 4 US communities: Forsyth County (North Carolina); Washington County (Maryland); Sacramento County (California); and Allegheny County (Penn). Potential participants were identified from a random sample stratified by age group (65-74, 75-84, and ≥85 years) from the Health Care Financing Administration Medicare Enrollment Lists. All persons thus identified and age-eligible household members who were planning to reside in the community for at least 3 years were eligible to participate. Exclusion criteria included being wheelchair bound in the home, being unable to participate in the examination at the field centers, or undergoing active treatment for cancer. Additional information regarding sampling and recruitment for the CHS has been published previously.[20,21] The length of follow-up for this group was 6 years for the analyses reported herein.

EVALUATION

Extensive demographic and health information was collected by trained interviewers or by clinical examination. Level of depressive symptoms at baseline was assessed with the 10-item version of the Center for Epidemiological Studies Depression Scale (CES-D[22,23]). Covariates to be included in the models tested were chosen from 4 categories—sociodemographic factors, prevalent clinical disease, subclinical disease, and biological or behavioral risk factors. For each of these categories, a subset of covariates was chosen based on previous findings in the CHS sample showing that these are important indicators of health status[19,24] within each of these categories. **Table 1** provides a listing of variables examined in this study and descriptive information for these variables.

Study participants were followed up for an average of 6 years. Deaths were confirmed through reviews of obituaries, medical records, death certificates, and the Health Care Financing Administration health care use database for hospitalizations. Through these methods, and interviews of contacts and proxies for participants unavailable for follow-up, there was 100% complete follow-up ascertainment of mortality status.

ANALYTIC METHODS

The major focus of the analyses was the relation between depression and 6-year mortality, after controlling for other known demographic and physical health status predictors. Depression and the other covariates were assessed at baseline. To better understand potential modifiers of the depression-mortality link, we tested a series of Cox proportional hazards regression models in which covariates of 4 general types were also controlled (Table 1). Survival time was coded as number of days between the baseline interview and death or the last follow-up visit. Five models were tested: (1) the sociodemographic model, controlling for age, sex, race, educational level, marital status, and stressful life events; (2) the prevalent disease model, controlling for objectively measured prevalent clinical disease such as diabetes, congestive heart failure, and stroke; (3) the subclinical disease model, controlling for subclinical indicators of prevalent clinical disease such as claudication, major electrocardiographic abnormalities, and carotid stenosis; (4) the risk factor model, controlling for known biological and behavioral risk factors for mortality such as smoking status, fasting glucose level, and body mass index; and (5) the combined model, which controlled for all variables in the previous 4 models. Models 2 through 4, which proceed from the most proximal to more distal predictors of mortality, also controlled for sociodemographic variables. Models 1 through 4 were tested by entering all variables into the equation on a single step. The combined model (model 5) was tested by entering all variables except for depression on a first step, with significant predictors determined using a forward selection procedure ($P = .05$ for entry and $P = .10$ for removal), then forcing depression into the equation on a second step. Table 1 presents information for all variables used in the analysis, including coding schemes and descriptive statistics. **Tables 2, 3, 4, 5**, and **6** present results for the 5 Cox proportional hazards regression models tested, and show adjusted and unadjusted relative risk (RR) ratios (from a Cox proportional hazards model with only that variable as a predictor). Depression scores were dichotomized with a cutoff of 8 or higher, which corresponds to the cutoff of 16 or higher for risk for clinical depression on the 20-item version of the CES-D.

As seen in Table 1, there were differing levels of missing data on the various baseline indicators, with higher rates for subclinical disease and risk factor variables. Fried et al[19] reported that variable estimates for their CHS mortality models were similar when using only participants with valid data vs replacing missing data and using all participants. Therefore, in the interests of clarity and simplicity, analyses were conducted only with participants who had no missing data, and thus the number of participants varies somewhat across models, ranging from 4710 (combined model) to 5173 (sociodemographic model). To test the proportional hazards assumption of the Cox proportional hazards model, the interaction of depression with survival time was computed and allowed to enter a model with all covariates. There was no violation of the assumption for depression.

els are tested. Models 1 through 4 examine depression as a predictor of mortality after controlling for (1) sociodemographics, (2) objectively measured prevalent clinical disease, (3) subclinical disease indicators, and (4) biological and behavioral risk factors for mortality. The fifth model examines the ability of depression to predict mortality after controlling for all variables in the previous 4 models.

The strength of this study lies in our ability to assess the relative risk of depression-related mortality in the context of specific classes of covariates that vary in their proximal relation to death, the careful measurement of predictors and outcome measures, and a large representative sample of community-residing older persons. In addition, 2 types of exploratory analyses are carried out to identify specific mecha-

Table 1. Variable Descriptions and Descriptive Statistics

Variable	Descriptive Statistics*	Comment
Sociodemographic (N = 5201)		
Age at baseline, y†	Mean, 72.8 (range, 65-100); SD, 5.6; median, 71.0	. . .
Sex‡		
Female	2962 (57.0)	. . .
Male	2239 (43.0)	. . .
Race‡		
White	4926 (94.7)	. . .
Nonwhite	275 (5.3)	. . .
Educational level, y (N = 5187)†	Mean, 13.9 (range, 0-21); SD, 4.7; median, 12.0	. . .
Marital status§		
Married (reference)	3596 (69.1)	. . .
Divorced or separated	196 (3.8)	. . .
Widowed	1197 (23.0)	. . .
Single or never married	212 (4.1)	. . .
Stressful life events†	Mean, 1.1 (range, 0-7); SD, 1.1; median, 1.0	Total of possible 10 stressful life events in past 6 mo
Depressive symptoms		
Center for Epidemiological Studies-Depression Scale (10-question version)‡	5192 (100.0)	. . .
Low (score, 0-7)	4156 (80.0)	. . .
High (score, ≥8)	1036 (20.0)	. . .
Prevalent clinical disease‡	5201 (100.0)	Present or absent for 6 primary disease end points (myocardial infarction, angina pectoris, congestive heart failure, intermittent claudication, stroke, or transient ischemic attack), required baseline self-reported diagnosis by physician plus the other criteria for the individual disease end point
Myocardial infarction	504 (9.7)	Either electrocardiographic evidence or medical record documentation
Angina pectoris	814 (15.7)	Medication use (nitroglycerin, β blocker, or calcium channel blocker), history of revascularization procedure, or medical record documentation
Congestive heart failure	217 (4.2)	Either medication use (diuretic and digitalis or another vasodilator) or medical record documentation
Intermittent claudication	135 (2.6)	Either ankle-arm ratio ≤.8 or history of lower extremity bypass, angioplasty, or amputation
Stroke	190 (3.7)	Medical record confirmation
Transient ischemic attack	130 (2.5)	Medical record confirmation
Diabetes‡	5201 (100.0)	. . .
Normal (reference)	2594 (49.9)	. . .
Impaired glucose tolerance	1434 (27.6)	(2-hr postload glucose level, >7.8-11.0 mmol/L [140-199 mg/dL])
Diabetic	1173 (22.6)	Fasting glucose level, >7.8 mmol/L (>140 mg/dL) or 2-hr drop in the glucose tolerance test of >11.1 mmol/L (>200 mg/dL), self-reported diagnosis by a physician, or self-reported insulin use or medication use (insulin or oral hypoglycemic)

Continued

nisms that might account for the depression-mortality effect.

RESULTS

For sociodemographic variables, participants ranged in age from 65 to 100 years at baseline (mean, 73 years); 57% were women, and 43% were men (Table 1). There was substantial variability on most of the prevalent disease, subclinical disease, and risk factor indicators. Approximately 20% of the sample met or exceeded the CES-D cutoff score for risk for clinical depression.

After 6 years of follow-up, there were 984 deaths, representing 18.9% of the total sample. There were 248 deaths (23.9%) among the 1036 participants with CES-D scores above the at-risk cutoff, while 734 (17.7%) of the 4156 participants below the cutoff had died within the follow-up period (unadjusted RR, 1.41; 95% confidence interval, 1.22-1.63). Depression scores for 2 of the persons who died were not available.

The sociodemographic model (Table 2) showed that participants who were older, male, less educated, and divorced, widowed, or separated were more likely to die. Controlling for sociodemographic characteristics, participants with a CES-D score higher than the cutoff score were also more likely to die. Similar to the unadjusted risk estimate, those with high depression scores had risks of mortality 43% higher than those with low depression scores. The prevalent disease model, shown in Table 3, revealed that participants with baseline angina, congestive heart failure, intermittent claudication, stroke, diabetes, and hypertension had higher mortality rates than

Table 1. Variable Descriptions and Descriptive Statistics (cont)

Variable	Descriptive Statistics*	Comment
Hypertension‡	5185 (100.0)	...
Normotensive (reference)	2273 (43.8)	...
Borderline hypertensive	774 (14.9)	Random zero sealed blood pressure: average systolic blood pressure of 140-159 mm Hg or diastolic blood pressure of 90-94 mm Hg
Hypertensive	2138 (41.2)	Random zero sealed blood pressure: average systolic blood pressure of >160 mm Hg or diastolic blood pressure of >95 mm Hg, or self-reported diagnosis by a physician and antihypertensive medication
Subclinical disease indicators (N = 5196)		
Rose questionnaire for claudication‡	100 (1.9)	Positive or negative result for claudication at baseline
Rose questionnaire for angina‡	320 (6.2)	Positive or negative result for angina at baseline
Forced expiratory volume at 1 s, mL (N = 5111)†	Mean, 2.1 (range, 0.3-4.5); SD, 0.7; median, 2.0	Measured during the baseline pulmonary function test
Ankle-arm ratio‖	5087 (100.0)	Minimum measure of right and left ankle-arm ratio measured in the clinic
0->0.9	4455 (87.6)	...
1-≤0.9	632 (12.4)	...
Left ventricular ejection fraction‖	5152 (100.0)	Based on echocardiographic readings by trained technicians
0 (normal or borderline)	4962 (96.3)	...
1 (abnormal)	190 (3.7)	...
Major electrocardiographic abnormality‡	1461/5028 (29.1)	Measured during the baseline electrocardiogram, any of the following: ventricular conduction defects, major Q- or QS-wave abnormalities, left ventricular hypertrophy, isolated major ST- or T-wave abnormalities, atrial fibrillation, or first-degree atrioventricular block
Carotid stenosis‡	2540/5171 (49.1)	Measured during baseline carotid ultrasonography as either of the following for left or right: carotid stenosis, >25th percentile
Biological or behavioral risk factors		
Systolic blood pressure, mm Hg (N = 5191)†	Mean, 135.8 (range, 77-230); SD, 21.5; median, 134	Average of 2 readings, zero muddler systolic blood pressure
Total cholesterol level, mmol/L (mg/dL) (N = 5173)†	Mean, 5.55 (214.6) (range, 62-433); SD, 1.02 (39.3); median, 5.51 (213.0)	...
Low-density lipoproteins, mg/dL (N = 5101)†	Mean, 133.1 (range, 28-340); SD, 35.7; median, 131.0	...
Fasting glucose level, mmol/L (mg/dL) (N = 5165)†	Mean, 6.1 (110.2) (range, 2.9-36.5 (53-657)); SD, 1.9 (34.6); median, 5.6 (101)	...
Triglyceride level, mmol/L (mg/dL) (N = 5173)†	Mean, 1.61 (142.70) (range, 0.42-14.94 (37-1323)); SD, 0.89 (78.5); median, 1.39 (123)	...
Smoking status§	5198 (100.0)	Self-report at baseline
Never smoker (reference)	2397 (46.1)	...
Former smoker	2200 (42.3)	...
Current smoker	601 (11.6)	...
Body mass index (N = 5185)†¶	Mean, 26.4 (range, 14.7-53.2), SD, 4.5; median, 25.9	...
Alcohol consumption, drinks per week	5183 (100.00)	Number of alcoholic beverages (beer, wine, or liquor) consumed per week at baseline
0 (reference)	2489 (48.0)	...
1-7	2026 (39.1)	...
>7	668 (12.9)	...

*Data are given as number (percentage) of participants unless otherwise indicated. Percentages may not total 100 because of rounding.
†Continuous variable.
‡Categorical or indicator variable.
§Categorical or dummy variable.
‖Dummy variable.
¶Calculated as weight in kilograms divided by the square of height in meters.

participants without prevalent disease. Controlling for sociodemographic variables and prevalent clinical disease, individuals with high levels of depressive symptoms were more likely to die (25% higher risk). The subclinical disease model (Table 4) revealed that 6 of 7 subclinical disease indicators were independently predictive of 6-year mortality. Individuals with intermittent claudication, a lower forced expiratory volume, lower ankle-arm ratios, abnormal left ventricular ejection fractions, a major electrocardiographic abnormality, or carotid stenosis were more likely to die. Once again, controlling for sociodemographic factors and subclinical

Table 2. Sociodemographic Model: Association of Sociodemographic Variables and Depressive Symptoms With 6-Year Mortality*

Variable	Unadjusted RR (95% CI)	Adjusted RR (95% CI)	Adjusted RR *P*
Sociodemographic factors			
Age (years)	1.11 (1.10-1.12)†	1.09 (1.08-1.10)	<.001
Sex‡	2.06 (1.81-2.34)†	2.28 (1.98-2.62)	<.001
Race§	1.26 (0.98-1.63)	1.09 (0.84-1.42)	.50
Educational level (years)	0.96 (0.94-0.97)†	0.97 (0.96-0.98)	<.001
Marital status‖			<.001
Divorced, separated, or widowed	1.49 (1.30-1.70)†	1.46 (1.25-1.69)	<.001
Single	1.12 (0.81-1.54)	1.21 (0.87-1.67)	.26
Stressful life events	0.94 (0.89-1.00)¶	0.95 (0.90-1.00)	.06
Depressive symptoms			
High CES-D score (≥8)	1.41 (1.22-1.63)†	1.43 (1.23-1.66)	<.001

*Adjusted model *N* = 5173; there were 979 deaths (18.9%). RR indicates relative risk; CI, confidence interval; and CES-D, Center for Epidemiological Studies Depression Scale.
†*P*<.001.
‡Female = 0, and male = 1.
§White = 0, and nonwhite = 1.
‖The reference category is married.
¶*P*=.04.

Table 3. Prevalent Disease Model: Association of Prevalent Clinical Disease and Depressive Symptoms With 6-Year Mortality*

Variable	Unadjusted RR (95% CI)	Adjusted RR (95% CI)	Adjusted RR *P*
Prevalent clinical disease			
Myocardial infarction	2.39 (2.04-2.81)†	1.15 (0.92-1.44)	.24
Angina pectoris	2.24 (1.96-2.56)†	1.30 (1.07-1.57)	.007
Congestive heart failure	4.27 (3.53-5.18)†	2.44 (1.98-2.99)	<.001
Intermittent claudication	3.16 (2.45-4.08)†	1.60 (1.22-2.09)	<.001
Stroke	3.06 (2.47-3.79)†	1.62 (1.04-2.53)	.03
Transient ischemic attack	2.64 (2.17-3.20)†	1.20 (0.80-1.79)	.37
Diabetes status‡			<.001
Impaired glucose tolerance	1.33 (1.14-1.55)†	1.12 (0.96-1.31)	.14
Diabetic	1.98 (1.71-2.30)†	1.54 (1.33-1.80)	<.001
Hypertension status§			<.001
Borderline hypertensive	1.37 (1.12-1.66)‖	1.17 (0.96-1.42)	.12
Hypertensive	1.66 (1.45-1.91)†	1.32 (1.14-1.52)	<.001
Depressive symptoms			
High CES-D score (≥8)	1.41 (1.22-1.63)†	1.25 (1.07-1.45)	.004

*Adjusted model *N* = 5166; there were 979 deaths (19.0%). The sociodemographic variables were controlled. RR indicates relative risk; CI, confidence interval; and CES-D, Center for Epidemiological Studies Depression Scale.
†*P*<.001.
‡The reference category is normal.
§The reference category is normotensive.
‖*P*=.002.

disease, a high baseline depression score was an independent predictor of 6-year mortality (35% higher risk than those with low depression scores). The biological and behavioral risk factors model (Table 5) showed that individuals with a higher systolic blood pressure, those with higher levels of fasting glucose, current and former smokers, those with a lower body mass index, and those who consumed no alcoholic beverages had higher 6-year mortality rates. Consistent with the previous 3 models, once sociodemographic and risk factor variables were controlled, high depression scores were predictive of mortality (42% higher risk). Results from the combined model, shown in Table 6, revealed that even after controlling for the best predictors from all 4 classes of covariates (selected using a Cox proportional hazards regression forward selection technique), a high baseline depression score was an independent risk factor for 6-year mortality (24% higher risk than those with low depression scores). Table 6 also serves as a summary of the best overall predictors of 6-year mortality across all classes of variables.

To further explore the depression-mortality link, the Cox proportional hazards models were run using the 10 individual items from the CES-D in place of the single dichotomous variable. Depressive symptoms are rated for their frequency of occurrence in the week before the interview on a 4-point scale ranging from 0 (rarely or none of the time) to 3 (most of the time). We were interested in whether there were specific aspects of depression that were more predictive of mortality. These models consistently showed that there were 2 CES-D items that were independently predictive of 6-year mortality: (1) "I felt that everything I did was an effort" was a significant predictor of mortality in all 5 models (RR range, 1.12-

Table 4. Subclinical Disease Model: Association of Subclinical Disease Indicators and Depressive Symptoms With 6-Year Mortality*

Variable	Unadjusted RR (95% CI)	Adjusted RR (95% CI)	Adjusted RR *P*
Subclinical disease indicators			
Intermittent claudication by Rose questionnaire	3.02 (2.24-4.07)†	1.56 (1.12-2.17)	.008
Angina by Rose questionnaire	1.69 (1.36-2.09)†	1.26 (1.00-1.59)	.05
Forced expiratory volume at 1 s	0.60 (0.55-0.67)†	0.57 (0.50-0.64)	<.001
Ankle-arm ratio	3.09 (2.68-3.58)†	1.51 (1.28-1.79)	<.001
Left ventricular ejection fraction	3.95 (3.20-4.88)†	2.02 (1.59-2.57)	<.001
Major electrocardiographic abnormality	2.62 (2.30-2.98)†	1.73 (1.50-1.99)	<.001
Carotid stenosis	2.32 (2.03-2.65)†	1.46 (1.26-1.69)	<.001
Depressive symptoms			
High CES-D score (≥8)	1.41 (1.22-1.63)†	1.35 (1.15-1.58)	<.001

Adjusted model N = 4756; there were 861 deaths (18.1%). The sociodemographic variables were controlled. RR indicates relative risk; CI, confidence interval; and CES-D, Center for Epidemiological Studies Depression Scale.

†P<.001.

Table 5. Risk Factor Model: Association of Biological or Behavioral Risk Factors and Depressive Symptoms With 6-Year Mortality*

Variable	Unadjusted RR (95% CI)	Adjusted RR (95% CI)	Adjusted RR *P*
Biological or behavioral risk factors			
Systolic blood pressure	1.01 (1.01-1.01)†	1.01 (1.00-1.01)	<.001
Total cholesterol level	0.99 (0.99-1.00)†	1.00 (0.99-1.00)	.48
Low-density lipoproteins	1.00 (0.99-1.00)†	1.00 (1.00-1.01)	.85
Fasting glucose level	1.01 (1.00-1.01)†	1.01 (1.00-1.01)	<.001
Triglycerides level	1.00 (1.00-1.00)‡	1.00 (1.00-1.00)	.20
Smoking status§			<.001
Former smoker	1.30 (1.13-1.49)†	1.28 (1.10-1.49)	.001
Current smoker	1.65 (1.37-1.99)†	2.15 (1.75-2.63)	<.001
Body mass index	0.97 (0.96-0.99)†	0.98 (0.96-0.99)	.006
Alcohol consumption, drinks/wk‖			.01
1-7	0.82 (0.72-0.94)‡	0.85 (0.74-0.98)	.03
>7	0.75 (0.61-0.93)‡	0.74 (0.58-0.93)	.009
Depressive symptoms			
High CES-D score (≥8)	1.41 (1.22-1.63)†	1.42 (1.22-1.65)	<.001

Adjusted model N = 5022; there were 941 deaths (18.7%). The sociodemographic variables were controlled. RR indicates relative risk; CI, confidence interval; and CES-D, Center for Epidemiological Studies Depression Scale.

†P<.001.

‡P<.05.

§*The reference category is never smoker.*

‖*The reference category is none.*

1.19), and (2) "I could not get going" was a significant independent predictor of mortality in 3 of the 5 models (RR range, 1.04-1.17). An additional attempt to help interpret the depression-mortality findings involved an exploratory analysis of other subjective self-assessments known to be related to mortality, such as self-assessed health status[25]: "How would you say your health is?" Possible answers were (1) excellent, (2) very good, (3) good, (4) fair, or (5) poor. Interestingly, when this single indicator was included as a covariate in the combined model, the depression effect disappeared (RR, 1.11, P=.21).

COMMENT

Using the most extensive array of sociodemographic and physical health control variables ever studied, to our knowledge, in a large population-based sample of elderly individuals, we show that depression is an independent risk factor for mortality in all 5 models tested. The risk of mortality was 25% to 43% higher among individuals with high levels of depressive symptoms in analyses examining the effects of depression on mortality in the context of sociodemographic factors, prevalent clinical disease, subclinical disease, and health risk factors, separately. When all predictors were combined, depression remained an independent risk factor for mortality (RR, 1.24). The full model showed that being older, male, less educated, and divorced, separated, or widowed were independent risk factors for mortality. Also, having hypertension, congestive heart failure, or stroke increased the risk of dying. Subclinical diseases, including intermittent claudication, a lower forced expiratory volume, a lower ankle-arm ratio, an abnormal left ventricular ejection fraction, a major electrocardiographic abnormality, and carotid stenosis, were also strong risk factors for mortality. Finally, 3 biological or behavioral risk factors, elevated fasting glucose level, being a current smoker, and low body mass index, were also risk factors for mortality.

Consistent with the observations of Lesperance and Frasure-Smith,[2] our data show that older individuals do not need to have major depression to be at increased risk

Table 6. Combined Model: Association of Sociodemographic Variables, Prevalent Clinical Disease, Subclinical Disease Indicators, Biological or Behavioral Risk Factors, and Depressive Symptoms With 6-Year Mortality*

Variable	Adjusted RR (95% CI)	P
Sociodemographics		
Age (years)	1.07 (1.06-1.08)	<.001
Sex†	2.42 (2.03-2.89)	<.001
Educational level (years)	0.98 (0.96-0.99)	.002
Marital status‡		.02
Divorced, separated, or widowed	1.26 (1.07-1.48)	.007
Single	1.05 (0.74-1.50)	.78
Prevalent clinical disease		
Hypertension status§		.01
Borderline hypertensive	1.08 (0.87-1.34)	.49
Hypertensive	1.26 (1.08-1.47)	.004
Congestive heart failure	1.96 (1.55-2.47)	<.001
Stroke	1.77 (1.39-2.26)	<.001
Subclinical disease indicators		
Intermittent claudication by Rose questionnaire	1.58 (1.14-2.20)	.007
Forced expiratory volume questionnaire at 1 s	0.62 (0.55-0.70)	<.001
Ankle-arm ratio	1.31 (1.10-1.55)	.002
Left ventricular ejection fraction	1.78 (1.38-2.29)	<.001
Major electrocardiographic abnormality	1.56 (1.34-1.81)	<.001
Carotid stenosis	1.38 (1.19-1.60)	<.001
Biological or behavioral risk factors		
Fasting glucose level	1.00 (1.00-1.01)	<.001
Smoking status‖		.002
Former smoker	1.14 (0.97-1.33)	.11
Current smoker	1.49 (1.19-1.87)	<.001
Body mass index	0.98 (0.96-1.00)	.01
Depressive symptoms		
High CES-D score (≥8)	1.24 (1.06-1.46)	.009

**N = 4710; there were 849 deaths (18.0%). Sociodemographic variables, prevalent clinical desease, subclinical disease indicators, and biological or behavioral risk factors shown were significant when all variables from these categories were entered into a Cox proportional hazards regression procedure using conditional forward selection. Depressive symptoms were forced into this best-fitting model on a second step. RR indicates relative risk; CI, confidence interval; and CES-D, Center for Epidemiological Studies Depression Scale.*

†Female = 0, and male = 1.

‡The reference category is married.

§The reference category is normotensive.

‖The reference category is never smoker.

of mortality. Even milder or subthreshold forms of depression increase the risk of death in older persons.

What might mediate the relation between depression and mortality? A follow-up analysis of specific items of our depression measure showed that the depression-mortality effect is accounted for by a few items reflecting motivational depletion (I could not get going and I felt that everything I did was an effort). Similar items were identified in a study by Anda et al,[26] who reported that wanting to give up and feeling that "I don't have what it takes anymore" were independent predictors of mortality. These findings are consistent with a growing number of reports in the literature suggesting that factors such as vital exhaustion[27] and decreased emotional vitality[28,29] are linked to functional decline and mortality in older persons. Behavioral and pathophysiological mechanisms are plausible explanations for the link between affective or motivational states and mortality. Individuals who "give up" are likely to disengage from preventive and potentially restorative health behaviors and supportive relations. At the same time, or as a consequence of these behavioral changes, the neuroendocrine system may become disregulated and homeostatic immune functioning may be compromised. It is important that we pursue the mechanisms that account for the depression-mortality effect, and our pursuit of this goal would be facilitated by a better understanding and measurement of the affective and motivational states that underlie the depression-mortality link.

Although our data clearly support a depression-mortality link, we were also interested in identifying factors that might explain why some studies do not find this relation. There are many reasons why a specific study may not find a relation between depression and mortality, including the sample size, mortality rate, method for assessing depression, completeness of follow-up, length of the follow-up period, and choice of covariates. Our data suggest that one overlooked factor concerns the extent to which other self-report measures of health and functioning are included in the analysis.[25] To the extent that the depression-mortality effect is driven by an underlying psychological state that includes elements of affect and motivation, we would expect its effects to be shared and diluted among a broad range of self-assessments, including perceived health, self-assessed functional status, and other indicators of subjective well-being. In general, studies[6,13-17,30] that fail to find a depression-mortality link include multiple self-report indicators of well-being and functioning. In contrast, studies[3,4,7,31-34] that show a significant association between depression and mortality typically rely on assessments of health and functioning based on relatively objective tests, ratings of study participants by an external evaluator, or both. This pattern is supported by our own data as well. As we would expect, once other self-report indicators of functioning and health are added to our multivariate model (eg, self-rating of health), the significant depression effect disappears. This does not mean that the depression-mortality link is a statistical artifact, but rather it suggests that depression is one of several interrelated constructs that reflect the motivational and affective status of the individual and that these factors are in turn related to mortality.

From a clinical perspective, the findings from this study indicate that subthreshhold levels of depression as measured by existing screening instruments should be taken seriously and further evaluated for possible treatment. Behavioral and medical interventions can be used to reduce these depressive symptoms and enhance quality of life and longevity in older persons.

Although this study represents a significant advance over existing literature in this area, it also has some limitations. First, we did not have available clinical diagnoses of depression or the psychiatric history of our respondents. The relation between clinical depression and mortality may actually be stronger than the relation between depressive symptoms and mortality observed in this study. Second, there is increasing evidence that depression may be linked specifically to cardiovascular mortality[3,26,32]; future analysis should focus on linking depression to specific causes of death, and this in turn will help us better understand the possible mechanisms linking depression to mortality. Finally, the limited psychosocial and behavioral data available in this study preclude a thorough exploration of the social and behavioral mechanisms underlying the depression-mortality effect. Identifying specific psychosocial and biological mechanisms that cause depressed persons to die prematurely should receive high priority in the next generation of studies in this area.

Accepted for publication November 1, 1999.

This article was supported in part by grants R01 MH 46015, R01 MH52247, and T32 MH19986 from the National Institute of Mental Health, grants AG13305 and AG01532 from the National Institute on Aging, and grant P50 HL65112 from the National Heart, Lung, and Blood Institute, Bethesda, Md; and the Petersen Endowed Chair Scholar Award from Oregon State University, Corvallis, Ore. The Cardiovascular Health Study is supported by contracts N01-HC-85079 through N01-HC-85086 from the National Heart, Lung, and Blood Institute.

The opinions and assertions expressed herein are those of the authors and should not be construed as reflecting those of the Uniformed Services University of the Health Sciences, Washington, DC, or the US Department of Defense.

Reprints: Richard Schulz, PhD, Department of Psychiatry and University Center for Social and Urban Research, University of Pittsburgh, 121 University Pl, Pittsburgh, PA 15260 (e-mail: schulz+@pitt.edu).

REFERENCES

1. Wulsin LR, Vaillant GE, Wells VE. A systematic review of the mortality of depression. *Psychosom Med.* 1999;61:6-17.
2. Lesperance F, Frasure-Smith N. The seduction of death [editorial comment]. *Psychosom Med.* 1999;61:18-20.
3. Barefoot JC, Scroll M. Symptoms of depression, acute myocardial infarction, and total mortality in a community sample. *Circulation.* 1996;93:1976-1980.
4. Penninx BWJH, Guralnik JM, Mendes de Leon CF, et al. Cardiovascular events and mortality in newly and chronically depressed persons >70 years of age. *Am J Cardiol.* 1998;81:988-994.
5. Rovner BW, German PS, Brant LJ, Clark R, Burton L, Folstein M. Depression and mortality in nursing homes. *JAMA.* 1991;265:993-996.
6. Yu ESH, Kean YM, Slymen CJ, Liu WT, Zhang M, Katzman R. Self-perceived health and 5-year mortality risks among the elderly in Shanghai, China. *Am J Epidemiol.* 1998;147:880-890.
7. Davidson IA, Dewey ME, Copeland JRM. The relationship between mortality and mental disorder: evidence from the Liverpool Longitudinal Study. *Int J Geriatr Psychiatry.* 1988;3:95-98.
8. Shah AK, Phongsathorn V, Geroge C, Bielawski C, Katona C. Psychiatric symptoms as predictors of mortality in continuing care geriatric patients. *Int J Geriatr Psychiatry.* 1994;9:695-702.
9. Koenig HG, Shelp F, Goli V, Cohen HJ, Blazer DG. Survival and health care utilization in elderly medical inpatients with major depression. *J Am Geriatr Soc.* 1989;37:599-606.
10. Evans ME. Depression in elderly physically ill inpatients: a 12-month prospective study. *Int J Geriatr Psychiatry.* 1993;8:587-592.
11. Murphy E, Smith R, Lindesay J, Slattery J. Increased mortality rates in late-life depression. *Br J Psychiatry.* 1988;152:347-353.
12. Callahan CM, Wolinsky FD, Stump TE, Nienaber NA, Hui SL, Tierney WM. Mortality, symptoms, and functional impairment in late-life depression. *J Gen Intern Med.* 1998;13:746-752.
13. Idler EL, Kasl SV. Health perceptions and survival: do global evaluations of health status really predict mortality? *J Gerontol.* 1991;46:S55-S65.
14. Thomas C, Kelman HR, Kennedy GJ, Ahn C, Yang CY. Depressive symptoms and mortality in elderly persons. *J Gerontol.* 1992;47:S80-S87.
15. Vogt T, Pope C, Mullooly J, Hollis J. Mental health status as a predictor of morbidity and mortality: a 15-year follow up of members of a health maintenance organization. *Am J Public Health.* 1994;84:227-231.
16. Jorm AF, Henderson AS, Kay DWK, Jacomb PA. Mortality in relation to dementia, depression, and social integration in an elderly community sample. *Int J Geriatr Psychiatry.* 1991;6:5-11.
17. Fredman L, Schoebarch VJ, Kaplan BH, et al. The association between depressive symptoms and mortality among older participants in the Epidemiologic Catchment Area–Piedmont Health Survey. *J Gerontol.* 1989;44:S149-S156.
18. Shah A. Can depression and depressive symptoms predict mortality at 18-month follow-up in acutely medically ill inpatients over the age of 80 years? *Int J Geriatr Psychiatry.* 1998;13:240-243.
19. Fried LP, Kronmal RA, Newman AB, et al. Risk factors for 5-year mortality in older adults: the Cardiovascular Health Study. *JAMA.* 1998;279:585-592.
20. Fried LP, Borhani NO, Enright P, et al. The Cardiovascular Health Study: design and rationale. *Ann Epidemiol.* 1991;1:263-276.
21. Tell GS, Fried LP, Hermanson B, Manolio TA, Newman AB, Borhani NO. Recruitment of adults 65 years and older as participants in the Cardiovascular Health Study. *Ann Epidemiol.* 1993;3:358-366.
22. Radloff LS. The CES-D scale: a self-report depression scale for research in the general population. *Appl Psychol Meas.* 1977;1:385-401.
23. Andersen EM, Marmgren JA, Carter WB, Patrick DL. Screening for depression in well older adults: evaluation of a short form of the CES-D. *Am J Prev Med.* 1994;10:77-84.
24. Kuller LH, Shemanski L, Psaty BM, et al. Subclinical disease as an independent risk factor for cardiovascular disease. *Circulation.* 1995;92:720-726.
25. Idler EL, Benyamini Y. Self-rated health and mortality: a review of twenty-seven community studies. *J Health Soc Behav.* 1997;38:21-37.
26. Anda R, Williamson D, Jones D, et al. Depressed affect, hopelessness, and the risk of ischemic heart disease in a cohort of US adults. *Epidemiology.* 1993;4:285-294.
27. Kop WJ, Appels AP, Mendes de Leon CF, de Swart HB, Bar FW. Vital exhaustion predicts new cardiac events after successful coronary angioplasty. *Psychosom Med.* 1994;56:281-287.
28. Penninx BW, Guralnik JM, Simonsick EM, Kasper JD, Ferrucci L, Fried LP. Emotional vitality among disabled older women: the Women's Health and Aging Study. *J Am Geriatr Soc.* 1998;46:807-815.
29. Schulz R. Remaining vital in the face of disability [editorial]. *J Am Geriatr Soc.* 1998;46:914-915.
30. Roberts RE, Kaplan GA, Camacho TC. Psychological distress and mortality: evidence from the Alameda County study. *Soc Sci Med.* 1990;31:527-536.
31. Pulska T, Pahkala K, Laippala P, Kivelä S-L. Major depression as a predictor of premature deaths in elderly people in Finland: a community study. *Acta Psychiatr Scand.* 1998;97:408-411.
32. Bruce ML, Leaf PJ. Psychiatric disorders and 15-month mortality in a community sample of older adults. *Am J Public Health.* 1989;79:727-730.
33. Bruce ML, Leaf PJ, Rozal GPM, Florio L, Hoff RA. Psychiatric status and 9-year mortality data in the New Haven Epidemiologic Catchment Area Study. *Am J Psychiatry.* 1994;151:716-721.
34. Aromaa A, Raitasalo R, Reunanen A, et al. Depression and cardiovascular diseases. *Acta Psychiatr Scand Suppl.* 1994:377:77-82.

MRI-Defined Vascular Depression

K. Ranga Rama Krishnan, M.D., Judith C. Hays, R.N., Ph.D., and Dan G. Blazer, M.D., Ph.D.

Objective: *The authors' goal was to characterize the clinical and demographic features of vascular depression.* *Method:* *They classified 89 depressed patients into two groups—those with vascular (N=32) and nonvascular (N=57) depression—on the basis of examination of brain magnetic resonance images. All of the patients were enrolled in the National Institute of Mental Health Clinical Research Center for the Study of Depression in Later Life, located at Duke University. The patients with vascular and nonvascular depression were compared on several clinical and demographic risk factors.* *Results:* *Bivariate analyses and a fully adjusted logistic regression model revealed that older age, late age at onset, and nonpsychotic subtype occurred more often in patients with vascular depression than in those with nonvascular depression. A family history of mental illness was found somewhat less often, and anhedonia and functional disability were seen somewhat more often in patients with vascular depression.* *Conclusions:* *The profile of patients with vascular depression needs to be developed further. This is likely to have important therapeutic and theoretical implications for the management of these patients.*

(Am J Psychiatry 1997; 154:497–501)

Risk factors for the onset of depression in late life are poorly understood. Genetic factors appear to be less important in late-onset depression than in early-onset depression (1). In contrast, structural changes in the brain, especially vascular or ischemic changes, appear to be of more importance (2, 3). Fujikawa et al. (4) used the term "silent cerebral infarction" to describe the pathology in these patients. We had introduced the term "arteriosclerotic depression" to denote depression in patients with cerebrovascular or ischemic changes in the brain (5). The term "vascular depression" may be more consistent with the current conceptualization of vascular dementia in, for example, DSM-IV, where the multiple cognitive deficits are judged to be related to multiple infarcts in the brain. We conceptualize vascular depression as depression related to multiple infarcts in the brain (we discussed this with George S. Alexopoulos, M.D., of Cornell University Medical College).

In this paper we used data from the National Institute of Mental Health (NIMH) Clinical Research Center for the Study of Depression in Later Life, located at Duke University, to further advance our understanding of vascular depression. Using brain magnetic resonance imaging (MRI), we identified depressed patients with vascular changes and compared them with depressed patients without vascular changes. The classification was based on a patients' scores on a modified Fazekas scale (6) (described in the Method section). Because depressive symptoms can occur quite often in the early stages of vascular dementia, we excluded patients whose mental status was compromised to safeguard against the confounding effect of cognitive impairment.

Five hypotheses were tested: patients with vascular depression would 1) be older, 2) have a later age at onset, 3) have less family history of mental illness, 4) report more apathy (based on our previous study noting greater loss of interest among patients with late-onset depression [7]), and 5) have more functional impairment than depressed patients without vascular changes.

METHOD

Subjects and Design

The study used a case-comparison group design. Clinical and phenomenological data for this study were obtained from patients treated at the NIMH Clinical Research Center for the Study of Depression in Later Life, located at Duke University (7). All patients with a diagnosis of major depressive disorder who had no comorbid dementia or other major neurological disorders, whose depression was not secondary to medications (e.g., steroids) or medical illnesses, and for whom brain MRI data were available were eligible for the study (N=156). As an additional safeguard against the confounding effect of cognitive impairment, patients with low-to-moderate scores on the Mini-Mental State scale (errors ≥4) (N=26) were removed from the study group. Data on age at onset were not available for 15 patients; these were dropped from further analysis. Missing values for age at onset were distributed similarly across patients with vascular and nonvascular depression. Of the remaining 115 patients, 89 had unipolar disorder and constituted the study group. Seventy-three of

Received July 15, 1996; revision received Nov. 4, 1996; accepted Nov. 11, 1996. From the Department of Psychiatry, Duke University Medical Center. Address correspondence to Dr. Krishnan, Box 3018, Duke University Medical Center, Durham, NC 27710.

Supported in part by NIMH grants MH-44716 and MH-51191.

TABLE 1. Risk Factors Among Patients With Vascular and Nonvascular Depression

Risk Factor	All Patients (N=89) N	All Patients (N=89) %	Patients With Vascular Depression (N=37) N	Patients With Vascular Depression (N=37) %	Patients With Nonvascular Depression (N=52) N	Patients With Nonvascular Depression (N=52) %	Analysis[a] Odds Ratio	Analysis[a] 95% Confidence Interval
Age (years)								
≥60	39	43.8	27	73.0	12	23.1		
<60	50	56.2	10	27.0	40	76.9		
Sex							0.87	0.30–2.51
Female	61	68.5	26	70.3	35	67.3		
Male	28	31.5	11	29.7	17	32.7		
Family history of mental illness							0.84	0.30–2.35
Yes	59	66.3	22	59.5	37	71.2		
No	30	33.7	15	40.5	15	28.8		
Family history of suicide							0.58	0.20–1.72
Yes	27	30.3	9	24.3	18	34.6		
No	62	69.7	28	75.7	34	65.4		
Family history of alcohol or drug use							1.53	0.55–4.29
Yes	45	50.6	18	48.6	27	51.9		
No	44	49.4	19	51.4	25	48.1		
Psychotic features							0.17	0.03–0.99
Yes	12	13.5	2	5.4	10	19.2		
No	77	86.5	35	94.6	42	80.8		
Loss of interest							1.40	0.45–4.34
Yes	66	74.2	29	78.4	37	71.2		
No	23	25.8	8	21.6	15	28.8		
Motor retardation							0.77	0.22–2.67
Yes	72	80.9	30	81.1	42	80.8		
No	17	19.1	7	18.9	10	19.2		
Guilt feelings							1.11	0.36–3.43
Yes	67	75.3	28	75.7	39	75.0		
No	22	24.7	9	24.3	13	25.0		
Age at onset (years)							3.35	1.02–10.97
>40 (late)	30	33.7	22	59.5	8	15.4		
≤40 (early)	59	66.3	15	40.5	44	84.6		
Number of episodes							1.66	0.52–5.32
>12	23	25.8	9	24.3	14	26.9		
≤12	66	74.2	28	75.7	38	73.1		
Montgomery-Åsberg Depression Rating Scale score							1.42	0.53–3.79
≥30	49	55.1	23	62.2	26	50.0		
<30	40	44.9	14	37.8	26	50.0		
Instrumental activities of daily living score							4.07	0.91–18.13
≥10	14	15.7	11	29.7	3	5.8		
<10	75	84.3	26	70.3	49	94.2		
Vascular symptoms							1.04	0.23–4.76
Yes	10	11.2	6	16.2	4	7.7		
No	79	88.8	31	83.8	48	92.3		

[a]Age-adjusted odds of risk factor among patients with vascular depression.

the 89 subjects had recurrent unipolar depression; 12 had psychotic features; six had a history of chronic obstructive pulmonary disease; six had a history of emphysema; none was diabetic; 15 had hypertension; 10 had cardiac disease; four had a history of alcohol dependence. The procedures and purpose of the study were explained to all patients and written informed consent was obtained from each.

Measures

Case status. MRI acquisition procedures were as follows: all subjects were screened by a technologist for presence of cardiac pacemakers, neurostimulators, metallic implants, metal in the orbit, aneurysm clips, or any other circumstance where MRI is contraindicated. Any such subjects were excluded from the study. Physicians (K.R.R.K. or another physician) conducted preliminary interviews with the screened subjects, explaining the MRI examination. The subjects wore patient gowns during scanning to eliminate any external ferromagnetic contaminants (e.g., snaps, zippers, hairpins, or bra underwire).

The standardized section of the MRI study used T_1- and T_2-weighted ^1H spin-echo pulse sequences to image the subject's brain in the head coil of the MRI system. The landmark of the imaging volume was the nasion. Calibration standards for T_2 (80- and 120-msec T_2 values) were included within the field of view. The first set of images were obtained with an axial multisection long TR (2500–3000 msec) double-echo (30–40 and 75–80 msec) spin-echo data-acquisition sequence with flow compensation gradients, 256 phase-encoding steps. To obtain enough sections to cover the whole brain, 5-mm-thick with 2.5-mm-gap acquisitions were used. Saturation of spins outside the imaging volume (standard gap=15 mm) and flow compensation (gradient moment nulling) were used routinely to eliminate artifacts due to flowing blood and CSF. This was followed by a series of T_1-weighted images (TR=500 msec, TE=20 msec) with a 256 × 192 matrix, 5-mm section thickness with 2.5-mm gap. Aliasing in the phase-encoding and frequency-encoding axes was eliminated if necessary by oversampling and filtration. These two sequences formed a "minimal" routine brain examination that is adequate for reference to clinical care standards and location of lesions but that needed additional sequences for good volume measurement and further characterization of lesions.

Lesions were classified according to a modified Fazekas classification system (8, 9), which provides a rough assessment of the extent of subcortical gray matter, deep white matter, and periventricular changes on brain MRI. Patients were classified as having vascular depression if they had a score of 2 or more on either deep white matter hyperintensity or subcortical gray matter ratings. Comparison subjects (those whose depression was nonvascular) had scores of 0 or 1 on both the deep white matter hyperintensity and subcortical gray matter ratings. A single punctate lesion in deep white matter reflects perivascular space and is considered normal; thus, the classification was based on a conservative interpretation. The large lesions correlated with areas of myelin pallor, infarcts, or lacunae (9). The ratings were conducted blind to clinical information. The intraclass correlation coefficient (ICC) for deep white matter hyperintensity was 0.85; for subcortical gray matter ICC=0.80.

Risk factors. All patients were given the Duke Depression Evaluation Schedule (7), a composite diagnostic interview instrument that includes the Center for Epidemiologic Studies Depression Scale, the Carroll Rating Scale, the NIMH Diagnostic Interview Schedule (DIS), and the Montgomery-Åsberg Depression Rating Scale. The instruments included were used separately and were enriched with items permitting diagnosis of all disorders in DSM-III and DSM-III-R, including major depressive episode, its subtypes, and comorbid psychiatric conditions (e.g., generalized anxiety, panic, and somatization disorders).

Data on all risk factors were taken from the Duke Depression Evaluation Schedule. Several of the clinical risk factors, such as age at onset, number of depressive episodes, symptoms of depression (apathy, guilt feelings, motor retardation), and subtype (psychosis), were obtained with the DIS section that assesses depression. The interrater reliability for most DIS items was 1.0, reflecting the extremely structured format of the Duke Depression Evaluation Schedule. Patients were subdivided into those with early-onset and late-onset depression by using age 40 as the cutoff. Cutoffs of 45 and 50 years were also examined. Excess risk for number of episodes was counted for patients with episodes in the highest quintile (>12). Information on family history of suicide, alcohol or drug abuse, and other mental illness was also obtained from the patients in the study. The reliability for family history of suicide was 0.83, based on a blind reassessment of videotaped interviews. Severity of depression was assessed by using the Montgomery-Åsberg Depression Rating Scale; patients were considered at high risk if their total score was 30 or higher.

Medical vascular risk was assessed as positive if the patient reported heart disease with history of hypertension or stroke or a history of hypertension and stroke. The measure of disability included nine self-reported instrumental activities of daily living items that assessed gross mobility and cognitive function (e.g., shopping and managing household finances). Instrumental activities of daily living risk was counted as positive for patients with disability scores in the highest quintile (≥10).

Analysis

Differences in risk factors between patients with vascular and nonvascular depression were examined initially with chi-square tests of differences in proportions and subsequently with logistic regression models of the vascular risk associated with each individual risk factor, adjusted for age only. No colinearity problems were evident among independent variables. A multivariable logistic regression model was also tested with all potential risk factors in the model. The relationship of risk factors to brain lesions measured as continuous variables was also examined.

TABLE 2. Multiple Logistic Regression Parameters for Comparison of 37 Patients With Vascular Depression and 52 Patients With Nonvascular Depression[a]

Risk Factor	Parameter Estimate	Standard Error	Odds Ratio	95% Confidence Interval
Age ≥60	–1.71	0.78	0.18	0.04–0.83
Female	0.03	0.65	1.03	0.29–3.72
Family history of mental illness	–1.02	0.72	0.36	0.09–1.48
Family history of suicide	–0.57	0.79	0.57	0.12–2.69
Family history of alcohol or drug use	1.49	0.79	4.42	0.94–20.88
Psychotic features	–2.52	1.16	0.08	0.01–0.79
Loss of interest	1.22	0.83	3.37	0.66–17.30
Motor retardation	–1.71	1.04	0.18	0.02–1.38
Guilt feelings	1.05	1.03	2.87	0.38–21.62
Late onset (>40 years)	1.97	0.87	7.16	1.30–39.45
Number of episodes >12	0.26	0.83	1.30	0.26–6.58
Montgomery-Åsberg Depression Rating Scale score ≥30	0.26	0.77	1.30	0.29–5.88
Instrumental activities of daily living score ≥10	1.40	0.93	4.04	0.65–25.08
Vascular symptoms	0.44	0.97	1.55	0.23–10.44

[a]–2 log likelihood χ^2=77.24, df=14, p=0.0001.

RESULTS

The distribution of risk factors in the patients with vascular and nonvascular depression is presented in table 1. Patients with vascular depression were more likely to be at least 60 years old than were patients with nonvascular depression (χ^2=21.9, df=1, p=0.001). In age-adjusted analyses, patients with vascular depression demonstrated higher odds of having nonpsychotic subtypes of depression and of having late-onset depression (>40 years) when the cutoff for age at onset was 40 years, but not when it was 45 or 50 years. In analyses adjusted only for age, vascular brain changes were not significantly disproportionate across the items of gender, family history of mental illness, depressive subtype, symptoms associated with the index episode, number of episodes, symptom severity, functional disability, or medical history of vascular problems. The relationship between age at onset and severity of hyperintensity was nonlinear when age was controlled for.

In fully controlled analyses (table 2), patients with vascular depression demonstrated significantly higher odds of being elderly, nonpsychotic, and having a late-onset depressive disorder. In addition, the odds of a family history of alcohol or drug abuse, functional disability, and anhedonia were greater than four or three times those of the patients with nonvascular depression (table 2). However, the confidence intervals associated with these odds ratios demonstrated that chance cannot be excluded as the reason for differences in the proportions. The number of subjects limits the precision of these estimates. Cognitively impaired subjects demonstrated more cardiovascular comorbidity and a trend toward more hyperintensities. Hyperintensities were more frequent in older men than in younger men or older women.

We also regressed continuously distributed scores for deep white matter hyperintensity over all risk factors in ordinary least squares models. Age, family history of alcohol use, and nonpsychotic subtype were strongly significant risk factors. Other risk factors were in the direction of hypothesized relationships (data not shown).

DISCUSSION

The present study of a relatively large number of depressed patients whose vascular or nonvascular depression was determined by MRI provides limited support for all five hypotheses. We found that both crude and adjusted risks of vascular depression were associated with age and late-onset depressive illness. These results validate earlier studies showing a link between vascular changes and late-onset depression (10–14). Lower risk of a family history of mental disorder or suicide and higher risk of anhedonia and functional disability were evident among patients with vascular depression, although chance cannot be ruled out as the explanation. The lack of significance may be related to an insufficient number of subjects and also the lack of clinically significant differences in these variables. The results of this study may reflect a unique group of patients who seek evaluation in a clinical research center. Further studies in larger numbers of patients are needed to expand on these initial results. The findings also suggest that depression—even in patients with cerebrovascular changes—is probably multifactorial and that genetic factors and life events continue to be important. The genetic factors in this group of patients may be different and could be related to the genetic risk factors for vascular disease.

The concept of vascular depression is subject to the same limitations as the concept of vascular dementia. The major problem with these concepts is that they presuppose that vascular factors are the sole cause of the syndrome. In the case of vascular dementia there is increasing recognition that vascular factors are often contributors even though they may not be the primary cause of the cognitive deficits (15–17). In a similar vein, we have speculated that depression in patients with cerebrovascular disease is also multifactorial in origin and that vascular factors are but one etiologic factor. In the case of vascular dementia, treatment of vascular risk factors has not been shown to provide cognitive improvement (18). To a certain extent, the findings affirm the effects of coexisting cerebrovascular disease, i.e., increased disability. At the current time there are limited data suggesting that treatment response is different in these patients (19). We are in the process of completing long-term outcome studies that could supplement the limited data now available. It is possible that treatment of vascular risk factors may be of benefit in patients with vascular depression.

We have suggested that depression in these patients may be the result of damage to the striato-pallido-thalamo-cortical pathways (20). The damage due to the lesions may cause depression either by means of direct disruption of the circuits regulating mood or disruption of the norepinephrine and serotonin circuits that regulate this system. Studies evaluating monoamine function and functional imaging studies may provide further exposition of the pathophysiology of vascular depression.

The concept of vascular depression may have diagnostic, prognostic, and treatment implications. Further studies are needed to evaluate if the cause of illness, disability, and cognitive impairment is different in these patients. The demonstration by recent epidemiologic studies that the type of vascular changes seen in the brain are related to carotid atherosclerosis, hypertension, and history of myocardial infarcts (21, 22) also points to the need for evaluating vascular risk more closely in these patients and designing suitable treatment regimens to reduce these risk factors. Treatment could include regimens such as a low-fat, low-salt diet, use of suitable pharmacological strategies to control high cholesterol or hypertension, and surgical techniques to treat carotid atherosclerosis.

REFERENCES

1. Mendlewicz J, Baron M: Morbidity risks in subtypes of unipolar depressive illness: differences between early and late onset forms. Br J Psychiatry 1981; 139:463–466
2. Coffey CE, Figiel GS, Djang WT: Leukoencephalopathy in elderly depressed patients referred for ECT. Biol Psychiatry 1988; 24:143–161
3. Lesser IM, Miller BL, Boone KB: Brain imaging and cognitive function in late-onset psychotic depression. J Neuropsychiatry 1991; 3:33–40
4. Fujikawa T, Yamawaki S, Touhouda Y: Incidence of silent cerebral infarction in patients with major depression. Stroke 1993; 24:1631–1634
5. Krishnan KRR, McDonald WM: Arteriosclerotic depression. Med Hypotheses 1995; 44:77–145
6. Fazekas F, Chawluk JB, Alavi A: MR signal abnormalities at 1.5T in Alzheimer's dementia and normal aging. AJNR Am J Neuroradiol 1987; 8:421–426
7. Krishnan KRR, Hays JC, Tupler LA, George LK, Blazer DG: Clinical and phenomenological comparisons of late-onset and early-onset depression. Am J Psychiatry 1995; 152:785–788
8. Greenwald BS, Kramer-Ginsberg E, Krishnan KRR, Ashtari M, Aupperle PM, Patel M: MRI signal hyperintensities in geriatric depression. Am J Psychiatry 1996; 153:1212–1215
9. Krishnan KRR, Boyko OB, McDonald WM, Charles HC, MacFall J, Tupler LA, Upchurch L: Magnetic resonance morphometry: image analysis methodology development for affective disorder. Depression 1993; 1:159–171
10. Coffey CE, Figiel GS, Djang WT, Saunders WB, Weiner RD: White matter hyperintensity on MRI clinical and neuroanatomic correlates in the depressed elderly. J Neuropsychiatry Clin Neurosci 1989; 1:135–144
11. Coffey CE, Figiel GS, Djang WT, Weiner RD: Subcortical hyperintensity on magnetic resonance imaging: a comparison of normal and depressed elderly subjects. Am J Psychiatry 1990; 147: 187–189
12. Figiel GS, Krishnan KRR, Doraiswamy PM, Rao VP, Nemeroff CB, Boyko OB: Subcortical hyperintensities on brain magnetic resonance imaging: a comparison between late age onset and early onset elderly depressed subjects. Neurobiol Aging 1991; 26:245–247
13. Zubenko GS, Sullivan P, Nelson JP, Belle SH, Huff FJ, Wolf GL: Brain imaging abnormalities in mental disorders of late life. Arch Neurol 1990; 47:1107–1113
14. Rabins PV, Pearlson GD, Aylward E, Kumar AJ, Dowell K: Cortical magnetic resonance imaging changes in elderly inpatients with major depression. Am J Psychiatry 1991; 148:617–620
15. Geldmacher DS, Whitehouse PJ: Multi infarct dementia, in Psy-

chopharmacology: The Fourth Generation of Progress. Edited by Bloom FE, Kupfer DJ. New York, Raven Press, 1993, pp 1513–1520
16. Brust JCM: Vascular dementia is overdiagnosed. Arch Neurol 1988; 45:799–801
17. O'Brien MD: Vascular dementia is underdiagnosed. Arch Neurol 1988; 45:797–798
18. Meyer JS, Judd BW, Tawakma T, Rogers RL, Mortel KF: Improved cognition after control of risk factors for MID. JAMA 1986; 256:2203–2209
19. Hickie I, Scott E, Mitchell P, Wilhelm K, Austin MP, Bennett B: Subcortical hyperintensities on magnetic resonance imaging: clinical correlates and prognostic significance in patients with severe depression. Biol Psychiatry 1995; 37:151–160
20. Krishnan KRR: Neuroanatomic substrates of depression in the elderly. J Geriatr Psychiatry Neurol 1993; 1:39–58
21. Bots ML, van Swieten JC, Breteler MM, de Jong PT, van Gijn J, Hofman A, Grobbee DE: Cerebral white matter lesions and atherosclerosis in the Rotterdam Study. Lancet 1993; 341:1232–1237
22. Manolio TA, Kronmal RA, Burke GL, Poirier V, O'Leary DH, Gardin JM, Fried LP, Steinberg EP, Bryan RN: Magnetic resonance abnormalities and cardiovascular disease in older adults: the Cardiovascular Health Study. Stroke 1994; 25:318–327

The Relationship of Depression to Cardiovascular Disease

Epidemiology, Biology, and Treatment

Dominique L. Musselman, MD; Dwight L. Evans, MD; Charles B. Nemeroff, MD, PhD

This article reviews the burgeoning literature on the relationship of mood disorders and heart disease. Major depression and depressive symptoms, although commonly encountered in medical populations, are frequently underdiagnosed and undertreated in patients with cardiovascular disease (CVD). This is of particular importance because several studies have shown depression and its associated symptoms to be a major risk factor for both the development of CVD and death after an index myocardial infarction. This review of the extant literature is derived from MEDLINE searches (1966-1997) using the search terms "major depression," "psychiatry," "cardiovascular disease," and "pathophysiology." Studies investigating pathophysiological alterations related to CVD in depressed patients are reviewed. The few studies on treatment of depression in patients with CVD are also described. Treatment of depression in patients with CVD improves their dysphoria and other signs and symptoms of depression, improves quality of life, and perhaps even increases longevity. Recommendations for future research are proposed.

Arch Gen Psychiatry. 1998;55:580-592

People never die of love or grief alone: though some die of inherent maladies, which the tortures of those passions prematurely force into destructive action.

Charlotte Bronte, Shirley, 1848

Depressive syndromes and major depression are exceedingly common. A recent comprehensive study, the National Comorbidity Study, reported lifetime prevalence rates of major depression and dysthymia of 13% and 5%, respectively.[1] Point prevalence rates of major depression in primary care outpatients range from 2% to 16% and from 9% to 20% for all depressive disorders[2-7] and are even higher in medical inpatients; 8% for major depression and 15% to 36% for all depressive disorders.[8,9]

Minor depressive disorder (depressive symptoms subthreshold in severity to major depression and dysthymia) is also common in the community[10-14] and in primary care clinics.[2,4,15-17] The Epidemiologic Catchment Area Study of more than 18 500 people reported the lifetime prevalence rate of subthreshold depressive symptoms to be 23%, in comparison with 6%, the sum of the prevalence rates of major depression and dysthymia.[14]

Though depression in patients with coronary artery disease (CAD) is rarely diagnosed by primary care physicians and cardiologists,[18-23] recognition and treatment of major depression is crucial, especially for patients after myocardial infarction (MI). Not only do depressed patients experience great difficulties in problem solving and coping with challenges, but depression adversely affects compliance with medical therapy[24] and rehabilitation[25,26] and increases medical comorbidity.[25] Minor depressive disorder is also associated with significant functional impairment and substantial increases in health care utilization.[13,14,27,28]

From the Department of Psychiatry and Behavioral Sciences, Emory University School of Medicine, Atlanta, Ga (Drs Musselman and Nemeroff); and the Department of Psychiatry, University of Pennsylvania School of Medicine, Philadelphia (Dr Evans).

This article is also available on our Web site: www.ama-assn.org/psych.

In patients with CAD, depression predicts future cardiac events[21,29,30] and hastens mortality.[23,31,32] Since the 1960s, multiple longitudinal and cross-sectional studies have scrutinized the association of cardiovascular disease (CVD), especially CAD, with depressive symptoms, as well as with major depression. This review of the extant literature is derived from MEDLINE searches (1966-1977), using the search terms "major depression," "psychiatry," "heart disease," and "pathophysiology."

EPIDEMIOLOGY

Depression and Cardiovascular Disease

Early studies reported the prevalence of depression to be from 18% to 60% in patients with CAD.[18,19,25,33,34] Later studies report relatively consistent prevalence rates of depression in patients with CVD, ranging from 16% to 23% (mean, 19%; median, 18%), despite the potential methodological weaknesses of some of the studies listed in **Table 1** (such as the use of unmodified psychiatric diagnostic instruments to determine the prevalence of depression, excluding patients because of severity of CVD, and measuring depressive symptoms at different times after hospital admission) and methodological differences among the studies (dissimilar patient populations, different diagnostic instruments, hospitalization status, or unspecified type of heart disease). Furthermore, structured clinical interviews such as the Diagnostic Interview Schedule[35] may not have the same validity in patients with CAD as in the general population.

Although severity of physical illness is one of the most important variables associated with depression in patients with other medical illnesses, studies of patients with CVD do not document a higher prevalence rate of depression in patients with measures of more advanced CVD or with a greater level of disability.[21-23,32]

Table 1. Prevalence of Major Depression in Patients With Cardiovascular Disease*

Study	No. and Type of Patients	Diagnostic Method	Prevalence, %
Carney et al[24]	52 patients with CAD undergoing elective cardiac catheterization	DIS	18
Schleifer et al[22]	283 patients hospitalized with MI	SADS	18
Frasure-Smith et al[23]	222 patients hospitalized with MI	DIS	16
Gonzalez et al[37]	99 patients hospitalized with CAD	DIS	23

*CAD indicates coronary artery disease; DIS, Diagnostic Interview Schedule, version III[35]; MI, myocardial infarction; and SADS, Schedule for Affective Disorders and Schizophrenia.[36]

Depression as a Risk Factor for Ischemic Heart Disease

The notion that having a psychiatric illness such as major depression increases one's risk for developing ischemic heart disease remains controversial and has been often intuitively "explained" by the hypothesis that persons with psychiatric disorders generally have other risk factors for the development of CAD.[38] **Table 2** contains studies with the most rigorous methods that are prospective in design, have used structured clinical interviews or diagnostic instruments, have included other risk factors for CVD in their analysis (such as hypertension, hypercholesterolemia, nicotine and other substance abuse, and physical inactivity), and controlled for demographic factors (such as age, sex, and socioeconomic status).

Nearly all the recent studies in Table 2 document increased cardiovascular morbidity and mortality in patients with depressive symptoms or major depression, thereby implicating depression as an independent risk factor in the pathophysiologic progression of CVD, rather than merely a secondary emotional response to the illness. Such large epidemiologic studies may use self-report instruments, rather than clinical interviews, to evaluate the importance of psychological factors in predicting CVD. Assessments of this type are typically added to large, multiple risk factor studies in which population-based samples are followed up prospectively.[38] The advantage of using "dimensional" measures of depression (rather than a categorical diagnosis of major depression) is the increased statistical power to detect smaller "effects." However, such epidemiologic data are not equivalent to clinical data.

A relatively large clinical study supporting depression as an independent risk factor for CVD observed that patients with major depression experience elevated mortality rates from CVD. Frasure-Smith and colleagues[23,32] found depression to be a significant predictor of mortality ($P<.001$) in 222 patients 6 months after MI. Depression remained a significant predictor of mortality ($P=.01$), even after multivariate statistical methodology was used to factor out the effects of left ventricular dysfunction and previous MI. Multiple logistic regression analyses revealed depression was significantly related to 18-month cardiac mortality, even after controlling for other significant multivariate predictors of mortality (previous MI, Killip class, frequency of premature ventricular contractions [PVCs]) ($P=.003$).

BIOLOGY

Hypothalamic-Pituitary-Adrenocortical and Sympathomedullary Hyperactivity

Recent advances in biological psychiatry have included the discoveries of numerous neurochemical, neuroendocrine, and neuroanatomic alterations in unipolar depression. Proposed as important adjuncts in the diagnosis of depressed subjects, certain of these biologic markers may reflect important pathophysiologic alterations that contribute to the increased vulnerability of depressed patients to CVD. These include sympathoadrenal hyperactivity, diminished heart rate variability (HRV), ventricular instability and myocardial ischemia in reaction to mental stress, and alterations in platelet receptors and/or reactivity (**Figure 1**).[61]

Two primary components central to the "fight or flight" stress re-

Table 2. Antecedent Depression and Subsequent Risk of Cardiovascular Disease (CVD)*

Source	No. and Type of Patients	Diagnostic Method	Relative Risk (RR) of Major Depression or Depressive Symptoms for CVD or CVD-Related Death
Ostfeld et al[39]	1990 male Western Electric employees	MMPI[40] 16 PF[41]	None
Brozek et al[42]	258 men	MMPI[43]	None
Goldberg et al[44]	82 pairs (male and female) of case/control subjects randomly selected from 2 communities	CES-D Scale[45] (plus 4 other depression scales)	None
Murphy et al[46]	1003 male and female subjects from the community	DPAX algorithm[47]	For CVD-related death, men = 2.5, women = 1.5
Anda et al[48]	2832 men and women (aged 45-77 y)	Depression subscale of GWS[49]	For IHD-related death, 1.5-2.1
Aromaa et al[50]	5355 men and women (aged 40-64 y)	PSE[50]	For MI, men = 2.62, women = 1.90
Ford et al[51]	1198 men	Depression questionnaire	For MI, 1.9
Vogt et al[52]	1187 men and 1386 women (aged ≥18 y) in an HMO	Depression scale[53]	Depressive symptoms not related to incidence of CVD
Simonsick et al[54]	1063 men and 2398 women (aged ≥65 y with hypertension	CES-D Scale[45]	Elevated rates of CVD-related death in women with high scores of depressive symptoms
Everson et al[55]	2428 men (aged 42-60 y)	Hopelessness self-report questionnaire	For CVD-related death, RH = 2.52 (with moderate hopelessness score); RH = 3.90 (with high hopelessness scores)
Barefoot and Schroll[56]	409 men and 321 women (all born in 1914)	MMPI[57]	For MI, 1.7
Pratt et al[58]	1551 men and women	DIS[35]	For MI, odds ratio = 2.07 (history of dysphoria); odds ratio = 4.54 (history of major depressive disorder)
Wassertheil-Smoller et al[59]	4736 men and women >60 y with hypertension	CES-D[60]	Baseline CES-D score ≥16 did not predict future MI; RR of future MI per 5-unit increase in CES-D score: women = 1.2

**MMPI indicates Minnesota Multiphasic Personality Inventory; PF, Personality Factor; CES-D, Center for Epidemiological Studies Depression Scale; DPAX, computer diagnosis of depression and anxiety; GWS, General Well-Being Schedule; IHD, ischemic heart disease; PSE, Present State Examination; MI, myocardial infarction; HMO, health maintenance organization; RH, relative hazard; and DIS, Diagnostic Interview Schedule.*

sponse observed by Cannon in 1911[62] and the "general adaptation syndrome" described by Selye[63] are the hypothalamic-pituitary-adrenocortical axis and sympathoadrenal system. In response to stress, hypothalamic neurons containing corticotropin-releasing factor (CRF) increase synthesis and release of corticotropin (ACTH), β-endorphin, and other pro-opiomelanocortin products from the anterior pituitary gland. Many studies have documented evidence of hypothalamic-pituitary-adrenocortical axis hyperactivity within medication-free patients with major depression, ie, elevated CRF concentrations in cerebrospinal fluid,[64-69] blunting of the ACTH response to CRF administration, nonsuppression of cortisol secretion following dexamethasone administration, hypercortisolemia, and pituitary and adrenal gland enlargement, as well as direct evidence of increased numbers of hypothalamic CRF neurons in the postmortem tissue of depressed patients as compared with controls.[70,71] Administered corticosteroids have long been known to induce hypercholesterolemia, hypertriglyceridemia, and hypertension. Other atherosclerosis-inducing actions of steroids include injury of vascular endothelial cells,[72] intima,[73-75] and inhibition of normal healing.[76] Indeed, elevated morning plasma cortisol concentrations have been significantly correlated with moderate to severe coronary atherosclerosis in young and middle-aged men.[77]

Many patients with major depression also exhibit dysregulation of the sympathoadrenal system. The adrenal medulla and sympathetic nervous system together comprise the sympathoadrenal system. Although the central nervous system regulation of the sympathoadrenal system is only partially characterized, hypothalamic CRF-containing neurons provide stimulatory input to several autonomic centers involved in regulating sympathetic activity.[78-80] Nerve impulses from regulatory centers in the central nervous system control catecholamine release from the sympathoadrenal system. Physiological and pathological conditions causing sympathoadrenal activation include physical activity, coronary ischemia, heart failure, and mental stress. Epinephrine in plasma is derived from the adrenal medulla whereas plasma norepinephrine (NE) concentrations reflect its secretion largely from sympathetic nerve terminals, with the remaining NE provided from the adrenal medulla and extra-adrenal chromaffin cells. Peripheral plasma NE concentrations are determined not only by rate of release from sympathetic nervous system nerve terminals, but also by reuptake into presynaptic terminals, local metabolic degradation, and redistribution into multiple physiological compartments.

Hypersecretion of NE in unipolar depression has been documented by elevated plasma NE and NE metabolite concentrations[81-84] and elevated urinary concentrations of NE and its metabolites. Not only do depressed patients exhibit higher basal plasma concentrations of NE but those with melancholia

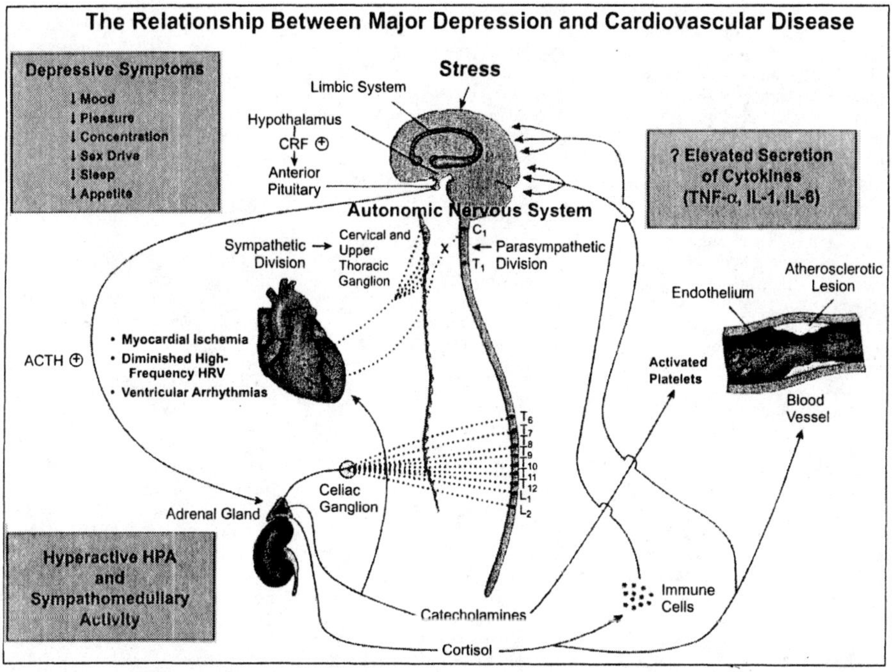

Figure 1. *Hypothetical schema of pathophysiologic alterations associated with depression that likely contribute to increased vulnerability to cardiovascular disease (CVD). Autonomic nervous system innervation of the heart via parasympathetic vagus (X) and sympathetic (postganglionic efferents from cervical and upper thoracic paravertebral ganglia) nerves is shown. CRF indicates corticotropin-releasing factor; ACTH, corticotropin; TNF-α, tumor necrosis factor α; IL-1, interleukin 1; IL-6, interleukin-6; HRV, heart rate variability; and HPA, hypothalamic-pituitary-adrenocortical axis.*

exhibit even greater elevations in plasma NE concentrations when subjected to orthostatic challenge than do normal control subjects and depressed patients without melancholia.[85] Furthermore, depressed patients who are dexamethasone test nonsuppressors exhibit significantly higher basal and cold-stimulated plasma concentrations of NE than depressed patients who are dexamethasone test suppressors.[85] Following treatment with tricyclic antidepresssants (TCAs), urinary excretion of NE and its metabolites diminish with plasma NE concentrations,[86-91] though Veith and colleagues[84] reported that long-term treatment with desipramine increased plasma concentrations of norepinephrine. Thus, sympathoadrenal hyperactivity seems to represent a state, rather than a trait, marker of depression, possibly reflecting increased CRF release within the central nervous system.

Sympathoadrenal hyperactivity contributes to the development of CVD through effects of catecholamines upon the heart, blood vessels, and platelets. Sympathoadrenal activation modifies the function of circulating platelets through direct effects on the platelet, catecholamine-induced changes of hemodynamic factors (increased shear stress), circulating lipids, and inhibition of vascular eicosanoid synthesis.[92] Arachidonic acid metabolites, such as prostaglandins and leukotrienes, contribute to diverse circulatory and hemostatic functions including inhibition of platelet aggregation and vascular contractility and permeability.[93] Elevations of plasma NE levels are found most frequently in young hypertensive patients[94] and subjects with high-cardiac-output borderline hypertension who later proceed to established high-resistance hypertension.[95]

Even normotensive depressed patients have been found to exhibit greater heart rates at rest, after orthostasis, and after exercise in comparison with normal controls. These depressed patients also exhibited increased plasma concentrations of NE and serotonin at rest.[96] Thus, the sympathoadrenal hyperactivity observed in many patients with major depression may contribute to the development of CVD via effects of catecholamines on cardiac function and platelets.

Diminished Heart Rate Variability

Alterations in autonomic nervous system activity, as demonstrated by reduced HRV, represent another potential mechanism contributing to the diminished survival of depressed patients with CVD. It is believed that the beat-to-beat fluctuations in hemodynamic parameters reflect the dynamic response of the cardiovascular control systems to a myriad of naturally occurring physiological perturbations, such as fluctuations in heart rate associated with respiration. Therefore, fluctuations in heart rate may provide a sensitive measure of the functioning of the rapidly reacting sympathetic, parasympathetic, and renin-angiotensin systems. Cardiovascular homeostasis is maintained by the parasympathetic and sympathetic nervous systems via afferent pressoreceptors and chemoreceptors and efferents that alter heart rate, atrioventricular conduction, and contractility and impinge on the peripheral vasculature, altering arterial and venous vasomotor tone.[97]

Heart rate variability is the standard deviation of successive intervals between 2 successive R waves (the first positive defelection of a QRS complex) on an electrocardiogram in sinus rhythm and reflects the interplay and balance between sympathetic and parasympathetic input on the cardiac pacemaker. Peripheral control of HRV is mainly via the parasympathetic cholinergic vagus nerve.[98] Central generation and control of heart rate is regulated by the hypothalamus, the limbic system, and the brainstem. Numerous central nervous system neurotransmitters are involved in modulating HRV, including acetylcholine, NE, serotonin, and dopamine.[99,100]

A high degree of HRV is observed in normal hearts with good cardiac function, whereas HRV can be significantly decreased in patients with severe CAD or heart failure.[101] Moreover, the relative risk of sudden death after acute MI is significantly higher in patients with decreased HRV.[102-107] Heart rate variability is one of many postinfarction prognostic factors (others include age, left ventricular ejection fraction, and frequency of arrythmias). Its positive predictive power is relatively modest when considered in isolation. Although positive predictive accuracy is not high when HRV is considered in combination with other prognostic factors,[108,109] clinically useful levels of negative predictive accuracy can be achieved.[108-110] Of the many arrhythmogenic factors, autonomic tone is the most difficult to measure,[110] and thus interest in HRV continues. Power spectral analysis measurements of HRV are often used because certain frequency bands of the heart period power spectrum have been associated with autonomic nervous system control of the sinus node.[111-113] The low-frequency power of the heart period power spectrum reflects modulation of sympathetic and vagal tone by baroreflex activity,[114] while high-frequency power reflects modulation of vagal tone, primarily by respiratory frequency and depth (the respiratory sinus arrhythmia).[115,116] The physiological mechanisms contributing to ultra low and very low-frequency power of the heart period spectrum (which account for >90% of the total power in a 24-hour period) remain obscure. In a study of 715 patients after MI, certain frequency bands (total, ultra low and very low-frequencies) of the heart period power spectrum were strongly associated with mortality during 4 years of follow up, even after adjustment for other major risk factors. Indeed, very low-frequency power was most strongly associated with death secondary to arrhythmia.[117]

Reduced high-frequency HRV has been observed in depressed patients in comparison with nondepressed groups,[101,118] though discrepant reports exist.[119,120] In patients with angiographically confirmed CAD, diminished HRV during 24-hour Holter monitoring was significantly more common in depressed patients than in matched nondepressed patients.[121] Diminished high-frequency HRV is thought to reflect decreased parasympathetic tone, possibly predisposing to ventricular arrhythmias and perhaps to the excessive cardiovascular mortality found in patients with CVD and comorbid major depressive disorder.[122] One study (without a placebo control group) revealed normalization of reduced HRV of depressed patients after effective treatment.[123] The prognostic importance of antidepressant-induced improvement in diminished HRV in depressed patients remains an intriguing area of research. Subsequent investigation will seek to determine the processes underlying ultralow and very low-frequency bands of the heart power spectrum; whether these bands are altered in depressed patients (with or without CVD) remains obscure.

Myocardial Ischemia and Ventricular Instability in Reaction to Mental Stress

It has long been thought that the combination of a vulnerable myocardium after MI, acute ischemia, and negative emotional arousal can trigger fatal ventricular arrhythmias.[124] The interplay of these factors in patients with CAD is being increasingly scrutinized. Jiang and colleagues[125] followed up 126 patients with CAD during a 5-year period. Mental stress–induced myocardial ischemia at baseline in patients with CAD was associated with significantly higher rates of subsequent fatal and nonfatal cardiac events, independent of age, baseline left ventricular ejection fraction, and previous MI. This study proposed that the relationship between psychological stress and adverse cardiac events is mediated by myocardial ischemia. Although myocardial ischemia is likely the most significant factor in predisposition to ventricular instability, other factors contribute. Central nervous system control mechanisms can significantly decrease the threshold for ventricular fibrillation.[126] Ventricular fibrillation is believed to be the mechanism underlying sudden cardiac death, the most common cause of fatality among patients with CAD.[127] Psychological stress predisposes to abnormal ventricular activity by lowering the ventricular vulnerable period threshold even to the point of fibrillation. The vagus nerve, however, exerts antiarrhythmic activity by direct action on the ventricular myocardium and interference with sympathetic activity.[128] Increased parasympathetic activity has a protective effect on myocardium electrically destabilized by increased adrenergic tone.[127]

Psychological and physical events can elicit a stress response; ie, the reaction of an organism to deleterious forces that disturb physiologic homeostasis.[129,130] Psychological stress in humans with CAD increases ventricular ectopic activity and increases the risk of ventricular fibrillation.[131,132] There are several similarities between the stress response and major depression. Both can be characterized by increased blood pressure and heart rate, as well as increased arousal and increased mobilization of energy stores.[133] Particularly relevant to both the stress response and depression are 2 critical brain structures, the locus coeruleus and the central nucleus of the amygdala, which are in turn both innervated by CRF-containing nerve terminals.[134,135] The stress response and major depression do differ, however, in some respects. In depression, some aspects of the normal stress response seem to escalate to a pathologic state[136] that fails to respond appropriately to usual counterregulatory responses, resulting in a sustained version of a usually transient phenomenon (such as hyperactivity of the hypothalamic-pituitary-adrenocortical axis or sympathoadrenal system). However, although many studies have linked stressful life events to onset of major depression,[137,138] some depressions are clearly endogeneous; ie, they have no obvious environmental precipitant.

Frasure-Smith and colleagues[32] proposed that depression worsens prognosis after MI via another mechanism, PVCs. The risk of sudden cardiac death associated with significant depressive symptoms was greatest among patients with 10 or more PVCs per hour (60% of these patients died within 18 months), suggesting arrhythmia as the link between depression and sudden cardiac death.[32] Depressed patients with CAD are not more likely to have arrhythmias than patients with CAD and no depression, but the risk associated with depression is largely confined to patients with PVCs. Patients who were not depressed experienced little increase in risk associated with PVCs, even in the presence of low left ventricular ejection fraction.[32] Thus, the prognostic impact of PVCs may be more related to depression than to PVCs per se. In the Cardiac Arrhythmia Supression Trial,[139] suppression of PVC frequency in post-MI patients did not reduce and actually increased mortality, even though previous studies revealed that PVCs are associated with increased mortality after MI. Treatment of depression may be the necessary component to improve survival in patients with PVCs.

Alterations in Platelet Receptors and/or Reactivity

The adverse effects of depression on cardiovascular disease may be also mediated via platelet mechanisms. Markovitz and Matthews[140] first proposed that enhanced platelet responses to psychological stress might trigger adverse coronary artery ischemic events. This association between platelet activation and vascular disease is indirectly supported by studies linking cerebrovascular disease and depression. The Established Populations for Epidemiologic Studies of the Elderly prospectively studied 10 294 persons aged 65 years and older for 6 years and determined that rates of stroke (adjusted for age, physical disability, and other medical disorders) were 2.3 to 2.7 times higher in persons designated with "high" vs "low" levels of depressive symptoms.[54] In another prospective study, 103 consecutive stroke patients[141] were assessed for major depression or dysthymia approximately 2 weeks after stroke. Patients with major depression or dysthymia were 3.4 times more likely to have died during the 10-year follow-up period than were nondepressed patients ($P = .007$), even after controlling for confounding variables (age, medical comorbidity, type of stroke, and lesion location) ($P = .03$).

Platelets play a central role in hemostasis, thrombosis, development of atherosclerosis, and acute coronary syndromes[142] through their interactions both with subendothelial components of damaged vessel walls and plasma coagulation factors, primarily thrombin. Human platelets contain adrenergic, serotonergic, and dopaminergic receptors. Through stimulation of the α_2-adrenoceptors on platelet membranes, increases in levels of circulating catecholamines (>4 nmol/L) potentiate the effects of other agonists and, at higher concentrations, initiate platelet responses, including secretion, aggregation, and activation of the arachidonate pathway. Following injury to vessel endothelium, platelets and circulating leukocytes attach to the newly exposed subendothelial layer. Platelet adhesion to collagen (and other components of the subendothelial matrix) exposed within a denuded area of the vascular endothelium and thrombin stimulates platelet activation. Activation converts platelet membrane GPIIb/IIIa complexes into functional receptors for fibrinogen. Activation is also accompanied by extrusion or secretion of platelet storage granule contents into the extracellular environment. Platelets activated at the interface with a vessel wall injury accelerate the local formation of thrombin and release a variety of products from their storage granules, including chemotactic and mitogenic factors inducing leukocyte migration from the blood stream and vascular cell proliferation. These secreted platelet products, such as platelet factor 4, β-thromboglobulin, and serotonin, stimulate and recruit other platelets and cause irreversible platelet-platelet aggregation, leading to formation of a fused-platelet thrombus. Platelets also contribute to vascular damage by stimulating lipoprotein uptake by macrophages and mediating vasoconstriction through the production and/or release of substances such as thromboxane A_2, platelet-activating factor, and serotonin.[96] Clinical trials have confirmed the importance of the platelet in vascular damage; antiaggregating medications are useful in secondary prevention[143-145] and delay progression of atherosclerotic lesions.[146] Many of these processes are depicted in **Figure 2**.

We wondered whether heightened susceptibility to platelet activation might be a mechanism by which depression in physically healthy young persons acts as a significant risk factor for heart and cerebrovascular disease and/or mortality after MI. Utilizing fluorescence-activated flow cytometric analysis, we discovered that, in comparison with 8 normal controls, 12 depressed patients exhibited enhanced baseline platelet activation and responsiveness.[147]

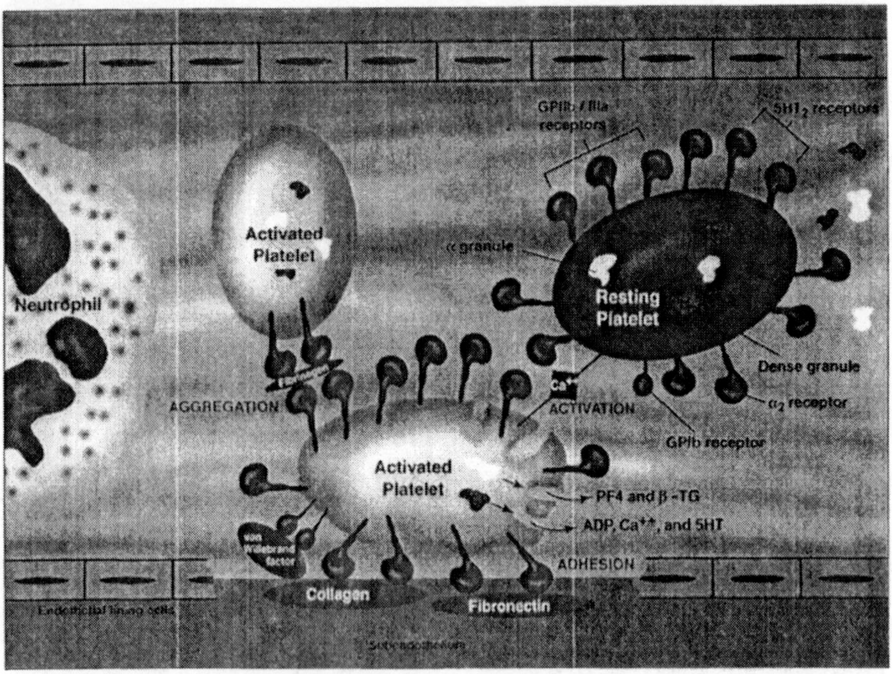

Figure 2. *Platelet adhesion to collagen exposed within the denuded area of vascular endothelium has stimulated platelet activation. Activation is accompanied by extrusion of platelet storage granule contents, which recruits other platelets, causes irreversible platelet-platelet aggregation, and forms a fused platelet thrombus. Ca++ indicates intracellular free calcium concentrations; PF4, platelet factor 4; β-TG, β-thromboglobulin; ADP, adenosine diphosphate; and 5HT, serotonin. Adapted from R&D Systems, Minneapolis, Minn. Used with permission.*

In another recent pilot study, 21 patients suffering from comorbid CVD and major depression exhibited increased platelet activation as measured by markedly elevated plasma concentrations of platelet secretion products platelet factor 4 and β-thromboglobulin when compared with 17 healthy control subjects and 8 nondepressed patients with CVD.[148] Although the mechanism(s) responsible remain unknown, we believe that heightened susceptibility to platelet activation and secretion underlies, at least in part, the increased vulnerability of depressed patients to CVD and/or mortality after MI.

Serotonin secreted by platelets induces both platelet aggregation and coronary vasoconstriction, both mediated by $5HT_2$ receptors. Vasoconstriction especially occurs when normal endothelial cell counterregulatory mechanisms of vascular relaxation are defective, as often occurs in patients with CAD.[148-150] Indeed, essential hypertension, elevated plasma cholesterol levels, older age, and smoking, well-known predisposing factors for development of CVD, all contribute to serotonin-mediated platelet activation. Moreover alterations of platelet serotonin-mediated activation have also been described in affective disorders, most notably major depression. Considerable evidence has accrued in the last 2 decades supportive of the hypothesis that alterations in central nervous system and platelet serotonergic function occur in depressed patients.[151]

Serotonin-mediated platelet activation can contribute to the development of atherosclerosis, thrombosis, and vasoconstriction. Even though serotonin itself is a weak platelet agonist, it markedly amplifies platelet reactions to a variety of other agonists such as adenosine diphosphate, thromboxane A_2, catecholamines, or thrombin. By an action on $5HT_2$ receptors, serotonin enhances the extent of platelet aggregation and the release of intragranular products and arachidonic acid metabolites in response to otherwise ineffective agonist concentrations.[150] Such serotonergic platelet amplification occurs at low concentrations attained when serotonin is released from seeping platelets subjected to shear stresses[152] and from platelet activation by contact with an arterial wall lesion.[153,154]

Several investigators have reported increases in platelet $5HT_2$ binding density in depressed patients.[155-159] Moreover, the changes seem to be state-dependent, in that $5HT_2$ binding-site density decreased to control values only in those patients who showed clinical improvement. Depressed patients have been found to exhibit significant reductions in the number of platelet and brain serotonin transporter sites as detected by [^{3}H]imipramine hydrochloride binding,[160-163] as well as the more selective ligand [^{3}H]paroxetine hydrochloride.[151,164] The increased $5HT_2$ receptor–binding density and decreased serotonin transporter sites suggest that depressed patients may be particularly susceptible to serotonin-mediated platelet activation and coronary artery vasoconstriction. Decreased numbers of platelet serotonin transporters would potentially hinder uptake and storage of periplatelet serotonin, exposing the increased numbers of $5HT_2$ receptors to serotonin.[165]

Platelets of depressed patients exhibit significantly increased elevations of intracellular free calcium concentrations after serotonin stimulation in comparison with controls.[166-168] Even functionally trivial increases in intraplatelet calcium "prime" the platelet secretion and aggregation response to stimulation by even a "weak" agonist (such as serotonin)[169] or in response to increased rate of blood flow. Thus, platelets with elevated intracellular free calcium concentrations, as observed in depressed patients, would likely exhibit increased activation in comparison with normal comparison subjects under basal conditions or in response to shear-induced aggregation (eg, following an orthostatic challenge). Future investigations will seek to confirm and interconnect the pathophysiological mechanisms of sympathoadrenal hyperactivity, exaggerated platelet reactivity, and alterations in the platelet serotonin system in depressed patients to their propensity for the development of CVD.

TREATMENT

Although some stress management or behavioral counseling programs with CVD patients have been associated with reduced risk of recurrent cardiovascular events[170] and increased rates of long-term (5-year) survival,[171-173] more recent studies report no benefit to patients[174,175] or an even worse outcome for women in comparison with usual care.[176]

Because of fewer potential adverse effects on the cardiovascular system and the lack of lethality in overdose, somatic treatment with selective serotonin reuptake inhibitors (SSRIs) or other atypical antidepressants (such as buproprion or nefazodone) may offer significant advantages in depressed patients with CVD. The cardiac toxic effects of the TCAs and related antidepressants limit their clinical use in patients with CVD. The reader is directed toward excellent reviews on the safety and efficacy of TCAs in patients with CVD.[177,178] Monoamine oxidase inhibitors and trazodone are generally free of effects on cardiac conduction, but, like the TCAs, may cause postural hypotension.[179] Because the SSRIs are newer than TCAs, little systematic research on their efficacy in elderly or CAD patients has been performed, including large-scale, randomized, treatment trials of post-MI patients with comorbid major depression.[180,181] A recent randomized, double-blind multicenter study compared the efficacy of nortriptyline and paroxetine in depressed patients with ischemic heart disease.[182] Both antidepressants were effective in the treatment of depression but, not surprisingly, there were more dropouts because of adverse effects and more cardiac-related effects with the TCA. The ongoing SADHART study, a randomized, multicenter, double-blind trial of sertraline vs placebo in the treatment of post-MI patients with comorbid major depression, seeks to determine the efficacy of this antidepressant in the depressed post-MI patient. Although these agents may be as effective as TCAs in depressed patients with CVD, their safety is not well established in this patient population.

Psychotherapeutic and/or psychopharmacologic treatment of the 15% to 23% of post-MI patients who fulfill the criteria for major depression, as well as those with significant dysphoria but subsyndromal depression, may have a significant effect (positive or negative) on both medical morbidity and mortality. Although the belief that the outcomes of CVD patients may be improved if their comorbid depressive symptoms are treated is tantalizing, the patient's perspective and preferences must be respected. Feelings of sadness are an expected response to painful life experiences, including being informed that one has a diagnosis of heart disease or has experienced an MI. These feelings may be coupled with reactions of shock, disbelief, anxiety, and other responses. Many patients would not agree that their persisting "sadness" or "loss of interest" constitutes a depressive syndrome. However, when these symptoms are of such a magnitude and duration that they fulfill *DSM-IV* criteria for major depression, a clinician's threshold for psychotherapeutic or psychopharmacologic intervention is reached, given the increased morbidity and mortality of depressed CVD patients. Because of advances in medical management of CVD patients, therapeutic trials determining improvement in survival must be quite large[176]; for example, the 22-month CAST trial was composed of 1489 subjects.[139] Such experience cautions against the raising of hopes toward demonstrating improving cardiac outcome via antidepressant treatment of depression in patients with CVD. Yet, awaiting the completion of a large-scale mortality trial similar to the CAST may not be appropriate given the interpersonal, social, and medical burden of depression and early indications of SSRI efficacy in depressed CVD patients. After short-term treatment with paroxetine or fluvoxamine, depressed patients exhibited no changes in HRV.[119] The only currently known cardiac effect of SSRIs is severe sinus node slowing, to date reported in only a few cases.[183,184] There have been some reports of alterations of hemostasis[185-187] and platelet aggregation[188] following treatment with fluoxetine. Because serotonin has been implicated both in platelet aggregation and coronary artery vasoconstriction, it is of paramount importance to determine whether the SSRIs, widely used to treat major depression, produce effects on platelet function. Because of inhibition of cytochrome P450 isoenzymes, SSRIs must be used with caution, particularly in those patients receiving medications metabolized by the P450 2D6 isoenzyme (such as lipophilic β-blockers and type 1C antiarrhythmics [encainide, flecainide, mexiletene, and propafenone]) and the P450 3A4 isoenzyme (such as calcium channel blockers and warfarin).[189]

FUTURE DIRECTIONS FOR RESEARCH

The principal unanswered questions in this field remain primarily prognostic, etiologic, and treatment-related: By what mechanisms does dysphoria and other depressive symptoms affect the cardiovascular and thrombotic systems—and will treatment of depression prevent or reduce CVD? Investigative strategies would include additional prospective studies of post-MI patients with comorbid depression. Because sociodemographic and medical variables do not reliably identify post-MI patients who are depressed while hospitalized nor predict those who will become depressed soon after hospital discharge,[190] identification of certain so-called biologic markers associated with depression (such as hypothalamic-pituitary-adrenocortical axis or sympathoadrenal system hyperactivity) might accurately identify those CVD patients with prodromal or subsyndromal depressive symptoms vulnerable to complications or even early death after MI. Certainly such investigations will determine whether such biologic alterations in depressed patients with CVD normalize after effective psychiatric treatment, and whether such change is associated with diminished morbidity and mortality of post-MI patients.

Other prospective studies might scrutinize biologic markers in depressed patients (without CVD); longitudinal follow-up of these patients (and fluctuations of such markers) over time could determine their utility as markers for the development of CVD. These biologic markers include platelet reactivity and markers of systemic inflammation,[191,192] as well as certain components of HRV, myocardial ischemia, or ventricular instability, particularly in those persons who respond to mental stress with depressive symptoms.[190]

Future studies should focus on women to assess gender-specific psychosocial and physiologic measures.[193,194] Despite the fact that women are more vulnerable to depression and that CVD is the leading cause of death among adult women in the United States, relatively little research has focused on the etiology and pathogenic mechanisms of major depression among women with CVD.[190,195] Which treatment modalities (psychotherapeutic vs psychopharmacologic or a combination) will be most effective in patients with recurrent or more severe depression remains to be determined. Commonly used SSRIs might be more effective and more easily tolerated than TCAs in patients with CVD, particularly in elderly patients. Treatment studies may also assess the relationship between depression and subsequent compliance with medication and risk factor modification for CVD.[32]

Illumination of the interplay between central nervous system, platelet, and cardiovascular processes, particularly in those patients with CVD and major depression, will undoubtedly lead to the development of new treatment modalities that will not only improve these patients' quality of life but potentially decrease their morbidity and improve long-term survival rates.

Accepted for publication February 20, 1998.

This research was supported by grants MH-01399, MH-42088, MH-49523, and RR-00039 from the National Institutes of Health, Bethesda, Md, and an Established Investigator Award from the National Alliance for Research on Schizophrenia and Depression, Chicago, Ill (Dr Nemeroff).

We are grateful for the assistance of James Browning, Laurence A. Harker, MD, Anne Griswell, Barbara J. Lewison, Bettina T. Knight, BSN, Drema Salvatore, David P. Schroeder, MD, and Paul Robinson, MD. We apologize to those colleagues whose work could not be cited due to space restraints.

Reprints: Charles B. Nemeroff, MD, PhD, Department of Psychiatry and Behavioral Sciences, Emory University School of Medicine, 1639 Pierce Dr, Suite 4000, Atlanta, GA 30322.

REFERENCES

1. Kessler RC, McGonagle KA, Zhao S, Nelson CB, Hughes M, Eshleman S, Wittchen HU, Kendler KS. Lifetime and 12-month prevalence of *DSM-III-R* psychiatric disorders in the United States: results from the National Comorbidity Survey. *Arch Gen Psychiatry.* 1994;51:8-19.
2. Hoeper EW, Nycz GR, Cleary PD. Estimated prevalence of RDC mental disorders in primary care. *Int J Ment Health.* 1979;8:6-15.
3. Leeper J, Badger L, Milo T. Mental disorders among physical disability determination patients. *Am J Public Health.* 1985;75:78-79.
4. Blacker CVR, Clare AW. Depressive disorder in primary care. *Br J Psychiatry.* 1987;150:737-751.
5. Barrett JE, Barrett JA, Oxman TE, Gerber PD. The prevalence of psychiatric disorders in a primary care practice. *Arch Gen Psychiatry.* 1988; 45:1100-1106.
6. Von Korff M, Shapiro S, Burke JD, Teitlebaum M, Skinner EA, German P, Turner RW, Klein L, Burns B. Anxiety and depression in a primary care clinic: comparison of Diagnostic Interview Schedule, General Health Questionnaire, and practitioner assessments. *Arch Gen Psychiatry.* 1987; 44:152-156.
7. Cohen-Cole SA, Kaufman KG. Major depression in physical illness: diagnosis, prevalence, and antidepressant treatment (a ten-year review: 1982-1992). *Depression.* 1993;1:181-204.
8. Magni G, Schifano F, DeLeo D. Assessment of depression in an elderly medical population. *J Affect Disord.* 1986;11:121-124.
9. Feldman E, Mayou R, Hawton K, Ardern M, Smith EB. Psychiatric disorder in medical inpatients. *QJM.* 1987;63:405-412.
10. Boyd JH, Weissman MM. Epidemiology of affective disorders. *Arch Gen Psychiatry.* 1981; 38:1039-1046.
11. Blazer D, Swartz M, Woodbury M, Manton KG, Hughes D, George LK. Depressive symptoms and depressive diagnoses in a community population: use of a new procedure for analysis of psychiatric classification. *Arch Gen Psychiatry.* 1988; 45:1078-1084.
12. Bebbington P, Katz R, McGuffin P, Tennant C, Hurry J. The risk of minor depression before age 65: results from a community survey. *Psychol Med.* 1989;19:393-400.
13. Broadhead WE, Blazer DG, George LK, Tse CK. Depression, disability days, and days lost from work in a prospective epidemiologic survey. *JAMA.* 1990;264:2524-2528.
14. Johnson J, Weissman MM, Klerman GL. Service utilization and social morbidity associated with depressive symptoms in the community. *JAMA.* 1992;267:1478-1483.
15. Shepherd M, Cooper B, Brown AC, Kalton GW. *Psychiatric Illness in General Practice.* London, England: Oxford University Press; 1966.
16. Kessler LG, Cleary PD, Burke JD Jr. Psychiatric disorders in primary care: results of a follow-up study. *Arch Gen Psychiatry.* 1985;42:583-587.
17. Ormel J, Koeter MWJ, van den Brink W, van de Willige G. Recognition, management, and course of anxiety and depression in general practice. *Arch Gen Psychiatry.* 1991;48:700-706.
18. Kurosawa H, Shimizu Y, Nishimatsu Y, Hirose S, Takano T. The relationship between mental disorders and physical severities in patients with acute myocardial infarction. *Jpn Circ J.* 1983; 47:723-725.
19. Wynn A. Unwarranted emotional distress in men with ischaemic heart disease. *Med J Aust.* 1967; 2:847-851.
20. Mayou R, Foster A, Williamson B. Medical care after myocardial infarction. *J Psychosom Res.* 1979;23:23-26.
21. Carney RM, Rich MW, teVelde A, Saini J, Clark K, Jaffe AS. Major depressive disorder in coronary artery disease. *Am J Cardiol.* 1987;60: 1273-1275.
22. Schleifer SJ, Macari-Hinson MM, Coyle DA,

Slater WR, Kahn M, Gorlin R, Zucker HD. The nature and course of depression following myocardial infarction. *Arch Intern Med.* 1989; 149:1785-1789.

23. Frasure-Smith N, Lesperance F, Talajic M. Depression following myocardial infarction: impact on 6-month survival. *JAMA.* 1993;270: 1819-1861.
24. Blumenthal JA, Williams RS, Wallace AG, Williams RB, Needles TL. Physiological and psychological variables predict compliance to prescribed exercise therapy in patients recovering from myocardial infarction. *Psychosom Med.* 1982;44:519-527.
25. Stern JJ, Pascale L, Ackerman A. Life adjustment post myocardial infarction: determine predictive variables. *Arch Intern Med.* 1977;137: 1680-1685.
26. Mayou R, Foster A, Williamson B. Psychosocial adjustment in patients one year after myocardial infarction. *J Psychosom Res.* 1978;22:447-453.
27. Skodol AE, Schwartz S, Dohrenwend BP, Levav I, Shrout PE. Minor depression in a cohort of young adults in Israel. *Arch Gen Psychiatry.* 1994;51: 542-551.
28. Wells KB, Stewart A, Hayes RD, Burnam MA, Rogers W, Daniels M, Berry S, Greenfield S, Ware J. The functioning and well-being of depressed patients: results of the Medical Outcomes Study. *JAMA.* 1989;262:914-919.
29. Carney RM, Rich MW, Freedland KE, Saini J. Major depressive disorder predicts cardiac events in patients with coronary artery disease. *Psychosom Med.* 1988;50:627-633.
30. Aromaa A, Raitasalo R, Reunanen A, Impivaara O, Heliovaara M, Kneckt P, Lehtinen V, Joukamaa M, Maatela J. Depression and cardiovascular diseases. *Acta Psychiatr Scand.* 1994;377: 77-82.
31. Ahern DK, Gorkin L, Anderson JL, Tierney C, Hallstrom A, Ewart C, Capone RJ, Schron E, Kornfeld D, Herd JA, Richardson DW, Follick MJ, for the CAPS Investigators. Biobehavioral variables and mortality or cardiac arrest in the Cardiac Arrhythmia Pilot Study (CAPS). *Am J Cardiol.* 1990;66:59-62.
32. Frasure-Smith N, Lesperance F, Talajic M. Depression and 18-month prognosis after myocardial infarction. *Circulation.* 1995;91:999-1005.
33. Hackett TP, Cassem, NH, Wishnie HA. The coronary-care unit: an appraisal of its psychologic hazards. *N Engl J Med.* 1968;279:1365-1370.
34. Cay EL, Vetter N, Philip AE, Dugard P. Psychological status during recovery from an acute heart attack. *J Psychosom Res.* 1972;16:425-436.
35. Robins LN, Helzer JE, Croughan JL, Williams JBW, Spitzer RL. The NIMH Diagnostic Interview Schedule, Version III. Public Health Service (HSS), ADM-T-42-3 (5-81, 8-81). Washington DC; 1981.
36. Endicott J, Spitzer RL. A diagnostic interview: the Schedule for Affective Disorders and Schizophrenia. *Arch Gen Psychiatry.* 1978;35:837-844.
37. Gonzalez MB, Snyderman TB, Colket JT, Arias RM, Jiang JW, O'Connor CM, Krishnan KR. Depression in patients with coronary artery disease. *Depression.* 1996;4:57-62.
38. Hayward C. Psychiatric illness and cardiovascular disease risk. *Epidemiol Rev.* 1995;17: 129-138.
39. Ostfeld AM, Lebovits BZ, Shekelle RB, Paul O. A prospective study of the relationship between personality and coronary heart disease. *J Chronic Dis.* 1964;17:265-276.
40. Hathaway SR, McKinley JC. *Minnesota Multiphasic Personality Inventory Manual (Revised Edition).* New York, NY: The Psychological Corporation; 1951.
41. Cattell, RB, Saunders DR, Stice G. *Handbook for the Sixteen Personality Factor Questionnaire.* Champaign, Ill: Institute for Personality and Ability Testing; 1957.
42. Brozek J, Keyes A, Blackburn H. Personality differences between potential coronary and noncoronary subjects. *Ann NY Acad Sci.* 1966;134: 1057-1064.
43. Dahlstrom WG, Welsh GS. *A MMPI Handbook: A Guide to Use in Clinical Practice and Research.* Minneapolis, Minn: University of Minnesota Press; 1960.
44. Goldberg EL, Comstock GW, Hornstra RK. Depressed mood and subsequent physical illness. *Am J Psychiatry.* 1979;136:530-534.
45. Radloff LS. The CES-D scale: a self-report depression scale for research in the general population. *J Applied Psychol Meas.* 1977;1:385-401.
46. Murphy JM, Monson RR, Olivier DC, Sobol AM, Leighton AH. Affective disorders and mortality. *Arch Gen Psychiatry.* 1987;44:473-480.
47. Murphy JM, Neff RK, Sobol AM, Rice JX, Olivier DC. Computer diagnosis of depression and anxiety: the Stirling County Study. *Psychol Med.* 1985;15:99-112.
48. Anda R, Williamson D, Jones D, Macera C, Eaker E, Glassman A, Marks J. Depressed affect, hopelessness, and the risk of ischemic heart disease in a cohort of U.S. adults. *Epidemiology.* 1993;4:285-294.
49. Dupuy HJ. A concurrent validational study of the NCHS General Well-Being Schedule. Vital Health Stat. 1977; No. 73.
50. Wing JK, Cooper JE, Sartorius N. The measurement and classification of psychiatric symptoms. London, England: Cambridge University Press; 1974.
51. Ford DE, Mead LA, Chang PP, Levine DM, Klag MJ. Depression predicts cardiovascular disease in men: the Precursors Study [abstract]. *Circulation.* 1994;90(Suppl I):614.
52. Vogt T, Pope C, Mullooly J, Hollis J. Mental heath status as a predictor of morbidity and mortality: a 15-year follow-up of members of a health maintenance organization. *Am J Public Health.* 1994;84:227-231.
53. McFarland BH, Freeborn DK, Mullooly JP, Pope CR. Utilization patterns among long-term enrollees in a prepaid group practice health maintenance organization. *Med Care.* 1985;23: 1221-1233.
54. Simonsick EM, Wallace RB, Blazer DG, Berkman LF. Depressive symptomatology and hypertension-associated morbidity and mortality in older adults. *Psychosom Med.* 1995;57: 427-435.
55. Everson SA, Goldberg DE, Kaplan GA, Cohen RD, Pukkala E, Tuomilehto J, Salonen JT. Hopelessness and risk of mortality and incidence of myocardial infarction and cancer. *Psychosom Med.* 1996;58:113-121.
56. Barefoot JC, Schroll M. Symptoms of depression, acute myocardial infarction, and total mortality in a community sample. *Circulation.* 1996; 93:1976-1980.
57. Greene RL. *The MMPI-2/MMPI: An Interpretive Manual.* Boston, Mass: Allyn and Bacon; 1991.
58. Pratt LA, Ford DE, Crum RM, Armenian HK, Gallo JJ, Eaton WW. Depression, psychotropic medication, and risk of myocardial infarction: prospective data from the Baltimore ECA follow-up. *Circulation.* 1996;94:3123-3129.
59. Wassertheil-Smoller S, Applegate WB, Berge K, Chang CJ, Davis BR, Grimm R, Kostis J, Pressel S, Schron E, for the SHEP Cooperative Research Group. Change in depression as a precursor of cardiovascular events. *Arch Intern Med.* 1996;156:553-561.
60. Berkman LF, Berkman CS, Kasl S, Freeman DH Jr, Ostfeld AM, Cornoni-Huntley J, Brody JA. Depressive symptoms in relation to physical health and functioning in the elderly. *Am J Epidemiol.* 1986;124:372-388.
61. Musselman DL, Knight BT, Baron A, Nemeroff CB. Further studies on altered platelet reactivity in major depression. Presented at Society of Biological Psychiatry Annual Meeting, May 27-31, 1998, Toronto, Canada.
62. Vingerhoets A. *Psychosocial Stress: An Experimental Approach.* Groningen, the Netherlands: Swets & Zeitlinger; 1985.
63. Selye H. *The Stress of Life.* New York, NY: McGraw-Hill; 1956.
64. Nemeroff CB, Widerlov E, Bissette G, Walleus H, Karlsson I, Eklund K, Kilts CD, Loosen PT, Vale W. Elevated concentrations of CSF corticotropin-releasing factor–like immunoreactivity in depressed patients. *Science.* 1984;226:1342-1344.
65. Arato M, Banki CM, Nemeroff CB, Bissette G, Hypothalamic-pituitary-adrenal axis and suicide. *Ann N Y Acad Sci.* 1986;487:263-270.
66. Banki CM, Bissette G, Arato M, O'Connor L, Nemeroff CB. Cerebrospinal fluid corticotropin-releasing factor-like immunoreactivity in depression and schizophrenia. *Am J Psychiatry.* 1987;144:873-877.
67. Banki CM, Karmasci L, Bissette G, Nemeroff CB. CSF corticotropin-releasing and somatostatin in major depression: response to antidepressant treatment and relapse. *Eur Neuropsychopharmacol.* 1992;2:107-113.
68. France RD, Urban B, Krishnan KRR, Bissett G, Banki CM, Nemeroff C, Spellman FJ. CSF corticotropin-releasing factor-like immunoreactivity in chronic pain patients with and without major depression. *Biol Psychiatry.* 1988;23:86-88.
69. Risch SC, Lewine RJ, Kalin NH, Jewart RD, Risby ED, Caudle JM, Stipetic M, Turner J, Eccard MB, Pollard WE. Limbic-hypothalamic-pituitary-adrenal axis activity and ventricular-to-brain ratio studies in affective illness and schizophrenia. *Neuropsychopharmacology.* 1992;6:95-100.
70. Raadsheer FC, Hoogendijk WJG, Stam FC, Tilders FJH, Swaab DF. Increased numbers of corticotropin-releasing hormone expressing neurons in the hypothalamic paraventricular nucleus of depressed patients. *Neuroendocrinology.* 1994;60:436-444.
71. Raadsheer FC, van Heerikhuize JJ, Lucassen PJ, Hoogendijk WJG, Tilders FJH, Swaab DF. Corticotropin-releasing hormone mRNA levels in the paraventricular nucleus of patients with Alzheimer's disease and depression. *Am J Psychiatry.* 1995;152:1372-1376.
72. Bjorkerud S. Effect of adrenocortical hormones on the integrity of rat aortic endothelium. In: Schettler G, and Weizel A, eds. *Proceedings of the 3rd International Symposium on Atherosclerosis.* Berlin, Germany: Springer-Verlag; 1973:245.
73. Nahas GG, Brunson JG, King WM, Cavert HM. Functional and morphologic changes in heart

lung preparations following administration of adrenal hormones. *Am J Clin Pathol.* 1958;34: 717-729.

74. Valigorsky JM. Metaplastic transformation of aortic smooth muscle cells in cortisone-induced dissecting aneurysms in hamsters. *Fed Proc.* 1969; 28:802.
75. Kemper JW, Baggenstoss AH, Slocumb CH. The relationship of therapy with cortisone to the incidence of vascular lesions in rheumatoid arthritis. *Ann Intern Med.* 1957;46:831-851.
76. Ross R, Harker L. Hyperlipidemia and atherosclerosis. *Science.* 1976;193:1094-1100.
77. Troxler RG, Sprague EA, Albanese RA, Fuchs R, Thompson AJ. The association of elevated plasma cortisol and early atherosclerosis as demonstrated by coronary angiography. *Atherosclerosis.* 1977;26:151-162.
78. Swanson LW, Sawchenko PE. Organization of ovine corticotropin-releasing factor immunoreactive cells and fibers in the rat brain: an immunohistochemical study. *Neuroendocrinology.* 1983;36:165-186.
79. Merchenthaler I, Vigh S, Petruscz P, Schally AV. Immunocytochemical localization of corticotropin-releasing factor (CRF) in the rat brain. *Am J Anatomy.* 1982;165:385-396.
80. Cummings S, Elde R, Ellis J, Lindall A. Corticotropin-releasing factor immunoreactivity is widely distributed with the central nervous system of the rat: an immunohistochemical study. *J Neurosci.* 1983;8:1355-1368.
81. Wyatt RJ, Portnoy B, Kupfer DJ, Snyder F, Engelman K. Resting plasma catecholamine concentrations in patients with depression and anxiety. *Arch Gen Psychiatry.* 1971;24:65-70.
82. Louis WJ, Doyle AE, Anavekar SN. Plasma noradrenaline concentration and blood pressure in essential hypertension, phaeochromocytoma and depression. *Clin Soc.* 1975;48:239S-242S.
83. Roy A, Pickar D, DeJong J, Karoum F, Linnoila M. Norepinephrine and its metabolites in cerebrospinal fluid, plasma, and urine: relationship to hypothalamic-pituitary-adrenal axis function in depression. *Arch Gen Psychiatry.* 1988;45: 849-857.
84. Veith RC, Lewis L, Linares OA, Barnes RF, Raskin MA, Villacres EC, Murburg MM, Ashleigh EA, Castillo S, Peskind ER, Pascualy M, Halter JB. Sympathetic nervous system activity in major depression: basal and desipramine-induced alterations in plasma norepinephrine kinetics. *Arch Gen Psychiatry.* 1994;51:411-422.
85. Roy A, Guthrie S, Pickar D, Linnoila M. Plasma NE responses to cold challenge in depressed patients and normal controls. *Psychiatry Res.* 1987; 21:161-168.
86. Charney DS, Menkes DB, Henninger GR. Receptor sensitivity and the mechanism of action of antidepressant treatment. *Arch Gen Psychiatry.* 1981;38:1160-1180.
87. Golden RN, Markey SP, Risby ED, Rudorfer MV, Cowdry RW, Potter WZ. Antidepressants reduce whole-body norepinephrine turnover while enhancing 6-hydroxymelatonin output. *Arch Gen Psychiatry.* 1988;45:150-154.
88. Linnoila M, Karoum F, Calil HM, Kopin IJ, Potter WZ. Alteration of NE metabolism with desipramine and zimelidine in depressed patients. *Arch Gen Psychiatry.* 1982;39:1025-1028.
89. Linnoila M, Guthrie S, Lane EA, Karoum F, Rudorfer M, Potter WZ. Clinical studies on NE metabolism: how to interpret the numbers. *Psychiatry Res.* 1986;17:229-239.
90. Scubee-Moreau JJ, Dresse AE. Effect of various antidepressant drugs on the spontaneous firing rate of locus coeruleus and raphe dorsalis neurons of the rat. *Eur J Pharmacol.* 1979; 57:219-225.
91. Sulser F, Vetulani J, Mobley PL. Mode of action on antidepressant drugs. *Biochem Pharmacol.* 1978;27:257-261.
92. Anfossi G, Trovati M. Role of catecholamines in platelet function: pathophysiological and clinical significance. *Eur J Clin Invest.* 1996;26:353-370.
93. Gerritsen ME. Physiological and pathophysiological roles of eicosanoids in the microcirculation. *Cardiovasc Res.* 1996;32:720-732.
94. Goldstein DS. Plasma catecholamines and essential hypertension: an analytical review. *Hypertension.* 1983;5:86-99.
95. Lund-Johansen P. Hemodynamic alterations in early essential hypertension: recent advances. In: Gross F, Strasser T, eds. *Mild Hypertension: Recent Advances.* New York, NY: Raven Press; 1983:237-249.
96. Lechin F, van der Dijs B, Orozco B, Lechin ME, Baez S, Lechin AE, Rada I, Acosta E, Arocha L, Jimenez V, Leon G, Garcia Z. Plasma neurotransmitters, blood pressure, and heart rate during supine-resting, orthostasis, and moderate exercise conditions in major depressed patients. *Biol Psychiatry.* 1995;38:166-173.
97. Akselrod S, Gordon D, Ubel FA, Shannon DC, Barger AC, Cohen RJ. Power spectrum analysis of heart rate fluctuation: a quantitative probe of beat-to-beat cardiovascular control. *Science.* 1981;213:220-222.
98. Low PA. Autonomic nervous system function. *J Clin Neurophysiol.* 1993;10:14-27.
99. Spyer KM. Central nervous system control of the cardiovascular system. In: Bannister, R, ed. *Autonomic Failure: A Textbook of Clinical Disorders of the Autonomic Nervous System.* Oxford, England: Oxford University Press; 1988:56-79.
100. Shields RW. Functional anatomy of the autonomic nervous system. *J Clin Neurophysiol.* 1993;10:2-13.
101. Dalack GW, Roose SP. Perspectives on the relationship between cardiovascular disease and affective disorder. *J Clin Psychiatry.* 1990;51 (suppl):4-9.
102. Wolf M, Varigos G, Hunt D, Sloman JG. Sinus arrhythmia in acute myocardial infarction. *Med J Aust.* 1978;2:52-53.
103. Billman GE, Schwartz PJ, Stone HL. Baroreceptor reflex control of heart rate: a predictor of sudden cardiac death. *Circulation.* 1982;66:874-880.
104. Kleiger RE, Miller PJ, Bigger TJ, Moss AJ, and the Multicenter Post-Infarction Research Group. Decreased heart rate variability and its association with increased mortality after acute myocardial infarction. *Am J Cardiol.* 1987;59: 256-262.
105. Bigger JT, Kleiger RE, Fleiss JL, Rolnitzky LM, Steinman RC, Miller JP. Components of HR variability measured during healing of acute myocardial infarction. *Am J Cardiol.* 1988;61: 208-215.
106. LaRovere MT, Specchia G, Mortana A, Schwartz PJ. Baroreflex sensitivity, clinical correlates, and cardiovascular mortality among patients with a first myocardial infarction: a prospective study. *Circulation.* 1988;78:816-824.
107. Cripps T, Malik M, Farrell T, Camm AJ. Prognostic value of reduced heart rate variability after myocardial infarction: clinical evaluation of a new analysis method. *Br Heart J.* 1991;65: 14-19.
108. Viskin S, Belhassen B. Noninvasive and invasive strategies for the prevention of sudden death after myocardial infarction: value, limitations and implications for therapy. *Drugs.* 1992;44: 336-355.
109. Araya-Gomez V, Gonzalez-Hermosillo J, Casanova-Garces J, Colin L, Kershenovich S, Iturralde P. Identification of patients at risk of malignant arrythmia in the 1st year after myocardial infarction [in Spanish]. *Arch Inst Cardiol Mex.* 1994; 64:145-159.
110. Campbell RWF. Can analysis of heart rate variability predict arrhythmias and antiarrhythmic effects? In: Oto AM, ed. *Practice and Progress in Cardiac Pacing and Electrophysiology.* Dordrecht, the Netherlands: Kluwer Academic Publishers; 1996:63-69.
111. Sayers BM. Analysis of heart rate variability. *Ergonomics.* 1973;16:17-32.
112. Pomeranz B, Macaulay RJB, Caudill MA, Kutz I, Adam D, Gordon D, Kilborn KM, Barger AC, Shannon DC, Cohen RJ, Benson H. Assessment of autonomic function in humans by heart rate spectral analysis. *Am J Physiol.* 1985;248: H151-H153.
113. Pagani M, Lombardi F, Guzzetti S, Rimoldi O, Furlan R, Pizzinelli P, Sandrone G, Malfatto G, Dell'Orto S, Piccaluga E, Turiel M, Baselli G, Cerutti S, Malliani A. Power spectral analysis of heart rate and arterial pressure variabilities as a marker of sympathovagal interaction in man and conscious dog. *Circ Res.* 1986;59: 178-193.
114. Koizumi K, Terui N, Kollai M. Effect of cardiac vagal and sympathetic nerve activity on heart rate in rhythmic fluctuations. *J Autonom Nerv Syst.* 1985;12:251-259.
115. Katona PG, Jih F. Respiratory sinus arrhythmia: noninvasive measure of the parasympathetic cardiac control. *J Appl Physiol.* 1975; 39:801-805.
116. Fouad FM, Tarazzi RC, Gerrario CM, Fighaly S, Alicandri C. Assessment of parasympathetic control of heart rate by a noninvasive method. *Am J Physiol.* 1984; 246:H838-842.
117. Bigger TJ Jr, Fleiss JL, Steinman RC, Rolnitzky LM, Kleiger RE, Rottman JN. Frequency domain measures of heart period variability and mortality after myocardial infarction. *Circulation.* 1992;85:164-171.
118. Miyawaki E, Salzman C. Autonomic nervous system tests in psychiatry: implications and potential uses of heart rate variability. *Integrated Psychiatry.* 1991;7:21-28.
119. Rechlin T, Weis M, Claus D. Heart rate variability in depressed patients and differential effects of paroxetine and amitriptyline on cardiovascular autonomic functions. *Pharmacopsychiatry.* 1994;27:124-128.
120. Yeragani VK, Pohl R, Ramesh C, Glitz D, Weinberg P, Merlos B. Effect of imipramine treatment on heart rate variability measures. *Neuropsychobiology.* 1992;26:27-32.
121. Carney RM, Saunders RD, Freedland KE, Stein P, Rich MW, Jaffe AS. Association of depression with reduced heart rate variability in coronary artery disease. *Am J Cardiol.* 1995;76: 562-564.
122. Roose SP, Glassman AH, Dalack GW. Depression, heart disease, and tricyclic antidepressants. *J Clin Psychiatry.* 1989;50(suppl 7):12-16.
123. Balogh S, Fitzpatrick DF, Hendricks SE, Paige SR. Increases in heart rate variability with success-

ful treatment in patients with major depressive disorder. *Psychopharmacol Bull.* 1993;29: 201-206.
124. Verrier RL. Behavioral stress, myocardial ischemia, and arrhthmias. In: Zipes DP, Jalife J, eds. *Cardiac Electrophysiology From Cell to Bedside.* Philadelphia, Pa: WB Saunders Co; 1990: 343-352.
125. Jiang W, Babyak M, Krantz DS, Waugh RA, Coleman RE, Hanson MM, Frid DJ, McNulty S, Morris JJ, O'Connor CM, Blumenthal JA. Mental stress-induced myocardial ischemia and cardiac events. *JAMA.* 1996;21:1651-1656.
126. Lown B, DeSilva RA, Reich P, Murawski BJ. Psychophysiologic factors in sudden cardiac death. *Am J Psychiatry.* 1980;137:1325-1335.
127. Lown B, Verrier RL. Neural activity and ventricular fibrillation. *N Engl J Med.* 1976;294:1165-1170.
128. Zaza A, Schwartz PJ. Role of the autonomic nervous system in the genesis of early ischemic arrhythmias. *J Cardiovasc Pharmacol.* 1985;7 (suppl 5):S8-S12.
129. *Stedman's Medical Dictionary.* Baltimore, Md: Williams & Wilkins; 1982.
130. Heit S, Owens MJ, Plotsky P, Nemeroff CB. Corticotropin-releasing factor, stress, and depression. *Neuroscientist.* 1997;3:186-194.
131. Tavazzi L, Zotti AM, Rondanelli R. The role of psychologic stress in the genesis of lethal arrhythmias in patients with coronary artery disease. *Eur Heart J.* 1986;7(suppl):99-106.
132. Follick MJ, Gorkin L, Capone RJ, Smith TW, Ahern DK, Stablein D, Niaura R, Visco J. Psychological distress as a predictor of ventricular arrhthmias in a post-myocardial infarction population. *Am Heart J.* 1988;116:32-36.
133. Gold PW, Gooodwin FK, Chrousos GP. Clinical and biochemical manifestations of depression: relation to the neurobiology of stress. *N Engl J Med.* 1988;319:413-420.
134. Valentino RJ, Foote SL, Page ME. The locus coeruleus as a site for integrating corticotropin-releasing factor and noradrenergic mediation of stress responses. *Ann N Y Acad Sci.* 1993;697: 173-188.
135. Curtis AL, Pavcovich LA, Grigoriadis DE, Valentino RJ. Previous stress alters corticotropin-releasing factor neurotransmission in the locus coeruleus. *Neuroscience.* 1995;65:541-550.
136. Chrousos GP, Gold PW. The concepts of stress and stress system disorders: overview of physical and behavioral homeostasis. *JAMA.* 1992; 267:1244-1252.
137. Paykel E. Causal relationships between clinical depression and life events. In: Barrett JE, ed. *Stress and Mental Disorder.* New York, NY: Raven Press; 1979.
138. Kendler KS, Kessler RC, Neale MC, Heath AC, Eaves LJ. The prediction of major depression in women: toward an integrated etiologic model. *Am J Psychiatry.* 1993;150:1139-1148.
139. Echt DS, Liebson PR, Mitchell LB, Peters RW, Obias-Manno D, Barker AH, Arensberg, D, Baker A, Friedman L, Greene HL, Huther ML, Richardson DW, and the CAST Investigators. Mortality and morbidity in patients receiving ecainide, flecenaide or placebo: the Cardiac Arrhythmia Suppression Trial. *N Engl J Med.* 1991;324:781-788.
140. Markovitz JH, Matthews KA. Platelets and coronary heart disease: potential psychophysiologic mechanism. *Psychosom Med.* 1991;53: 643-668.
141. Morris PLP, Robinson RG, Andrzejewski P, Samuels J, Price TR. Association of depression with 10-year poststroke mortality. *Am J Psychiatry.* 1993;150:124-129.
142. Lefkovits J, Plow EF, Topol EJ. Platelet glycoprotein IIb/IIIa receptors in cardiovascular medicine. N Engl J Med. 1995;332:1553-1559.
143. Hess H, Mietaschk A, Deichsel G. Drug-induced inhibition of platelet function delays progression of peripheral occlusive arterial disease: a prospective double-blind arteriographically controlled trial. *Lancet.* 1985;1:415-419.
144. Antiplatelet Trialists' Collaboration. Secondary prevention of vascular disease by prolonged antiplatelet treatment. *BMJ.* 1988;296:320-331.
145. Verstraete M. Risk factors, interventions and therapeutic agents in the prevention of artherosclerosis-related ischaemic diseases. *Drugs.* 1991;42(suppl 5):22-38.
146. Ridker PM, Manson JE, Burning JE, Goldhaber SZ, Hennekens CH. The effect of chronic platelet inhibition with low-dose aspirin on atherosclerotic progression and acute thrombosis: clinical evidence from the Physicians' Health Study. *Am Heart J.* 1991;122:1588-1592.
147. Musselman DL, Tomer A, Manatunga AK, Knight BT, Porter MR, Kasey S, Marzec U, Harker LA, Nemeroff CB. Exaggerated platelet reactivity in major depression. *Am J Psychiatry.* 1996;153: 1313-1317.
148. Laghrissi-Thode F, Wagner WR, Pollock BG, Johnson PC, Finkel MS. Elevated platelet factor 4 and β-thromboglobulin plasma levels in depressed patients with ischemic heart disease. *Biol Psychiatry.* 1997;42:290-295.
149. Weyrich AS, Solis GA, Li KS, Tulenko TN, Santamore WP. Platelet amplification of vasospasm. *Am J Physiol.* 1992;263(suppl):H349-H358.
150. DeClerck F. Effects of serotonin on platelets and blood vessels. *J Cardiovasc Pharmacol.* 1991; 17(suppl 5):S1-S5.
151. Owens MJ, Nemeroff CB. Role of serotonin in the pathophysiology of depression: focus on the serotonin transporter. *Clin Chem.* 1994;40:288-295.
152. Osim EE, Wyllie JH. Evidence for loss of 5-hydroxytryptamine from circulating platelets. *J Physiol (Lond).* 1982;326:25P-26P.
153. Ashton JH, Benedict CR, Fitzgerald C, Raheja S, Taylor AL, Campbell WB, Buja LM, Willerson JT. Serotonin as a mediator of cyclic flow variations in stenosed canine coronary arteries. *Circulation.* 1986;73:572-578.
154. Ashton JH, Ogletree ML, Michel IM, Golino P, McNatt JM, Taylor AL, Raheja S, Schmitz J, Buja LM, Campell WB, Willerson JT. Cooperative mediation by serotonin S2 and thromboxane A2/ prostaglandin H2 receptor activation of cyclic flow variation in dogs with severe coronary artery stenosis. *Circulation.* 1987;76:952-959.
155. Biegon A, Weizman A, Karp L, Ram A, Iano S, Wolff M. Serotonin 5-HT2 receptor binding on blood platelets: a peripheral marker for depression? *Life Sci.* 1987;41:2485-2492.
156. Biegon A, Grinspoon A, Blumenfelt B, Bleich A, Apter A, Mester R. Increased serotonin 5-HT2 receptor binding on blood platelets in suicidal men. *Psychopharmacology.* 1990; 100:165-167.
157. Biegon A, Essar N, Israeli M, Elizur A, Bruch S, Bar-Nathan AA. Serotonin 5-HT2 receptor binding on blood platelets as a state dependent marker in major affective disorder. *Psychopharmacology.* 1990;100:73-75.
158. Arora RC, Meltzer HY. Increased serotonin (5-HT2) receptor binding as measured by 3H-LSD in the blood platelets of depressed patients. *Life Sci.* 1989;44:725-734.
159. Pandey GN, Pandey SC, Janicak PG. Platelet serotonin-2 binding sites in depression and suicide. *Biol Psychiatry.* 1990;28:215-222.
160. Briley MS, Langer SZ, Raisman R, Sechter D, Zarifian E. Tritiated imipramine binding sites are decreased in platelets of untreated depressed patients. *Science.* 1980;209:303-315.
161. Langer SZ, Arifian E, Briley MS, Raisman R, Sechter D. High-affinity binding of 3H-imipramine in brain and platelets and its relevance to the biochemistry of affective disorders. *Life Sci.* 1981;29:211-218.
162. Paul SM, Rehavi M, Skolnick P, Ballenger JC, Goodwin FK. Depressed patients have decreased binding of titrated imipramine to platelet serotonin "transporter." *Arch Gen Psychiatry.* 1981;38:1315-1317.
163. Nemeroff CB, Knight DL, Krishnan KRR, Slotkin TA, Bissette G, Melville ML, Blazer DG. Marked reduction in the number of platelet [^{3}H]imipramine binding sites in geriatric depression. *Arch Gen Psychiatry.* 1988;45:919-923.
164. Nemeroff CB, Knight DL, Franks J, Craighead WE, Krishnan KRR. Further studies on platelet transporter binding in depression. *Am J Psychiatry.* 1994;151:1623-1625.
165. Cerrito F, Lazzaro MP, Gaudio E, Arminio P, Aloisi G. 5HT2-receptors and serotonin release: their role in human platelet aggregation. *Life Sci.* 1993;53:209-215.
166. Kusumi I, Koyama T, Yamashita I. Serotonin-stimulated Ca2 + response is increased in the blood platelets of depressed patients. *Biol Psychiatry.* 1991;30:310-312.
167. Mikuni M, Kusumi I, Kagaya A, Kuroda Y, Mori H, Takahashi K. Increased 5-HT$_2$ receptor function as measured by serotonin-stimulated phosphoinositide hydrolosis in platelets of depressed patients. *Prog Neuropsychopharmacol Biol Psychiatry.* 1991;15:49-61.
168. Eckert A, Gann H, Riemann D, Aldenhoff J, Muller WE. Elevated intracellular calcium levels after 5-HT2 receptor stimulation in platelets of depressed patients. *Biol Psychiatry.* 1993;34: 565-568.
169. Ware JA, Smith M, Salzman EW. Synergism of platelet aggregating agents: role of elevation of cytoplasmic calcium. *J Clin Invest.* 1987;80: 267-271.
170. Friedman M, Thoresen CE, Gill JJ, Ulmer D, Powell LH, Price VA, Brown B, Thompson L, Rabin DD, Breall WS, Bourg E, Levy R, Dixon T. Alteration of type A behavior and its effect on cardiac recurrences in post myocardial infarction patients: summary results of the Recurrent Coronary Prevention Project. *Am Heart J.* 1986;112:653-665.
171. Frasure-Smith N, Prince R. The ischemic heart disease life stress monitoring program: impact on mortality. *Psychosom Med.* 1985;47: 431-445.
172. Frasure-Smith N. In-hospital symptoms of psychological stress as predictors of long-term outcome after acute myocardial infarction in men. *Am J Cardiol.* 1991;67:121-127.
173. Frasure-Smith N, Lesperance F, Juneau M. Differential long-term impact of in-hospital symptoms of psychological stress after non-Q-wave and Q-wave myocardial infarction. *Am J Cardiol.* 1992;69:1128-1134.
174. Jones DA, West RR. Psychological rehabilitation after myocardial infarction: multicentre randomised

controlled trial. *BMJ.* 1996;313:1517-1521.
175. Taylor CB, Miller NH, Smith PM, DeBusk RF. The effect of a home-based, case-managed, multifactorial risk-reduction program on reducing psychological distress in patients with cardiovascular disease. *J Cardiopulm Rehabil.* 1997;17:157-162.
176. Frasure-Smith N, Lesperance F, Prince RH, Verrier P, Garber RA, Juneau M, Wolfson C, Bourassa MG. Randomised trial of home-based psychosocial nursing intervention for patients recovering from myocardial infarction. *Lancet.* 1997;350:473-479.
177. Muskin PR, Glassman AH. The use of tricyclic antidepressants in a medical setting. In: Finkel JB, ed. *Consultation-Liason Psychiatry: Current Trends and Future Perspectives.* New York, NY: Grune & Stratton; 1983:137-158.
178. Roose SP, Dalack GW. Treating the depressed patient with cardiovascular problems. *J Clin Psychiatry.* 1992;53:25-31.
179. Arana GW, Hyman SE. *Handbook of Psychiatric Drug Therapy, Second Edition.* Boston, Mass: Little Brown & Co; 1991:61.
180. Roose SP, Dalack GW, Glassman AH, Woodring S, Walsh T, Giardina GV. Cardiovascular effects of buproprion in depressed patients with heart disease. *Am J Psychiatry.* 1991b;148:512-516.
181. Roose SP, Glassman AH, Attia E, Woodring S. Comparative efficacy of selective serotonin reuptake inhibitors and tricyclics in the treatment of melancholia. *Am J Psychiatry.* 1994;151:1735-1739.
182. Roose SP, Laghrissi-Thode F, Kennedy J, Nelson C, Bigger JT Jr, Pollock B, Gafney A, Narayan M, Finkel MS, McCafferty J, Gergel I. Comparison of paroxetine and nortriptyline in depressed patients with ischemic heart disease. *JAMA.* 1998;279:287-291.
183. Ellison JM, Milofsky JE, Ely E. Fluoxetine-induced bradycardia and syncope in two patients. *J Clin Psychiatry.* 1990;51:385-386.
184. Enemark B. The importance of ECG monitoring in antidepressant treatment. *Nord J Psychiatry.* 1993;47(suppl):57-65.
185. Humphries JE, Wheby MS, VandenBerg SR. Fluoxetine and the bleeding time. *Arch Pathol Lab Med.* 1990;114:727-728.
186. Evans TG, Buys SS, Rodgers GM. Acquired abnormalities of platelet function. *N Engl J Med.* 1991;324:1671.
187. Yaryura-Tobias JA, Kirschen H, Ninan P, Mosberg HF. Fluoxetine and bleeding in obsessive-compulsive disorder. *Am J Psychiatry.* 1991;148:949.
188. Alderman CP, Moritz CK, Ben-Tovim DI. Abnormal platelet aggregation associated with fluoxetine therapy. *Ann Pharmacother.* 1992;26:1517-1519.
189. Callahan AM, Marangell LB, Ketter TA. Evaluating the clinical significance of drug interactions: a systematic approach. *Harvard Rev Psychiatry.* 1996;4:153-158.
190. Lesperance F, Frasure-Smith N, Talajic M. Major depression before and after myocardial infarction: its nature and consequences. *Psychosom Med.* 1996;58:99-110.
191. Ridker PM, Cushman M, Stampfer MJ, Tracy RP, Hennekens CH. Inflammation, aspirin, and the risk of cardiovascular disease in apparently healthy men. *N Engl J Med.* 1997;336:973-979.
192. Musselman DL, Lewison BJ, Porter MR, Pearce BD, McDaniel JS, Miller AH, Nemeroff CB. HPA axis hyperactivity and interleukin-6 plasma concentrations in cancer patients with depression. Paper presented at: the 36th meeting of the American College of Neuropsychopharmacology; December 10, 1997; Waikoloa, Hawaii.
193. Grodstein F, Stampfer MJ. The epidemiology of coronary heart disease and estrogen replacement in postmenopausal women. *Prog Cardiovasc Dis.* 1995;38:199-210.
194. Kon Koh K, Mincemoyer R, Bui MN, Csako G, Pucino F, Guetta V, Maclawiw M, Cannon RO. Effects of hormone-replacement therapy on fibrinolysis in postmenopausal women. *N Engl J Med.* 1997;336:683-690.
195. Eaker ED, Packard B, Thom TJ. Epidemiology and risk factors for coronary heart disease in women. *Cardiovasc Clin.* 1989;9:129-145.

Symptoms of Anxiety and Symptoms of Depression

Same Genes, Different Environments?

Kenneth S. Kendler, MD; Andrew C. Heath, DPhil; Nicholas G. Martin, PhD; Lindon J. Eaves, DSc

• While traditional multivariate statistical methods can describe patterns of psychiatric symptoms, they cannot provide insight into why certain symptoms tend to co-occur in a population. However, this can be achieved using recently developed methods of multivariate genetic analysis. Examining self-report symptoms in a clinically unselected twin sample (3798 pairs), traditional factor analysis indicates that symptoms of depression and anxiety tend to form separate symptom clusters. Multivariate genetic analysis shows that genes act largely in a nonspecific way to influence the overall level of psychiatric symptoms. No evidence could be found for genes that specifically affect symptoms of depression without also strongly influencing symptoms of anxiety. By contrast, the environment seems to have specific effects, ie, certain features of the environment strongly influence symptoms of anxiety while having little impact on symptoms of depression. These results, which are replicated across sexes, suggest that the separable anxiety and depression symptom clusters in the general population are largely the result of environmental factors.

(*Arch Gen Psychiatry* 1987;44:451-457)

Individual psychiatric symptoms are not independently distributed in the population. Rather, symptoms tend to cluster to form recognizable psychiatric syndromes. Although initially the province of the diagnostician, the task of recognizing and describing clinical syndromes has been supplemented, for several decades, by multivariate statistical methods.[1,2] These methods can identify syndromes by showing that certain symptoms often occur together in individuals in a population; however, they provide no insight into why these symptoms tend to covary.

In this article, we apply newly developed methods of multivariate genetic analysis[3] that can move beyond traditional factor analysis to clarify why certain symptoms tend to cluster. We apply these methods to self-report symptoms of anxiety and depression from a large clinically unselected twin sample.[4] Our goal is to understand why certain individuals display depressive symptoms, while for others the symptoms of anxiety are more pronounced.[5-13]

We wish to test two major hypotheses. The first is that certain genes specifically influence the liability to depressive symptoms and other genes specifically influence the liability to symptoms of anxiety. The second hypothesis is that certain environmental factors are specifically depressogenic and others are specifically anxiogenic.

METHODS

Sample

This study is based on completed postal questionnaires, mailed during the period from 1980 to 1982, received from 1978 same-sex female, and 918 same-sex male, and 902 opposite-sex volunteer twin pairs older than the age of 18 years from the Australian National Health and Medical Research Council (NHMRC) Twin Register, Canberra. As described elsewhere,[4] zygosity was determined by questionnaire items shown to be at least 95% accurate. The questionnaire contained a seven-item anxiety and a seven-item depression subscale from the Delusions-Symptoms-States Inventory (DSSI), developed and validated by Bedford et al.[14] Respondents were asked to indicate whether they had experienced symptoms "recently": 1, not at all; 2, a little; 3, a lot; and 4, unbearably. The prevalence of symptoms of anxiety and depression as assessed by this scale was similar in the twin sample and in general population samples from Australia.[4] Frequency of contact among members of a twin pair was shown to be unrelated to concordance for symptoms. To simplify the analyses, the 902 opposite-sex twin pairs were excluded from the multivariate genetic analyses.

Because few individuals checked the most extreme response (unbearably), response categories 3 and 4 were collapsed into a single category for the purposes of these analyses. Furthermore, because of the low response rate, the last item of the depression scale (depressed, thoughts of suicide) was eliminated from the multivariate analysis. Since the full text of these items has been presented previously,[4] in this report, we will use the abbreviated item versions.

Data Analysis: An Overview

Because of the statistical complexity of some of the material in this article, in this section, a relatively nontechnical overview of the methods of data analysis is presented. More technical aspects are outlined in the "Data Analysis: Methods" section. Finally, the first paragraph of the "Comment" section contains a nontechnical summary of the important results.

There are three major steps to the data analysis presented in this article. First, a traditional factor analysis of the twin responses to the DSSI items is presented. Second, the fit of various models to these responses is examined using multivariate genetic analysis. Third, after the determination of the most appropriate multivariate genetic model, the results of that model are presented in detail.

Factor analysis attempts to account for the observed correlations between a relatively large number of symptoms in terms of the effects of a small number of latent dimensions or factors. Factor analysis utilizes as "raw" data only the cross-correlations of symptoms within individuals. Thus, factor analysis is purely a descriptive technique that can succinctly summarize patterns of symptom covariation. For example, if the DSSI items are providing only a gross measure of overall "psychiatric distress," we would expect a single-factor solution. If the items are able to discriminate between two dimensions of symptomatology (eg, symptoms of anxiety vs depression), at least two factors would be needed to explain the observed pattern of symptoms correlations.

The next step in the data analysis is multivariate genetic

Accepted for publication Aug 29, 1986.

From the Departments of Psychiatry (Dr Kendler) and Human Genetics (Drs Kendler, Heath, Martin, and Eaves), Medical College of Virginia, Virginia Commonwealth University, Richmond. Dr Martin is now with Queensland Institute for Medical Research, Herston, Queensland, Australia.

Reprint requests to Department of Psychiatry, Medical College of Virginia, Virginia Commonwealth University, PO Box 710, Richmond, VA 23298 (Dr Kendler).

Relationship, as depicted by schematic path diagrams, among hypothesized genetic factors (G_1 and G_2), hypothesized environmental factors (E_1 or E_1 and E_2), two hypothesized symptoms of anxiety (Anx 1 and Anx 2), and two hypothesized symptoms of depression (Dep 1 and Dep 2). Strong relationships among variables are represented by black arrows and weak relationships by gray arrows. In common-pathway model, genetic and environmental factors affect symptoms by both acting on same latent variable. That is, one genetic (G_1) and one environmental (E_1) factor specifically influence latent variable anxiety (Anx), while second genetic (G_2) and second environmental (E_2) factor specifically influence latent variable depression (Dep). Individual symptoms are in turn influenced by latent variables. In this model, genes and environment, by their influence on latent variables, are equally specific (or nonspecific) in their influence on symptoms of anxiety and depression. In independent-pathway model, genes and environment directly and separately influence individual symptoms. One of many possible configurations is depicted here with this model in which two genetic factors (G_1 and G_2) and one environmental factor (E_1) directly influence the four symptoms. G_1 is relatively specific for symptoms of anxiety and G_2 for symptoms of depression, but E_1 is nonspecific and influences approximately equally symptoms of both anxiety and depression. Thus, in this specific configuration, genes and not environment are responsible for tendency of symptoms of anxiety to correlate more highly with other symptoms of anxiety than with symptoms of depression, and vice versa. In another possible configuration of independent-pathway model, and one more consistent with results of this article, environmental factors would be relatively specific in their impact on symptoms of anxiety and symptoms of depression while a genetic factor would nonspecifically influence both sets of symptoms.

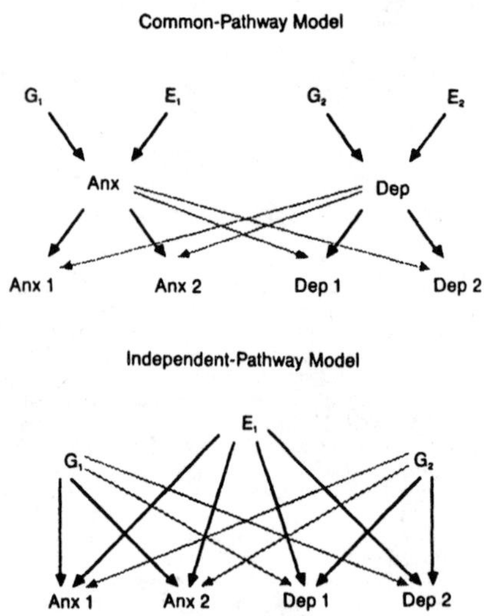

analysis. This technique can be understood as a generalization of factor analysis that permits the estimation of separate genetic and environmental factors. By using information from the correlations between monozygotic (MZ) and dizygotic (DZ) twin pairs for the same symptom and cross-correlations between and within twins for different symptoms, multivariate genetic analysis permits the separation of the genetic from the environmental impact on symptom covariation.

We wish to test two models in our multivariate genetic analysis that represent different ways in which genes and environment might affect multiple symptoms (Figure). The first, or "common-pathway," model assumes that genes and environment both contribute to one or more intermediate latent variables (eg, liability to "anxiety" and liability to "depression," denoted as "Anx" and "Dep" in the upper section of the Figure), which are in turn responsible for the observed pattern of symptom covariation. In other words, this model assumes that genes and environment act on symptom covariation by a final common pathway.

Under the second, or "independent-pathway," model, genes and environment may have different effects on the pattern of symptom covariation. For example (as pictured in the bottom section of the Figure), there could be two sets of genes—one of which was relatively selective for symptoms of anxiety and the other for symptoms of depression—but environmental influences that predispose equally to both sets of symptoms. It can be shown algebraically that the common-pathway model can be subsumed as a submodel of the independent-pathway model, so that the fit of the two models can be tested statistically (by means of a likelihood ratio χ^2 test).[13]

The final step in the "Results" section is to present in detail the findings of the most appropriate multivariate genetic model. This presentation permits a detailed comparison of results between the conventional and multivariate genetic factor analyses and an examination of the consistency of the findings across sexes.

Data Analysis: Methods

Methods of data summary and analysis designed for continuous variables are inappropriate for discontinuous variables, such as our item scores, which have only three-point scales. The approach that we have used assumes the existence, for each item, of a normally distributed liability that determines the probability of response to that item. The observed distribution is related to the latent distribution by abrupt "thresholds" superimposed on the latent distribution. With multicategory data as those used in this article, it is possible to test statistically the validity of these assumptions. As described previously,[4] the fit of this "threshold" model to the observed data was good.

The first step in our data analysis was a traditional factor analysis of the twin responses. The sample was subdivided by sex and then into first and second members from each twin pair. A factor analysis was performed separately for each of the four resulting subsamples. Factor loadings were estimated by the unweighted least-squares method.[14] In each analysis, the number of factors extracted was determined by the number of eigenvalues greater than unity. We estimated uncorrelated ("orthogonal") factors for comparability with the multivariate genetic analysis. To select for study one of the infinite number of statistically equivalent solutions ("factor rotations"), we used the simplest technique of fixing to 0 the loadings of one depression item ("lost interest in everything") on the second and third factors, and of an anxiety item ("pain or tension in head") on the third factor.[15] This method of rotation ensured comparability of factor rotations between sexes, between first and second twins, and between the traditional and multivariate genetic factor analyses. These items were chosen by performing varimax rotations[16] on the results from the four subsamples and then selecting the items for which the mean-squared factor loadings were highest on the observed depression and anxiety factors. In fitting three factors, this traditional factor analysis required the estimation of 36 common factor loadings for 13 items on the first latent factor, 12 on the second, and 11 on the third. Item-specific factor loadings, which explain the variance not accounted for by the common factors loadings, were obtained by subtracting from unity the variance accounted for by the common factor loadings. By convention, these item-specific loadings are not tabulated.

Although solutions that permit correlated ("oblique") factors are sometimes preferred for descriptive purposes, our chief interest was in causal analysis for which uncorrelated factors are much simpler to interpret. This is particularly true with respect to the action of different genes that, in the absence of gametic-phase disequilibrium, should be uncorrelated in the population.

Theoretically, the best data summaries for multivariate analysis

Table 1.—Factor Loadings (×100) of Symptoms of Anxiety and Depression on Phenotypic Factors in Females and Males*

	Females						Males					
	Twin 1			Twin 2			Twin 1			Twin 2		
Item	I	II	III	I	II	III	I	II	III	I	II	III
Anxiety subscale												
1. Worried about everything	62	37	16	63	28	22	55	37	20	55	33	29
2. Breathless or heart pounding	37	34	0	42	42	−8	43	44	1	35	55	0
3. Worked up, can't sit still	57	44	3	61	34	11	50	50	23	57	37	19
4. Feelings of panic	66	40	−8	72	27	0	71	29	1	63	42	7
5. Pain or tension in head	41	44	0†	41	44	0†	49	45	0†	38	59	0†
6. Worrying kept me awake	58	31	39	60	25	51	54	25	58	55	27	56
7. Anxious, can't make up my mind	78	32	−7	79	21	−2	73	16	14	74	34	6
Depression subscale												
1. Miserable difficulty with sleep	68	31	74	72	24	63	68	27	52	68	29	57
2. Depressed without knowing why	70	23	−3	71	18	−2	72	19	−2	72	22	1
3. Gone to bed not caring	84	1	7	85	7	2	83	−3	−4	83	11	4
4. Low in spirits, just sat	80	6	1	80	10	2	76	5	−5	78	7	2
5. Future seems hopeless	83	−3	8	85	−6	9	83	−18	7	84	10	4
6. Lost interest in everything	89	0†	0†	92	0†	0†	86	0†	0†	91	0†	0†

*Orthogonal factors.
†Parameter fixed to 0.

of our discontinuous data would be 13-way contingency tables, cross-classifying the scores of individuals on each of the 13 items, for factor analysis, or 26-way tables, cross-classifying responses of first and second twins on each of the 13 items, for multivariate genetic analysis. In practice, fitting models to such contingency tables, which would require the repeated numerical integration of the multivariate normal distribution, would be infeasible with current computer resources. Instead, we have obtained maximum likelihood estimates of the "polychoric correlation"[17] between every pair of variables, separately for each twin group (male and female first and second twins for factor analysis; male and female MZ and DZ pairs for the multivariate genetic analysis). We then fitted models to 13×13 or 26×26 matrices of polychoric correlations. The factor analyses were performed separately on each 13×13 matrix, but the multivariate genetic analysis involved simultaneous analysis of two matrices, one for MZ pairs and the other for DZ pairs of a given sex. Models were fitted by unweighted least squares, in the case of the factor analysis, but by weighted least squares, using estimates of the reciprocal of the sampling variance of each polychoric correlation as noniterative weights,[18-20] for the multivariate genetic analysis. The latter approach gives us an approximate χ^2 goodness-of-fit test of the absolute fit of the model with the number of degrees of freedom equal to the number of unique correlations (650 if we are analyzing two 26×26 correlation matrices) minus the number of estimated parameters. We can also compute an approximate likelihood ratio χ^2 (or "χ^2 difference") test of the relative fit of each model compared with more complete models. For the full model, only a goodness-of-fit test is available. For subsidiary models, the likelihood ratio χ^2 provides a more powerful test. Thus, it is possible that by a goodness-of-fit test a model may provide an acceptable fit to the data, yet be rejected in favor of a different model by a likelihood ratio test.

In our multivariate genetic analysis using the independent-pathway model, we estimated simultaneously item loadings on the common genetic factors, the common (nonfamilial) environmental factors, and item-specific genetic factors. Loadings on the common genetic factors contribute both to the within-individual and to the between-twin cross-correlations between items. Loadings on the common (nonfamilial) environmental factors contribute to the within-individual but not to the between-twin item cross-correlations. Loadings of the item-specific genetic factors contribute to the correlation between twins for a specific item, but not the cross-correlations between items. Finally, item-specific environmental factors, which explain the residual variance, are obtained by subtraction. Both common and item-specific loadings are expected to be the same for both members of a twin pair. An independent-pathway model that allows for three common genetic, three common environmental, and item-specific genetic factors requires the estimation of 85 parameters: 36 (13+12+11) common genetic factor item loadings, 36 common environmental factor loadings, and 13 item-specific genetic factor loadings.

Using the common-pathway model, we estimated as before common genetic, item-specific genetic, and item-specific environmental loadings. However, under this model, the item loadings of each common environmental factor are expected to be a constant multiple of the loadings on the corresponding common genetic factor. Therefore, it was necessary to estimate only a single scalar multiplier for each common genetic factor from which loadings on the corresponding common environmental factor could be derived. In the three-factor common-pathway model, it was therefore necessary to estimate only 52 parameters: 36 common genetic loadings, three scalar multipliers, and 13 item-specific genetic loadings.

The previous univariate analysis[4] indicated that the overall effect of common environmental or genetic dominance on symptoms of anxiety and depression in this sample was small or undetectable. If a variable accounts for a small proportion of variance in an item, statistical principles dictate that it cannot make a major contribution to the covariation of that item with other items. Therefore, our multivariate analyses considered only additive genetic and nonfamilial (or random) environmental effects, both of which were shown, in our univariate analysis, to have a large impact on symptoms of anxiety and depression.[4]

For an estimate of the similarity of factor loadings obtained on different samples (eg, twin 1 vs twin 2 or males vs females), the congruency coefficient (r_c) was used.[21]

RESULTS

Factor Analysis

Using the eigenvalue criterion, three orthogonal factors were extracted in each case for the first and second members of the male and female twin pairs. The results of this traditional, or phenotypic, factor analysis are seen in Table 1. Factor loadings (which, in an orthogonal solution, are equivalent to the correlation of an item with the underlying latent factor) are given for the rotated solution.

The first phenotypic factor, which accounted for between 45.8% and 50.5% of the total variation, was similar across groups. The congruency coefficients were above .99 for all six possible compari-

Table 2.—Factor Loadings (×100) of Symptoms of Anxiety and Depression on Genetic and Environmental Factors in Female and Male Twins*

	Genetic Factors				Environmental Factors			
Item	I	II	III	Specific	I	II	III	Specific
Females								
Anxiety subscale								
1. Worried about everything	51	2	10	33	40	32	21	56
2. Breathless or heart pounding	31	39	−9	25	29	25	−1	73
3. Worked up, can't sit still	50	11	2	35	36	37	8	59
4. Feelings of panic	59	14	1	20	41	26	−3	60
5. Pain or tension in head	33	34	0†	34	28	34	0†	68
6. Worrying kept me awake	40	13	29	29	43	25	39	50
7. Anxious, can't make up my mind	68	−2	−10	0	45	25	6	51
Depression subscale								
1. Miserable, difficulty with sleep	46	10	45	0	51	28	50	0‡
2. Depressed without knowing why	53	2	13	21	47	21	−16	61
3. Gone to bed not caring	51	18	13	43	71	−2	1	17
4. Low in spirits, just sat	60	1	17	32	53	9	−11	46
5. Future seems hopeless	53	2	1	34	69	−11	14	32
6. Lost interest in everything	63	0†	0†	17	66	0†	0†	37
Males								
Anxiety subscale								
1. Worried about everything	33	8	46	0	40	35	3	63
2. Breathless or heart pounding	42	44	7	0	14	28	−2	73
3. Worked up, can't sit still	38	22	19	36	31	45	13	58
4. Feelings of panic	74	1	15	0	17	31	−5	55
5. Pain or tension in head	32	34	0†	37	24	44	0†	63
6. Worrying kept me awake	44	6	23	29	29	25	72	0‡
7. Anxious, can't make up my mind	60	13	18	6	45	25	1	57
Depression subscale								
1. Miserable, difficulty with sleep	44	4	29	9	48	32	37	50
2. Depressed without knowing why	57	−7	5	23	39	35	−8	58
3. Gone to bed not caring	57	−4	12	5	56	−3	4	59
4. Low in spirits, just sat	65	1	−16	0	48	10	4	55
5. Future seems hopeless	51	−1	7	32	68	−2	2	41
6. Lost interest in everything	62	0†	0†	0	64	0†	0†	45

*Orthogonal factors, weighted least-square solution.
†Parameter fixed to 0.
‡Parameter value constrained to be positive.

sons across the four groups. The highest factor loadings in all groups were found on four core depression items: "gone to bed not caring," "low in spirits, just sat," "future seems hopeless," and "lost interest in everything." However, the factor was not highly specific for depression as all items loaded positively (ie, > +0.30) on this factor. This factor was termed "depression-distress" to signify that depression items consistently loaded highest on this factor, but it was also, in part, a general psychiatric distress factor.

The second phenotypic factor, which accounted for between 6.5% and 10.9% of the total variation, was also quite similar in the four groups. Five of the six possible congruency coefficients were above .96 and the sixth (between male twin 1 and male twin 2) was .93. The four highest loadings in all groups were from among five anxiety items: "worried about everything," "breathless or heart pounding," "worked up, can't sit still," "feelings of panic," and "pain or tension in head." Unlike the first factor, the second factor was relatively specific. The loadings of all anxiety items except "anxious, can't make up my mind" were in excess of .25, while the loadings for the four core depression items never exceeded .11. This factor was termed "general anxiety."

A third factor, which accounted for between 5.6% and 5.9% of the total variation, had in all four groups by far the highest loading on the two insomnia items: "worrying kept me awake" and "miserable, difficulty with sleep." Five of the six possible congruency coefficients were above .90 and the sixth (between female twin 1 and male twin 1) was .87. This factor was termed "insomnia."

A useful way to quantify the contribution of the first two phenotypic factors to the original anxiety and depression subscales is to compare the proportion of total variance accounted for in the two subscales by the first two factors. Across all four groups, the mean (±SD) proportion of variance in the anxiety and depression subscales accounted for by the "depression-distress" factor was, respectively, 33.8% ± 2.8% and 63.4% ± 1.9%. In other words, the "depression-distress" factor accounted for one third of the total variance of the anxiety subscale, but for nearly two thirds of the total variance for the depression subscale. The mean proportion of variance in the anxiety and depression subscales accounted for by the "general anxiety" factor was, respectively, 14.1% ± 3.0% and 2.4% ± 0.4%. The "general anxiety" factor accounted for over five times as much variance in the anxiety as in the depression subscale.

Multivariate Genetic Analysis: Model Fitting

We considered two major multivariate models: the common-pathway and independent-pathway models (Figure). By a χ^2 goodness-of-fit test, the fit of a "full" independent-pathway model with three genetic and three environmental factors was excellent for both females ($\chi^2 = 470.8$; $df = 565$; $P = .98$) and males ($\chi^2 = 556.8$; $df = 565$; $P = .59$). For females, all subsidiary models with fewer than three genetic and three environmental factors could be rejected by likelihood ratio χ^2 tests. For males, all subsidiary models could also be rejected except that which contained all three environmental factors and only the first two genetic factors ($\chi^2=16.3$; $df=11$; $P=.13$).

The two- and one-factor common-pathway models could be rejected at high levels of statistical significance ($P<.00001$) for both males and females. However, the three-factor common-pathway model produced a reasonable fit in both females ($\chi^2=550.0$; $df=598$; $P=.92$) and males ($\chi^2=638.4$; $df=598$; $P=.12$). However, compared with the full independent-pathway model, the three-factor common-pathway model could be rejected by likelihood ratio tests at high levels of significance for both females ($\chi^2=79.3$; $df=33$; $P<.0001$) and males ($\chi^2=81.6$; $df=33$; $P<.0001$).

Finally, we fitted the full independent-pathway model to both sexes simultaneously. The likelihood ratio test of heterogeneity was very highly significant ($\chi^2=222.9$; $df=85$; $P<.0001$), indicating that although this model was appropriate for each sex, the factor loadings differed significantly between females and males.

Results of Best-Fitting Model

Genetic and environmental factor loadings are given under the full independent-pathway model separately for females and for males (Table 2). Although a slightly simpler model also provided an adequate fit in males (ie, two genetic and three environmental factors), the full model was somewhat superior in fit and had the advantage of simplifying the comparison of the results across sexes. In comparing these results with the phenotypic factor loadings shown in Table 1, it should be remembered that we are now fitting a total of six (three genetic and three environmental) factors rather than three phenotypic factors, so that the individual factor loadings will, in almost all cases, be lower in Table 2 than in Table 1. A comparison of these tables should focus on the pattern rather than the absolute value of the factor loadings.

The first genetic factor, which accounted for 26.7% of the total phenotypic variance in females and 27.3% in males, was very similar in both sexes ($r_c=.986$). The four items with highest loading in both sexes were two anxiety items, "feelings of panic" and "anxious, can't make up my mind," and two depression items, "low in spirits, just sat" and "lost interest in everything." Like the first phenotypic "depression-distress" factor, all items tended to load highly and positively on this factor. Unlike the first phenotypic factor, the average loading for anxiety items was almost as high as that found for depression items. Because of the apparent lack of specificity of this factor, it was termed the "genetic distress" factor.

The second genetic factor accounted for 2.8% of the total variance in females and 3.0% in males and was reasonably similar across sexes ($r_c=.837$). In both sexes, only two items had substantial loadings on this factor: "breathless or heart pounding" and "pain or tension in head." This factor differed from the second phenotypic "general anxiety" factor in having low loadings for other anxiety items, especially "worried about everything" and "feelings of panic." Therefore, this factor was termed the "genetic somatic anxiety" factor.

The third genetic factor, which accounted for 2.9% of the total variation in females and 3.8% in males, was only modestly stable across sexes ($r_c=.510$). In females, substantial loadings were seen only for the two insomnia items. In males, the highest loading was seen on the first anxiety item "worried about everything," followed by the two insomnia items. This factor was broadly similar to the third phenotypic factor and, hence, was termed the "genetic insomnia" factor. The second and third genetic factors, although statistically significant because of the large size of the sample, account for a small proportion of total variance in liability to symptoms in the twin population. The genetic specific loadings, which reflect the genetic influences unique to each symptom, were, on the average, relatively modest, accounting for only 7.8% of the total variation in liability to symptoms in females and 4.0% in males. These results suggest that the majority of genetic variance in these symptoms is accounted for by the three extracted factors.

The first environmental factor, which accounted for 24.5% of the total phenotypic variance in females and 18.8% in males was similar across sexes ($r_c=.984$). In both sexes, the four highest loadings were on the core depression items: "gone to bed not caring," "low in spirits, just sat," "future seemed hopeless," and "lost interest in everything." This factor was relatively similar to the first phenotypic "depression-distress" factor, but the specificity for depressive symptoms was somewhat greater. Therefore, this factor was termed the "environmental depression" factor.

The second environmental factor, which accounted for 5.8% of the phenotypic variance in females and 8.1% in males, was also very similar in the two sexes ($r_c=.986$). In both sexes, the three highest loadings were on the core anxiety symptoms "worried about everything," "worked up, can't sit still," and "pain or tension in head." This factor was quite similar to the second phenotypic "general anxiety" factor in loading more equally on all the anxiety items and hence was termed the "environmental general anxiety" factor.

The third environmental factor, which accounted for 4.0% of the total variance in females and 5.3% in males, was also reasonably similar in males and females ($r_c=.835$). In both sexes, this factor had substantial loadings on only the two insomnia items. This factor was broadly similar to both the "insomnia" and "genetic insomnia" factors and was termed the "environmental insomnia" factor.

For almost all the items, item-specific environmental loadings that represent environmental effects (including measurement error) influencing one item but no others, accounted for a substantial proportion of the total variation. For all items, specific environmental variation accounted for 26.0% of the total phenotypic variation in females and 30.0% in males.

A useful way to contrast the contribution of the first genetic and environmental factors to the anxiety and depression subscales is to compare the proportion of variance accounted for in these subscales by the two factors. The "genetic-distress" factor contributed more to the total variation in the depression than to the anxiety subscale in both females (29.8% vs 24.1%) and males (31.8% vs 23.3%), but the differences were quite small. This is in contrast to the "environmental depression" factor, which contributed more than 2½ times the total variance to the depression than to the anxiety subscale in females (36.3% vs 14.4%). In males, this ratio was over 3:1 (30.0% vs 9.3%). These results support the conclusion that the first genetic factor is nonspecific, while the first environmental factor is relatively specific for symptoms of depression.

COMMENT

This article represents, to our knowledge, the first application of multivariate genetic methods to individual psychiatric symptoms. We analyzed responses of 3978 twin pairs to the anxiety and depression subscales of the DSSI. Our major goal was to clarify the role of genes vs the environment in the etiology of separable anxiety and depression symptom clusters in the general population. Three major results are noteworthy. First, a traditional factor analysis consistently identified two important factors termed "depression-distress" and "general anxiety." Second, in fitting multivariate genetic models, the common-pathway model could be clearly rejected in favor of the independent-pathway model. Third, fitting the full independent-pathway model produced three factors of particular interest, termed: "genetic distress," "environmental depression," and "environmental anxiety." We could find little evidence that genes influenced specifically either symptoms of depression or symptoms of anxiety. However, certain environments appeared to be specifically depressogenic and others anxiogenic.

Phenotypic Factor Analysis

In this large volunteer twin sample, the traditional eigenvalue criterion readily identified three phenotypic factors that were stable across four groups (ie, twin 1 and 2 in females and males). After rotation, the first of these phenotypic factors, termed "depression-distress," accounted for about half of the total variation. As the name implies, this factor loaded substantially on almost all items, but loadings were consistently highest on the depression items. The second phenotypic factor, which accounted for between 6% and 11% of the total variance, was termed a "general anxiety" factor. Loadings for this factor were both relatively specific for the anxiety subscale, and were similar for almost all the anxiety items. The third or "insomnia" factor had highest loadings on the two insomnia items with only quite modest loadings on all other items.

Controversy over the discrimination between symptoms of anxiety and depression has a long history.[6,12,22] Two major viewpoints, which have been termed the "distinct-syndrome" and "unitary-syndrome" positions,[6] have been articulated. The distinct-syndrome position views depression and anxiety as qualitatively distinct, albeit with some overlap of symptomatology. The unitary-syndrome viewpoint, by contrast, argues that these two states are on a single continuum, and that any differences between them are basically quantitative and not qualitative. As recently reviewed,[12,13] empirical studies using a variety of multivariate techniques have tended to support the distinct-syndrome position, although these results are not unequivocal. In addition, follow-up studies have strongly supported the discrimination between anxiety states and depression.[10,23]

Previous multivariate studies of the relationship between anxiety and depression have, with rare exception,[24] been performed on samples obtained in a treatment setting. Such an approach introduces an important possible bias. Individuals with symptoms of both disorders are more likely to present for treatment than those with symptoms from only one disorder. This bias can create a spurious covariation of symptoms. By contrast, no such bias can be operating in the general population sample studied in this article.

The Australian NHMRC Twin Registry represents a large, volunteer twin population, in which reported levels of anxiety and depression do not differ from those observed in the general Australian population.[4] Results from this sample provide some support for the "distinct-syndrome" position in that two phenotypic factors that could be identified as depression and anxiety were extracted from each of the four subject groups. However, these symptom dimensions were not completely independent, as anxiety items consistently loaded positively on the first "depression-distress factor." By contrast, most depression items had very low loadings on the second "general anxiety" factor.

Contrary to expectation, consistent evidence was found for a third "insomnia" factor. We are unaware of any similar results that suggest an insomnia factor can be discriminated from anxiety and depression in the general population. These insomnia items, along with other questionnaire data about sleep duration and quality, are the focus of another report in preparation.

Multivariate Genetic Model Fitting

Three aspects of model fitting were examined: (1) the best-fitting model, (2) the required number of genetic and environmental factors, and (3) the consistency of results across sexes. We considered two different models of how genetic and environmental factors might influence symptom covariation. The first, or common-pathway model, assumed that both genes and environment act on symptoms by influencing the same latent variables. The second, or independent-pathway model, permitted genes and environment to influence symptom covariation in different ways. The common-pathway model could be clearly rejected in favor of the independent-pathway model. These findings indicate that in this sample genes and environment are influencing the pattern of covariation of individual symptoms of anxiety and depression in qualitatively different ways.

The previously reported univariate analysis of these symptoms included an examination of the genetic and environmental correlation of liability between sexes.[4] These analyses required the consideration of opposite-sex DZ twin pairs, the inclusion of which in the present multivariate analysis would have been extremely cumbersome. In the multivariate genetic analyses, our consideration of sex differences was limited to showing that, although the same model produced the best fit in both sexes, the individual factor loadings differed significantly between the sexes. These results required the separate analysis of results in females and males, which had the advantage of permitting an assessment of the similarity of results across sexes.

Results of Best-Fitting Multivariate Genetic Model

The results of the best-fitting multivariate model gave a striking confirmation of the previous finding that genes and environment were influencing symptom covariation in a qualitatively different fashion. Of the three genetic factors, the first two were relatively stable across sexes, while the third was only modestly so. The first "genetic-distress" factor was so named because factor loadings were high on all items with relatively little difference found between depression and anxiety items. Compared with the first phenotypic factor, the first genetic factor was substantially less specific for depression. This "genetic-distress" factor, which accounted for around 27% of the total phenotypic variance and over two thirds of the total genetic variance in both sexes, indicated that genes were largely acting nonspecifically to influence the predisposition to symptoms of psychiatric distress.

The second and third genetic factors were quite minor, each accounting for less than 4% of the total phenotypic variance. The second, or "genetic somatic anxiety" factor, loaded highly on only two anxiety items, both of which reflected the somatic symptoms of anxiety. This factor differed from the phenotypic "general anxiety" factor in the low loadings found for several key symptoms reflecting cognitive aspects of anxiety. Although genes seem to "code" specifically for symptoms of anxiety to a modest degree, they apparently influence only the somatic symptoms of anxiety.

The third, or "genetic insomnia" factor, was broadly similar to the third phenotypic factor in loading most prominently on the two insomnia items. Genetic factors that influence complaints of insomnia are, at least in part, separable from those that influence general levels of distress or symptoms of physical anxiety.

Of the three environmental factors, the first two were stable and the third relatively stable across sexes. The first or "environmental depression" factor loaded consistently highest on four core depression items. This factor was more specific for depression than the first phenotypic "depression-distress" factor, as reflected by the fact that the "environmental depression" factor accounted for over 2½ times the total variance in the depression subscale than in the anxiety subscale.

The second, or "environmental general anxiety" factor, was quite similar to the phenotypic "general anxiety" factor. Loadings were consistently highest on both physical and cognitive symptoms of anxiety, while loadings were low on the core depression symptoms. The third, or "environmental insomnia" factor, like the two other insomnia factors, had highest loadings on the two insomnia items. The environmental factors that influence insomnia also appear to be in part separable from those that cause anxiety and depression. This is not surprising in that nighttime noise might be expected to produce precisely this effect.

Limitations

One potential limitation of this report is noteworthy. The symptoms studied were obtained by self-report from the general population. As noted above, this has distinct advantages for the kind of multivariate analyses performed. The use of a population-based sample avoids the possible bias associated with help-seeking behavior. However, it does mean that the results obtained here on symptoms of anxiety and depression cannot necessarily be extrapolated to clinical syndromes. For example, if there were genes specific for panic disorder, individuals with such genes could be rare enough in our sample to prevent detection of a separable "panic" genetic factor.

Significance

The results of this study suggest that the tendency in the general population for symptoms of anxiety to co-occur with other symptoms of anxiety and symptoms of depression to co-occur with other symptoms of depression is largely the result of environmental factors. Contrary to our expectation, genetic influences on these symptoms were largely nonspecific. That is, while genes may "set" the vulnerability of an individual to symptoms of psychiatric distress, they do not seem to code specifically for symptoms of depression or anxiety. These findings are consistent with a previous analysis of the total anxiety and depression scale scores performed with the Australian NHMRC Twin Registry data analyzed here.[25] In that report, high genetic correlations were found between transformed total scores on the anxiety and depression subscales, indicating that the same genes were largely responsible for genetic variation in the two subscales.

The one notable exception to the apparent nonspecificity of gene action on symptoms of anxiety and depression was the consistent emergence of a minor "genetic somatic anxiety" factor. These results suggest that genes may be responsible for the frequently observed partial independence of "somatic" from "psychic" symptoms of anxiety.[26]

Because measures of relevant environmental variables were not obtained on twins from the Australian NHMRC Twin Registry, little further information can be extracted from the registry regarding the particular environmental variables that predispose to symptoms of anxiety vs symptoms of depression. However, as indicated by the results of the univariate genetic analyses of these data,[4] these environmental variables were not shared by members of a twin pair. Therefore, the environmental effects that specifically predispose to symptoms of anxiety vs symptoms of depression could not plausibly be parental characteristics, to which both members of a twin pair would be exposed.[27-29] By contrast, since most life events, except death or illness in relatives, are not shared by members of an adult twin pair, the results of this study are consistent with findings that certain classes of life events specifically precipitate either depression or anxiety.[30-32] This study demonstrates that genetically informative designs such as MZ and DZ twins, when appropriately analyzed, can not only provide insight into the role of genetic and environmental factors in the etiology of individual psychiatric symptoms, but can also clarify the degree to which the clustering of individual psychiatric symptoms into syndromes is the result of genetic vs environmental influences.

This study was supported in part by the Department of Mental Health and Mental Retardation, Commonwealth of Virginia, and by National Institutes of Health grants AG04954, GM30250, GM32732, HD15838, HL28922, HL31010, and MH40828.

The data on which this report is based were collected with support from the National Health and Medical Research Council of Australia who also support the Australian NHMRC Twin Registry. We acknowledge the roles of J. D. Mathews, MD, PhD, in establishment of the Register and of A. S. Henderson, MD, in collection of the psychiatric symptoms data. We thank Rosemary Jardine, PhD, and Marilyn Olsen for substantial help in preparation of the data.

References

1. Fleiss JL, Gurland BJ, Cooper JE: Some contributions to the measurement of psychopathology. *Br J Psychiatry* 1971;119:647-656.
2. Paykel ES: Have multivariate statistics contributed to classification? *Br J Psychiatry* 1981;139:357-362.
3. Martin NG, Eaves LJ: The genetical analysis of covariance structure. *Heredity* 1977;38:79-95.
4. Kendler KS, Heath A, Martin NG, Eaves LJ: Symptoms of anxiety and depression in a volunteer twin population: The etiologic role of genetic and environmental factors. *Arch Gen Psychiatry* 1986;43:213-221.
5. Fahy TJ, Brandon S, Garside RF: Clinical syndromes in a sample of depressed patients: A general practice material. *Proc R Soc Med* 1969;62:331-335.
6. Derogatis LR, Klerman GL, Lipman RS: Anxiety states and depressive neurosis: Issues in nosologic discrimination. *J Nerv Ment Dis* 1972;155:392-403.
7. Derogatis LR, Lipman RS, Covi L, Rickels K: Factorial invariance of symptom dimensions in anxious and depressive neuroses. *Arch Gen Psychiatry* 1972;27:659-665.
8. Mendels J, Weinstein N, Cohrane C: The relationship between depression and anxiety. *Arch Gen Psychiatry* 1972;27:649-653.
9. Roth M, Gurney C, Garside RF, Kerr TA: Studies in the classification of affective disorders: The relationship between anxiety states and depressive illnesses—I. *Br J Psychiatry* 1972;121:147-161.
10. Gurney C, Roth M, Garside RF, Kerr TA, Schapira K: Studies in the classification of affective disorders: The relationship between anxiety states and depressive illnesses—II. *Br J Psychiatry* 1972;121:162-166.
11. Prusoff B, Klerman GL: Differentiating depressed from anxious outpatients. *Arch Gen Psychiatry* 1974;30:302-308.
12. Roth M, Mountjoy CQ: The distinction between anxiety states and depressive disorders, in Paykel ES (ed): *Handbook of Affective Disorders.* New York, Guilford Press, 1982, pp 70-92.
13. Mullaney JA: The relationship between anxiety and depression: A review of some principal component analytic studies. *J Affect Dis* 1984;7:139-148.
14. Bedford A, Foulds GA, Sheffield BF: A new personal disturbance scale (DDSI/SAD). *Br J Soc Clin Psychiatry* 1976;15:387-394.
15. Joreskog KG, Sobrom D, Lisrel VI: *Analysis of Linear Structural Relationships by the Method of Maximum Likelihood.* Chicago, International Educational Services, 1983.
16. Harman HH: *Factor Analysis*, ed 3. Chicago, University of Chicago Press, 1976.
17. Olsson U: Maximum likelihood estimation of the polychoric correlation coefficient. *Psychometrika* 1979;44:443-460.
18. Heath AC, Berg K: Effects of social policy on the heritability of education achievement, in Berg K (ed): *Medical Genetics: Past, Present, Future.* New York, Alan R Liss Inc, 1985.
19. Heath AC, Berg K, Eaves LJ, Solaas MH, Sundet J, Nance WE, Corey LA, Magnus P: No decline in assortative mating for education level. *Behav Genet* 1985;15:349-369.
20. Heath AC, Berg K, Eaves LJ, Solaas MH, Corey LA, Sundet J, Magnus P, Nance WE: Education policy and the heritability of educational attainment. *Nature* 1985;314:734-736.
21. Derogatis LR, Serio JC, Cleary PA: An empirical comparison of three indices of factorial similarity. *Psychol Rep* 1972;30:791-804.
22. Mapother E: Discussion on manic-depressive psychosis. *Br Med J* 1926;2:872-879.
23. Kerr TA, Roth M, Schapira K, Gurney C: The assessment and prediction of outcome in affective disorders. *Br J Psychiatry* 1972;121:167-174.
24. Murphy JM, Neff RK, Sobol AM, Rice JX, Olivier DC: Computer diagnosis of depression and anxiety: The Stirling Country Study. *Psychol Med* 1985;15:99-112.
25. Jardine R, Martin NG, Henderson AS: Genetic covariation between neuroticism and the symptoms of anxiety and depression. *Genet Epidemiol* 1984;1:89-107.
26. Schalling D, Cronholm B, Asberg M, Espmark S: Ratings of psychic and somatic anxiety indicants: Interrater reliability and relations to personality variables. *Acta Psychiatr Scand* 1973;49:353-368.
27. Parker G: Reported parental characteristics in relation to trait depression and anxiety levels in a non-clinical group. *Aust NZ J Psychiatry* 1979;13:260-264.
28. Parker G: Parental characteristics in relation to depressive disorders. *Br J Psychiatry* 1979;134:138-147.
29. Parker G: Parental representations of patients with anxiety neurosis. *Acta Psychiatr Scand* 1981;63:33-36.
30. Barrett JE: The relationship of life events to the onset of neurotic disorders, in Barrett JE (ed): *Stress and Mental Disorder.* New York, Raven Press, 1979, pp 87-109.
31. Finlay-Jones R, Brown GW: Types of stressful live events and the onset of anxiety and depressive disorders. *Psychol Med* 1981;11:803-815.
32. Torgersen S: Developmental differentiation of anxiety and affective neuroses. *Acta Psychiatr Scand* 1985;71:304-310.

Stressful Life Events, Genetic Liability, and Onset of an Episode of Major Depression in Women

Kenneth S. Kendler, M.D., Ronald C. Kessler, Ph.D., Ellen E. Walters, M.S., Charles MacLean, Ph.D., Michael C. Neale, Ph.D., Andrew C. Heath, D.Phil., and Lindon J. Eaves, Ph.D., D.Sc.

Objective: This study was undertaken to clarify how genetic liability and stressful life events interact in the etiology of major depression. Method: Information about stressful life events and onset of major depressive episodes in the past year was collected in a population-based sample of female-female twin pairs including 2,164 individuals, 53,215 person-months of observation, and 492 onsets of depression. Results: Nine "personal" and three aggregate "network" stressful events significantly predicted onset of major depression in the month of occurrence, four of which predicted onset with an odds ratio of >10 and were termed "severe": death of a close relative, assault, serious marital problems, and divorce/breakup. Genetic liability also had a significant impact on risk of onset of depression. For severe stressful events, as well as for 10 of the 12 individual stressful events, the best-fitting model for the joint effect of stressful events and genetic liability on onset of major depression suggested genetic control of sensitivity to the depression-inducing effects of stressful life events. In individuals at lowest genetic risk (monozygotic twin, co-twin unaffected), the probability of onset of major depression per month was predicted to be 0.5% and 6.2%, respectively, for those unexposed and exposed to a severe event. In those at highest genetic risk (monozygotic twin, co-twin affected), these probabilities were 1.1% and 14.6%, respectively. Linear regression analysis indicated significant Genotype by Environment interaction in the prediction of onset of major depression. Conclusions: Genetic factors influence the risk of onset of major depression in part by altering the sensitivity of individuals to the depression-inducing effect of stressful life events.
(Am J Psychiatry 1995; 152:833–842)

According as the humour itself is intended or remitted in men [and] their . . . rational soul is better able to make resistance; so are they more or less affected [by adversity]. For that which is but a flea-biting to one, causeth insufferable torment to another; and which one by his singular moderation and well-imposed carriage can happily overcome, a second is no whit able to sustain, but upon every small occasion of misconceived abuse, injury, grief, disgrace [and] loss . . . yields so far to passion, that . . . his digestion hindered, his sleep gone, his spirits obscured, and his heart heavy . . . he himself [is] overcome with melancholy.

—R. Burton (1)

There is . . . a group of depressive illnesses in which the psychological impetus is of prime importance . . . . These depressive states are constitutionally based: they occur in individuals who from youth onward are inclined to take

Received May 20, 1994; revision received Nov. 18, 1994; accepted Dec. 1, 1994. From the Department of Psychiatry and the Department of Human Genetics, Medical College of Virginia/Virginia Commonwealth University. Address reprint requests to Dr. Kendler, Box 980710, Medical College of Virginia, Richmond, VA 23298-0710.
Supported by NIMH grant MH-40828. The Virginia Twin Registry, established and maintained by W. Nance, M.D., Ph.D., and L. Corey, Ph.D., is supported by NIH grants HD-26746 and NS-31564.
The authors thank Pak Sham, M.D., for comments on an earlier version of the manuscript.

things badly, whose depressive reaction [to "psychological upsets"] is generally severe and of more than average duration.

—K. Bonhoeffer (2)

The concept that depression commonly arises when a vulnerable individual confronts adversity is not new. However, surprisingly little progress has been made in confirming or refuting this plausible and widely held belief by rigorous hypothesis testing. Although substantial evidence now exists that adversity (3, 4), especially stressful life events, and genetic predisposition (5, 6) are important risk factors for major depression, we still know little about how these two risk factors interact. Previous studies of this question have suffered from methodologic limitations, including small sample size, indirect methods of assessment, simplistic analytic strategies, and an inability to separate genetic from familial/environmental effects.

In 1922 Strecker (7) examined the family histories of "mental disease" of patients with manic-depressive psychosis and noted that the proportion of patients with a positive family history was lowest among those whose onset was associated with severe stress. He concluded that "extraneous" factors are of less etiologic importance in cases of manic-depressive illness when the family background is "defective." Using family history information, Pollitt (8) found that the risk of major depression in relatives was 50% lower when the patient's onset was associated with a severe stressful life event. Perris et al. (9), however, found no difference in the number of stressful life events prior to a depressive episode among patients with family histories of major depression and those without. Phelan et al. (10) examined depressive symptoms and found that individuals with positive family histories were more sensitive to the depression-inducing effects of certain stressful life events than those who had no family history of major depression. In contrast, McGuffin et al. (11) examined the impact of recent stressful life events and family background on the risk of current depression and found that individuals at high familial risk for major depression were *less* sensitive to the depressive effects of stressful life events than were individuals at low familial risk.

If both genetic and environmental risk factors are of etiologic importance in major depression, they may interact in disease etiology in potentially complex ways (12, 13). Of the possible models, we emphasize two: *additive* and *genetic control of sensitivity to the environment.* In the additive model, the increase in risk associated with exposure to stressful life events is similar for individuals with low-risk and high-risk genotypes; this model predicts that the impact of stressful life events and genetic risk factors on liability to major depression are independent. In genetic control of sensitivity to the environment, the increase in risk of major depression associated with exposure to stressful life events is *greater* for those with a high genetic risk than for those with a low genetic risk; that is, genes have an impact on the risk of major depression in part by altering the individual's sensitivity to the depression-inducing effect of stressful life events.

In this report we examine how stressful life events and genetic vulnerability influence the risk of onset of an episode of major depression in a population-based sample of personally interviewed female twins. We address the following specific questions:

1. What are the magnitude and duration of the impact of stressful life events on the risk of onset of major depression?
2. What is the magnitude of the impact of genetic factors on the risk of onset of major depression?
3. What is the nature of the interaction between stressful life events and genetic factors in the risk of onset of major depression? Specifically, can we find evidence in support of an additive model or a model of genetic control of sensitivity to the environment?

METHOD

We studied female-female Caucasian twin pairs ascertained from the population-based Virginia Twin Registry (6, 14, 15) whose mean age at first interview was 30.1 years (SD=7.6). Twin pairs were enrolled if both individuals responded to a mailed questionnaire, the individual response rate to which was 64%. Personal interviews were then conducted with 93% of this group (N=2,164 individuals) (92% face to face and 8% by telephone), which included both members of 1,033 pairs. Follow-up interviews were then conducted with 2,002 of the twins initially interviewed (93% of the 2,164), including both members of 938 pairs. Unlike the initial interviews, nearly all of the follow-up interviews were conducted by telephone. After an explanation of the research procedure, written informed consent was obtained from all subjects before the personal interviews. For telephone interviews, verbal assent was obtained.

The mean number of months between these two interviews was 17.3 (SD=3.8). Both interviews were conducted by individuals with a master's degree or doctorate in social work or psychology or a bachelor's degree and at least 2 years of clinical experience. The same interviewer never interviewed both members of a twin pair. As outlined in detail elsewhere (6), zygosity was determined from a set of interview questions and photographs, and when these were not definitive, from DNA polymorphisms, producing an error rate in zygosity assignment that can be estimated to be under 2%. Final determinations of zygosity yielded 590 monozygotic and 440 dizygotic twin pairs as well as three pairs of unknown zygosity.

Included in both interviews was an identical section that assessed episodes of major depression, defined according to the DSM-III-R criteria, and a series of stressful life events over the month of the interview and the 12 preceding months. These were assessed in different portions of the interview to reduce retrospective reporting bias. Specifically, we assessed the occurrence over the past year of 14 individual symptoms that represented the disaggregated nine "A" criteria for major depression in DSM-III-R (including two items for criterion A4 to assess separately insomnia and hypersomnia). For each symptom reported as present, interviewers probed to ensure that it was not due to physical illness or medication. Respondents then had to aggregate reported symptoms over the past year into co-occurring syndromes. If depressive syndromes occurred, respondents were asked when they occurred, and their onset and end were recorded to the nearest month.

The months of occurrence of all stressful life events were also recorded. At both interviews we assessed nine "personal" events (events that happened primarily to the informant: assault (assault, rape, or mugging), serious marital problems, divorce/breakup (divorce, marital separation, broken engagement, or breakup of other romantic relationship), job loss (being laid off from a job or fired), loss of a confidant (separation from other loved one or close friend), serious illness, major financial problem, being robbed, and serious legal problem. We also assessed 22 "network" events, i.e., events that occurred primarily to, or in interaction with, an individual in the respondent's social network, including death or severe illness of the respondent's spouse, child, parent, co-twin, other sibling, other relative, or "other individual close to you" and serious trouble getting along with the respondent's parent, child, twin, sibling, in-laws, other relative, neighbor, or close friend. Because of the large sample size and limited time in the interview, we assessed neither the contextual aspects nor the putative independence of the life events (3). Interrater reliability for determining the occurrence and dating of our stressful life event categories was assessed for 53 jointly interviewed twins and found to be in the good to excellent range, with kappas equaling 0.93 and 0.82, respectively.

The diagnosis of major depression was made by computer algorithm incorporating the DSM-III-R criteria except for criterion B2 (which excludes depressive syndromes considered to be uncomplicated bereavement). For the 53 jointly interviewed twins, the 1-year prevalence of major depression was assessed with perfect agreement (kappa=1.00). We assessed the reliability of our dating of depressive episodes by examining raters' agreement on the respondent's having had a depressive episode in the 689 (53×13) assessed months. Reliability was excellent (kappa=0.97). The details of our statistical analyses are outlined in appendix 1.

TABLE 1. Frequency of Occurrence of Individual Personal Stressful Life Events and Associated Odds Ratios for Onset of Major Depression in 2,164 Female Twins

Event	Number of Person-Months Containing Event	Odds Ratio for Onset of Major Depression: In Month of Event	One Month After Event	Two Months After Event
Assault	48	12.1*	1.4	—[a]
Serious marital problems	506	11.7*	1.0	1.3
Divorce/breakup	629	11.5*	0.7	1.4
Job loss	149	6.0*	0.5	0.5
Loss of confidant	562	4.6*	1.2	1.1
Serious illness	877	3.7*	1.2	1.4
Major financial problem	1,420	2.4*	0.6	1.2
Being robbed	182	1.1	1.2	0.4
Serious legal problem	24	—[a]	—[a]	—[a]

[a]Stable estimate could not be obtained because of small number of occurrences.
*p<0.0001.

RESULTS

Our total sample contained 53,215 person-months of exposure among 2,164 individuals. Four hundred ninety-two separate onsets of major depression were recorded, for an uncorrected monthly risk of 0.92%. These 492 onsets occurred in 312 individuals (or 14% of the entire sample of 2,164). Of those reporting at least one episode of major depression over the period of ascertainment, 189 (61%) had a single episode, 78 (25%) had two episodes, and 45 (14%) had three or more episodes.

Stressful Life Events

Personal. Table 1 lists the number of occurrences of each of the nine assessed personal stressful life events and the odds ratio for the onset of major depression in the month in which the event occurred and 1 and 2 months afterward. Serious legal problems were too rare to obtain stable estimates.

The odds ratio for major depression was significantly increased in the month of occurrence of seven of the remaining eight life events; the exception was being robbed. The odds ratios ranged from 2.4 for major financial problems to 12.1 for assault. None of these personal stressful life events significantly increased the risk of major depression 1 or 2 months after their occurrence. Similar results were found for 3 months after occurrence.

Network. The frequency of individual network stressful life events varied widely (table 2). While death of a spouse, co-twin, child, or other sibling was very rare, serious illness in individuals in the respondent's social network and serious trouble getting along with them were considerably more common. The impact of network events on the odds ratios for major depression in the month of the events' occurrence is also shown in table 2. For death of major network figures, only in the case of parents, other relatives, and "other individuals close to you" were there enough events to obtain a stable estimate. The odds ratio for major depression upon the death of a parent (21.3) was the highest noted for any stressful life event. A serious illness of a parent, co-twin, child, other sibling, other relative, or "other individual close to you" significantly but modestly increased the odds ratio for major depression in the month of its occurrence. Trouble getting along with others significantly increased the odds ratio for major depression in the month of its occurrence in all categories of the social network except other sibling. For the seven most common individual network events, where we could obtain stable estimates, we examined the odds ratios for major depression 1–3 months after their occurrence. Only three of these 21 individual analyses yielded significant results (none below p=0.02), with no evident pattern.

To produce more stable estimates and reduce the number of categories for subsequent analyses, we created the categories death of, serious illness of, and serious trouble getting along with a close relative. For death and serious illness, a close relative was defined as a parent, spouse, child, co-twin, or other sibling. For trouble getting along, a close relative was defined as a parent, child, co twin, or other sibling.

Table 3 shows the results for these combined network event categories, all three of which strongly predicted the risk of major depression in the month of their occurrence. The odds ratio for major depression within a month of the death of a close relative (20.5) was higher than that found for illness of or trouble getting along with a close relative. With the exception of serious illness in a close relative, these stressful life events did not increase the risk of major depression 1, 2, or 3 months after their occurrence.

TABLE 2. Frequency of Occurrence of Individual Network Events and Associated Odds Ratios for Onset of Major Depression in the Month of the Event's Occurrence Among 2,164 Female Twins

	Death of Relative		Serious Illness of Relative		Serious Trouble Getting Along With Relative	
Relative	N	Odds Ratio in Month of Event	N	Odds Ratio in Month of Event	N	Odds Ratio in Month of Event
Parent	88	21.3†	481	4.4†	192	10.8†
Spouse	1	0.0[a]	52	1.7	—[b]	—[b]
Co-twin	0	0.0[a]	95	5.8***	148	5.0†
Child	6	0.0[a]	66	3.6*	148	9.4†
Other sibling	12	—[c]	72	6.6†	137	1.9
In-laws	—[b]	—[b]	—[b]	—[b]	169	5.8†
Other relative	742	2.0*	600	1.9*	83	4.4**
"Other individual close to you"	428	2.7***	225	2.8*	218	4.1†

[a]Odds ratio is 0.0 because no month contained both the event and an onset of major depression.
[b]Not inquired about, except for trouble getting along with spouse, which was assessed separately as marital problems.
[c]Stable estimate could not be obtained because of small number of occurrences.
*$p<0.05$. **$p<0.01$. ***$p<0.001$. † $p<0.0001$.

TABLE 3. Frequency of Occurrence of Combined Categories of Stressful Life Events and Associated Odds Ratios for Onset of Major Depression in the Month of the Event's Occurrence and One and Two Months Afterward Among 2,164 Female Twins

		Odds Ratio for Onset of Major Depression		
Event	N	In Month of Event	One Month After Event	Two Months After Event
Death of close relative	107	20.5**	1.3	1.4
Serious illness of close relative	755	4.3**	1.0	2.2*
Serious trouble getting along with close relative	625	7.2**	0.9	1.2
Any severe stressful event	1,228	12.2**	0.9	1.2

*$p<0.05$. **$p<0.0001$.

Severe. We created a post hoc category of severe stressful life events that included the four events that produced odds ratios for major depression in excess of 10: death of a close relative, assault, serious marital problems, and divorce/breakup. A total of 1,228 person-months contained a severe stressful life event, and the odds for onset of a depressive episode in the month in which the event occurred were increased 12.2-fold (table 3). No significant increased risk of major depression 1–3 months after the severe stressful event was found.

Genetic Risk Factors

Subsequent analyses were restricted to members of the 1,030 twin pairs of known zygosity both members of which were assessed at the first personal interview. This subsample contained 51,268 person-months at risk and 476 onsets of major depression. By logistic regression, controlling for age and zygosity, we found that the rates of onset of major depression and severe life events were similar in the twins included in this subsample and those excluded from it (χ^2=0.60, df=1, n.s., and χ^2=1.66, df=1, n.s., respectively).

The impact of genetic factors on onset of an episode of major depression in this sample was assessed using a single variable termed "genetic risk" (appendix 1). Using all control variables, we found that this index highly significantly predicted onset of an episode of major depression (χ^2=65.85, df=1, $p<0.001$). If we assign the lowest risk group (monozygotic twin with co-twin unaffected) a risk of 1.0, then the odds ratio for major depression in any given month is 1.3 when there is an unaffected dizygotic co-twin, 2.0 when there is an affected dizygotic co-twin, and 2.6 when there is an affected monozygotic co-twin.

Stressful Life Events and Genetic Risk Factors

Table 4 presents results of the analyses that examined jointly the main effects of environmental risk factors (stressful life events), genetic risk factors, and their interaction in the prediction of onset of major depression in the month of the stressful life event. We examined the individual personal stressful life events that had previously been shown to be significant predictors of major depression, the three aggregate network events, and the combined category of any severe stressful life event. In all of these analyses, both the main effect of stressful life events and the main effect of genetic risk factors on the onset of major depression were highly significant. However, in these 11 separate analyses, the interaction term was significant only once, and in seven of them, the chi-square value of the interaction term was <1.0. Furthermore, in the category of any severe stressful life event, despite an extremely high level of statistical significance for the main effect of stressful events (environmental factors), the interaction term between stressful life events and genetic risk factors was ***nonsignificant.***

We then calculated the risk of illness in the eight relevant categories of twins (four levels of genetic risk with and without exposure to the stressful life event) predicted from the best-fitting model for the various categories of stressful life events. Except for "serious trouble getting along with a close relative," all of these

TABLE 4. Results of Logistic Regression Analyses Predicting Onset of Major Depression From Environmental Risk Factors (Stressful Life Events), Genetic Risk Factors, and Their Interaction in Both Members of 1,030 Female-Female Twin Pairs

	Regression Results					
	Environmental Factors		Genetic Factors		Interaction of Genetic and Environmental Factors	
Event	Odds Ratio	χ^2 (df=1)	Odds Ratio	χ^2 (df=1)	Odds Ratio	χ^2 (df=1)
Assault	15.0	34.8**	1.6	62.3**	1.5	0.5
Serious marital problems	12.3	214.8**	1.6	60.9**	0.7	2.9
Divorce/breakup	12.3	269.3**	1.6	62.6**	0.7	3.4
Job loss	6.8	29.5**	1.6	63.8**	0.7	0.6
Loss of confidant	4.9	51.6**	1.6	61.4**	1.0	0.0
Serious illness	4.3	57.5**	1.6	62.8**	0.8	0.9
Major financial problem	2.5	21.8**	1.6	61.0**	0.9	0.2
Death of close relative	16.0	86.9**	1.6	63.8**	0.8	0.6
Serious trouble getting along with close relative	8.4	148.0**	1.6	59.6**	0.6	4.5*
Serious illness of close relative	4.9	67.6**	1.6	62.2**	0.9	0.2
Any severe stressful event	13.3	492.2**	1.6	57.4**	0.8	2.7

*p=0.03. **p<0.0001.

models included only the main effects of stressful life events and genetic risk factors.

Figure 1 shows the results of these calculations for the category of severe stressful life events. While differing in quantitative terms, the figures looked similar for the individual stressful life events. Three major conclusions can be reached from these results. First, even in the presence of high genetic risk and severe stressful life events, the majority of individuals *do not* develop an episode of major depression. Second, genetic factors are important in influencing the risk of major depression both in the presence *and* in the absence of stressful life events. Put another way, environmental risk factors influence the risk of major depression in individuals at both low and high genetic risk. Third, the impact of environmental factors on the risk of major depression is substantially *greater* for individuals at high genetic risk than for those at low genetic risk. For example, in those at lowest genetic risk (monozygotic twins whose co-twins are unaffected), the risk of onset of an episode of major depression in a month without a severe stressful life event is estimated at 0.5%. In the month of a severe stressful life event, the risk of onset of major depression in these individuals is predicted to be 6.2%. That is, in individuals at low genetic risk, the predicted *increase* in risk of a depressive episode associated with a severe stressful life event is 5.7%. However, for those at highest genetic risk (monozygotic twins whose co-twins are affected), the risk of onset of an episode of major depression in the absence and in the presence of a severe stressful life event is predicted to be 1.1% and 14.6%, respectively. That is, for genetically predisposed individuals, exposure to a severe stressful life event is associated with a 13.5% increase in the risk of a depressive episode. As predicted by the model of genetic control of sensitivity to the environment, the increased risk of onset of major depression with exposure to a severe stressful life event is 2.4 times *greater* for those at highest genetic risk than for those at lowest genetic risk.

Using logistic regression, we found no evidence of an interaction between stressful life events and genetic factors in predicting the onset of an episode of major depression. However, what is additive on a logistic scale should be approximately multiplicative on the scale of probabilities (appendix 1 includes a brief discussion of scales of measurement). To test this hypothesis, we conducted a discrete-time survival linear regression predict-

FIGURE 1. Risk of Onset of Major Depression per Person-Month as a Function of Genetic Liability and the Presence or Absence of a Severe Stressful Life Event in That Month Among 2,060 Female Twins[a]

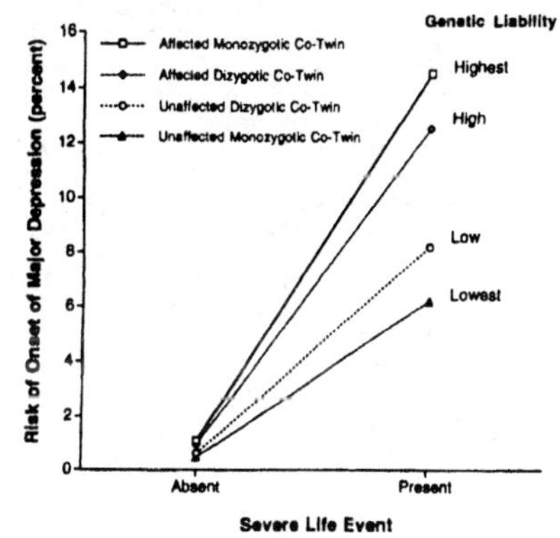

[a]Genetic liability is reflected by both the zygosity of the twin and the lifetime history of major depression in her co-twin. The results presented here are those predicted by the best-fitting logistic regression equation that contains the control variables outlined in the text and the main effects of the life event and genetic risk factors. A severe life event is defined as assault, serious marital problems, divorce/breakup, or death of a close relative.

ing onset of major depression. Consistent with the results of the logistic regression, both severe stressful life events (beta=0.095, t=12.47, df=48117, $p<0.0001$) and genetic risk factors (beta=0.004, t=6.88, df=48117, $p< 0.0001$) had highly significant main effects. However, in contrast to the results with logistic regression, the interaction term was both positive and statistically significant (beta=0.020, t=2.32, df=48115, p=0.02). On the scale of probabilities, as predicted by the model of genetic control of sensitivity to the environment, the increased risk of onset of major depression associated with exposure to a stressful life event was significantly greater for those at high genetic risk than for those at low genetic risk for major depression.

DISCUSSION

We sought to clarify in this report the interaction between stressful life events and genetic predisposition in the etiology of major depression in a population-based sample of female twins. We discuss our major results in turn.

Stressful Life Events

In this sample, all personal and aggregate network stressful life events except being robbed were significantly related to the onset of episodes of major depression in the month of the events' occurrence. The odds ratio for major depression given these events ranged from 2.4 to 20.5. For our category of severe events, the odds ratio was 12.2. The magnitude of the effect of stressful life events on onset of major depression in our data is toward the upper range of that found by previous researchers (3, 16–19), most of whom examined the impact of stressful life events over longer time periods (e.g., 3–6 months).

We consistently found that the odds ratio for major depression was increased only in the month of occurrence of the stressful life event. In their influential report, Brown and Harris (3) noted a large increase in the rate of severe stressful life events in the first 3 weeks prior to onset of major depression, with much smaller increases seen in the second and third 3-week periods prior to onset. They concluded that "severe events usually lead fairly quickly to depression—most often within nine weeks." Other researchers have also noted that the depression-inducing impact of stressful life events tends to occur quickly (18, 20).

There have been several previous attempts to describe the class of stressful life events that is potent in precipitating major depression, with descriptions containing terms such as "loss," "exit," "assault on self-esteem," and "long-term contextual threat" (3, 4, 21–23). Three of the six stressful life events with an odds ratio of >5 for onset of depression were directly related to "loss": death of a close relative, divorce/breakup, and job loss. However, the other three events (assault, serious marital problems, and serious trouble getting along with a close relative) are probably more accurately seen as threatening and/or reflecting loss of self-esteem and support.

Another major issue in life event research has been the characterization of stressful life events as putatively independent versus dependent on the respondent's behavior (3, 4). We did not assess the independence/dependence of individual stressful life events. Of the six events most potent in precipitating major depression, only one (death of a close relative) is unambiguously independent. Depending on individual circumstances, two other event categories (assault and job loss) might be either independent or dependent. However, in most circumstances, the three remaining potent events (serious marital problems, divorce/breakup, and serious trouble getting along with a close relative) would be considered, at least in part, dependent on the respondent's own behavior. These results are consistent with previous findings that most depression-inducing stressful life events are in part dependent on the individual's behavior (4). Because the single stressful life event category that most strongly predicted the onset of major depression, death of a close relative, was clearly independent of the respondent's own behavior, our results suggest that the association between stressful life events and major depression cannot be entirely due to individuals precipitating their own stressful life events.

Genetic Risk Factors

Using discrete-time survival analysis, we found that genetic risk factors strongly predicted onset of an episode of major depression. The individuals at highest risk (monozygotic twins with affected co-twins) had a risk of depression that was 2.6 times greater than that of those with the lowest genetic risk (monozygotic twins with unaffected co-twins). These results are consistent with the results in most, but not all, of the previous twin and adoption literature (5), as well as with results obtained in this twin sample with the use of more traditional analyses of both lifetime (6) and 1-year (14) prevalence of major depression.

Interaction of Genetic and Environmental Risk Factors

Our major goal was to clarify how genetic and environmental (stressful life events) risk factors interact in the etiology of major depression. Our initial analyses, using logistic regression, found strong evidence for a main effect of stressful life events and a main effect for genetic risk factors in influencing onset of episodes of major depression, but no evidence for an interaction. Because logistic regression utilizes the logarithm of the probability of a depressive episode, the absence of an interaction indicates that the impact of genetic and environmental risk factors on major depression was multiplicative in nature. When we examined the predicted risks from the best-fitting logistic models, we found that the impact of stressful life events on the risk of onset of depression was much greater for individuals at high genetic risk than for those at low genetic risk. These results were consistent with the expectations of the model of genetic control of sensitivity to the environment and not with the additive model.

To test formally for the presence of an interaction on the scale of probabilities (rather than the log of probabilities), we used linear regression to examine the impact of severe stressful life events and genetic factors on onset of major depression. These analyses showed statistically significant evidence of positive interaction between genotype and environment. That is, the net increase in risk of onset of major depression associated with a severe stressful life event was significantly greater for individuals with a high genetic liability to major depression than for those with a low genetic liability. These results suggest that genetic factors influence the risk of major depression in part by influencing the susceptibility of individuals to the depressive effect of stressful life events (12).

However, in all of the regression analyses examining interactions, both genetic effects and stressful life events continued to have substantial and significant main effects. These results suggest that 1) even in the absence of the assessed stressful life events, the risk of onset of depression was influenced by genetic factors, and 2) even in the absence of high genetic risk, stressful life events continued to be significant predictors of onset of major depression.

Previous attempts to rigorously examine the interrelation of genetic and environmental factors in the etiology of psychiatric illness have been rare and restricted to adoption studies of alcoholism (24, 25), antisocial personality (26, 27), and schizophrenia (28). All of these studies examined the interaction between genetic risk factors and the rearing environment in the adoptive home. To our knowledge, no previous study has examined the interrelation between genetic factors and environmental risk factors that occur close to the onset of an episode of psychiatric illness in adulthood.

We are aware of five studies that have examined the relation between family history of major depression and exposure to stressful life events in governing the risk of major depression or depressive symptoms. Of these studies, three (7, 8, 10) found results broadly consistent with those reported here—that individuals with a familial "loading" for major depression are more sensitive to the depression-inducing effects of stressful events—while two (9, 11) did not.

Issues of Scale

All statistical interactions are scale dependent. In this study, with the use of a logistic scale, no statistical interaction was found between stressful life events and genetic predisposition in the prediction of onset of major depression. However, when these results are examined on the scale of true probability, a substantial interaction is evident. Which scale is correct?

Unfortunately, no definitive answer to this question is available. In the biological and social sciences, there is rarely strong a priori evidence for the validity of one scale of measurement over another. Some persons have argued that a logarithmic scale is more appropriate and statistically convenient (29). We choose to emphasize the scale of true probability for three reasons. First, most clinicians think in terms of probabilities and not logarithms of probabilities. Second, Rothman (13) argued persuasively that causal assumptions about the independence of the effect of multiple risk factors can only be rigorously evaluated by using the scale of true probabilities. Biological effects are, he argued, more likely to increase the *probability* of onset rather than the *odds* of onset. Third, public health officials implicitly use the scale of probabilities in their efforts to identify individuals at increased risk for a disorder because of exposure to a given risk factor. Only by using this scale is it possible to identify individuals who, when exposed to a given environmental agent, have a particularly large *absolute* increase in risk of illness.

Implications and Limitations

Etiologic models for psychiatric illness in which genetic and environmental risk factors act additively are easy to understand and to analyze statistically. However, the results of this and other studies (24–27) suggest that despite their intuitive appeal, such models are unlikely to be correct. While our findings complicate the task of understanding the etiology of mental illness, they are exciting because they force us to confront the *dynamic* nature of our genetic endowment. Gene expression as it influences risk of psychiatric illness is not static but, rather, reacts to and interacts with environmental experiences.

The results of this study should be interpreted in the context of six potentially significant methodologic limitations. First, the analyses assume that observations in twin pairs are independent. This is not precisely true. However, the tetrachoric correlation (0.17) in all twin pairs for onset of major depression in a given month is so small that correcting for it (30) would produce no substantial change in the findings. Second, our logistic regression discrete-time survival analysis modeled genetic effects in a way that is less elegant and immediately interpretable than it would be with structural equations (31). However, under most realistic conditions, this approach produces little distortion in the estimation of genetic effects (32).

Third, the discrete-time survival model, as well as all continuous-time survival models, treats each individual's history as if it were a set of independent observations (33). Violations of this assumption will result in standard error estimates that are biased downward, while parameter estimation is not affected. However, we included control variables in our model that indexed the prior occurrence of stressful life events and episodes of major depression during the period of observation. Furthermore, only a small proportion of the twins with major depression in our sample reported multiple episodes over the period of ascertainment. It is therefore unlikely that this problem produced substantial distortions in our pattern of results.

Fourth, time was too limited in our interviews to assess contextual information for each individual life event that would have allowed judgments of severity or "degree of threat" (3). Therefore, the life events analyzed in each category are probably heterogeneous with respect to contextual severity. Such heterogeneity would more likely attenuate than exaggerate effects.

Fifth, since both stressful life events and onsets of major depression were assessed to the nearest month, we assumed that when both occurred in the same month, the stressful life event preceded and influenced the onset of major depression. We tested the validity of this key assumption in two ways. First, in a section of the interview separate from that which evaluated stressful life events, respondents with a depressive syndrome in the past year were asked, "Did something happen to make you feel that way or did the feeling just come on you 'out of the blue'?" There were 96 twins who reported a severe stressful life event and onset of depression occurring in the same month and who answered this question in sufficient detail. In 81 (84%) of these cases, the twins answered this question with the same life event they had previously reported as occurring in the same month and which we had scored as "severe." In 11 cases (11%), two or more stressful life events had occurred together in a single causal sequence in 1 month, and one was considered by us to be "severe" while the twin listed another as "causing" the major depression. In only four cases (4%), did the twin state that her major depression was "caused" by something other than the severe stressful life event that occurred in the same month as the onset of the depression. Validating the assumptions of our analysis, our results suggest that in 96% of cases, when a severe stressful life event and onset of depression occurred in the same month, the respondent considered the stressful life event to precede and either directly or indirectly contribute to the onset of major depression.

We then examined whether onset of depression significantly predicted stressful life events in the subsequent month. Of the 11 categories of stressful life events examined in table 4 (including the aggregate measure of any severe stressful life event), we could obtain stable estimates for nine (no onset of serious marital problems or death of a close relative occurred in the month following onset of a depressive episode). In none of these analyses did the onset of major depression significantly predict the occurrence of stressful life events in the succeeding month. These findings further support the hypothesis that the tendency for onset of major depression and stressful life events to co-occur in the same month is due mostly to stressful life events predisposing to onset of depression.

Sixth, in this sample, both the risk of major depression (6, 14) and the probability of experiencing certain stressful life events (34) were influenced by genetic factors. We have not considered here whether these genetic factors are correlated—whether genes that increase the risk of major depression might also predispose individuals to stressful life events. In a standard linear regression, this phenomenon, termed "genotype-environment correlation" or "genetic control of exposure to the environment" (12), would not influence estimates of genotype-environment interaction. We further addressed this issue by assessing, in two different ways, the strength of the possible genetic correlation between major depression and stressful life events. First, adding to our model the co-twin's history of stressful life events in the past 2 years neither significantly predicted onset of major depression nor changed any of the other parameter estimates. Second, we examined how much of the impact of stressful life events on major depression might be noncausal and mediated through common genetic influences. Examining severe stressful life events, we found that the odds ratio in predicting onset of depression declined 5% when the co-twin's history of major depression was added to the model. These analyses suggest that if any genetic correlation exists between major depression and stressful life events, it is modest and explains very little of the impact of stressful life events on onset of major depression. Our assessment of genotype-environment interaction in this sample was, therefore, unlikely to be substantially biased by a correlation between genetic risk factors for major depression and stressful life events.

APPENDIX 1. Statistical Analysis

We conducted an event history analysis using a discrete-time approach (35, 36), examining each "person-month" of observation. This usually meant 26 months of observation for individuals who were interviewed initially and at follow-up, and 13 for those not successfully interviewed at follow-up. Each person-month record contained information about whether an episode of major depression started in that month, whether a given stressful life event occurred in that month, or whether that stressful life event occurred in the previous 3 months. Each observation record also showed the relevant covariates, which included age, previous history of that stressful life event or major depression within the time frame of the study, and the year of the study (first versus second). The hazard rate for major depression for that month (as measured from the time of the interview) was also included as a control variable, since episodes of major depression were not uniformly distributed over the period of study. When a twin experienced an episode of major depression, she was censored from the sample until she was again at risk, having recorded an end to that depressive episode. She then re-entered the sample with the variable "previous history of major depression" updated. We had, in our sample, a number of women who reported chronic depressions that began prior to our period of ascertainment. These individuals were *not* considered to have an onset of major depression in the first study month and were censored from the sample for the entire period they reported meeting criteria for major depression. Our discrete-time survival model assumed that if the same individual experienced multiple onsets of major depression within the study period, the same underlying processes operated in all onsets. Analyses that included history of major depression *prior* to the observation period as a covariate were also completed. Little change in results was found.

These analyses treat each individual person-month as an independent observation. The risk of having an onset of major depression is modeled as the dependent variable in a logistic regression. A weighted sum of the independent variables is transformed to a predicted risk (or probability of onset) by a logistic function. The effects of independent variables are therefore linear on the logistic scale but usually nonlinear on the scale of probability. Allison (35) has shown that under the assumption of independence of the individual observations, such a model produces the true maximum-likelihood estimators and artifactually inflates neither the sample size nor the test statistic.

Previous analyses in this sample suggested that the familial aggregation of both lifetime and 1-year prevalence of major depression was due to additive genetic factors (6, 14). Given these results, all twins could be conveniently assigned to one of four categories of increasing "genetic risk" of major depression on the basis of their co-twins' lifetime history of major depression: 1) monozygotic twin and co-twin unaffected, 2) dizygotic twin and co-twin unaffected, 3) dizygotic twin and co-twin affected, and 4) monozygotic twin and co-twin affected. For the present analysis, we assume that the genetic effects in these four groups are proportional to –1.0, –0.5, 0.5, and 1.0, respectively. The magnitude of the estimated regression coefficient therefore reflects the importance of additive genetic effects (37, 38).

This parsimonious model has potential limitations. First, there is no simple relation between the estimated logistic regression coefficient for genetic effects and heritability as determined by the liability-threshold model (39). However, there is a surprising degree of correspondence between the two over the range of parameters utilized in this study (32).

Second, this model does not contain measures of family environment or genetic dominance. In fitting a full twin regression model to our data (38), which include such effects, modest evidence was found for genetic dominance but not for family environment. However, we chose not to include dominance in our final models for three reasons. First, previous analyses indicate that in studies restricted to twins, additive and dominance variance are highly confounded (31). Second, inclusion of dominance would considerably complicate the analyses, requiring the estimation of two separate genotype-environment interactions. Third, the exclusion of genetic dominance leads to a conservative estimate of the impact of genetic effects.

The odds ratio for major depression given stressful life events and a high genetic risk of illness is calculated from the logistic regression coefficient, controlling for all of the covariates outlined above.

Interactions and Scale

In these analyses the dependent variable, the presence or absence of onset of major depression in a given person-month, is dichotomous. This fact introduces unavoidable practical and conceptual complexity into our analyses because 1) we are primarily interested in clarifying the nature of the interaction between genetic and environmental risk factors and 2) *from a statistical perspective, any interaction is scale dependent.* In regression analysis, dichotomous dependent variables have two unattractive properties. First, true probabilities that would be used to predict such variables have floor and ceiling effects (probabilities of illness must range from 0 to 1). Second, such probabilities would not be homoscedastic (have equal variance at any point on the scale). Therefore, the most popular regression method for the analysis of dichotomous dependent variables is now logistic regression (40). In logistic regression, instead of the probability of a given outcome *p*, the model predicts the logistic function of *p*, which equals $\ln p/(1-p)$, where ln equals the natural logarithm. The logistic function has a number of important advantages, including homoscedasticity and a range from $-\infty$ to ∞. However, it has one important disadvantage. With the inclusion of a logarithmic function in the dependent variable, the nature of what an interaction means has been dramatically changed. ***What is a multiplicative interaction in the probability model becomes (to a first approximation) simply additive in the logistic model.*** What is additive in the probability model usually becomes a ***negative*** interaction in the logistic model.

Because of the ease and wide acceptability of logistic regression, most of our analyses used this method. However, we recognized a priori that evidence for an additive model in logistic regression is, in fact, usually evidence for a multiplicative interaction on the scale of simple probabilities. To confirm this, we implemented a cumbersome regression method on the scale of simple probabilities using standard linear regression (40). To correct for unequal error variances due to the dichotomous dependent variable, iterated weighted regressions were carried out (41, 42). For each iteration, each observation was weighted by the inverse of the binomial variance of the observation plus a small adjustment factor that allowed observations with a predicted value of 0 or 1 to be included in the next iteration. Observations with a predicted value of <0 or >1 were excluded from subsequent analyses, resulting in a loss of power. The variance was calculated with the use of the predicted value of the previous regression. Iteration was continued until improvement in heteroscedasticity was no longer obtained.

REFERENCES

1. Burton R: The Anatomy of Melancholy, vol 1 (1621). New York, EP Dutton, 1932
2. Bonhoeffer K: How far should all psychogenic illnesses be regarded as hysterical? (1909), in Themes and Variations in European Psychiatry: An Anthology. Edited by Hirsch SR, Shepherd M. Charlottesville, University Press of Virginia, 1974
3. Brown GW, Harris T: Social Origins of Depression: A Study of Psychiatric Disorder in Women. New York, Free Press, 1978
4. Thoits PA: Dimensions of life events that influence psychological distress: an evaluation and synthesis of the literature, in Psychosocial Stress: Trends in Theory and Research. Edited by Kaplan HB. New York, Academic Press, 1983
5. Tsuang MT, Faraone SV: The Genetics of Mood Disorders. Baltimore, Johns Hopkins University Press, 1990
6. Kendler KS, Neale MC, Kessler RC, Heath AC, Eaves LJ: A population-based twin study of major depression in women: the impact of varying definitions of illness. Arch Gen Psychiatry 1992; 49:257–266
7. Strecker EA: A preliminary study of the precipitating situation in two hundred cases of mental disease. Am J Psychiatry 1922; 78: 503–536
8. Pollitt J: The relationship between genetic and precipitating factors in depressive illness. Br J Psychiatry 1972; 121:67–70
9. Perris H, von Knorring L, Perris C: Genetic vulnerability for depression and life events. Neuropsychobiology 1982; 8:241–247
10. Phelan J, Schwartz JE, Bromet EJ, Dew MA, Parkinson DK, Schulberg HC, Dunn LO, Blane H, Curtis EC: Work stress, family stress and depression in professional and managerial employees. Psychol Med 1991; 21:999–1012
11. McGuffin P, Katz R, Bebbington P: The Camberwell Collaborative Depression Study, III: depression and adversity in the relatives of depressed probands. Br J Psychiatry 1988; 152:775–782
12. Kendler KS, Eaves LJ: Models for the joint effect of genotype and

environment on liability to psychiatric illness. Am J Psychiatry 1986; 143:279–289
13. Rothman KJ: Modern Epidemiology. Boston, Little, Brown, 1986
14. Kendler KS, Neale MC, Kessler RC, Heath AC, Eaves LJ: A longitudinal twin study of 1-year prevalence of major depression in women. Arch Gen Psychiatry 1993; 50:843–852
15. Kendler KS, Kessler RC, Neale MC, Heath AC, Eaves LJ: The prediction of major depression in women: toward an integrated etiologic model. Am J Psychiatry 1993; 150:1139–1148
16. Paykel ES: Contribution of life events to causation of psychiatric illness. Psychol Med 1978; 8:245–253
17. Costello CG: Social factors associated with depression: a retrospective community study. Psychol Med 1982; 12:329–339
18. Surtees PG, Miller PM, Ingham JG, Kreitman NB, Rennie D, Sashidharan SP: Life events and the onset of affective disorder: a longitudinal general population study. J Affect Disord 1986; 10: 37–50
19. Bebbington PE, Sturt E, Tennant C, Hurry J: Misfortune and resilience: a community study of women. Psychol Med 1984; 14: 347–363
20. Bebbington PE, Tennant C, Hurry J: Adversity and the nature of psychiatric disorder in the community. J Affect Disord 1981; 3: 345–366
21. Finlay-Jones R, Brown GW: Types of stressful life events and the onset of anxiety and depressive disorders. Psychol Med 1981; 11:803–815
22. Gilbert P: Depression: The Evolution of Powerlessness. New York, Guilford Press, 1992
23. Brown GW, Harris TO: Depression, in Life Events and Illness. Edited by Brown GW, Harris TO. New York, Guilford Press, 1989
24. Bohman M, Sigvardsson S, Cloninger CR: Maternal inheritance of alcohol abuse: cross-fostering analysis of adopted women. Arch Gen Psychiatry 1981; 38:965–969
25. Cloninger CR, Bohman M, Sigvardsson S: Inheritance of alcohol abuse: cross-fostering analysis of adopted men. Arch Gen Psychiatry 1981; 38:861–868
26. Cadoret RJ, Troughton E, O'Gorman TW: Genetic and environmental factors in alcohol abuse and antisocial personality. J Stud Alcohol 1987; 48:1–8
27. Cadoret RJ, Cain CA, Crowe RR: Evidence for gene-enviroment interaction in the development of adolescent antisocial behavior. Behav Genet 1983; 13:301–310
28. Tienari P: Interaction between genetic vulnerability and family environment: the Finnish Adoptive Family Study of Schizophrenia. Acta Psychiatr Scand 1991; 84:460–465
29. Everitt BS, Smith AMR: Interactions in contingency tables: a brief discussion of alternative definitions. Psychol Med 1979; 9: 581–583
30. Kish L, Frankel MR: Inferences from complex samples. J Royal Statistical Society Series B 1974; 36:1–37
31. Neale MC, Cardon LR: Methodology for Genetic Studies of Twins and Families. Dordrecht, The Netherlands, Kluwer Academic, 1992
32. Sham PC, Walters EE, Neale MC, Heath AC, MacLean CJ, Kendler KS: Logistic regression analysis of twin data: estimation of parameters of the multifactorial liability-threshold model. Behav Genet 1994; 24:229–238
33. Allison PD: Event History Analysis. Beverly Hills, Calif, Sage, 1984
34. Kendler KS, Neale MC, Kessler RC, Heath AC, Eaves LJ: A twin study of recent life events and difficulties. Arch Gen Psychiatry 1993; 50:589–596
35. Allison PD: Discrete-time methods for the analysis of event histories, in Sociological Methodology. Edited by Leinhardt S. San Francisco, Jossey-Bass, 1982
36. Laird N, Olivier D: Covariance analysis of censored survival data using log-linear analysis techniques. J Am Statistical Assoc 1981; 76:231–240
37. Falconer DS: Introduction to Quantitative Genetics, 3rd ed. New York, John Wiley & Sons, 1989
38. DeFries JC, Fulker DW: Multiple regression analysis of twin data. Behav Genet 1985; 15:467–474
39. Falconer DS: The inheritance of liability to certain diseases, estimated from the incidence among relatives. Ann Hum Genet 1965; 29:51–76
40. SAS/STAT User's Guide, version 6, 4th ed, vols 1, 2. Cary, NC, SAS Institute, 1990
41. Cox DR: The Analysis of Binary Data. London, Methuen, 1970
42. Fleiss J: Statistical Methods for Rates and Proportions, 2nd ed. New York, John Wiley & Sons, 1981

The Genetics of Major Depressive Disorder

Gin S. Malhi, MB, MRCPsych, Janette Moore, MB, MRCPsych, and Peter McGuffin, MB, PhD, FRCP, FRCPsych

Address
SGDP Research Centre, Institute of Psychiatry, DeCrespigny Park, Denmark Hill, London SE5 8AF, UK.
E-mail: p.mcguffin@iop.kcl.ac.uk

Current Psychiatry Reports 2000, **2**:165–169
Current Science Inc. ISSN 1523-3812

There is consistent evidence that major depression is familial and population-based twin studies as well as hospital register-based twin studies find substantial heritability. However, there is also a large proportion of variation in liability left to be explained by nongenetic factors. Although there seems little doubt that life events play a role in precipitating depression, studies that have attempted to examine familial liability along with social adversity find that environmental measures tend to be contaminated by genetic effects. Thus, the tendency to experience (or report) life events appears to be influenced by shared family environment, and for certain types of events there is a genetic component. The molecular genetic basis of liability to depression is an under-researched area, but some candidate gene studies show potentially promising results. Systematic mapping studies aiming to cover the entire genome are currently being launched.

Introduction

Compared with the general population, the relatives of depressed probands have at least a three-fold increase in their risk of developing major depressive disorder (MDD) [1]. In a recent study using narrow ICD-10 (International Classification of Diseases of the World Health Organization, edn 10) criteria, depression was nine times as frequent in the siblings of depressed probands compared with siblings of healthy controls [2•]. Some family studies have also shown that the prevalence of MDD is greater among the relatives of those who experience their first depressive episode before the age of 20 [3], and childhood onset was recently reported as being associated with an increased familial risk [4]. However, the relationship between age of onset and family loading for depression is by no means clear. For example, in one study very early onset (before puberty) was associated with a high rate of antisocial behavior among relatives, rather than "pure" depression [5], and a twin study of depressive symptoms in childhood found that they were familial, but in children below age 11; this resulted from shared environment rather than shared genes [6].

Twin Studies

Broadly speaking, twin studies of MDD in adults suggest that genes and specific environmental factors are important, and that shared environmental factors, although important in less severe subtypes of depression, are perhaps of less significance in this patient group [7]. It is of interest to note that the heritability of unipolar depression appears to be higher than was once thought, with estimates in the region of 40% to 70%.

Recent large twin registry studies have explored the influence of genetic factors on major depression in male twins [8•,9•]. In both studies, the best fitting biometric twin model for major depression again contained only genetic and nonshared environmental factors. Lyons *et al.* [9•] in a further analysis stratified the diagnosis of major depression according to severity and found that this particular model held only for severe or psychotic depression. Dysthymia, as well as mild and moderate depression, were best explained by a nongenetic model containing only common family environment and nonshared environment. This is further evidence that perhaps more severe forms of depression differ in their etiology from milder disorders. Kendler *et al.* [8•] used an approach based on bivariate path analysis to further explore the genetic correlation in the liability to major depression in men and women, and found it to be +0.57. They concluded that although major depression is equally heritable in men and women and most genetic risk factors influence liability to major depression similarly in both sexes, genes may exist that act differently on the risk for the disorder between the two sexes.

Multivariate approaches have also been applied to the investigation of the genetic origins of comorbidity in disorders such as panic disorder, phobia, bulimia, and alcoholism, as well as major depression and generalized anxiety disorder (GAD) [10]. Two sets of shared genetic factors have been suggested by this analysis. The first contributes to major depression and GAD, and the second to phobia, panic disorder, and bulimia. Genetic effects for alcoholism appear to be specific in nature. It is not clear, however, whether these findings can be extrapolated to clinical samples, given the somewhat more liberal interpretation of the diagnostic criteria that suggest the lifetime prevalence of major depression and GAD as 31% and 24%, respectively. There is also evidence that the covariation of anxiety and depressive symptoms in childhood (maternally rated) may be explained by a common set of genes [6]. However, this study also suggested a role for nonshared environmental factors in the comorbidity of these symptoms and the influence of specific genetic effects for depressive symptomatology.

Gene-Environment Interplay

Although older terminology suggested that some forms of depression were *reactive* and others *endogenous*, there is little genetic evidence to support such a separation. A recent twin-family analysis showed that it is unlikely that there are two broad subtypes of depression, one mainly genetic and the other mainly nongenetic [11]. Rather, it seems probable that depression generally results from a combination of genetic liability and environmental adversity. However, the relationship between these factors is complicated. One of the first studies to explore gene–environment interplay found an increased rate not only of depression among relatives of depressive probands [12], but also an increase in reported life events. The authors suggested that part of the association between life events and depression may be due to this familial aggregation. Such findings suggest the possibility that familial factors may be influencing the liability to major depression indirectly, by predisposing an individual to a more aversive environment [13••]. Several studies have supported the surprising proposition that life events may be partly genetically influenced [13••,14]. Kendler [13] categorized life events, according to their likely range of impact, into *personal events*, which focused primarily on the proband, and *network events* where the impact extended to other individuals in the proband's social circle. For network events twin resemblance appeared to result purely from common environmental effects, whereas for personal events twin resemblance appeared to be due to genetic influence only. In a third category, *interpersonal difficulties*, both genetic and common environmental factors appeared to operate. The distinct familial origins of different categories of events are underlined by a recent sib pair study [2•]. This study showed positive correlations between siblings for events classified as *independent* (that is, not likely to result from the subject's deliberate actions), but this was almost entirely explained by *shared* events such as death or illness of a parent. Nevertheless, it remains that some life events (or how they are reported) are influenced by genetic factors, and there is evidence that the genetic factors operating in depression and in the predisposition to life events are positively correlated, thereby implying an association via a common set of genes [15,16•,17•]. To what degree, therefore, is the relationship between stressful life events and depression due to a causal relationship, with life events contributing directly to the onset of major depression? Kendler *et al.* [18] explored this question in their population-based sample of female twins and found strong evidence that the observed association was, at least in part, causal.

Molecular Genetics

Having demonstrated a genetic contribution to anxiety and depressive disorders, the next stage of the investigation draws on molecular genetic methods in an attempt to locate and identify the genes involved. Depression does not follow mendelian segregation patterns, thereby indicating a complex mode of inheritance. It is likely that the genetic influences on these disorders are multigenic in nature, acting in concert with environmental factors. Segregation analyses have been unable to confirm specific modes of inheritance. Given that the genome contains 3 billion base pairs and over 100,000 genes, the task of locating a susceptibility gene for a particular disease is formidable. Linkage analysis, by detecting the co-inheritance of chromosomal regions and disorder within families, offers a possibility of achieving this.

Linkage Studies

Linkage studies of affective disorder have primarily focused on the bipolar phenotype and there have been few recent linkage studies of major depression. Older studies, predating the availability of DNA markers, made use of classical genetic markers such as blood group antigens and protein polymorphisms with inconclusive results. More recently analyses using DNA polymorphisms have concentrated on excluding linkage to chromosomal regions known to contain possible candidate genes, such as those involved in neuroendocrine or neurotransmitter systems [19,20], or those implicated in bipolar disorder [21]. These have employed parametric linkage methods. Such conventional lod score linkage analysis requires precise knowledge of the disease mode of transmission and assumes a gene of major effect is operating [22]. As stated previously, the mode of inheritance is unknown for depressive disorders, and parametric linkage analysis requires reasonably accurate specification of parameters such as gene frequency and penetrance. Mis-specification of the parameters of such a model introduces the possibility of error. An alternative linkage strategy requiring no information about the mode of inheritance, and useful in disease involving several (oligogenic) or many genes (polygenic), is the affected sib pair method. This nonparametric linkage method is associated with some loss of statistical power. Although such analysis has been used in linkage studies of depression [23] only a small number of pedigrees were involved, whereas very large samples sizes (many hundreds of families) are likely to be required to detect genes of small effect [24]. Genome-wide screens of several hundred roughly evenly spaced DNA markers are commencing in a number of centers. These should be successful if there are relatively common genes that contribute at least a moderate relative risk of around 2 or more, but if depression turns out to be highly polygenic other methods will be required [24].

Association Studies

This method allows the detection of much smaller effects (relative risks of less than 2) but is limited by the fact that allelic association results either from very tight linkage between a marker and a disease susceptibility locus (resulting in linkage disequilibrium) or from the marker locus itself conferring susceptibility. This means that until recently it has not been feasible to consider a whole genome scan for association (although methods are now emerging to accomplish this [24]. Therefore, research has focused on candidate genes. Candidate genes for major depression and anxiety disorders have primarily been suggested by the molecular mechanisms implicated in the action of therapeutic drugs and the putative pathophysiology for these disorders. Of particular interest are genes associated with neurotransmitter systems. Many of the association studies associated with these phenotypes have focused on the serotonergic system and in particular the serotonin transporter gene located on chromosome 17 (17q11.1-17q12). Many antidepressant and anxiolytic drugs such as tricyclic antidepressants and the newer serotonin selective reuptake inhibitors influence the transporter facilitated uptake of serotonin. Several polymorphisms of the serotonin transporter (*SERT*) gene have been described.

A 44 bp insertion/deletion polymorphism in the transcriptional control region of the gene has been described by Heils *et al.* [25]. The short version of this promoter polymorphism was shown to be associated with decreased transcriptional efficiency resulting in reduced serotonin transporter expression. Since an original report of association between this genetic variant and personality traits that are likely to be relevant to vulnerability to depression [26], various studies have explored this further. Katsuragi *et al.* [27] replicated the finding in a Japanese sample but several other studies have failed to do so [28–30]. Ohara *et al.* [31] described a tendency for the shorter variant of this polymorphism to be more frequent in patients diagnosed with an anxiety disorder using DSM-IV (Diagnostic and Statistical Manual of Mental Disorders, edn 4) criteria. Associations of this polymorphism with affective disorders have also been described [32]. Similar associations have been shown for both unipolar and bipolar subtypes separately [33], although this too has not been replicated [34].

A further variable number tandem repeat polymorphism, in the second intron of the serotonin transporter gene, has also been described [35]. Several variants of this polymorphism were found to be associated with affective disorder [36,37]. In particular an association of the nine copy variant with unipolar depression has been reported [38,39]. However, this has not been replicated in independent studies [40]. Gelernter *et al.* [41•] investigated the range of allele frequency variation for both the promoter and second intron polymorphisms of the serotonin transporter gene in seven different populations and found significant global variation. Linkage disequilibrium varied among the populations suggesting a large potential for population stratification in association studies employing population controls; as the majority of studies exploring depressive and anxiety related phenotypes have done. Taken as a whole, therefore, the various association findings suggest that polymorphic variation at this gene results in some phenotypic effect but it is unclear at present what phenotypic construct best captures this [30].

Other candidate gene association studies in depression and anxiety have investigated the dopamine receptor genes [42], the tryosine hydroxylase gene [43], genes related to the gamma-aminobutyric acid system [44], and the catechol-O-methyltransferase gene [45,46]. Candidate gene approaches are limited in that they are only as good as the current understanding of the disease pathophysiology [47]. However, the possibility of a genome-wide search for association, similar to that for linkage studies, is increasingly feasible with the development of high throughput genotyping techniques such as DNA pooling [48]. In order to scan systematically for allelic association, however, a much denser map of polymorphic markers would be required and biallelic single nucleotide polymorphisms are likely to provide this in the near future [24].

Conclusions

The genetics of unipolar depression is a neglected area in comparison with bipolar disorder or schizophrenia despite being a much more common disorder. This may be because the role of psychosocial adversity has seemed so obviously important and depression appears as an understandable reaction to stress. However familial aggregation is a consistent finding and recent twin studies suggest that heritability is substantial. Studies trying to incorporate environmental measures within a genetic design have only really taken place in the past 10 to 15 years and suggest a complicated picture where measures of stress are actually confounded by familial or genetic effects. The future is likely to see an increasing emphasis on trying to elucidate gene–environment interplay. Molecular genetic studies of unipolar disorder have scarcely begun and have so far been mainly restricted to candidate genes but is likely that more systematic approaches using linkage and linkage disequilibrium mapping will identify susceptibility loci within the foreseeable future.

References and Recommended Reading

Papers of particular interest, published recently, have been highlighted as:

- • Of importance
- •• Of major importance

1. McGuffin P, Katz R: **Nature , nurture and affective disorder.** In *The Biology of Depression.* Edited by Deakin JWF. London: Gaskell; 1986:26–51.
2.• Farmer A, Harris T, Redman K, *et al.*: **The Cardiff Depression Study: a sib pair study of life events and familiality in major depression.** *Br J Psychiatry* 2000, **176**:150–155.

The most recent attempt to study the familiality of both depression and social adversity with in a clinically ascertained sample. Depressive disorder as defined by ICD 10 was highly familial. Independent life events were also familial but this largely resulted from both members of sib pairs sharing the same events.

3. Weissman MM, Warner V, Wickramaratne P, Prusoff BA: **Early-onset major depression in parents and their children.** *J Affect Disord* 1988, **15**:269–277.
4. Kovacs M, Devlin B, Pollock M, *et al.*: **A controlled family history study of childhood-onset depressive disorder.** *Arch Gen Psychiatry* 1997, **54**:13–623.
5. Harrington RC, Rutter M, Weissman M, *et al.*: **Psychiatric disorders in the relatives of depressed probands I: comparison of pre- pubertal, adolescent and early adult onset cases.** *J Affect Disord* 1997, **42**:9–22.
6. Thapar A, McGuffin P: **Anxiety and depressive symptoms in childhood - a genetic study of comorbidity.** *J Child Psychol Psychiatry* 1997, **38**:651–656.
7. McGuffin P, Katz R, Watkins S, Rutherford J: **A hospital-based twin register of the heritability of DSM-IV unipolar depression.** *Arch Gen Psychiatry* 1996, **53**:129–136.
8.• Kendler KS, Prescott CA: **A population based twin study of lifetime major depression in men and women.** *Arch Gen Psychiatry* 1999, **56**:39–44.

The first large scale population-based twin study to examine the extent to which the same genes influence depression in the two sexes. In both men and women depression showed substantial and significant heritability, but there was evidence of both common genetic effects and genetic effects that differ between the sexes.

9.• Lyons MJ, Eisen SA, Goldberg J, *et al.*: **A registry-based twin study of depression in men.** *Arch Gen Psychiatry* 1998, **55**: 468–472.

A large scale study confirming that major depression in men is substantially heritable but that certain affective disorder subtypes such as dythysmia may be largely environmental in origin.

10. Kendler KS, Walters EE, Neale MC, *et al.*: **The structure of the genetic and environmental risk factors for six major psychiatric disorders in women. Phobia, generalised anxiety disorder, panic disorder, bulimia, major depression and alcoholism.** *Arch Gen Psychiatry* 1995, **52**:374–383.
11. Andrew M, McGuffin P, Katz R: **Genetic and non-genetic subtypes of major depressive disorder.** *Br J Psychiatry* 1998, **173**:523–526.
12. McGuffin P, Katz R, Bebbington P: **The Camberwell Collaborative Study III. Depression and adversity in the relatives of depressed probands.** *Br J Psychiatry*, 1988, **152**:775–782.
13.•• Kendler K: **Major depression and the environment: a psychiatric genetic perspective.** *Pharmacopsychiatry* 1998, **31**:5–9.

A masterly account of the ways in which genes and environment are likely to co-act and interact to cause depression.

14. Plomin R, Lichtensein P, Pedersen NL, *et al.*: **Genetic influence on life events during the last half of the life span.** *Psychol Ageing* 1990, **5**:25–30.
15. Kendler KS, Karkowski-Shuman L: **Stressful life events and genetic liability to major depression: genetic control of exposure to the environment?** *Psychol Med* 1997, **27**:539–547.
16.• Silberg J, Pickles A, Rutter M, *et al.*: **The influence of genetic factors and life stress on depression among adolescent girls.** *Arch Gen Psychiatry* 1999, **56**:225–232.

This paper, like the paper by Thapar *et al.* [17•], is an important attempt to study depression and life events in the context of a twin study.

17.• Thapar A, Harold G, McGuffin P: **Life events and depressive symptoms in childhood - shared genes or shared adversity? A research note.** *J Child Psychol Psychiatry* 1998, **39**:1153–1158.

The focus here is on depressive symptoms rather than disorder. There is evidence that life events, at least when reported by questionnaire, are in part influenced by the same genes that are associated with reporting depressive symptoms.

18. Kendler KS, Karkowski LM, Prescott CA: **Causal relationship between stressful life events and the onset of major depression.** *Am J Psychiatry* 1999, **156**:837–841.
19. Neiswanger K, Zubenko GS, Giles DE, *et al.*: **Linkage and association analysis of chromosomal regions containing genes related to neuroendocrine or serotonin function in families with early-onset, recurrent major depression.** *Am J Med Genet* 1998, **81**:443–439.
20. Wang Z, Crowe RR, Tanna VL, Winokur G: **Alpha 2 adrenergic receptor subtypes in depression: a candidate gene study.** *J Affect Disord* 1992, **25**:191–196.
21. Balciuniene J, Yuan QP, Engstrom C, *et al.*: **Linkage analysis of candidate loci in families with recurrent major depression.** *Mol Psychiatry* 1998, **3**:162–168.
22. McGuffin P, Owen MJ: **Molecular Genetic Studies of Schizophrenia.** *Cold Spring Harbor Symposia on Quantitative Biology* 1996, **61**:815–822.
23. Wilson AF, Elston RC, Mallott DB, *et al.*: **The current status of genetic linkage studies of alcoholism and unipolar depression.** *Psychiatr Genet* 1991, **2**:107–124.
24. McGuffin P, Martin N: **Behaviour and Genes.** *Br Med J* 1999, **319**:37–40.
25. Heils A, Teufel A, Petri S, *et al.*: **Allelic variation of human serotonin transporter gene expression.** *J Neurochem* 1996, **66**:2621–2624.
26. Lesch KP, Bengel D, Heils A, *et al.*: **Association of anxiety-related traits with a polymorphism in the serotonin transporter gene regulatory region.** *Science* 1996, **274**:1527–1531.
27. Katsuragi S, Kunugi H, Sano A, *et al.*: **Association between serotonin transporter gene polymorphism and anxiety-related traits.** *Biol Psychiatry* 1999, **45**:368–370.
28. Ball D, Hill L, Freeman B, *et al.*: **The serotonin transporter gene and peer-rated neuroticism.** *Neuroreport* 1997, **8**:1301–1304.
29. Ebstein RP, Gritsenko I, Nemanov L, *et al.*: **No association between the serotonin transporter gene regulatory region polymorphism and the Tridimensional Personality Questionnaire (TPQ) temperament of harm avoidance.** *Mol Psychiatry* 1997, **2**:224–226.
30. Gelernter J, Kranzler H, Coccaro EF, *et al.*: **Serotonin transporter protein gene polymorphism and personality measures in African American and European American subjects.** *Am J Psychiatry* 1998, **155**:1332–1338.
31. Ohara K, Nagai M, Suzuki Y, *et al.*: **Association between anxiety disorders and a functional polymorphism in the serotonin transporter gene.** *Psychiatry Res* 1998, **81**:277–279.
32. Collier DA, Stober G, Li T, *et al.*: **A novel functional polymorphism within the promoter of the serotonin transporter gene: possible role in the susceptibility to affective disorder.** *Mol Psychiatry* 1996, **1**:453–460.
33. Furlong RA, Ho L, Walsh C, *et al.*: **Analysis and meta-analysis of two serotonin transporter gene polymorphisms in bipolar and unipolar affective disorders.** *Am J Med Genet* 1998, **81**:58–63.
34. Ohara K, Nagai M, Tsukamoto T, *et al.*: **Functional polymorphism in the serotonin transporter promoter at the SLC6A4 locus and mood disorders.** *Biol Psychiatry* 1998, **44**:550–554.

35. Lesch KP, Balling U, Gross J, *et al.*: **Organisation of the human serotonin transporter gene.** *J Neural Transmission* 1994, **95**:157–162.
36. Collier DA, Arranz MJ, Sham P, *et al.*: **The serotonin transporter is a potential susceptibility factor for bipolar affective disorder.** *Neuroreport* 1996, **7**:1675–1679.
37. Rees M, Norton N, Jones I, *et al.*: **Association studies of bipolar disorder at the human serotonin transporter gene (hSERT; 5HTT).** *Molecular Psychiatry* 1997, **2**:398–402.
38. Battersby S, Ogilvie AD, Smith CAD, *et al.*: **Structure of a variable number tandem repeat of the serotonin transporter gene and association with affective disorder.** *Psychiatr Genet* 1996, **6**:177–181.
39. Ogilvie AD, Battersby S, Bubb VJ, *et al.*: **Polymorphism in serotonin transporter gene associated with susceptibility to major depression.** *Lancet* 1996, **347**:731–733.
40. Kunugi H, Hattori M, Kato T, *et al.*: **Serotonin transporter gene polymorphisms: ethnic difference and possible association with bipolar affective disorder.** *Mol Psychiatry* 1997, **2**:457–462.
41.• Gelernter J, Cubells JF, Kidd JR, *et al.*: **Population studies of polymorphisms of the serotonin transporter protein gene.** *Am J Med Genet* 1999, **88**:61–66.
An attempt to explicate the population genetics of the serotonin transporter gene, a candidate gene that has provoked much interest and controversy in association studies of depression.
42. Serretti A, Macciardi F, Cusin C, *et al.*: **Dopamine receptor D4 gene is associated with delusional symptomatology in mood disorders.** *Psychiatry Res* 1998, **80**:129–136.
43. Serretti A, Macciardi F, Verga M, *et al.*: **Tyrosine hydroxylase gene associated with depressive symptomatology in mood disorder.** *Am J Med Genet* 1998, **81**:127–130.
44. Oruc L, Verheyen GR, Furac I, *et al.*: **Positive association between the GABRA5 gene and unipolar recurrent major depression.** *Neuropsychobiology* 1997, **36**:62–64.
45. Ohara K, Nagai M, Suzuki Y, *et al.*: **No association between anxiety disorders and catechol-o-methyltransferase polymorphism.** *Psychiatry Res* 1998, **80**:145–148.
46. Kunugi H, Vallada HP, Hoda F, *et al.*: **No evidence for an association of affective disorders with high or low activity allele of catechol-o-methyltransferase gene.** *Biol Psychiatry* 1997, **42**:282–285.
47. Craddock N, Owen MJ: **Modern molecular genetic approaches to psychiatric disease.** *Br Med Bull* 1996, **52**:434–452.
48. Daniels J, Holmans P, Williams N, *et al.*: **A simple method for analyzing microsatellite allele image patterns generated from DNA pools and its application to allelic association studies.** *Am J Hum Genet* 1998, **62**:1189–1197.

Genetic Epidemiology of Major Depression: Review and Meta-Analysis

Patrick F. Sullivan, M.D., F.R.A.N.Z.C.P.

Michael C. Neale, Ph.D.

Kenneth S. Kendler, M.D.

Objective: The authors conducted a meta-analysis of relevant data from primary studies of the genetic epidemiology of major depression.

Method: The authors searched MEDLINE and the reference lists of previous review articles to identify relevant primary studies. On the basis of a review of family, adoption, and twin studies that met specific inclusion criteria, the authors derived quantitative summary statistics.

Results: Five family studies met the inclusion criteria. The odds ratios for proband (subjects with major depression or comparison subjects) versus first-degree relative status (affected or unaffected with major depression) were homogeneous across the five studies (Mantel-Haenszel odds ratio=2.84, 95% CI=2.31–3.49). No adoption study met the inclusion criteria, but the results of two of the three reports were consistent with genetic influences on liability to major depression. Five twin studies met the inclusion criteria, and their statistical summation suggested that familial aggregation was due to additive genetic effects (point estimate of heritability of liability= 37%, 95% CI=31%–42%), with a minimal contribution of environmental effects common to siblings (point estimate=0%, 95% CI=0%–5%), and substantial individual-specific environmental effects/measurement error (point estimate=63%, 95% CI=58%–67%). The literature suggests that recurrence best predicts the familial aggregation of major depression.

Conclusions: Major depression is a familial disorder, and its familiality mostly or entirely results from genetic influences. Environmental influences specific to an individual are also etiologically significant. Major depression is a complex disorder that does not result from either genetic or environmental influences alone but rather from both. These findings are notably consistent across samples and methods and are likely to be generally applicable.

(Am J Psychiatry 2000; 157:1552–1562)

Major depression, a common (1–4), costly (5), and recurrent disorder (6), is associated with considerable morbidity (7–10) and excess mortality (11). Major depression has been projected to become the second leading cause of disability worldwide by 2020 (second to ischemic heart disease) (12). Moreover, major depression is of increasing importance in clinical psychiatry (13).

There are many primary studies of the genetic epidemiology of major depression, and a number of excellent reviews are available (14–17). However, to our knowledge, no single source has provided a quantitative summation of these data, which have been gathered through considerable effort by many teams of researchers worldwide over the past three decades. We believe that this area of research is sufficiently mature to warrant meta-analysis.

This synthetic meta-analysis addressed three questions. First, to what extent is major depression familial? Second, if major depression is familial, what are the relative contributions of genes and environment in the etiology of the disorder? Third, are there clinical features of major depression that predict familial aggregation?

Method

The key advantage of synthetic meta-analysis over traditional literature review is the potential to yield a less biased quantitative summary of the findings of many primary empirical studies (18–21). In performing this meta-analysis, we attempted to apply principles similar to those customarily applied to considerably larger bodies of literature (e.g., randomized clinical trials for common medical illnesses such as myocardial infarction).

First, to identify all relevant primary studies, we performed computerized MEDLINE searches for an inclusive list of descriptors and searched the reference lists of prior reviews of major depression to identify any reports that were not retrieved in the MEDLINE search. Second, we created an a priori set of criteria for studies' inclusion in the meta-analysis. To be included, a study had to possess features essential to interpretability, such as 1) explicit distinction between unipolar major depression and bipolar disorder, 2) systematic proband recruitment and ascertainment of relatives, 3) direct collection of diagnostic data from all or nearly all subjects (by using direct interview or, in one instance [22], by using questionnaires), 4) use of operationalized diagnostic criteria, and 5) diagnostic determination by assessors who were blind to ascertainment source and diagnoses of other relatives. For family studies, we also required a comparison group that was studied in a similar manner. For twin studies, we also required that zygosity was estimated with reasonable accuracy and blind to diagnoses.

More than half of the extant family and twin studies did not meet one or more of these criteria (most were unblinded and/or uncontrolled). If relative or co-twin diagnoses are assigned without "blindfolding," it is impossible to know the degree to which the results are contaminated by experimental bias. For archival purposes, we provide the citations for the family (23–30) and twin studies (31–34) that were not included.

We considered each family study as a two-by-two contingency table of proband diagnosis (major depression or comparison) versus relative diagnosis (affected or unaffected with major depression), with the odds ratio as a summary statistic (35). Assuming a fixed-effects model, each of the two-by-two tables for the five family studies forms a stratum. To pool these data, we used the Mantel-Haenszel method after first assessing the homogeneity of the data with the Breslow-Day chi-square test (21, 36).

No adoption study met our inclusion criteria, so the three published reports were considered qualitatively. We include these reports for three reasons. First, adoption studies have a fundamentally different set of assumptions than do twin studies. Consistent results from adoption and twin studies increase the likelihood that the conclusions more accurately reflect an underlying reality. Second, although adoption studies are theoretically elegant, they contain a host of practical and ethical difficulties: adoption studies are rather rare, and there may be few additional adoption studies of major depression in the future. Third, the results of adoption studies of major depression are often described in the literature as ambiguous or inconsistent with family and twin studies; we believe that this interpretation is incorrect.

For the twin studies, we first used structural equation modeling to perform univariate analysis of the primary studies (37). Briefly, by comparing the similarity of monozygotic twins with the similarity of dizygotic twins, it is possible to partition the variance in liability (38) to major depression into three components: additive genetic influences (a^2), environmental influences shared by members of a twin pair (c^2), and environmental influences specific to one or the other member of a twin pair (e^2). (The abbreviations a^2, c^2, and e^2 refer to quantitative estimates of the three components.) We used the structural equation modeling package Mx (39, 40) for these analyses. These statistical models can be fit to the raw contingency table data, and 95% confidence intervals (CIs) can be calculated for the relevant parameters (41). Mx is available on the World Wide Web at http://views.vcu.edu/mx.

After computing the estimates for each study, we created a more complex model that included the data from all of the twin studies. This model necessitated a series of assumptions: that prevalences of major depression were similar across studies, that the prevalences among monozygotic and dizygotic twins were similar, that the model parameters could be equated across studies, and that the data were similar across ascertainment methods and gender. We tested these assumptions by using the likelihood ratio chi-square difference test. For these tests, we in effect compared two models. For example, one model might allow a set of parameters to vary freely across studies, generating a goodness-of-fit chi-square with a certain number of degrees of freedom. A submodel might constrain these parameters to be equal, generating a goodness-of-fit chi-square with fewer degrees of freedom. The difference between the chi-square values of these two models is also a chi-square test. If the chi-square difference is large, the model fit worsens when moving from the unconstrained model to the submodel, indicating that the submodel provides a poorer representation of the data. On the other hand, a small chi-square difference suggests that the submodel provides a reasonable representation of the data.

On the basis of prior data about the biology of twinning (i.e., that monozygotic twins are, for most purposes, genetically identical and that dizygotic twins share half of their genes identical by descent) and assuming that etiologically relevant environmental factors are similar across monozygotic and dizygotic twins, a set of expectations can be generated. Comparing the experimental data to these expectations allows assessment of the goodness-of-fit of the observed data to the expectations.

Results

Familial Aggregation

Family studies can be conceptualized as a type of case-control study, as described in detail elsewhere (42, 43). In these studies, probands have major depression and comparison subjects have no history of major depression and are usually matched with probands on potentially confounding variables such as age and gender, and the outcome of interest is the prevalence of major depression in biological relatives (usually first-degree relatives).

Table 1 summarizes data from the five family studies of major depression that met our inclusion criteria for the meta-analysis (44–48). Only the study by Gershon et al. (44) did not match comparison subjects to probands by age and gender. All five studies showed evidence in support of the familial aggregation of major depression in probands, compared with comparison subjects. Across the five studies, there was strong evidence for an association between major depression in the proband and major depression in first-degree relatives (χ^2=97.7, df=1, p<0.00005). In addition, the hypothesis that the odds ratios were homogeneous across the five studies could not be rejected (Breslow-Day χ^2=5.22, df=4, p=0.27), and the summary Mantel-Haenszel odds ratio across the five studies was 2.84 (95% CI=2.31–3.49). Thus, in aggregate, these five studies provided strong and consistent evidence in support of the familiality of major depression.

These findings have two important potential limitations. First, all extant studies recruited most or all subjects with major depression from clinical sources. If having a family history of major depression increases the chance of clinical referral, then the overall odds ratio will be biased upward. One study did not find evidence for this potential bias (48), although two others did (49, 50). The overall impact of this potential bias is unclear, although it may not materially alter the conclusions (49).

Second, screening comparison subjects for the presence of psychopathology (other than major depression) generally leads to lower morbidity risks of major depression in first-degree relatives in comparison subjects and biases the overall odds ratio upward (51–53). This effect is evident in Table 1, which shows that the two studies with unscreened comparison subjects had lower odds ratios (45, 46) than the three studies with comparison subjects who were screened for psychopathology (44, 47, 48). When the data were analyzed more formally, there were indications (of marginal statistical significance) that the odds ratios from studies with screened and unscreened comparison samples were heterogeneous (Breslow-Day χ^2=3.75, df=1, p=0.053). However, it is critical to note that although the summary Mantel-Haenszel odds ratio from the studies

TABLE 1. Results of Family Studies of Major Depression

		Subjects With Major Depression		Comparison Subjects			
Study	Country	Source of Subjects	Morbidity Risk[a]	Source of Subjects[b]	Morbidity Risk[a]	Odds Ratio[c]	95% CI
Gershon et al., 1982 (44)	United States	Clinical setting	16.6	Screened medical patients	5.8	3.23	1.59–6.58
Maier et al., 1993 (45)	Germany	Clinical setting	21.6	Unscreened general population	10.6	2.32	1.62–3.33
Tsuang et al., 1980 (46)	United States	Clinical setting	15.2	Unscreened surgical patients	7.5	2.21	1.35–3.62
Weissman et al., 1984 (47)[d]	United States	Clinical setting	17.6	Screened general population	5.9	3.41	2.23–5.20
Weissman et al., 1993 (48)[e]	United States	Clinical plus general population	21.0	Screened general population	5.5	4.57	2.43–8.60

[a] Morbidity risk of major depression in first-degree relatives calculated by using the Strömgren method, except for studies by Maier et al. (45) and Weissman et al. (48), which used proportional hazards analysis.
[b] Screening excluded subjects with any diagnosed lifetime psychopathology.
[c] Summary Mantel-Haenszel odds ratio=2.84, 95% CI=2.31–3.49.
[d] Subjects with major depression included subjects with severe and mild major depression. Some subjects were also included in the group studied by Gershon et al. (44).
[e] Subjects had early-onset (age ≤30 years) major depression. Fifty-eight percent of subjects with major depression were drawn from the general population, and 42% from clinical sources.

with screened comparison samples was greater (odds ratio=3.62, 95% CI=2.65–4.97), the summary odds ratio from the unscreened studies (odds ratio=2.38, 95% CI=1.78–3.17) was still significantly greater than 1. Hence, even if screening comparison subjects for psychopathology results in bias toward greater familiality of major depression, the basic conclusion that major depression is familial appears to be correct.

Taken together, these methodologically rigorous studies demonstrate that major depression is a familial disorder (i.e., that it "runs" in families). Family studies cannot, however, distinguish genetic influences from environmental risk factors that are also familial. Accomplishing this aim requires other methodological approaches.

Genetic and Environmental Influences

Adoption and twin studies are the two principal approaches to delineating genetic and environmental effects in humans. Adoption studies are social quasi-experiments in which the offspring of one set of parents are reared from early in life by unrelated strangers. In contrast, twin studies are biological quasi-experiments that contrast genetically identical monozygotic twins with dizygotic twins who share many environment features while sharing half their genes on average. One analytic approach to adoption and twin data yields a partition of the etiological sources of variation into three types of causes. These are additive genetic effects, environmental effects common to both members of a twin pair, and environmental effects unique to an individual. The approach is described briefly (54) and in detail elsewhere (17, 37).

Adoption studies. The three adoption studies of major depression that we are aware of (55–57) did not meet our inclusion criteria for the meta-analysis, for the following reasons.

The study by von Knorring et al. (55) did not find evidence for a genetic influence on major depression. However, the diagnoses of major depression in that study were based on indirect sources (i.e., sick leave registrations and evidence of clinical treatment) that may underestimate the true lifetime prevalence of major depression, as only a subset of those with major depression seek treatment (58, 59). The odds ratio from this matched design was 0.71 (95% CI=0.16–2.94) (35, pp. 209–211).

The study by Cadoret et al. (56) had markedly limited data on biological parents and limited statistical power. This study is widely regarded as not supporting the hypothesis of genetic influences on major depression because the results were nonsignificant when they were analyzed separately by gender. However, the trend-level relationship evident in both genders became significant when the data were combined (χ^2=3.87, df=1, p=0.05; odds ratio=2.54, 95% CI=1.00–6.47, calculations ours).

The large study by Wender et al. (57) found evidence for a genetic effect on the transmission of major depression (χ^2=4.73, df=1, p=0.03; odds ratio=7.24, 95% CI=1.21–43.20). However, the diagnoses of major depression in that study were based on indirect sources rather than personal interviews.

In summary, two of these three adoption studies provided qualitative evidence consistent with the existence of significant genetic factors in the etiology of major depression.

Twin studies. The data from the twin studies of major depression that met our inclusion criteria are summarized in Table 2. At the time of this writing, the twin data and the principal Mx script are available on the World Wide Web at http://views.vcu.edu/pub/mx/examples/mdreview. More than 21,000 individuals have been included in these studies, and, notably, all of the studies used the DSM-III-R criteria for major depression. Four studies included community samples (22, 60–62), and two included clinical samples (22, 63). The original paper by Kendler and Prescott (61) has been amended (64), and the amended rather than the original data were analyzed for this report. Two published reports are not shown in Table 2. The limited data presented in one of those reports, by Andrews et al. (65), precluded critical evaluation of the claim that there were no important genetic effects for major depression. In addition, their sample partially overlapped with the larger

TABLE 2. Estimates of Concordance for Major Depression and of the Components of a Full Model of Variance in Liability to Major Depression From Studies of Male and Female Twins[a]

Source of Subjects	Study	Country	Subjects' Sex	Concordance[b] Monozygotic	Concordance[b] Dizygotic	Tetrachoric Correlation Monozygotic	Tetrachoric Correlation Dizygotic	a^2	95% CI	c^2	95% CI	e^2	95% CI
Community	Bierut et al., 1999 (60)	Australia	Male	0.34	0.30	0.24	0.09	24	0–39	0	0–26	76	61–91
			Female	0.50	0.37	0.47	0.09	44	29–53	0	0–12	56	47–65
Community	Kendler et al., 1995 (22)[d]	Sweden	Male	0.40	0.33	0.57	0.39	57	0–96	2	0–73	41	4–100
			Female	0.67	0.32	0.82	0.24	78	18–94	0	0–42	22	6–55
Community	Kendler and Prescott, 1999 (61)	United States	Male	0.41	0.34	0.32	0.12	31	5–41	0	0–22	69	59–79
			Female	0.47	0.43	0.39	0.17	38	1–50	0	0–31	62	50–75
Community	Lyons et al., 1998 (62)[e]	United States	Male	0.23	0.14	0.37	0.13	36	11–47	0	0–20	64	53–75
Clinical setting	Kendler et al., 1995 (22)[d,f]	Sweden	Male	0.50	0.33	—	—	49	0–99	21	0–89	30	1–93
			Female	0.32	0.20	—	—	17	0–55	0	0–38	83	45–83
Clinical setting	McGuffin et al., 1996 (63)[f]	United Kingdom	Male	0.46	0.15	—	—	58	4–81	0	0–40	42	19–72
			Female	0.46	0.22	—	—	38	14–61	0	0–24	62	39–86
Summary[g]	Full model							37	31–42	0	0–5	63	58–67
	Best-fitting model							37	33–42	—	—	63	58–67

Components of Full Model of Variance in Liability to Major Depression[c]: a^2, 95% CI, c^2, 95% CI, e^2, 95% CI.

[a] These data are available on the World Wide Web at http://views.vcu.edu/pub/mx/examples/mdreview.
[b] Probandwise concordance in studies with community as source of subjects; pairwise concordance in studies with clinical settings as source of subjects.
[c] In the full model, a^2=proportion of variance due to genetic effects, c^2=proportion of variance due to shared environmental effects, and e^2= proportion of variance due to individual-specific environmental effects plus measurement error.
[d] Unipolar "intermediate" major depression diagnoses determined on the basis of responses to mailed questionnaire.
[e] Vietnam era twin registry, which included twin pairs concordant for military service from 1965 to 1975.
[f] Modeling assumes lifetime prevalence of major depression of 12.7% for males and 21.3% for females, as determined in the National Comorbidity Survey (4). Kendler et al. (22) and McGuffin et al. (63) used different lifetime prevalence estimates and reported different parameter estimates.
[g] Summary full model consists of the aggregate values across studies of a^2, c^2, and e^2. The best-fitting model consists of aggregate values across studies of a^2 and e^2.

sample studied by Bierut et al. (60). We present the most recent data from the longitudinal cohort first reported by Kendler et al. (3).

The results from the community and clinical studies summarized in Table 2 (also depicted in Figure 1) broadly support five conclusions. First, consistent with theoretical work on the statistical power of the classic twin study for discrete traits like major depression (66), the 95% CIs for the parameter estimates from these twin studies were fairly broad. One key purpose of a meta-analysis is to combine data across studies in an attempt to narrow the CIs on a parameter and thereby to increase precision. Second, the CIs for a^2 (heritability in liability) did not include 0 for seven of 11 of these studies, suggesting that the aggregate value of a^2 across the studies would be nonzero. Third, the 95% CIs for c^2 (proportion of trait variance due to shared environmental factors) included 0 in all of the twin studies, indicating that environmental influences shared by members of a twin pair are unlikely to have substantial impact on the liability to major depression. Fourth, heritability point estimates from community and clinically ascertained samples were not markedly discrepant. Finally, there were no consistent gender differences across the twin studies.

Before summary estimates of these twin data could be generated, it was necessary to test a number of critical hy-

FIGURE 1. Estimates of the Heritability in Liability to Major Depression in Studies of Male and Female Twins[a]

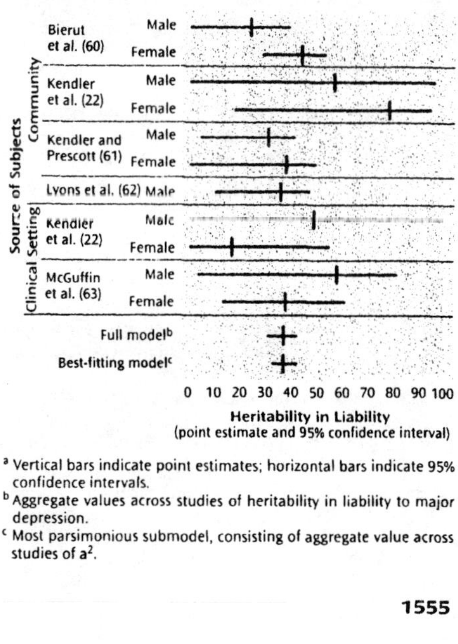

[a] Vertical bars indicate point estimates; horizontal bars indicate 95% confidence intervals.
[b] Aggregate values across studies of heritability in liability to major depression.
[c] Most parsimonious submodel, consisting of aggregate value across studies of a^2.

potheses and assumptions under which the data might be combined. First, it was necessary to allow the individual studies to have different major depression liability thresholds (i.e., prevalences) because equating the thresholds across studies led to an enormous worsening of the fit of the statistical model (χ^2=739.5, df=10, p≈0). Possible explanations for these differences include cross-cultural differences in major depression prevalence (67), age cohort effects (2), and differences in diagnostic approaches. Second, unexpectedly, it was necessary to allow same-sex dizygotic twins to have higher liability thresholds for major depression than same-sex monozygotic twins because equating the thresholds led to a worsening of the fit of the statistical model (χ^2=31.96, df=7, p=0.00004). Slight monozygotic-dizygotic differences have been observed for a number of traits; speculations about these findings generally focus on differential recruitment bias or a subtle protective effect of being a particular type of twin. Third, given the higher prevalence of major depression in women than in men, equating the thresholds for opposite-sex dizygotic pairs led to a considerable further worsening of fit (χ^2=47.13, df=2, p<0.0001). Fourth, when we tested whether the a^2, c^2, and e^2 parameters could be equated versus whether it was necessary for them to be free to vary across studies, we found that it was reasonable to equate the parameters (χ^2=7.86, df=8, p=0.45). This was a critical step in the goal of aggregating data from the published twin studies of major depression. Fifth, we also found that it was reasonable to equate the a^2, c^2, and e^2 parameters for studies from clinical and community sources (χ^2=5.10, df=4, p=0.28). Sixth and finally, it was reasonable to equate the a^2, c^2, and e^2 parameters across gender (χ^2= 3.23, df=2, p=0.20).

Although the principal reason for these comparisons was to establish the validity of our meta-analytic procedure, they also allow a substantiative conclusion that is important to our understanding of major depression. Despite the many differences across these twin studies in the prevalence of major depression, ascertainment, methods, ethnicity, and geographic location, the fundamental genetic architecture of major depression appears homogeneous across samples and across gender.

The next step was to generate the 95% CIs of the parameter estimates of the full model (bottom of Table 2 and Figure 1). These CIs suggest that the variance in liability to major depression is mostly due to individual-specific environmental effects (58%–67%) and additive genetic effects (31%–42%), with a negligible contribution by environmental effects shared by siblings (0%–5%). It is critical to note that the individual-specific environment includes the effects of measurement error and gene-environment interactions. As this meta-analysis had particular power to detect common environmental effects, it is notable that these effects accounted for a small proportion of variance.

In addition to estimating parameters under a full model, it is useful to investigate whether simpler models offer a more parsimonious explanation of the data (37). Fitting submodels reduces the number of parameters and leads to narrower CIs. As might be predicted from the summary results in Table 2, the best-fitting and most parsimonious submodel contained only additive genetic (a^2=37%, 95% CI 33%–42%) and individual-specific environmental effects (e^2=63%, 95% CI=58%–67%).

We investigated the heritability of major depression in community and clinical studies separately because of suggestions that clinically ascertained major depression might be "more genetic." Estimates of heritability were similar in subjects ascertained from community (a^2=37%, 95% CI=28%–42%) and clinical (a^2=43%, 95% CI=21%–58%) sources.

Gender. There is strong evidence that the risk of depression is greater in women than in men (67–69). These findings raise two questions. First, is the relative importance of genetic effects in the etiology of major depression the same in males and females? Four studies found no gender difference in heritability (22, 61–63), although one study did (60). Unsurprisingly, our meta-analysis did not find substantial differences in heritability in liability for major depression between men and women. In addition, the adoption study by Cadoret et al. (56) reported similar odds ratios in men (2.5) and women (2.4). Thus, the weight of the evidence suggests similar genetic effects on liability to major depression in males and females.

Second, even if genetic influences are equivalent in males and females, to what extent do these pools of genes overlap? One study estimated the correlation between genetic effects for males and females (r_a) to be 0.57 (61), and another study estimated the correlation to be 1.0 (22). Family data are consistent with partial overlap (70–72). Although the data are limited, the most parsimonious explanation appears to be that men and women share most but not all genetic influences for major depression. Possible reasons for these differences are discussed elsewhere (61, p. 43).

Assumptions. There are several potential threats to the interpretation of these studies. First, the critical equal-environment assumption posits that monozygotic and dizygotic twins are equally correlated in their exposure to environmental events of etiologic relevance to major depression. If this were not true, the greater similarity between monozygotic versus dizygotic twins for major depression could result from environmental and not genetic factors. The equal-environment assumption has been examined repeatedly, and there is considerable evidence supporting its validity for major depression (73, 74). Second, conclusions about major depression from twins may not generalize to singletons if there are protective or risk factors specifically associated with twins. Moreover, twins are distinctive from singletons in a number of potentially important ways (75); however, the incidence of treated major depression is similar in singletons, monozygotic

TABLE 3. Results of Studies of Clinical Indices Associated With Familial Aggregation of Major Depression[a]

	Significance of Clinical Index						
Study	Early Onset	Recurrent	Impairment	Duration	Number of Symptoms	Symptom Pattern	Comorbidity
Cadoret et al., 1977 (79)	*						
Gershon et al., 1986 (80)		*	*				
Kendler et al., 1994 (81)	n.s.[b]	**	*	n.s.	n.s.	n.s.	*[c]
Kendler et al., 1999 (82)	n.s.[b,d]	***	*	**	n.s.	**[e]	
Leckman et al., 1984 (83)						*[f]	
Leckman et al., 1984 (84)						*[g]	
Lyons et al., 1998 (62)	—[h]				—[h]		
McGuffin et al., 1987 (25)	n.s.						
McGuffin et al., 1996 (63)	n.s.	—[h]		—[h]		*[i]	
Mendlewicz and Baron, 1981 (85)	*						
Stancer et al., 1987 (29)	*						
Weissman et al., 1986 (86)	**[b]	n.s.[d]				n.s.	**[j]

[a] A blank cell indicates the study did not investigate the clinical index.
[b] Controlled for age at interview or year of birth.
[c] Bulimia and, separately, panic disorder.
[d] Clinical index was significantly associated with familial aggregation of major depression in univariate but not in multivariate analyses.
[e] Thoughts of death.
[f] Autonomous depression.
[g] Appetite change and guilt.
[h] Heritability in liability to major depression was greater when the study group was stratified by clinical index.
[i] Endogenous depression.
[j] Anxiety disorder and, separately, alcoholism.
*p<0.05. **p<0.01. ***p<0.0001.

twins, and dizygotic twins (see reference 76 for review), as are the mean levels of current depressive symptoms (77).

Finally, some unknown or poorly measured bias may be responsible for the results from twin studies. Estimates of heritability in liability from an alternative design can provide an important cross-check of this possibility. We computed tetrachoric correlations from the results of the controlled family studies of major depression in Table 1 (38). If a set of fairly restrictive assumptions are met, these tetrachoric correlations multiplied by 2 estimate heritability in liability to major depression (78). These assumptions are distinct from those of twin studies' design, and convergent results from different methodological approaches suggest that the assumptions of both methods are problematic or, more parsimoniously, that the results reflect the fundamental nature of major depression. From the family studies summarized in Table 1, the weighted mean heritability in liability to major depression was 58% (95% CI=42%–74%). Given that probands in all family studies were clinically ascertained, this result is in reasonable agreement with the heritability in liability from clinically ascertained twin studies (a^2=43%, 95% CI=21%–58%).

Without recourse to a more formal experimental design, it is not possible to prove that the results from twin studies are uncontaminated by all conceivable biases and violations of critical assumptions. However, given the available data, there is no reason at present to question the validity of the conclusions about major depression from twin studies.

Clinical Indices of Familial Aggregation

Table 3 summarizes data from studies of the clinical indices that predict familial aggregation of major depression (25, 29, 62, 63, 79–86). Given the biases possible with clinical ascertainment (87, 88), it is notable that only a few of these studies were based on community samples (62, 81, 82). Several of these reports are based on partially or wholly overlapping samples (80–84, 86).

Given the diversity of these studies and of the analytic methods used, we are limited to qualitative comparisons. The most widely studied clinical feature is early-onset major depression, although there are two critical conceptual difficulties. First, comparison across studies is problematic, as early onset has been defined in many different ways (e.g., onset at age <30, <32, <36, <40, or <52.2 years). Second, only a few studies (81, 82, 86) controlled for confounding between age at onset and age cohort effects for major depression (89), without which the analyses are difficult to interpret. Among the community-based studies we reviewed, a study of one twin cohort found that age at onset of major depression did not predict familial aggregation (81, 82), but another twin study found that age at onset was related to increased heritability (62). Early onset of major depression predicted increased familial risk in four other studies (29, 79, 85, 86) (only one of these controlled for year of birth [86]), but not in two others (25, 63).

The overall picture for recurrent major depression is clearer: recurrence has predicted familial aggregation in every study in which it was investigated (25, 63, 80–82, 86). In one study, however, recurrence was a significant predictor in univariate but not in multivariate analyses (86). It is critical to note, however, that groups defined by early onset of major depression and by recurrent major depression overlap considerably.

Other clinical features have been found to be associated with increased familiality of major depression. Impairment associated with major depression was a significant predictor of familial aggregation in the three studies in which it was examined (80–82). The duration of the longest episode was associated with familiality of major depression in two studies (63, 82), but not in an overlapping cohort in a third report (81). Number of symptoms was associated with familiality in one study (62), but not in two others (81, 82). Finally, a number of specific depression symptoms and comorbid disorders have been investigated without the emergence of any clear pattern of results.

In conclusion, recurrent major depression appears to be the subtype of major depression that most consistently identifies increased familial risk. We are aware that early onset of major depression is prominently viewed as the clinical feature associated with familial aggregation (90), although this view is not entirely consistent with findings reported in the literature. Several other features warrant further investigation, including: 1) impairment associated with major depression, 2) atypical major depression with reversed vegetative features (91), 3) mood response to tryptophan depletion (92), and 4) several EEG sleep measures (93).

Discussion

The results of this synthetic meta-analysis of the literature on the genetic epidemiology of major depression support six conclusions.

Findings of the Meta-Analysis

Aggregation of major depression in families. Five large and carefully conducted family studies each demonstrated the familiality of major depression. Aggregating these data yielded a summary odds ratio of 2.84 (95% CI=2.31–3.49).

Genetic influences and familial aggregation. The conclusion that genetic influences are the most important contributor to familial aggregation is supported by two of the three adoption studies and all of the twin studies of major depression we reviewed. The heritability of major depression is likely to be in the range of 31%–42%. This is probably the lower bound, and the level of heritability is likely to be substantially higher for reliably diagnosed major depression or for subtypes such as recurrent major depression. In comparison, the heritabilities of schizophrenia and bipolar disorder are estimated to be approximately 70% (94).

Etiological importance of environmental influences. Environmental influences that are etiologically important appear to be specific to an individual. There was little evidence that environmental influences common to family members (e.g., general parenting style, socioeconomic status, or local environmental qualities) were important. The large sample size of the twin meta-analysis should have afforded reasonable power to detect common environmental effects. If these effects are in fact nonzero, their magnitude is quite small (less than 5%).

Major depression as a complex disorder. Data from the studies we reviewed are consistent with the conceptualization of major depression as a complex disorder (95) that does not result from either genetic or environmental influences alone but rather from both.

Consistency. The consistency of a finding across samples and methodologies is a key element for determining causation (96, 97). In psychiatric research, consistency of research findings has often been elusive. The four conclusions discussed above are remarkably consistent across three quite different methodological approaches (five of five family studies, two of three adoption studies, and all twin studies). In addition, the estimates of heritability in liability from clinically ascertained family and twin studies are quite similar.

Generalizability. The first three conclusions above are likely to generalize to groups other than those studied. The studies included in the meta-analysis used different methodologies and had as subjects men and women from diverse cultures. Yet nearly all supported the same conclusions. This finding is particularly relevant for heritability of liability to major depression, which is a population-specific statistic. When nearly all twin studies suggest essentially the same heritability figure, it is considerably more likely to reflect the fundamental nature of major depression.

Individual-Specific Environment

Measurement error inflates estimates of individual-specific environmental effects (e^2) at the expense of additive genetic (a^2) and/or shared environmental influences (c^2) (37). Measurement error was a concern for all the types of studies discussed here. The test-retest reliability (one type of measurement error) of a lifetime history of major depression has not been impressive in community samples (98, 99), although it has been somewhat higher in clinical samples (100). However, if two or more assessments are conducted over time, measurement error can be parsed out of the analysis (99, 101). In the longitudinal sample of female twins studied by Kendler et al. (3, 61, 99), the heritability of reliably diagnosed major depression was 66% (95% CI=53%–78%) (102). This finding strongly suggests that the true heritability of liability of major depression is substantially greater than the point estimate of 37% reported in Table 2.

Gene-environment interactions have been hypothesized to be of importance in the etiology of major depression. For example, a genetic vulnerability to major depression might be expressed only if an individual is exposed to stressful life events (103). Twin studies generally have poor power to resolve gene-environment interactions, and the presence of these interactions will lead to an increase in the estimate of individual-specific environmental effects. These more complex, but perhaps more likely, etiological pathways could lead to an overall underestimate of the importance of genetic effects in the etiology of major depression.

Clinical Implications

The results of this meta-analysis have implications for how clinicians conceptualize the etiology of major depression and how they might answer the question commonly encountered clinically, What causes major depression? The answer remains regrettably imprecise and has three components: 1) major depression results from both genetic and environmental factors, 2) major depression is heterogeneous, and 3) it is likely that a number of pathways lead to the common endpoint of major depression. Because of the astonishing complexity of major depression—and despite a broad array of research efforts—more precise explanations are not currently possible.

The second implication relates to how clinicians conceptualize the etiology of major depression in a particular patient, as exemplified by the question, Why do I have major depression? Overtly or covertly imbedded in this question is the complex question of who or what is to blame. Although the studies summarized here add weight to our understanding of the etiology of major depression at the level of large groups of individuals, the relevance of these findings to a particular patient is difficult to determine. Indeed, a key task in many types of clinical work—from pharmacological management to intensive psychotherapy—is to develop an individualized understanding of etiology. Our conclusions are relevant, but an important role for the clinician is to attempt to avoid a number of common misinterpretations (see reference 104 for review). The following points may help clinicians in their work with individual patients:

1. Heritability of liability applies to groups, not individuals. We cannot now state with confidence that a particular person's major depression is or is not genetic in origin, much less that some percentage of the disorder is "due to genes."

2. The causation of major depression is probabilistic, not deterministic. If we could measure liability to major depression directly, we would find substantial numbers of people with high liability who are not affected with major depression and people with low liability who are affected. Individuals' life experiences, intentions, choices, and actions are critically important.

3. Environmental influences are important. Even if heritability of liability to major depression is predominant in the etiology of the disorder, environmental events account for substantial portions of the variance in liability. The absence of shared environmental effects does not mean that the influences of parents and other family members are irrelevant. The most parsimonious explanation may be one that is familiar to clinicians: it is not the general qualities of some facet of the environment (e.g., a parent's rearing style, neighborhood, poverty) but rather how these qualities influence an individual and how he or she interacts with this part of the environment across developmental stages.

Research Implications

Although the conclusions summarized above constitute an important step in conceptualizing the nature of major depression, they do not immediately lead to the essential goal of a clear understanding of the pathophysiology of major depression. We submit, however, that these conclusions have the following implications for research on major depression:

1. These conclusions are consistent with efforts to identify susceptibility loci for major depression, as noted in an NIMH report on genetics and mental disorders (www.nimh.nih.gov/research/genetics.htm). We are aware of three major efforts to identify susceptibility loci that began in early 2000 and could yield results within 4–5 years.

2. If certain depressive features (i.e., recurrence) predict familiality of major depression, it may be useful to investigate the rationality of family-based screening as a primary and secondary preventive measure. Moreover, for clinical and biological studies, it may be possible to stratify heterogeneous samples to identify more homogeneous subsamples. Recurrence and family history of major depression are two variables that could be used to stratify samples. However, the most efficient means of obtaining these data (i.e., using the major depression proband as informant) may not be sufficiently sensitive (105–108) to be applied with confidence.

3. The finding that the prevalence of major depression was higher in dizygotic than monozygotic twins was unexpected but intriguing. Possible explanations include differential cooperation in monozygotic versus dizygotic twins in the presence of major depression, a protective effect of being a monozygotic twin, and/or a predisposing effect of being a dizygotic twin.

Limitations

This review has three general limitations. First, there may be published or unpublished family, adoption, or twin studies that were not included in this analysis. We attempted to limit the impact of this problem as described in the Method section. Second, the extant studies focused on predominantly Caucasian subjects from developed nations. It is not known whether the results generalize worldwide or across time cohorts. Third, although it is reassuring that the extant data support the validity of the equal-environment assumption in twin studies of major depression, it is impossible to prove that all potential violations have been assessed. Therefore, we cannot exclude the possibility that a cryptic violation of the equal-environment assumption could influence the results.

Received Sept. 3, 1999; revision received Mar. 23, 2000; accepted May 10, 2000. From the Department of Psychiatry, Virginia Institute for Psychiatric and Behavioral Genetics, Virginia Commonwealth University. Address reprint requests to Dr. Sullivan, Department of Psychiatry, Virginia Institute for Psychiatric and Behavioral Genetics, P.O. Box 980126, Richmond, VA 23298-0126; sullivan@psycho.psi.vcu.edu (e-mail).

This work was supported by National Institute of Mental Health grants MH-59160, A138429, MH-01458, MH-40828, MH/AA-49492, and MH-01277. The authors thank Laura Bierut, M.D., and Andrew Health, Ph.D., for providing the raw data on major depression from the Australian Twin Registry.

References

1. Wells JE, Bushnell JA, Hornblow AR, Joyce PR, Oakley-Browne MA: Christchurch psychiatric epidemiology study, part I: methodology and lifetime prevalence for specific psychiatric disorders. Aust NZ J Psychiatry 1989; 23:315–326
2. Weissman MM, Bruce ML, Leaf PJ, Florio LP, Holzer C III: Affective disorders, in Psychiatric Disorders in America: The Epidemiologic Catchment Area Study. Edited by Robins LN, Regier DA. New York, Free Press, 1991, pp 53–80
3. Kendler K, Neale MC, Kessler RC, Heath AC, Eaves LJ: A population-based twin study of major depression in women: the impact of varying definitions of illness. Arch Gen Psychiatry 1992; 49:257–266
4. Kessler RC, McGonagle KA, Zhao S, Nelson CB, Hughes M, Eshleman S, Wittchen H-U, Kendler KS: Lifetime and 12-month prevalence of DSM-III-R psychiatric disorders in the United States: results from the National Comorbidity Survey. Arch Gen Psychiatry 1994; 51:8–19
5. Greenberg PE, Stiglin LE, Finkelstein SN, Berndt ER: The economic burden of depression in 1990. J Clin Psychiatry 1993; 54:405–418
6. Piccinelli M, Wilkinson G: Outcome of depression in psychiatric settings. Br J Psychiatry 1994; 164:297–304
7. Wells KB, Stewart A, Hays RD, Burnam MA, Rogers W, Daniels M, Berry S, Greenfield S, Ware J: The functioning and well-being of depressed patients: results from the Medical Outcomes Study. JAMA 1989; 262:914–919
8. Broadhead WE, Blazer DG, George LK, Tse CK: Depression, disability days, and days lost from work in a prospective epidemiologic survey. JAMA 1990; 264:2524–2528
9. Judd LL, Paulus MP, Wells KB, Rapaport MH: Socioeconomic burden of subsyndromal depressive symptoms and major depression in a sample of the general population. Am J Psychiatry 1996; 153:1411–1417
10. Ustun TB, Rehm J, Chatterji S, Saxena S, Trotter R, Room R, Bickenbach J (WHO/NIH Joint Project CAR Study Group): Multiple-informant ranking of the disabling effects of different health conditions in 14 countries. Lancet 1999; 354:111–115
11. Harris EC, Barraclough BB: Excess mortality of mental disorder. Br J Psychiatry 1998; 173:11–53
12. Murray CJL, Lopez AD: Evidence-based health policy: lessons from the Global Burden of Disease Study. Science 1996; 274:740–743
13. Pincus HA, Tanielian TL, Marcus SC, Olfson M, Zarin DA, Thompson J, Magno Zito J: Prescribing trends in psychotropic medications: primary care, psychiatry, and other medical specialties. JAMA 1998; 279:526–531
14. McGuffin P, Katz R: The genetics of depression and manic-depressive disorder. Br J Psychiatry 1989; 155:294–304
15. Tsuang MT, Faraone SV: The Genetics of Mood Disorders. Baltimore, Johns Hopkins University Press, 1990
16. Merikangas KR, Kupfer DJ: Mood disorders: genetic aspects, in Comprehensive Textbook of Psychiatry, 6th ed, vol 1. Edited by Kaplan HI, Sadock BJ. Baltimore, Williams & Wilkins, 1995, pp 1102–1116
17. Plomin R, DeFries JC, McClearn GE, Rutter M: Behavioral Genetics. New York, WH Freeman, 1997
18. Glass GV, McGaw B, Smith ML: Meta-Analysis in Social Research. Beverly Hills, Calif, Sage Publications, 1981
19. Smith ML, Glass GV, Miller TI: The Benefits of Psychotherapy. Baltimore, Johns Hopkins University Press, 1980
20. Thacker SB: Meta-analysis: a quantitative approach to research integration. JAMA 1988; 259:1685–1689
21. Petitti DB: Meta-Analysis, Decision Analysis, and Cost-Effectiveness Analysis. New York, Oxford University Press, 1994
22. Kendler KS, Pedersen NL, Neale MC, Mathé A: A pilot Swedish twin study of affective illness including hospital- and population-ascertained subsamples: results of model fitting. Behav Genet 1995; 25:217–232
23. Angst J, Frey R, Lohmeyer B, Zerbin-Rüdin E: Bipolar manic-depressive psychosis: results of a genetic investigation. Hum Genet 1980; 55:237–254
24. Gershon ES, Mark A, Cohen N, Belizon N, Baron M, Knobe KE: Transmitted factors in the morbid risk of affective disorders: a controlled study. J Psychiatr Res 1975; 12:283–299
25. McGuffin P, Katz R, Bebbington P: Hazard, heredity, and depression: a family study. J Psychiatr Res 1987; 4:365–375
26. Perris C: A study of bipolar (manic-depressive) and unipolar recurrent depressive psychoses. Acta Psychiatr Scand Suppl 1966; 194:1–188
27. Scharfetter C: Subdividing the functional psychoses: a family hereditary approach. Psychol Med 1981; 11:637–640
28. Smeraldi E, Negri F, Melica AM: A genetic study of affective disorders. Acta Psychiatr Scand 1977; 56:382–398
29. Stancer HC, Persad E, Wagener DK, Jorna T: Evidence for homogeneity of major depression and bipolar affective disorder. J Psychiatr Res 1987; 21:37–53
30. Winokur G, Cadoret R, Dorzab J, Baker M: Depressive disease: a genetic study. Arch Gen Psychiatry 1971; 24:135–144
31. Allen MG, Cohen S, Pollin W, Greenspan SI: Affective illness in veteran twins: a diagnostic review. Am J Psychiatry 1974; 131:1234–1239
32. Bertelsen A, Harvald B, Hauge M: A Danish twin study of manic-depressive disorders. Br J Psychiatry 1977; 130:330–351
33. Slater E, Shields J: Psychotic and Neurotic Illnesses in Twins. London, Her Majesty's Stationery Office, 1953
34. Torgersen S: Genetic factors in moderately severe and mild affective disorders. Arch Gen Psychiatry 1986; 43:222–226
35. Schlesselman JJ: Case-Control Studies: Design, Conduct, Analysis. New York, Oxford University Press, 1982
36. SAS/STAT Software: Changes and Enhancements Through Release 6.11. Cary, NC, SAS Institute, 1996
37. Neale MC, Cardon LR: Methodology for the Study of Twins and Families. Dordrecht, the Netherlands, Kluwer, 1992
38. Falconer DS: The inheritance of liability to certain diseases, estimated from the incidence among relatives. Ann Hum Genet (London) 1965; 29:51–76
39. Neale MC, Boker S, Xie G, Maes H: Mx: Statistical Modeling. Richmond, Medical College of Virginia, Department of Psychiatry, 1999
40. Hamagami F: A review of the Mx computer program for structural equation modeling. Structural Equation Modeling 1997; 4:157–175
41. Neale MC, Miller MB: The use of likelihood-based confidence intervals in genetic models. Behav Genet 1997; 27:113–120
42. Weissman MM, Merikangas KR, John K, Wickramaratne P, Prusoff BA, Kidd KK: Family-genetic studies of psychiatric disor-

ders: developing technologies. Arch Gen Psychiatry 1986; 43: 1104–1116
43. Khoury MJ, Beaty TH, Cohen BH: Fundamentals of Genetic Epidemiology. New York, Oxford University Press, 1993
44. Gershon ES, Hamovit J, Guroff JJ, Dibble E, Leckman JF, Sceery W, Targum SD, Nurnberger JI Jr, Goldin LR, Bunney WE Jr: A family study of schizoaffective, bipolar I, bipolar II, unipolar, and normal control probands. Arch Gen Psychiatry 1982; 39: 1157–1167
45. Maier W, Lichtermann D, Minges J, Hallmayer J, Heun R, Benkert O, Levinson DF: Continuity and discontinuity of affective disorders and schizophrenia: results of a controlled family study. Arch Gen Psychiatry 1993; 50:871–883
46. Tsuang MT, Winokur G, Crowe RR: Morbidity risks of schizophrenia and affective disorders among first-degree relatives of patients with schizophrenia, mania, depression, and surgical conditions. Br J Psychiatry 1980; 137:497–504
47. Weissman MM, Gershon ES, Kidd KK, Prusoff BA, Leckman JF, Dibble E, Hamovit J, Thompson WD, Pauls DL, Guroff JJ: Psychiatric disorders in the relatives of probands with affective disorders: the Yale University-NIMH Collaborative Study. Arch Gen Psychiatry 1984; 41:13–21
48. Weissman MM, Wickramaratne P, Adams PB, Lish JD, Horwath E, Charney D, Woods SW, Leeman E, Frosch E: The relationship between panic disorder and major depression: a new family study. Arch Gen Psychiatry 1993; 50:767–780
49. Kendler KS: Is seeking treatment for depression predicted by a history of depression in relatives? implications for family studies of affective disorder. Psychol Med 1995; 25:807–814
50. Sullivan PF, Wells JE, Joyce PR, Bushnell JA, Mulder RT, Oakley-Browne MA: Family history of depression in clinic and community samples. J Affect Disord 1996; 40:159–168
51. Tsuang MT, Fleming JA, Kendler KS, Gruenberg AS: Selection of controls for family studies: biases and implications. Arch Gen Psychiatry 1988; 45:1006–1008
52. Schwartz S, Link BG: The "well control" artefact in case/control studies of specific psychiatric disorders. Psychol Med 1989; 19: 737–742
53. Kendler KS: The super-normal control group in psychiatric genetics: possible artifactual evidence for coaggregation. Psychiatr Genet 1990; 1:45–53
54. Kendler KS: Twin studies of psychiatric illness: current status and future directions. Arch Gen Psychiatry 1993; 50:905–915
55. von Knorring A-L, Cloninger CR, Bohman M, Sigvardsson S: An adoption study of depressive disorders and substance abuse. Arch Gen Psychiatry 1983; 40:943–950
56. Cadoret RJ, O'Gorman TW, Heywood E, Troughton E: Genetic and environmental factors in major depression. J Affect Disord 1985; 9:155–164
57. Wender PH, Kety SS, Rosenthal D, Schulsinger F, Ortmann J, Lunde I: Psychiatric disorders in the biological and adoptive families of adopted individuals with affective disorders. Arch Gen Psychiatry 1986; 43:923–929
58. Regier DA, Goldberg ID, Taube CA: The de facto US mental health services system: a public health perspective. Arch Gen Psychiatry 1978; 35:685–693
59. Regier DA, Narrow WE, Rae DS, Manderscheid RW, Locke BZ, Goodwin FK: The de facto US mental and addictive disorders service system: Epidemiologic Catchment Area prospective 1-year prevalence rates of disorders and services. Arch Gen Psychiatry 1993; 50:85–94
60. Bierut LJ, Heath AC, Bucholz KK, Dinwiddie SH, Madden PAF, Statham DJ, Dunne MP, Martin NG: Major depressive disorder in a community-based twin sample: are there different genetic and environmental contributions for men and women? Arch Gen Psychiatry 1999; 56:557–563
61. Kendler KS, Prescott CA: A population-based twin study of lifetime major depression in men and women. Arch Gen Psychiatry 1999; 56:39–44; correction, 2000; 57:94–95
62. Lyons MJ, Eisen SA, Goldberg J, True W, Lin N, Meyer JM, Toomey R, Faraone SV, Merren J, Tsuang MT: A registry-based twin study of depression in males. Arch Gen Psychiatry 1998; 55:468–472
63. McGuffin P, Katz R, Watkins S, Rutherford J: A hospital-based twin register of the heritability of DSM-IV unipolar depression. Arch Gen Psychiatry 1996; 53:129–136
64. Kendler KS, Gardner CO, Prescott CA: Corrections to two prior published articles (letter). Arch Gen Psychiatry 2000; 57:94–95
65. Andrews G, Stewart G, Allen R, Henderson AS: The genetics of six neurotic disorders: a twin study. J Affect Disord 1990; 19: 23–29
66. Neale MC, Eaves LJ, Kendler KS: The power of the classical twin study to resolve variation in threshold traits. Behav Genet 1994; 24:239–258
67. Weissman MM, Bland R, Joyce PR, Newman S, Wells JE, Wittchen H-U: Sex differences in rates of depression: cross-national perspectives. J Affect Disord 1993; 29:77–84
68. Kessler RC, McGonagle KA, Swartz M, Blazer DG, Nelson CB: Sex and depression in the National Comorbidity Survey, I: lifetime prevalence, chronicity and recurrence. J Affect Disord 1993; 29:85–96
69. Gater R, Tansella M, Korten A, Tiemens BG, Mavreas VG, Olatawura MO: Sex differences in the prevalence and detection of depressive and anxiety disorders in general health care settings. Arch Gen Psychiatry 1998; 55:405–413
70. Faraone SV, Lyons MJ, Tsuang MT: Sex differences in affective disorder: genetic transmission. Genet Epidemiol 1987; 4:331–343
71. Merikangas KR, Weissman MM, Pauls DL: Genetic factors in the sex ratio of major depression. Psychol Med 1985; 15:63–69
72. Reich T, Van Eerdewegh P, Rice J, Mullaney J, Endicott J, Klerman GL: The familial transmission of primary major depressive disorder. J Psychiatr Res 1987; 21:613–624
73. Kendler KS, Neale MC, Kessler RC, Heath AC, Eaves LJ: Parental treatment and the equal environment assumption in twin studies of psychiatric illness. Psychol Med 1994; 24:579–590
74. Kendler KS, Gardener CO: Twin studies of adult psychiatric and substance dependence disorders: are they biased by differences in the environmental experiences of mono- and dizygotic twins in childhood and adolescence? Psychol Med 1998; 28:625–633
75. Bryan E: Twins and Higher Multiple Births: A Guide to Their Nature and Nurture. London, Edward Arnold, 1992
76. Kendler KS, Pedersen NL, Farahmand BY, Persson P-G: The treated incidence of psychotic and affective illness in twins compared to population expectation. Psychol Med 1996; 26: 1135–1144
77. Kendler KS, Martin NG, Heath AC, Eaves LJ: Self-report psychiatric symptoms in twins and their non-twin relatives: are twins different? Am J Med Genet Neuropsychiatr Genet 1995; 60: 588–591
78. Reich T, Cloninger CR, Guze SB: The multifactorial model of disease transmission, I: description of the model and its use in psychiatry. Br J Psychiatry 1975; 127:1–10
79. Cadoret RJ, Woolson R, Winokur G: The relationship of age of onset in unipolar affective illness to risk of alcoholism and depression in parents. J Psychiatr Res 1977; 13:137–142
80. Gershon ES, Weissman MM, Guroff JJ, Prusoff BA, Leckman JF: Validation of criteria for major depression through controlled family study. J Affect Disord 1986; 11:125–131
81. Kendler KS, Neale MC, Kessler RC, Heath AC, Eaves LJ: The clinical characteristics of major depression as indices of the familial risk to illness. Br J Psychiatry 1994; 165:66–72

82. Kendler KS, Gardner CO, Prescott CA: Clinical characteristics of major depression that predict risk of depression in relatives. Arch Gen Psychiatry 1999; 56:322–327; correction, 2000; 57: 94–95
83. Leckman JF, Weissman MM, Prusoff BA, Caruso KA, Merikangas KR, Pauls DL, Kidd KK: Subtypes of depression. Arch Gen Psychiatry 1984; 41:833–838
84. Leckman JF, Caruso KA, Prusoff BA, Weissman MM, Merikangas KR, Pauls DL: Appetite disturbance and excessive guilt in major depression. Arch Gen Psychiatry 1984; 41:839–844
85. Mendlewicz J, Baron M: Morbidity risks in subtypes of unipolar depressive illness: differences between early and late onset forms. Br J Psychiatry 1981; 139:463–466
86. Weissman MM, Merikangas KR, Wickramaratne P, Kidd KK, Prusoff BA, Leckman JF, Pauls DL: Understanding the clinical heterogeneity of major depression using family data. Arch Gen Psychiatry 1986; 43:430–434
87. Berkson J: Limitations of the application of fourfold table analysis to hospital data. Biometrics Bull 1946; 2:47–53
88. Cohen P, Cohen J: The clinician's illusion. Arch Gen Psychiatry 1984; 41:1178–1182
89. Klerman GL, Weissman MM: Increasing rates of depression. JAMA 1989; 261:2229–2235
90. NIMH Genetics Workgroup: Genetics and Mental Disorders. Bethesda, Md, National Institute of Mental Health, 1998
91. Kendler KS, Eaves LJ, Walters EE, Neale MC, Heath AC, Kessler RC: The identification and validation of distinct depressive syndromes in a population-based sample of female twins. Arch Gen Psychiatry 1996; 53:391–399
92. Benkelfat C, Ellenbogen MA, Dean P, Palmour RM, Young SN: Mood-lowering effect of tryptophan depletion. Arch Gen Psychiatry 1994; 51:687–697
93. Giles DE, Kupfer DJ, Rush AJ, Roffwarg HP: Controlled comparison of electrophysiological sleep in families of probands with unipolar depression. Am J Psychiatry 1998; 155:192–199
94. Kendler KS: Overview: a current perspective on twin studies of schizophrenia. Am J Psychiatry 1983; 140:1413–1425
95. Lander ES, Schork NJ: Genetic dissection of complex traits. Science 1994; 265:2037–2048
96. Hill AB: The environment and disease: association or causation. Proc R Soc Med 1965; 58:295–300
97. Rothman KJ: Modern Epidemiology. Boston, Little, Brown, 1986
98. Bromet EJ, Dunn LO, Connell MM, Dew MA, Schulberg HC: Long-term reliability of diagnosing lifetime major depression in a community sample. Arch Gen Psychiatry 1986; 43:435–440
99. Kendler KS, Neale MC, Kessler RC, Heath AC, Eaves LJ: The lifetime history of major depression in women: reliability of diagnosis and heritability. Arch Gen Psychiatry 1993; 50:863–870
100. Keller MB, Klein DN, Hirschfeld RMA, Kocsis JH, McCullough JP, Miller I, First MB, Holzer CP III, Keitner GI, Marin DB, Shea T: Results of the DSM-IV mood disorders field trial. Am J Psychiatry 1995; 152:843–849
101. Bulik CM, Sullivan PF, Kendler KS: Heritability and reliability of binge-eating and bulimia nervosa. Biol Psychiatry 1998; 44: 1210–1218
102. Foley DL, Neale MC, Kendler KS: Reliability of a lifetime history of major depression: implications for heritability and co-morbidity. Psychol Med 1998; 28:857–870
103. Kendler KS, Kessler RC, Walters EE, MacLean CJ, Neale MC, Heath AC, Eaves LJ: Stressful life events, genetic liability, and onset of an episode of major depression in women. Am J Psychiatry 1995; 152:833–842
104. Rutter M, Plomin R: Opportunities for psychiatry from genetic findings. Br J Psychiatry 1997; 171:209–219
105. Andreasen NC, Rice J, Endicott J, Reich T, Coryell W: The family history approach to diagnosis: how useful is it? Arch Gen Psychiatry 1986; 43:421–429
106. Chapman TF, Mannuzza S, Klein DF, Fyer AJ: Effects of informant mental disorder on psychiatric family history data. Am J Psychiatry 1994; 151:574–579
107. Orvaschel H, Thompson WD, Belanger A, Prusoff BA, Kidd KK: Comparison of the family history method to direct interview: factors affecting the diagnosis of depression. J Affect Disord 1982; 4:49–59
108. Thompson WD, Orvaschel H, Prusoff BA, Kidd KK: An evaluation of the family history for ascertaining psychiatric disorders. Arch Gen Psychiatry 1982; 39:53–58

Childhood Sexual Abuse as a Risk Factor for Depression in Women: Psychosocial and Neurobiological Correlates

Erica L. Weiss, M.D., James G. Longhurst, M.D., and Carolyn M. Mazure, Ph.D.

Objective: Depression is twice as common in women as in men, but the reason for this sexual dimorphism is unknown. This article reviews recent studies of the role of childhood sexual abuse in the subsequent development of major depressive disorder, and the biological and psychosocial mechanisms by which early stressors may contribute to adult-onset depression in women. Particular attention is paid to investigations of the long-term effects of early stress on hypothalamic-pituitary-adrenal (HPA) axis function. **Method:** Studies were identified by means of computerized and manual searches; further references were obtained from the bibliographies of reviewed articles. **Results:** Childhood sexual abuse is associated with adult-onset depression in both men and women, and occurrence of such abuse is more common in girls than in boys. There is evidence from both animal and human studies that early stressors produce long-term dysregulation of the HPA axis similar to that seen in depressed patients and that such dysregulation results in a differential response to stressors in adulthood. In addition, it appears that the HPA axis in females may be more susceptible to stress-induced dysregulation, which might contribute to an increased vulnerability to depression in adulthood. **Conclusions:** Childhood sexual abuse is an important early stressor that may predispose individuals to adult-onset depression by means of dysregulation of the HPA axis. Investigation of the mechanisms mediating the relationship between childhood sexual abuse and adult-onset depression, and the study of gender differences in exposure to this and other stressors, may improve our understanding of the etiology of depressive illness in general.

(Am J Psychiatry 1999; 156:816–828)

It is well known that depression is twice as common in women as in men, but the origins of this dramatic difference remain obscure (1). Life stressors have long been hypothesized to be risk factors for depression (2), and contemporary theories continue to emphasize the role of psychological stress in the etiology of major depressive disorder (3–6). Empirical studies support these theoretical formulations; in both case-control comparisons and recent studies of multiple risk factors, exposure to stressful life events is a strong predictor of liability for major depression (7, 8). Despite the importance of life stressors in predicting depression and the higher rates of depression in women, few studies have directly examined whether stress accounts, at least in part, for the high rates of depression in women. In order to address this issue, it is important to determine whether women are exposed to more stressors, have greater exposure to certain types of stressors, or respond differently to stressors than do men.

The purpose of this article is to examine the empirical data regarding the role of exposure to the specific stressor of childhood sexual abuse in the adult onset of depression, with particular emphasis on whether higher rates of childhood sexual abuse in girls may in

Received Nov. 26, 1997; revision received Oct. 26, 1998; accepted Dec. 7, 1998. From the Department of Psychiatry, Yale University School of Medicine. Address reprint requests to Dr. Mazure, Yale-New Haven Hospital, 10-520 East Pavilion, 20 York St., New Haven, CT 06504; carolyn.mazure@yale.edu (e-mail).
James G. Longhurst, M.D., is deceased.

part account for the higher incidence of depression in women. Sexual abuse during childhood is a stressor experienced more frequently by girls than boys, with estimates of the incidence of childhood sexual abuse in girls varying from 6% to 62% (9). This wide range is related to disparate definitions of childhood sexual abuse and differing methods of data collection, but most studies estimate the incidence to be at least 6%–15% (9). Childhood sexual abuse is considerably less common in males, with the ratio of female to male victims estimated to be as high as 12:1 (10). There is also some evidence that childhood sexual abuse may be particularly pernicious in its effects and that it is more likely to predict the subsequent development of psychiatric illness than does sexual assault occurring in adulthood (11).

We begin by examining the literature regarding the relationship between childhood sexual abuse and the development of depression in adult women, which demonstrates an association between the two. Next, we present studies comparing the relative impact of childhood sexual abuse on the occurrence of adult-onset depression in women and men, which suggest that boys who are victims of childhood sexual abuse may be less likely to become depressed subsequently than abused girls. We then briefly consider which characteristics of childhood sexual abuse may influence the likelihood of depressive episodes in adulthood.

In the second half of the article, our focus turns to factors, both psychosocial and neurobiological, that may mediate the observed relationship between childhood sexual abuse and adult-onset depression. In particular, we review the evidence suggesting that early stress induces permanent changes in the regulation of the hypothalamic-pituitary-adrenal (HPA) axis, which may result in an increased vulnerability to depression following stress in adulthood. Finally, we hypothesize that there is a sexual dimorphism in the HPA axis response to stress that may create a higher biological vulnerability to depression in women.

EFFECT OF CHILDHOOD SEXUAL ABUSE ON ADULT-ONSET DEPRESSION IN WOMEN

Most studies aimed at understanding the relationship between childhood sexual abuse and adult-onset depression have used all-female study groups. Of these, seven were derived from community populations, five from college women, and nine from clinical populations. The incidence of childhood sexual abuse ranged from 6% to 46% in studies of nonclinical study groups and from 7% to 43% in studies using patient groups for which subjects were not selected on the basis of childhood sexual abuse. Although the retrospective design in all but one of these studies confers methodological limitations, the pattern of results across studies is remarkably consistent. Only one study did not find a higher incidence of adult-onset depression in women who had been abused as children than in women who had not been abused.

Community Studies

All seven studies using various groups of community-based subjects found a significantly higher occurrence of adult-onset depression in women who reported histories of childhood sexual abuse when compared to those without reported childhood abuse. Although the incidence of depression varied across groups because of differences in population characteristics, ascertainment methods, assessment instruments, and diagnostic criteria, the pattern of results remained the same. Table 1 summarizes the features and findings of these studies conducted across several different countries.

Two investigations from Britain used randomly selected community samples to study the relationship between childhood sexual abuse and adult-onset depression in working-class mothers. In the first of these studies (N=286) (12), 64% of women who reported childhood sexual abuse before age 17 years were diagnosed with adult-onset depression during the 3-year study period, whereas 26% of the nonabused women suffered from a major depressive episode. This study attempted to control for the possibility that the presence of depression influenced the reporting of childhood sexual abuse by excluding those subjects who were depressed at the time that a history of childhood sexual abuse was determined. The relationship between childhood sexual abuse and adult-onset depression was maintained in this second analysis (50% versus 15%) (Yates-corrected $\chi^2=7.50$, df=1, $p<0.01$). In the second random sample of working-class British mothers (N=101) (13), subjects with a history of childhood sexual abuse were also more likely to be diagnosed with depression during a 12-month period, compared to those without such a history (29% versus 10%). The presence of childhood sexual abuse was identified in both of these studies by using two screening questions, followed by further questioning for those subjects with positive responses. The five community studies described below employed more rigorous methods to determine a history of childhood sexual abuse by means of detailed questioning of all subjects (14) and use of structured sexual abuse interviews (15–18).

In a random sample of 314 women selected from Dunedin, New Zealand (15), 20.7% of women with a history of childhood sexual abuse met lifetime diagnostic criteria for an adult psychiatric disorder (mostly depressive), but only 6.3% of those not abused met such criteria. These investigators defined childhood sexual abuse as some form of genital contact before age 12, which represented the youngest cutoff age among the community study groups. In a second randomly selected sample of urban New Zealand women, 298 subjects reporting childhood sexual abuse were compared with 298 subjects without reported childhood sexual abuse (16). A history of major depression

TABLE 1. Community Studies Examining the Relationship of Childhood Sexual Abuse and Adult-Onset Depression in Women

				Diagnostic Tools			Childhood Sexual Abuse			Chi-Square Analysis[b] (df=1 unless otherwise specified)		
								% Depressed				
Study	Year	N	Country	Depression Measures[a]	Childhood Sexual Abuse Assessment	Depression Assessment Period	% of Subjects	With Abuse	Without Abuse	χ^2	p	Definition of Child Sexual Abuse
Bifulco et al. (12)	1991	286	Britain	PSE	Two screening questions and additional questions for positive responses	3 years	9	64	26	14.46	<0.001	Any sexual contact before age 17 years, excluding willing contact in teens and with nonrelated peers
Andrews et al. (13)	1995	101	Britain	PSE	Two screening questions and additional questions for positive responses	12 months	12	29	10	4.49	<0.05	Any sexual contact before age 17 years, excluding willing contact in teens and with nonrelated peers
Mullen et al. (14)	1988	314	New Zealand	GHQ; PSE	Two screening questions and semistructured interview for positive responses	Lifetime	13[c]	20.7	6.3	6.92	<0.01	Some form of genital contact before age 12 years
Mullen et al. (15)	1993	596	New Zealand	GHQ; PSE	Semistructured interview with detailed questions about childhood sexual abuse	Lifetime	32	13	5	7.70	<0.01	At least genital contact before age 16 years, excluding noncoercive actions with peers
Bushnell et al. (16)	1992	301	New Zealand	DIS-3A	Five questions about childhood sexual abuse	Lifetime	13	—[d]	—	—	—	Intrafamilial
Bagley and Ramsey (17)	1985	377	Canada	CES-D, Middlesex	Modified Finkelhor Childhood Sexual Abuse Survey	Current	22	16	3	16.48	<0.001	Before age 16 years
Peters (18)	1988	119	United States	SADS-L, DIS, Beck	Childhood sexual abuse semistructured interview	Lifetime	—[e]	—[f]	66	6.88, df=2	<0.05	Noncontact abuse before age 18 years or contact abuse before age 18 years involving intentional, unambiguous behavior of physical nature with perpetrator who was more than 5 years older or used coercion

[a] PSE=Present State Examination. GHQ=General Health Questionnaire. DIS=National Institute of Mental Health Diagnostic Interview Schedule. DIS-3A=National Institute of Mental Health Diagnostic Interview Schedule, version 3A. CES-D=Center for Environmental Studies Depression Scale. Middlesex=Middlesex Hospital Questionnaire. SADS-L=Schedule for Affective Disorders and Schizophrenia—Lifetime Version. Beck=Beck Depression Inventory Short Form.
[b] Yates corrected.
[c] General population estimate, 9.9%.
[d] Childhood sexual abuse examined as a function of depression; odds ratio=2.0.
[e] Noncontact abuse, 14%; contact abuse, 46%.
[f] Noncontact abuse, 59%; contact abuse, 85%.

was again found to be more common in women who reported past abuse than in those who denied childhood abuse (13% versus 5%). A third study, by Bushnell and colleagues (14), examined the rates of childhood sexual abuse in 301 urban New Zealand women who met lifetime criteria for an affective disorder, eating disorder, and/or substance use disorder. This study, the only investigation that focused on intrafamilial childhood sexual abuse, found that women with a lifetime diagnosis of depression were twice as likely to report a history of intrafamilial childhood sexual abuse as women who had never been depressed.

TABLE 2. Studies of College Women Examining the Relationship of Childhood Sexual Abuse and Adult-Onset Depression

Study	Year	N	Childhood Sexual Abuse Assessment[a]	Depression Assessment Period	% of Subjects With Childhood Sexual Abuse	Depression Measure[b]	Relation of Depression to Childhood Sexual Abuse	Definition of Abuse
Briere and Runtz (19)	1988	278	Finkelhor survey	12 months	15	HSCL[c]	F=4.21, df=1, 222, p<0.04	Sexual contact (touching through intercourse) between girl under age 15 and individual at least 5 years older
Gold (20)	1986	191	Screening questions and Finkelhor survey	—	50	Beck, HSCL	Univariate F test—Beck: F=17.33, df=1, 164, p<0.001; HSCL: F=11.44, df=1, 164, p<0.001	Sexual contact before age 12 with postpubertal person at least 5 years older; or sexual contact at age 12–16 with person 10 years older; or any contact before age 16 with person who used physical force
Sedney and Brooks (21)	1984	301	—	Lifetime	16	Clinical diagnosis[d]	χ^2=5.52, df=1, p<0.05, Yates corrected	Some sexual experience with another person while growing up (ranging from single exposure to forced intercourse)
Yama et al. (22)	1993	149	Finkelhor survey	Current	—	Beck	F=6.24, df=1, 133, p<0.03	Age <13 years: sexual contact with person(s) ≥5 years older; age 13–16 years: sexual contact with person(s) ≥10 years older[e]
Fromuth (23)	1986	383	Questionnaire, Finkelhor survey	Current	22	Beck, HSCL	Beck: r=0.01 (n.s.); HSCL: r=0.04 (n.s.)	Age <12 years: partner had to be 16 years old and ≥5 years older; age 13–16 years: sexual contact with person ≥10 years older (ranging from exhibitionism to physical contact)

[a] Finkelhor survey=modified version of the Finkelhor Childhood Sexual Abuse Survey.
[b] HSCL=Hopkins Symptom Checklist. Beck=Beck Depression Inventory.
[c] Subjects with childhood sexual abuse had a mean depression score of 22.8; subjects without abuse had a mean score of 20.7.
[d] Of the subjects with childhood sexual abuse, 65% were diagnosed as depressed; 43% of those without abuse were diagnosed as depressed.
[e] Exclusion criteria for comparison subjects: age <13 years: sexual contact with person(s) ≥ 3 years older; age 13–15 years: sexual contact with person(s) ≥7 years older.

Both of the studies from North America examined the lifetime incidence of major depression in community-based study groups. In the first, in which the study group was drawn from a large Canadian city, Bagley and Ramsey (17) found depression to be significantly more common in women with a history of childhood sexual abuse than women who had not been abused (16% versus 3%). In the second study, the study group was culled from a large sample of Los Angeles county women (18). Results showed that a significantly greater proportion of women who reported histories of childhood sexual abuse had experienced at least one depressive episode than had women who did not report abuse (85% versus 66%). The high percentage of depressed subjects in this study is likely due to the fact that the subjects were selected from those participating in a larger study of sexual socialization and sexual experiences. In fact, this study reported a 60% incidence of childhood sexual abuse, which was markedly greater than the incidence rates in any of the other six studies.

Studies of College Women

Five studies used nonclinical study groups composed of college students to examine the relationship between childhood sexual abuse and adult onset depression in a high-functioning group. It has been suggested that investigations of college women who report a history of sexual abuse selects for "healthy survivors"—i.e., those who have coped well enough with the effects of past abuse to achieve academic standing at a college level. Nonetheless, four of these studies found a significantly greater incidence of depressive symptoms in those women who reported a history of childhood sexual abuse than those who did not (19–22). All five studies assessed depressive symptoms (unlike the community studies, most of which required a diagnosis of depression) and used a variety of symptom checklists. Table 2 summarizes the features and findings of these studies composed of college women. Symptom severity, as evidenced by itemized or mean scores on symptom scales, was provided only in the study by Briere and Runtz (19) (table 2).

The one study that failed to find a significant relationship between past sexual abuse and depression (23) used a relatively broad definition for past abuse. For example, this study classified subjects who reported a one-time "exhibition" as having been sexually abused. Use of this broad definition may have contributed to the lack of an observed correlation between abuse and adult symptoms. However, the study by Sed-

TABLE 3. Clinical Studies on the Relationship of Childhood Sexual Abuse and Adult-Onset Depression in Women

Study	Year	Subjects	Childhood Sexual Abuse Assessment	Depression Assessment Period	% of Subjects With Childhood Sexual Abuse
Bagley and McDonald (24)	1984	87 girls followed prospectively: 20 with childhood sexual abuse and separated, 37 without childhood sexual abuse and separated, and 30 without childhood sexual abuse and not separated	Verified by the child and report of an adult familiar with household	Current	—
Bryer et al. (25)	1987	66 female psychiatric inpatients	Single screening question	Current	21
Vize and Cooper (26)	1995	180 psychiatric inpatients and outpatients: 40 with anorexia, 60 with bulimia, 40 with major depression, and 40 comparison subjects	Childhood Experience of Care and Abuse Measure	Current	Anorexia=35; bulimia=25; depressed=25; comparison=8
Gorcey et al. (27)	1986	97 psychiatric outpatients: 41 with and 56 without childhood sexual abuse	Self-report	Current	—
Priber and Dinwiddie (28)	1992	78 psychiatric outpatients: 52 with and 26 without childhood sexual abuse	Set of questions	Lifetime	—
Felitti (29)	1991	231 general medical patients: 131 with and 100 without childhood sexual abuse	One screening question	Chronic	—
Walker et al. (30)	1992	100 patients scheduled for diagnostic laparoscopy	14-question sexual assault instrument	Lifetime	44
McCauley et al. (31)	1997	1,931 women from primary care practices	Single screening question	Current	7.2
Cheasty et al. (32)	1998	1,189 women from general medical practices screened: 132 were depressed; 105 nondepressed subjects were used for comparison	Semistructured interview	Current	37 of the depressed women; 23 of the comparison subjects

[a] Middlesex=Middlesex Hospital Questionnaire. SADS=Schedule for Affective Disorders and Schizophrenia. SADS-L=Schedule for Affective Disorders and Schizophrenia—Lifetime Version. Beck=Beck Depression Inventory. DIS=National Institute of Mental Health Diagnostic Interview Schedule. DIS-3A=National Institute of Mental Health Diagnostic Interview Schedule, version 3A. HSCL=Hopkins Symptom Checklist.

ney and Brooks (21) also used a broad definition of sexual abuse ("some kind of sexual experience with another person while growing up"), yet found a greater likelihood of depressive symptoms in those with past "sexual experiences." In contrast, the most stringent definition of childhood sexual abuse was required in the study by Briere and Runtz (19); these authors found a significant relationship between a history of childhood sexual abuse and a higher rate of chronic depressive symptoms.

Clinical Studies

Nine studies used subjects from clinical settings to examine the relationship between childhood sexual abuse and adult-onset depression. Although rates of reported childhood sexual abuse might have been higher when studying individuals seeking help, all nine investigations found a significant relationship between a history of childhood sexual abuse and adult-onset depression. The features and findings of these studies examining clinical study groups are summarized in table 3.

The only prospective study to investigate the relationship between childhood sexual abuse and adult-onset depression identified and followed a group of girls removed from their homes because of known sexual abuse and compared them with girls separated from their homes (because of disorganization in the home, absence of the mother, physical neglect or abuse) who had not been sexually abused (24). At follow-up, a group of women who were neither separated nor abused as girls was added as another comparison group. As adults, the women with histories of childhood sexual abuse had more depressive symptoms than both comparison groups.

Two studies used groups composed totally, or in part, of psychiatric inpatients. Bryer et al. (25) reviewed consecutively admitted female psychiatric inpatients with a variety of psychiatric diagnoses and found that women with a reported history of abuse (sexual or physical) before age 16 years had significantly more depressive symptoms than did those who did not report abuse. Since over half of those who reported childhood sexual abuse before age 16 years also reported subsequent sexual abuse as adults, revictimization may have played a role in these findings. Vize and Cooper (26) examined the rates of childhood sexual abuse in female inpatients and outpatients with diagnoses of major depressive disorder, anorexia nervosa, and bulimia nervosa compared with normal subjects. They found that there was a significantly greater rate of childhood sexual abuse in the clinical groups than in

Depression Measure[a]	Rate of Depression (%): Subjects With Childhood Sexual Abuse	Rate of Depression (%): Subjects Without Childhood Sexual Abuse	Analysis	Definition of Abuse
Middlesex	—	—	r=0.60, $p<0.01$	Manipulation or interference with unclothed genitals of a female child under age 14, by a closely related male over age 18 living in the same household, more than three times over more than 3 months
Chart review, SCL-90-R	—[b]	—[b]	F=5.77, df=3, 62, $p<0.002$	Positive response to screening question: Before age 16, did (father, mother, brother, sister, friend, acquaintance) ever pressure you into doing more sexually than you wanted to?
SADS-L, Beck	—	—	χ^2=15.1, df=3, $p<0.01$, Yates corrected[c]	Unwanted sexual activity before age 17
Beck	—	—	t test, $p<0.01$	Not defined (all subjects reported abuse before age 14)
Computerized version of DIS	89	57	χ^2=7.88, df=1, $p<0.01$, Yates corrected	Unwanted sexual contact between interviewee and a relative too close to marry
Interview	83	32	χ^2=58.24, df=1, $p<0.001$, Yates corrected	Incest (sexual events between direct relatives or step-relatives) or molestation (sexual events outside the family) or rape (forced sexual events); childhood age not given
DIS-3A	86	36	Odds ratio=10.6, 95% CI=2.2–50.7	Less severe: exhibitionism or aborted attempts before age 14; more severe: incest, rape, oral contact, or repeated fondling before age 14
HSCL	45[d]	26[d]	t=5.7, df=1290, $p<0.001$	Positive response to screening question: Were you ever sexually abused before age 18?
Beck, HSCL, SADS	67	51	χ^2=4.93, df=1, $p<0.03$, Yates corrected	Involvement of child under 16 years old in sexual activity involving contact child did not fully understand, was not in a position to give informed consent for, and was intended to gratify or satisfy the needs of another person

[b] The mean HSCL depression scores were 49.71 (SD=8.72) and 45.04 (SD=9.94) for the subjects with and without childhood sexual abuse, respectively.
[c] Rate of childhood sexual abuse higher in clinical groups than comparison subjects.
[d] High HSCL depression score.

the comparison groups but no difference in rates between the three clinical groups.

Two studies examined childhood sexual abuse in women seeking outpatient treatment. In the first study, a group of women with a history of sexual abuse before age 14 years scored significantly higher on the Beck Depression Inventory than did patients who had not been abused (27). The second study focused specifically on the effects of incest occurring before age 14 years (28). It found that the lifetime incidence of major depression was significantly higher in women who had been victims of incest than in female patients who had not been victims of incest (89% versus 57%).

Study groups of women drawn from general medical practices were used in the remaining four studies. A total of 131 consecutive women outpatients who gave a history of childhood incest, molestation, or rape described themselves as depressed more often than did nonabused comparison subjects (83% versus 32%) (29). In a group of 100 women scheduled for diagnostic laparoscopy, the risk for lifetime diagnosis of major depression was higher for those who gave a history of severe sexual abuse (incest, rape, oral contact, or repeated fondling) than for those with less severe abuse (exhibitionism or aborted attempts) or no abuse (86% versus 36%) (30). A series of patients from four community-based primary care practices composed the largest clinical study group examined (N=1,931) (31). Despite the use of a single screening question to define a history of childhood sexual abuse, those subjects with childhood sexual abuse demonstrated a significantly higher mean score on the depression subscale of the Hopkins Symptom Checklist-90 than did those without childhood sexual abuse. A rigorous screening method was utilized to identify depressed subjects and to define the history of childhood sexual abuse in another large study group drawn from a general medical practice (N=1,189) (32). These investigators considered the history of childhood sexual abuse in women who were depressed versus those who were not depressed and discovered that whereas 37% of the depressed women reported childhood sexual abuse, only 23% of the nondepressed comparison subjects reported childhood sexual abuse.

RELATIONSHIP OF CHILDHOOD SEXUAL ABUSE TO ADULT-ONSET DEPRESSION IN MEN COMPARED WITH WOMEN

A review of the literature identified three studies that provide data on the relationship between childhood abuse and adult-onset depression in men versus women. Only two of these focused specifically on the impact of childhood sexual abuse on adult-onset depression (33, 34), whereas the third defined past abuse as sexual or physical (35).

All three studies found a strong positive correlation between reported childhood abuse and adult-onset depression when the data were analyzed without regard to gender. When the data for each gender were examined independently, one study found no difference in the strength of this relationship between women and men, but 168 women were compared to only 20 men (33). However, results from two studies raised the possibility that this relationship may be greater for women than for men (34, 35). The first of these studies (35) found that female subjects with a history of childhood abuse were more than twice as likely to have depressive symptoms as males with childhood abuse histories (69% versus 27%). The second study, by Stein and colleagues (34), which reanalyzed data from a community study of 3,132 adults (11), excluded those subjects whose first incident of sexual abuse occurred after the age of 16 years. In this study, female victims had a significantly higher lifetime prevalence and current incidence rates of major depressive disorder when compared with female nonvictims, whereas male victims failed to demonstrate significantly higher rates of major depressive disorder when compared with male nonvictims (34).

CHARACTERISTICS OF CHILDHOOD SEXUAL ABUSE AND SUBSEQUENT ADULT-ONSET DEPRESSION

The relationship between a number of characteristics of childhood sexual abuse and its psychological sequelae have been examined in order to establish which aspects of abuse are most deleterious. The data strongly suggest that greater severity, frequency, and duration of abuse results in an increased likelihood of subsequently developing depression (15, 19, 21, 36). For example, Bifulco et al. (12) found the incidence of depression to be 100% in women who suffered forced intercourse, 78% in those with repeated abuse not involving intercourse, and 30% in those with a single episode of abuse not involving intercourse.

While there have been mixed findings regarding the impact of the age at which childhood sexual abuse takes place on the subsequent development of adult-onset depression, the majority of studies have failed to demonstrate a clear relationship (12, 15, 19, 21, 37). Similarly conflicting findings have also emerged regarding the effect of the relationship between the victim and the perpetrator (14, 21, 23, 38). While no consistent pattern has been observed for abuse by a relative versus a nonrelative, a stranger versus an acquaintance, or incest versus nonincest, it has been suggested that father-daughter incest may be more damaging than other sorts of abuse (38, 39).

FACTORS MEDIATING THE RELATIONSHIP BETWEEN CHILDHOOD SEXUAL ABUSE AND MAJOR DEPRESSIVE DISORDER

The evidence just presented suggests that childhood sexual abuse in girls is a risk factor for adult-onset depression in women. We now consider the mechanisms, both psychosocial and neurobiological, by which such early traumatic experiences may result in psychiatric disorders in adulthood.

Psychosocial Factors

It has been suggested that there may be a direct causal relationship between childhood sexual abuse and adult-onset depression. However, it is also possible that other variables, such as poor parenting, may increase the likelihood of both childhood sexual abuse and adult-onset depression. There is a large collection of literature offering theoretical explanations for the connection between childhood sexual abuse and depression (39, 40), but few of these theories are based on empirical data. Areas in which empirical studies have been performed include the effects of parenting, cognitive style, and lifestyle on the long-term consequences of childhood sexual abuse.

Parenting. It has been suggested that poor parenting may either independently increase the risk of both childhood sexual abuse and adult-onset depression or that it may act to increase the likelihood of subsequent depression in children who have been abused (24).

Eight studies have examined the relationship between family dysfunction, childhood sexual abuse, and adult-onset depression (12, 15, 17, 18, 20, 22, 23, 41). Of these, four found a positive correlation between childhood sexual abuse and various markers of familial dysfunction, including early parental separation, family violence, physical punishment, and lack of parental warmth (12, 17, 20, 22). Indeed, evidence suggests a positive correlation between poor parenting and adult-onset depression, even in the absence of childhood sexual abuse (12, 18, 22, 23), and one study found that poor parental support was a better predictor of subsequent impaired psychological functioning than childhood sexual abuse (23). However, in the four studies in which the variables related to family dysfunction or poor parenting were controlled, the relationship between childhood sexual abuse and adult-onset depression was maintained (12, 15, 17, 41). When considering all eight studies together, the weight of evidence suggests that there is a relationship between childhood sexual abuse and adult-onset depression in women, even when controlling for poor parenting as a risk factor for later depression.

Cognition. Gold has pointed out that studies directed at understanding the long-term effects of childhood sexual abuse tend to consider variables surrounding the abuse event and do not address ways in which the cognitive characteristics of the victim, or the victim-environment interaction, might predict outcome (20). Gold stated the hypothesis that a person's "causal attributions and expectancies" are critical in his or her response to the environment and, therefore, in how he or she is affected by a stressful event such as sexual abuse during childhood. Empirical work by Gold showed that attributional style (measured in terms of internal-external, stable-unstable, and global-specific attributions) was related to adult functioning. Specifically, those women who had been sexually abused as children and also had high scores on psychological distress scales (such as the Beck Depression Inventory) tended to have internal, stable, and global attributional styles when confronted with adverse events. However, it is not clear whether these attributional styles preceded the abusive event or resulted from it. These findings generate further questions about the role of predisposing cognitive factors and reflect the difficulty in determining the long-term effects of early abuse by means of retrospective investigation, with all of its associated methodological difficulties (such as recall bias and the problem of distinguishing cause and effect).

Lifestyle. A number of studies have found that women with histories of childhood sexual abuse lead more disadvantaged lives in general, with a greater incidence of teenage marriage, divorce or separation, lower socioeconomic status, and higher rates of various other life stressors than women without abuse histories (12, 14, 17). Although data are not available to show the role of these psychosocial variables in the childhood sexual abuse-adult depression relationship, one might postulate that these life circumstances are mediating factors between childhood sexual abuse and adult-onset depression.

Neurobiological Factors

Neurobiological hypotheses regarding the relationship between childhood stressors and adult-onset depression have generally focused on the HPA axis. Particular emphasis has been placed on the increased levels of corticotropin-releasing hormone (CRH), adrenocorticotropic hormone (ACTH), and corticosteroids seen both following early stress and in patients with depression.

A number of investigators have demonstrated that early stressors may result in both acute and chronic changes in the activity and regulation of the HPA axis, chiefly in the form of hypersecretion of CRH. This has led to the hypothesis that such CRH hypersecretion may create a biological vulnerability to the subsequent development of depression, either directly or by means of an increased sensitivity to stressors in adulthood (42–50).

There are two main lines of evidence supporting this hypothesis. First, the HPA axis is known to be hyperactive in depression, with higher production and secretion of CRH. Second, data from animal and human studies suggest that early stress produces both acute HPA hyperactivity (by means of increases in CRH) and long-term changes in HPA activity, resulting in a differential response to stressors in adulthood. Thus, both the effects of stress and the pathophysiology of depression are associated with similar changes in HPA axis activity.

In addition to providing a possible explanation for the association of stress and depression, both the magnitude and the nature of the stress-induced changes in the HPA axis may differ between the sexes. The mechanism of these differences may be particularly important in understanding the disparity between the genders in both the response to stress and the prevalence of depression. Of special relevance to this review is the increased frequency and impact of one particular early stressor in females—childhood sexual abuse—and how HPA axis dysregulation induced by childhood sexual abuse might provide a biological basis for vulnerability to adult-onset depression in women.

HPA AXIS IN DEPRESSION

Major depressive disorder is associated with hyperactivity of the HPA axis (51). Abnormalities documented in patients with depression include an elevation in urinary free cortisol and basal plasma cortisol and failure to suppress endogenous cortisol secretion in response to dexamethasone administration. In addition, it is likely that there is centrally mediated hypersecretion of CRH in subjects with major depressive disorder. This is reflected in a blunted ACTH response to stimulation with exogenous CRH (51, 52). Further evidence in support of hypersecretion of hypothalamic CRH in patients with major depression includes the findings that increased concentrations of CRH are found in the CSF of depressed subjects (53, 54), that healthy subjects given infusions of CRH display a similar pattern of cortisol hypersecretion to that seen in depressed subjects (51), and that there is a decreased density of CRH-binding sites in the frontal cortex of suicide victims (55). In addition, glucocorticoids stimulate serotonin breakdown, hippocampal serotonergic projections reduce hypothalamic CRH secretion, and compounds with proserotonergic effects (such as selective serotonin reuptake inhibitors and L-tryptophan) have antidepressant activity (56).

Effects of Stress on the HPA Axis

There is considerable experimental evidence that the physiologic response to stress is largely mediated by an increase in CRH production and secretion, resulting in an increased release of ACTH and cortisol (57). These increases are usually transient, but certain acute stressors, when acting on the subject during particular periods in early life, appear to cause chronic hypersecretion of CRH and ACTH, with accompanying adrenal and pituitary hypertrophy. This chronic hyperactivity of the HPA axis following early stress is likely to be mediated, at least in part, by changes in gene expression, as demonstrated by higher CRH mRNA levels in the paraventricular nucleus neurons (58).

It has been theorized that early stress, such as maternal deprivation or childhood sexual abuse, may produce a biological vulnerability to depression that can become manifest in response to adult stress (42, 44). Although few studies address this issue directly, both animal and human data may be helpful in clarifying the neurobiological relationship between early stress and adult-onset depression.

Animal studies. Animal studies have been important in delineating the neuroendocrine response to stress, and some lend support to the notion that the stress response is associated with hypersecretion of CRH (59–61). Although most animal studies have focused on responses to stress in rats at a single point in time, several studies have shown chronic changes in the HPA axis in response to the early stress of mother-infant separation (44, 62–64). Of particular relevance are the following three studies that examined the response of the HPA axis to stress in adults who had been exposed to stress as infants.

A group of adult, nonhuman primates exposed to early stress (rearing by mothers exposed to environmental unpredictability) were found to have elevated concentrations of CRH in their CSF when compared to a group not exposed to early stress (65). These findings suggest long-term hyperactivity of the HPA axis following early stress that persists into adulthood.

Ladd and colleagues hypothesized that early stress could affect CRH neurons in a manner that would neurochemically predispose animals to a particular stress response in adulthood (44). Accordingly, they administered a foot shock to two groups of adult rats—those that had been maternally deprived as pups and those that had not. When the neurochemical responses of these two groups were compared, adult rats that had been maternally deprived had higher basal ACTH concentrations, a greater ACTH response to stress, fewer CRH binding sites in the anterior pituitary, more CRH binding sites in the rapine nucleus, and higher CRH concentrations in the parabrachial nucleus and the median eminence. Similarly, Plotsky and Meaney (66) found elevations in baseline hypothalamic CRH mRNA in adult male rats that had experienced early maternal separation when compared with adult rats that had not. In response to restraint stress, adult rats that had been maternally separated had higher plasma cortisol responses than did comparison animals. These animal data suggest that there are long-term effects of early stress on the neurophysiological status of the HPA axis in male rats and nonhuman primates and that these effects may produce hypersecretion of CRH in response to stress in adulthood. Furthermore, the lasting neurochemical changes seen following early stress appear to be similar to those found in patients with depression.

Human studies. In a study of men and women who had experienced parental loss before age 17 years, Briere et al. (67) assessed the quality of the subjects' home lives following their loss and their adult psychiatric status; measured their resting levels of plasma cortisol, β-endorphin, and ACTH; and performed dexamethasone suppression tests. Those individuals with adult psychopathology had significantly higher levels of plasma cortisol and β-endorphin than did subjects without psychopathology; these plasma levels were inversely correlated with the quality of childhood home life following parental loss. Another group found significantly lower basal and CRH-stimulated ACTH levels in a group of girls aged 7–15 years who had been sexually abused when compared with matched comparison girls who had not (68). The subjects were not depressed at the time of the study, and a mean of 4.7 years had elapsed following the abuse. While there were no group differences in free cortisol levels or CRH cortisol stimulation, it was notable that the decreased ACTH response to CRH stimulation in these girls was similar to the blunted ACTH response to CRH previously demonstrated in adult depressed subjects. In contrast, Kaufman et al. (69) compared depressed prepubertal children with a history of abuse to depressed, nonabused children and normal comparison subjects and found a significantly greater ACTH response to exogenous CRH in those subjects with a history of abuse.

These six studies (44, 65–69) offer preliminary evidence that early stress results in long-term changes in HPA axis function and regulation similar to those believed to be important in the pathophysiology of depression. These similarities lend support to the hypothesis that a significant adverse event during childhood may contribute to depressive illness during adulthood by means of chronic dysregulation of the HPA axis.

Sex Differences in HPA Axis Response to Stress

Considerable human and animal data suggest that the HPA axis is more reactive to stress in females than in males (70–74). These studies examine the effects of sex on the response of the HPA axis to a wide variety of stressors. The study most relevant to this review is that of McCormick et al. (75), who found that female rats exposed to prenatal stress developed greater ACTH and corticosteroid levels in response to restraint as adults, whereas similarly exposed male rats did not.

In considering what might account for the sex differences in the HPA axis response to stress, some groups have examined the possible role of gonadal steroids. It has been demonstrated that castration results in an increase in the adrenal response to stress in adult male rats and hamsters, and estrogen administration in both sexes causes an increase in basal cortisol secretion, accompanied by a greater ACTH and cortisol response to stress (70, 71). Following exposure to exogenous glucocorticoids, male rats have a diminished ACTH response to restraint stress, whereas, by contrast, intact female rats maintain an ACTH response similar to that before glucocorticoid exposure; ovariectomized female rats show an intermediate ACTH response (76). Finally, a direct effect of estrogen on parvocellular hypothalamic CRH cells has been suggested by the localization of estrogen receptor mRNA within these cells (71), and evidence has been found for an estrogen-responsive portion of the promoter region of the CRH gene (77). Thus, these studies suggest that neurochemical changes occurring as a result of childhood stress may be long lasting, may appear to differ between women and men, and may create a greater biological vulnerability to depression in women.

DISCUSSION

There is considerable evidence that childhood sexual abuse has long-term effects. Studies of community, college, and clinical groups of women demonstrate a clear relationship between childhood sexual abuse and adult-onset depression, and this relationship appears to persist even when controlling for other variables that may be independently associated with adult-onset depression. In addition, there is a positive correlation between the severity of sexual abuse in childhood and the incidence of subsequent adult-onset depression. Studies including both men and women have shown less consistent results, but some evidence suggests that women with histories of childhood sexual abuse may be more likely to suffer from depression in adulthood than men who have been victims of childhood sexual abuse.

A small but growing body of evidence from both animal and human studies suggests that a neurobiological mechanism may explain the link between the trauma of childhood sexual abuse and adult-onset depression. The pathophysiological similarities observed in both the stress response and depressive illness, together with the evidence linking the clinical experience of stress and depression, suggest a neurophysiological relationship between the two. Of particular interest here is the chronic dysregulation of the HPA axis sometimes induced by early stress, as well as the apparent sexual dimorphism in the HPA axis response to stress. Such dimorphism may produce sex differences in the neurobiological response to stress and perhaps, therefore, in the incidence of depression.

We suggest that gonadal steroids have some role in the modulation of the HPA axis and thus may be important in the higher sensitivity of the HPA axis to stress in females. In apparent contrast, other work has shown that the use of estrogen as augmentation to serotonin-promoting drugs results in a therapeutic effect on mood symptoms (78). These two findings may not be incompatible, since gonadal steroids may play a role in early sensitization to extreme stress and thereby increase the possibility of a stress-induced mood syndrome. At the same time, estrogen may be important in the regulation of mood by means of other mechanisms outside the stress-related pathways. In addition, recent preclinical evidence suggests that stress can elevate gonadal steroids and estrogen, which may be protective when it occurs in moderation but lead to dysfunction when exaggerated (79). Moreover, it is clear that the etiology and pathophysiology of depression are complex, and there exist a number of critical factors beyond the scope of this article. Those most relevant here include the neuroendocrinologic interactions between estrogen and serotonin (80), cultural responses (which may lead victimized women toward depression and victimized men toward alcoholism) (81), and hereditary factors (7) (some of which have been hypothesized to be associated with abnormalities in the serotonin system passed from abusive alcoholic fathers to their daughters who develop depression [82]).

While the focus of this review is on the relationship of childhood sexual abuse to adult-onset depression, some studies report on the impact of childhood sexual abuse with regard to the subsequent development of other psychiatric conditions. For example, there is evidence that a number of psychiatric disorders may be higher in populations of women who have been sexually abused in childhood (25). Bulimia nervosa (13), panic disorder with agoraphobia (83), generalized anxiety disorder (84), somatization disorder (84), and borderline personality disorder (85) have each been found not only to be associated with childhood sexual abuse but to be more prevalent in women than in men (DSM-IV). Although Wexler et al. (86) found a specific association between childhood abuse and adult-onset depression as compared with other disorders, it is important to recognize that while depression may be the most common negative long-term effect of early sexual abuse, it is not the only possible negative outcome.

Additionally, it is possible that other severe early traumas may increase the risk for adult-onset depression or other psychiatric syndromes. We have focused on childhood sexual abuse in this review since it is the form of childhood trauma that has been investigated far more than any other. Other types of childhood trauma examined include parental loss (67), poor parenting (87), parental drinking, family violence, and parental mental illness (88).

The studies reviewed here only begin to shed light on questions about why some abused girls and not others develop a depressive illness later in life. Investigations have begun to consider the type of sexual abuse encountered, the environmental factors that accompany abuse (such as parenting), and attributional styles. However, these variables need further study, as do predictors of depression that may have existed before the abuse, such as genetic loading and temperament. In addition, particular attention to self-concept, core beliefs, and coping style would be useful, as recent literature suggests that these may play a role in mediating the onset of adult disorders after exposure to early adversity (89, 90). It is possible that there are victims who were already more vulnerable to injury or less able to adapt in the face of an early trauma. Further research needs to be conducted to understand the nature of this relationship. Such research should include studies of the mediating factors between childhood sexual abuse and adult-onset depression and, in particular, the effects of sex on stress-induced dysregulation of the HPA axis.

REFERENCES

1. Weissman MM, Bruce ML, Leaf PJ, Florio LP, Holzer C: Affective disorders, in Psychiatric Disorders in America: The Epidemiological Catchment Area Study. Edited by Robins LN, Regier DA. New York, Free Press, 1991, pp 53–80
2. Freud S. Mourning and melancholia (1917 [1915]), in Complete Psychological Works, standard ed, vol 14. London, Hogarth Press, 1957, pp 243–258
3. Beck A: Cognitive therapy of depression: new perspectives, in Treatment of Depression: Old Controversies and New Approaches. Edited by Clayton PJ, Barrett JE. New York, Raven Press, 1983, pp 265–290
4. Beck AT: Cognitive models of depression. J Cognitive Psychotherapy 1987; 1:5–37
5. Brown GW, Harris T: Social Origins of Depression: A Study of Psychiatric Disorder in Women. New York, Free Press, 1978
6. Shrout PE, Link BG, Dohrenwend BP, Skodol AK, Stueve A, Mirotznik J: Characterizing life events as risk factors for depression: the role of fateful loss events. J Abnorm Psychol 1989; 95:460–467
7. Kendler KS, Kessler RC, Neale MC, Heath AC, Eaves LJ: The prediction of major depression in women: toward an integrated etiologic model. Am J Psychiatry 1993; 150:1139–1148
8. Mazure CM: Life stressors as risk factors in depression. Clin Psychol Science and Practice 1998; 5:291–313
9. Finkelhor K: The sexual abuse of children: current research reviewed. Psychiatr Annals 1987; 17:233–241
10. Silverman AB, Reinherz HZ, Giaconia RM: The long-term sequelae of child and adolescent abuse: a longitudinal community study. Child Abuse Negl 1996; 20:709–723
11. Burnam MA, Stein JA, Golding JM, Siegel JM, Sorenson SB, Forsythe AB, Telles CA: Sexual assault and mental disorders in a community population. J Consult Clin Psychol 1988; 56: 443–450
12. Bifulco A, Brown GW, Adler Z: Early sexual abuse and clinical depression in adult life. Br J Psychiatry 1991; 159:115–122
13. Andrews B, Valentine R, Valentine JD: Depression and eating disorders following abuse in childhood in two generations of women. Br J Clin Psychol 1995; 34:37–52
14. Mullen PE, Romans-Clarkson SE, Walton VA, Herbison GP: Impact of sexual and physical abuse on women's mental health. Lancet 1988; 1:841–845
15. Mullen PE, Martin JL, Anderson JC, Romans SE, Herbison GP: Childhood sexual abuse and mental health in adult life. Br J Psychiatry 1993; 163:721–732
16. Bushnell JA, Wells JE, Oakley-Brown MA: Long-term effects of intrafamilial sexual abuse in childhood. Acta Psychiatr Scand 1992; 85:136–142
17. Bagley C, Ramsey R: Sexual abuse in childhood: psychosocial outcomes and implications for social work practice. J Social Work and Human Sexuality 1985: 4:33–48
18. Peters SD: Child sexual abuse and later psychological problems, in Lasting Effects of Child Abuse. Edited by Wyatt GE, Powell GJ. Beverly Hills, Calif, Sage Publications, 1988, pp 101–117
19. Briere J, Runtz M: Symptomatology associated with childhood sexual victimization in a nonclinical adult sample. Child Abuse Negl 1988; 12:51–59
20. Gold ER: Long-term effects of sexual victimization in childhood: an attributional approach. J Consult Clin Psychol 1986; 54:471–475
21. Sedney MA, Brooks B: Factors associated with a history of childhood sexual experience in a nonclinical female population. J Am Acad Child Adolesc Psychiatry 1984; 23:215–218
22. Yama MF, Tovey SL, Fogas BS: Childhood family environment and sexual abuse as predictors of anxiety and depression in adult women. Am J Orthopsychiatry 1993; 63:136–141
23. Fromuth ME: The relationship of childhood sexual abuse with later psychological and sexual adjustment in a sample of college women. Child Abuse Negl 1986; 10:5–15
24. Bagley C, McDonald M: Adult mental health sequels of child sexual abuse, physical abuse and neglect in maternally separated children. Can J Community Ment Health 1984; 3:15–26
25. Bryer JB, Nelson BA, Miller JB, Krol PA: Childhood sexual and physical abuse as factors in adult psychiatric illness. Am J Psychiatry 1987; 144:1426–1430
26. Vize CM, Cooper PJ: Sexual abuse in patients with eating disorders, patients with depression and normal controls: a comparative study. Br J Psychiatry 1995; 167:80–85
27. Gorcey M, Santiago JM, McCall-Perez F: Psychological consequences for women sexually abused in childhood. Soc Psychiatry 1986; 21:129–133
28. Pribor EF, Dinwiddie SH: Psychiatric correlates of incest in childhood. Am J Psychiatry 1992; 149:52–56
29. Felitti VJ: Long-term medical consequences of incest, rape and molestation. South Med J 1991; 84:328–331
30. Walker EA, Katon WJ, Hansom J, Harrop-Griffiths J, Holm L, Jones ML, Hickok L, Jemelka RP: Medical and psychiatric symptoms in women with childhood sexual abuse. Psychosom Med 1992; 54:658–664
31. McCauley J, Kern DE, Kolodner K, Dill L, Schroeder AF, DeChant HK, Ryden J, Derogatis LR, Bass EB: Clinical characteristics of women with a history of childhood abuse. JAMA 1997; 277:1362–1368
32. Cheasty M, Clare AW, Collins C: Relation between sexual abuse in childhood and adult depression: case control study. BMJ 1998; 316:198–201
33. Roesler TA, McKenzie N: Effects of childhood trauma on psychological functioning in adults sexually abused as children. J Nerv Ment Dis 1994; 182:145–150
34. Stein JA, Golding JM, Seigel JM, Burnam MA, Sorenson SB: Longterm psychological sequelae of child sexual abuse, in Lasting Effects of Child Abuse Edited by Wyatt GE, Powell GJ. Beverly Hills, Calif, Sage Publications, 1988, pp 135–154
35. Carmen E(H), Rieker PP, Mills T: Victims of violence and psychiatric illness. Am J Psychiatry 1984; 141:378–383
36. Murphy SM, Kilpatrick DG, Amick-McMullan A, Veronen LJ, Paduhovich J, Best CL, Villeponteaux LA, Saunders BE: Current psychological functioning of child sexual assault survivors: a community study. J Interpersonal Violence 1988; 3: 55–79
37. Browne A, Finkelhor D: Impact of child sexual abuse: a review of the research. Psychol Bull 1986; 99:66–77
38. Tsai M, Feldman-Summers S, Edgar M: Childhood molestation: variables related to differential impacts on psychosexual functioning in adult women. J Abnorm Psychol 1979; 88:407–417
39. Bowlby J: Maternal Care and Mental Health. Geneva, World Health Organization, 1951
40. Breuer J, Freud S: Studies on Hysteria (1895 [1893–1895]): Complete Psychological Works. standard ed, vol 2. London, Hogarth Press, 1955
41. Fergusson DM, Horwood LJ, Lyndkey MT: Child sexual abuse and psychiatric disorder in young adulthood, II: psychiatric outcomes of childhood sexual abuse. J Am Acad Child Adolesc Psychiatry 1996; 35:1365–1374
42. Nemeroff CB: The corticotropin-releasing factor (CRF) hypothesis of depression: new findings and new directions. Mol Psychiatry 1996; 1:336–342
43. Heit S, Owens MJ, Plotsky P, Nemeroff CB: Corticotropin-releasing factor, stress, and depression. Neuroscientist 1997; 3: 186–194
44. Ladd CO, Owens MJ, Nemeroff CB: Persistent changes in corticotropin-releasing factor neuronal systems induced by maternal deprivation. Endocrinology 1996; 137:1212–1218

45. Romero LM, Sapolsky RM: Patterns of ACTH secretagog secretion in response to psychological stimuli. J Neuroendocrinol 1996; 8:243–258
46. Sapolsky RM: Why stress is bad for your brain. Science 1996; 276:749–750
47. Sapolsky RM: The physiological relevance of glucocorticoid endangerment of the hippocampus. Ann NY Acad Sci 1994; 746:294–304
48. Liu D, Diorio J, Tannenbaum B, Caldji C, Francis D, Freedman A, Sharma S, Pearson D, Plotsky PM, Meaney MJ: Maternal care, hippocampal glucocorticoid receptors and hypothalamic-pituitary-adrenal responses to stress. Science 1997; 277:1659–1662
49. Heinrichs SC, Stenzel-Poore MP, Gold LH, Battenberg E, Bloom FE, Koob GF, Vale WW, Pich EM: Learning impairment in transgenic mice with central overexpression of corticotropin-releasing factor. Neuroscience 1996; 74:303–311
50. Sapolsky RM: The importance of a well-groomed child. Science 1997; 277:1620–1621
51. Gold PW, Goodwin FK, Chrousos GP: Clinical and biochemical manifestations of depression in relation to the neurobiology of stress. N Engl J Med 1988; 319:413–420
52. Lesch M, Laux G, Schulte HM, Pfuller H, Beckmann H: Corticotropin and cortisol response to human CRH as a probe for HPA system integrity in major depressive disorder. Psychiatry Res 1988; 24:25–34
53. Nemeroff CB, Widerlov E, Bissette G, Walleus H, Karlsson I, Eklund K, Kilts C, Loosen PT, Vale W: Elevated concentrations of CSF corticotropin-releasing factor-like immunoreactivity in depressed patients. Science 1984; 226:1342–1344
54. Owens MJ, Plotsky PM, Nemeroff CB: Peptides and affective disorders, in Biology of Schizophrenia and Affective Disease. Edited by Watson SJ. Washington, DC, American Psychiatric Press, 1996, pp 259–293
55. Nemeroff CB, Owens MJ, Bissette G, Andorn AC, Stanley M: Reduced corticotropin releasing factor binding sites in the frontal cortex of suicide victims. Arch Gen Psychiatry 1988; 45:577–579
56. Maes M, Meltzer HY: The serotonin hypothesis of major depression, in Psychopharmacology: The Fourth Generation of Progress. Edited by Bloom FE, Kupfer DJ. New York, Raven Press, 1995, pp 933–944
57. Stratakis CA, Chrousos GP: Neuroendocrinology and pathophysiology of the stress system. Ann NY Acad Sci 1995; 771:1–18
58. Herman JP, Adams D, Prewitt C: Regulatory changes in neuroendocrine stress-integrative circuitry produced by a variable stress paradigm. Neuroendocrinology 1995; 61:180–190
59. Chappell PB, Smith MA, Kilts CD, Bissette G, Ritchie J, Anderson C, Nemeroff CB: Alterations in corticotropin-releasing factor-like immunoreactivity in discrete rat brain regions after acute and chronic stress. J Neurosci 1986; 6:2908–2914
60. Fuchs E, Flugge G: Modulation of binding sites for corticotropin-releasing hormone by chronic psychosocial stress. Psychoneuroendocrinology 1995; 20:33–51
61. Swiergiel AH, Takahashi LK, Kalin NH: Attenuation of stress-induced behavior by antagonism of corticotropin-releasing factor receptors in the central amygdala in the rat. Brain Res 1993; 623:229–234
62. Levine S, Huchton DM, Wiener SG, Rosenfeld P: Time course of the effect of maternal deprivation on the hypothalamic-pituitary-adrenal axis in the infant rat. Dev Psychobiol 1992; 24:547–558
63. Kuhn CM, Pauk J, Schanberg SM: Endocrine responses to mother-infant separation in developing rats. Dev Psychobiol 1990; 23:395–410
64. Stanton ME, Gutierrez YR, Levine S: Maternal deprivation potentiates pituitary-adrenal stress responses in infant rats. Behav Neurosci 1988; 102:692–700
65. Coplan JD, Andrews MW, Rosenblum LA, Owens MJ, Friedman S, Gorman JM, Nemeroff CB: Persistent elevations of cerebrospinal fluid concentrations of corticotropin-releasing factor in adult nonhuman primates exposed to early-life stressors: implications for the pathophysiology of mood and anxiety disorders. Proc Natl Acad Sci USA 1996; 93:1619–1623
66. Plotsky PM, Meaney MJ: Early postnatal experience alters hypothalamic corticotropin-releasing factor (CRF) mRNA, median eminence CRF content and stress-induced release in adult rats. Brain Res Mol Brain Res 1993; 18:195–200
67. Briere A, Kelsoe JR, Kirwin PD, Beller SA, Wolkowitz OM, Pickar D: Early parental loss and development of adult psychopathology. Arch Gen Psychiatry 1988; 45:987–993
68. De Bellis MD, Chrousos GP, Dorn LD, Burke L, Helmers K, Kling MA, Trickett PK, Putnam FW: Hypothalamic-pituitary-adrenal axis dysregulation in sexually abused girls. J Clin Endocrinol Metab 1994; 78:249–255
69. Kaufman J, Birmaher B, Perel J, Dahl RE, Moreci P, Telson B, Weiss W, Ryan ND: The corticotrophin-releasing hormone challenge in depressed abused, depressed nonabused, and normal control children. Biol Psychiatry 1997; 20:669–679
70. Ogilvie KM, Riview C: Gender difference in alcohol-evoked hypothalamic-pituitary-adrenal activity in the rat: ontogeny and role of neonatal steroids. Alcohol Clin Exp Res 1996; 20:255–261
71. Handa RJ, Burgess LH, Kerr JE, O'Keefe JA: Gonadal steroid hormone receptors and sex differences in the hypothalamo-pituitary-adrenal axis. Horm Behav 1994; 28:464–476
72. Kant GJ, Lenox RH, Bunnell BN, Mougey EH, Pennington LL, Meyerhoff JL: Comparison of stress response in male and female rats: pituitary cyclic AMP and plasma prolactin, growth hormone and corticosterone. Psychoneuroendocrinology 1983; 8:421–428
73. Spinedi E, Salas M, Chisari A, Perone M, Carino M, Gaillard RC: Sex differences in the hypothalamo-pituitary-adrenal axis response to inflammatory and neuroendocrine stressors. Neuroendocrinology 1994; 60:609–617
74. Greenspan SL, Rowe JW, Maitland LA, McAloon-Dyke M, Elahi D: The pituitary-adrenal glucocorticoid response is altered by gender and disease. J Gerontol 1993; 48:M72–M77
75. McCormick CM, Smythe JW, Sharma S, Meaney MJ: Sex-specific effects of prenatal stress on hypothalamic-pituitary-adrenal responses to stress and brain glucocorticoid receptor density in adult rats. Brain Res Dev Brain Res 1995; 84:55–61
76. Young EA: Sex differences in response to exogenous corticosterone: a rat model of hypercortisolemia. Mol Psychiatry 1996; 1:313–319
77. Vamvakopoulos NC, Charousos GP: Evidence of direct estrogenic regulation of human corticotropin-releasing hormone gene expression. J Clin Invest 1993; 92:1896–1902
78. Schneider LS, Small GW, Hamilton SH, Bystritsky A, Nemeroff CB, Meyers BS, Fluoxetine Collaborative Study Group: Estrogen replacement and response to fluoxetine in a multicenter geriatric depression trial. Am J Geriatr Psychiatry 1997; 5:97–106
79. Shors TJ: Stress and sex effects on associative learning: for better or for worse. Neuroscientist 1998; 4:353–364
80. Halbreich U, Lumley LA: The multiple interactional biological processes that might lead to depression and gender differences in its appearance. J Affect Disord 1993; 29:159–173
81. Holmes SJ, Robins LN: The role of parental disciplinary practices in the development of depression and alcoholism. Psychiatry 1988; 51:24–36
82. Jarmas AL, Kazak AE: Young adult children of alcoholic fathers: depressive experiences, coping styles, and family systems. J Consult Clin Psychol 1992; 60:244–251
83. Stein MB, Walker JR, Anderson G, Hazen AL, Ross CA, Eldridge G, Forde DR: Childhood physical and sexual abuse in patients with anxiety disorders and in a community sample. Am J Psychiatry 1996; 153:275–277
84. Poregijs PJ, Jeuken FM, van der Horst FG, Kraan HF, Knottnerus JA: A troubled youth: relations with somatization, depression and anxiety in adulthood. Fam Pract 1996; 13:1–11
85. Zanarini MC, Williams AA, Lewis RE, Reich RB, Vera SC, Marino MF, Levin A, Yong L, Frankenburg FR: Reported pathological childhood experiences associated with the devel-

opment of borderline personality disorder. Am J Psychiatry 1997; 154:1101–1106
86. Wexler BE, Lyons L, Lyons H, Mazure CM: Physical and sexual abuse during childhood and development of psychiatric illness during adulthood. J Nerv Ment Dis 1997; 185:522–524
87. Oakley-Browne MA, Joyce PR, Wells JE, Bushnell JA, Hornblow AR: Adverse parenting and other childhood experiences as risk factors for depression in women aged 18–44 years. J Affect Disord 1995; 34:13–23
88. Kessler RC, Magee WJ: Childhood adversities and adult depression: basic patterns of association in a US national survey. Psychol Med 1993; 23:679–690
89. Mannarino AP, Cohen JA, Berman SR: The relationship between preabuse factors and psychological symptomatology in sexually abused girls. Child Abuse Negl 1994; 18:63–71
90. Wyatt GE, Newcomb M: Internal and external mediators of women's sexual abuse in childhood. J Consult Clin Psychol 1990; 58:758–767

NEWS AND VIEWS

Is Depression an Adaptation?

Randolph M. Nesse, MD

Many functions have been suggested for low mood or depression, including communicating a need for help, signaling yielding in a hierarchy conflict, fostering disengagement from commitments to unreachable goals, and regulating patterns of investment. A more comprehensive evolutionary explanation may emerge from attempts to identify how the characteristics of low mood increase an organism's ability to cope with the adaptive challenges characteristic of unpropitious situations in which effort to pursue a major goal will likely result in danger, loss, bodily damage, or wasted effort. In such situations, pessimism and lack of motivation may give a fitness advantage by inhibiting certain actions, especially futile or dangerous challenges to dominant figures, actions in the absence of a crucial resource or a viable plan, efforts that would damage the body, and actions that would disrupt a currently unsatisfactory major life enterprise when it might recover or the alternative is likely to be even worse. These hypotheses are consistent with considerable evidence and suggest specific tests.

Arch Gen Psychiatry. 2000;57:14-20

Pain or suffering of any kind, if long continued, causes depression and lessens the power of action; yet it is well adapted to make a creature guard itself against any great or sudden evil.
The Life and Letters of Charles Darwin,
Charles Darwin, 1887

Some manifestations of disease arise directly from a defect in the body's machinery while others are defenses or dysregulations of defenses.[1,2] Manifestations of disease that arise directly from defects, such as jaundice or seizures, have no utility. However, defenses such as pain or diarrhea are adaptations shaped by natural selection. Dysregulated or extreme defenses cause many diseases, such as chronic pain or dehydration from diarrhea. Distinguishing manifestations of disease that arise from these 3 causes is important. Correcting a defect is almost always useful, but blocking a defense can be harmful. For instance, drug treatment of *Shigella*-induced diarrhea often causes complications.[3] Searching for the cause of a defect starts with the defect itself, but the cause of a defense, such as cough, is sought in the abnormality that arouses it, not in its mediating mechanisms.

Is depression an adaptation, an adaptation gone awry, or a pathological state unrelated to any function? Opinions range from dismissal of the possibility that depression or low mood could be useful to the conviction that even severe depression is an adaptation with a specific function.[4] These opinions have important practical consequences. Patients who believe that depression is normal may refuse drug treatment for fear of "covering up the real problem," while those who believe depression is purely a product of brain pathology may be reluctant to examine how their relationships may contribute to their symptoms. Clinicians who believe depression is an adaptation may spend years trying to help a patient understand its significance, while other clinicians actively discourage such inquiry. The physiological changes associated with depression are assumed to be defects by many researchers, while others see them as merely reflecting the activity of mood regulation mechanisms. Despite huge advances in our ability to treat depression and growing rec-

From the Department of Psychiatry, University of Michigan, Ann Arbor.

ognition that it is often a medical disease resulting from multiple pathways,[5] fundamental disagreements continue about its adaptive significance.

Terminology is inconsistent in this area. Those who see depression as intrinsically pathological tend to reserve the word for severe states that are mostly unrelated to ordinary mood variation, while those who see it as a defense use the same word to cover a wide range of normal and abnormal states. In this article, *depression* will refer to severe states of negative affect that are often but not necessarily pathological, and *low mood* will refer to states in the common range of normal experience. Low mood and depression have been difficult to distinguish from each other and from related states such as sadness, grief, demoralization, guilt, and boredom. This difficulty may reflect the nature of the organism. Natural selection may have gradually and partially differentiated a generic state of inhibition into subtypes specialized to cope with particular kinds of situations. Sadness, depression, guilt, and grief may be partially differentiated members of a "fuzzy set"[6,7] whose commonalities are explained partially by phylogeny and partially by the benefits certain responses offer in any unpropitious situation.

Many people believe that low mood is normal and probably useful in certain situations, but when excessive, prolonged, or expressed in the wrong situation, it becomes pathological depression. This plausible starting position gives rise to several questions: In what situations is low mood useful? How does it give a selective advantage? At what level of severity does low mood become pathological depression? Is some depression unrelated to low mood? Firm answers to these questions will not be possible until we better understand the evolutionary origins and functions of low mood. These questions about why the capacity for mood exists at all are separate and distinct from proximate questions about the psychological and brain mechanisms that cause low mood, and from the question of why people differ in their vulnerability to low mood or depression.

GLOBAL EVIDENCE

The match between the eye's complex form and its function demonstrates that it is an adaptation, while seizures are obviously a defect. Do the global characteristics of low mood or depression give clues to their adaptive significance? Depression is painful and interferes with normal function, so it seems obviously maladaptive. However, other useful capacities, such as pain, nausea, and fatigue, are also aversive and disruptive. In fact, their very aversiveness is likely a product of natural selection, probably because they promote escape and avoidance of situations that decrease fitness. From this perspective, the intrinsic aversiveness of most low mood and depression suggests that they may be related to a defense.

The epidemiology of mood disorders offers other clues. If depression were rare, like schizophrenia, and had symptoms unrelated to the experiences of most people, this would suggest it was a disease unrelated to any defense. In fact, major depressive disorder affects about 10% of the US population in a year.[8] Depressive syndromes that do not meet diagnostic criteria are even more common.[9,10] Furthermore, there is no point of rarity in the distribution that can differentiate pathologic from nonpathologic depression,[11] and subjects move frequently between syndromal and subthreshold depression over time.[12-14] Also, the incidence of depression is highest at the ages where reproductive value peaks, a pattern characteristic of few diseases.

Defenses are regulated by cues associated with situations in which they are useful; defects are not.[15-17] The regularity of the relationship between loss and negative affect and the proportionality of low mood to the magnitude of a loss[18,19] imply that mood is regulated. However, the relationship of depression to events is less consistent. While about 80% of first episodes in women are preceded by a severe life event,[18,20] only about one sixth of previously well women develop a depression after a severe life event.[21] For third and subsequent episodes of endogenous depression, onset is unrelated to life events,[22] suggesting that many depressive episodes are not defenses.

The global evidence undermines the idea that low mood and depression are defects unrelated to a defense but is insufficient to support any firm conclusion about their adaptive significance. Just as for most other traits, any conclusion about their utility requires consideration of specific hypotheses about how they could have offered a selective advantage.

POSSIBLE FUNCTIONS OF LOW MOOD AND DEPRESSION

Signaling benefits of several kinds have been attributed to low mood or depression.[23] An infant's crying motivates its mother to help, an essential mechanism shaped by kin selection.[24,25] While crying makes a strong link to adult depression, it is less clear that states of passive withdrawal benefit infants.[26] Lewis[27] suggested that depression in adults is a plea for help. This view remains prevalent, but the evidence is mixed. The capacity to arouse pity in others may be helpful, but there are few data to support this. However, reactions to patients with chronic depression are mainly negative.[28] Depression has also been interpreted as a communication designed to manipulate others into providing resources.[29,30] Following Lewis[27] and Meyer,[31] and citing studies of infants, Klerman concluded: "depression is clearly adaptive, especially for infant primates, including man,"[32(p135)] but, "My current view is that the adult depressive episode represents an attempt at adaptation that has failed,"[32(p143)] presumably because help was not forthcoming.

Engel and Schmale[33,34] used the phrase *conservation-withdrawal* to refer to the presumed utility of the "despair" phase of the behavior pattern of a lost infant monkey. Depression in adults after a loss has been interpreted as analogous to this pattern of infant behavior, and many authors,[35] including Beck,[36] emphasize a role for depression in conserving resources. However, unlike hibernation, depression is rarely a state of calm conservation, does not affect all individuals in a group synchronously, and, with the possible exception of seasonal depression,[37] is not usually corrected by the mere passage of time. While conserving energy during bad times is sensible, depression seems poorly designed for this purpose.

Bowlby[38] emphasized the value of attachment and of aversive feelings when an attachment is threatened or lost. He and his followers have generally treated grief and depression in adults as an epiphenomenon of attachment.[39] However, it remains to be determined whether grief is merely a design constraint or an adaptation in its own right.[40]

Price and others[41,42] have suggested the utility of depression as a yielding signal in hierarchy conflicts. Basing their theory on animal models, they recognized that many of their patients with depression were unwilling to yield to a more powerful adversary. If they did finally yield, this signaled to the dominant figure that the person was no longer a threat, ended the conflict, and resolved the depression.[43] This theory suggests a possible role for high as well as low mood in negotiating hierarchies[44] and is supported by clinical evidence of episodes of depression precipitated by social competition and resolved by reconciliation.[20,45] Hartung[46] has suggested a variation in which self-deception about one's abilities ("deceiving down") lulls superiors into thinking one is no threat.

Clinicians have long noted that depression is common in people who are pursuing unreachable goals.[47,48] "Failure to yield" may be an example, in the status competition domain, of this more general situation. When current life plans are not working, the distress and lack of motivation that characterize depression may motivate planning and reassessment[49] or escape, even by suicide.[50] Hamburg summarized possible functions of depression, saying,

> [when] the subject estimates the probability of effective action is low . . . the depressive responses can be viewed as adaptive. . . . Feelings of sadness and discouragement may be a useful stimulus to consider ways of changing [the] situation. . . . Moreover, [the] state of sadness may elicit heightened interest and sympathetic consideration on the part of significant other people.[51(p240)]

The helplessness literature takes a related view but emphasizes the frequency and costs of incorrect perceptions of lack of control instead of the benefits of a passive strategy.[52-54] Tiger[55] offers an explicitly evolutionary view of optimism.

The role of depression in disengaging motivation from an unreachable goal was specified more explicitly in the incentive-disengagement theory of Klinger.[56,57] If a commitment to pursue a goal encounters an obstacle, efforts increase and become aggressive. If the obstacle cannot be overcome, low mood helps to disengage the commitment and end the cycle. If the individual cannot disengage, low mood escalates. Klinger concludes, "depression is ordinarily, therefore, a normal, adaptive part of disengaging oneself from an incentive."[56(p21)] Many other researchers also see a close relationship between depression and difficulty in disengaging from major commitments.[58,59]

This position has been elaborated in the framework of control theory, which suggests that low mood motivates consideration of alternative strategies when the distance from the goal is being reduced more slowly than anticipated.[60-62] Several related theories have led to evidence that low mood is aroused by a mismatch between achievements and expectations.[45,63-65] Closely related is work on the information functions of mood.[64] Low mood shifts cognition to the more systematic[66] and perhaps the more realistic.[67,68] Many studies support the relationship of goal pursuit to low mood,[69] but few have addressed clinical depression.

My previous attempts to explain mood have emphasized the benefits of regulating investment strategies as a function of changes in anticipated levels of payoffs.[70-72] In a propitious situation, organisms gain by upregulating effort and risk taking. In an unpropitious situation, downregulation of effort and risk taking is adaptive. Mood thus regulates the allocation of effort and resources—toward enterprises, strategies, and times likely to give a high payoff and away from unprofitable enterprises and times when efforts will likely be wasted or dangerous. As Wender and Klein put it,

> . . . biologically based self-esteem—and mood in general—seems to us to have evolutionary utility . . . If one is subject to a series of defeats, it pays to adopt a conservative game plan of sitting back and waiting and letting others take the risks. Such waiting would be fostered by a pessimistic outlook. Similarly if one is raking in the chips of life, it pays to adopt an expansive risk taking approach, and thus maximize access to scarce resources.[73(p204)]

IN WHAT SITUATIONS IS LOW MOOD USEFUL?

Most attempts to explain low mood have been formulated in terms of specific functions, especially communication, motivation, and regulation of effort. However, a single emotional state may serve several different functions, and different emotions have functions in common. Emotions differ from one another not because they have different functions, but because they were shaped to cope with different situations.[64,70,74-78] After all, the global function of an emotion or affect is to create a special state in an organism that allows it to cope effectively with the adaptive challenges characteristic of some situation that has recurred and influenced fitness over the course of many generations. Thus, the crucial question about low mood is not its function but in what situations its various characteristics offers fitness advantages.

The characteristics of low mood and the situations that arouse it offer clues to when and how it has been useful. Decreased motivation and activity would obviously be useful mainly in situations in which action would be futile or dangerous. Organisms carefully regulate when and where they exert effort; foraging theory offers robust predictions for one such kind of effort.[79,80] As the food in a patch is depleted, organisms give up on that patch at close to the optimal time, namely, when the rate of return in the current patch declines below the average rate of return over all patches. If the overall rate of return from all patches drops below the cost, foraging stops. When the snow is deep and the temperature is low, foraging may cost a deer more energy per hour than it can gain, so its best option, even if it is starving, is to stand still and wait.[35]

Human behavior is far more complex and is organized around the pursuit of personal goals. In recent years, psychologists have increasingly viewed emotions as arising from an individual's appraisal of how an event will influence goal attainment.[75,81,82] An enormous body of literature now describes the role of affect in regulating goal pursuit,[65,66,83-85] but little of this work has made its way into psychiatry and even less is grounded in evolutionary biology. Specific emotions have been matched to particular situations,[6] and control theorists have documented how emotions are influenced by success or failure in the pursuit of goals.[69] Situations that regularly arise in the pursuit of goals arouse special states ("mind sets") to deal with them effectively.[86] Failing to reach a goal is an especially potent elicitor of negative affect.[56,59] There is considerable agreement that low mood helps to disengage individuals from unproductive efforts.

ARE THE CORE ASPECTS OF DEPRESSION EVER USEFUL?

It is easy to see how lack of motivation for one activity could free effort for something more productive, but depression is characterized by a more pervasive pessimism, low self-esteem, and reduced initiative. These characteristics pose the core conundrum of depression. They are the exact opposite of the optimism, energy, and a willingness to make changes that would help a person get out of a bad situation. However, there are situations in which active efforts just make things worse. One, well described by Price,[41] is when challenging a dominant figure starts fights that cannot be won. In this situation, it is far better to inhibit striving and signal submission and a wish for reconciliation.[87] Another situation is the failure of a major life enterprise. The pursuit of large goals requires constructing expensive social enterprises that are difficult to replace—marriages, friendships, careers, reputation, status, and group memberships. Major setbacks in these enterprises precipitate life crises. In such situations, it is often useful to inhibit any tendency to shift quickly to a different endeavor. The start-up costs for a new enterprise are huge, there is often no certainty that another enterprise can be found at all, and the attractiveness of alternatives may be illusory. Hastily giving up on an unsatisfying marriage or job often takes a person out of the frying pan and into the fire. In this situation, pessimism, lack of energy, low self-esteem, lack of initiative, and fearfulness can prevent calamity even while they perpetuate misery. There are also many other kinds of unpropitious situations, such as lacking a viable life plan or some crucial resource or being so stressed that striving would cause bodily damage. Just as anxiety inhibits dangerous actions, depression inhibits futile efforts.

This seems to contradict the idea that depression facilitates disengagement from unreachable incentives. Which is it? Does depression foster giving up and moving on when efforts to reach a goal are not working, or does it motivate persisting despite little likelihood of success? This apparent contradiction arises from trying to frame the explanation in terms of one function. When depression is instead seen as a state shaped to cope with unpropitious situations, it is clear how it could be useful, both to decrease investment in the current unsatisfying life enterprise and also to prevent the premature pursuit of alternatives. Failure to disengage can cause depression, and depression can make it harder to disengage. This may explain why the low-mood system is so prone to getting stuck in positive feedback loops.[88-91] Mood dysregulation may now be so prevalent because we are bereft of kin, beliefs, and rituals that routinely extracted our ancestors from such cycles.[92] Also, the costs of low mood may be small compared with those of inappropriate high mood, so in certain situations the "smoke detector principle" biases the system toward low mood.[1]

Usually, the dilemma is resolved by changing or accepting the current situation or by moving on. When it is not, serious pathology may arise. The argument in this article has so far been presented in the cold quasieconomic terms of behavioral ecology. However, for most people the resources at issue are relationships that are mediated not by calculated reciprocity, but by powerful emotional commitments. To break such commitments and turn energies elsewhere is far different from just moving to a different foraging patch. At least as important as the risks and costs of making a change is the threat to the person's identity, reputation, and sense of a secure place in a social network and the cosmos. As a result, most people do not treat others as objects, to be exploited optimally and then replaced when convenient. Instead, despite the difficulties, they persist in their relationships, for better and for worse. Ambivalent relationships can cause vast suffering.[93]

TESTS

The several theses presented herein require different kinds of assessment.[94,95] The first, that it is important to determine if depression is a defense, a dysregulated defense, or a defect, extends a well-recognized distinction from the rest of medicine to psychiatry. The second, that evolutionary hypotheses about low mood and depression are better formulated in terms of the situations that shaped them instead of just their functions either will or will not prove itself useful. The third, that generic low mood and related negative affect have been shaped to deal with unpropitious situations, predicts that the effect of a life event on mood will depend primarily on how it changes the anticipated payoff of future efforts. Many data exist to test this proposal, and initial forays have been made. For instance, depression is precipitated not so much by life events that involve loss, but by those that are humiliating or entrapping.[20,96] Life events research has moved steadily from lists of events to examination of the individual context of the event.[19] A further step in this direction is to assess an individual's major life goals and ability to achieve them. This requires the ideographic study of why an individual is committed to certain goals and that individual's values, relationships, enterprises, strategies, obstacles, anticipated success or failure, strategic conflicts and trade-offs, and decisions about what to do next in life.[84]

A related thesis, that natural selection has partially differentiated several negative affects to deal with different kinds of unpropitious situations, predicts substantial overlap for the characteristics of low mood, depression, anxiety, guilt, and grief. Likewise, the brain mechanisms that mediate them should be tightly intertwined parts of the behavioral inhibition system.[97] Drugs that relieve depression should (and do) also relieve anxiety. Substantial comorbidity of depression and anxiety disorders[98] is expected, not only because related brain mechanisms give shared diatheses, but also because situations that involve persistence in futile efforts also involve risk and loss. Much work remains to consider how subtypes of negative affects may match certain situations, such as seasonal low mood in cold, dark seasons and grief after a loss.

The simplest untested prediction is that depression should be common in people who are unable to disengage from unreachable goals. Graduate students who are failing and faculty who are unlikely to make tenure are obvious candidates for study, but other situations are far more common: unrequited love, inability to get work, pursuing an elusive large life goal, or trying to lose weight, stop using drugs, satisfy a fetish, be morally exemplary, get famous, or please a critical parent. Ability to repress such wishes should prevent depression.

Negative thinking and lack of motivation should be especially common in situations characterized by temptation to challenge a dominant figure, failure of a major life enterprise, or lack of a viable life plan. They should be less common after discrete losses, even large ones. Low self-esteem should be an especially prominent part of those depressions that arise from inability to yield in a status competition. Furthermore, if negative thinking functions partly to keep people from prematurely leaving bad situations, then antidepressant treatment should increase the proportion of people who leave. It would be interesting to see if drug treatment of spouses who are abused and have depression makes them more likely to leave or to tolerate a bad situation. The benefits of cognitive therapy should be mediated not just by correcting negative distortions, but more specifically by increasing the person's expectations of the effectiveness of future actions.

This perspective also suggests animal and neural models. If the brain mechanisms that regulate foraging are related to those that mediate depression, then antidepressants should change the duration of foraging time in a depleted patch and the willingness to exert effort even when the net rate of return is negative. They might also change preferences for working hard for a large intermittent reward vs easily getting small, frequent rewards. If low mood is an active coordinated state, then the brain mechanisms that mediate it can be blocked at different points, so antidepressants should be effective via multiple mechanisms.

This perspective predicts that depression should be frequent in people who are anxious, duty-bound, ambitious, or lacking alternatives because such individuals are especially likely to get themselves into situations in which they are unable to give up a major goal.[99] People who lack the resources or power to accomplish their goals may be especially vulnerable.[100] Subjective well-being should be (and is) lower in those pursuing large longer-term projects,[101,102] especially conflicting ones.[103] It is interesting, in this context, to note that some of the genetic predisposition to depression is mediated by differential exposure to severe life events.[104,105]

Finally, this perspective predicts that social factors should influence rates of depression. Depression should be more common in cultures with rigid hierarchies and in those in which life enterprises tend to be huge, vulnerable, and irreplaceable. Media exposure should increase depression, not just by fostering negative social comparisons, but also by motivating the pursuit of unreachable goals. Relevant here are cross-cultural data that find subjective well-being to be higher in societies with greater income equality[106] and data showing increasing rates of depression in developed societies.[107]

CONCLUSIONS

Is depression an adaptation? At present, we do not have the evidence needed to say for sure. However, it seems likely that low mood and related negative affects were shaped to help organisms cope with unpropitious situations. Some negative and passive aspects of depression may be useful because they inhibit dangerous or wasteful actions in situations characterized by committed pursuit of an unreachable goal, temptations to challenge authority, insufficient internal reserves to allow action without damage, or lack of a viable life strategy. However, it is essential to emphasize that many depressions are clearly disease states: some caused by dysregulations of negative affect and others by brain defects unrelated to low mood. The fact that low mood, and perhaps some depression, may be useful should not distract attention from recognition that depression is one of humanity's most serious medial problems.[108] A deeper understanding of the adaptive significance of low mood and depression will improve our ability to prevent and relieve both mood disorders and low moods that are normal, but unnecessary.

Accepted for publication September 28, 1999.

Preparation of this article was made possible by a grant from the Kaplan Foundation, Englewood, NJ, and by support from the Department of Psychiatry and the Institute for Social Research, University of Michigan, Ann Arbor.

I thank Linda Brakel, MD, Deborah Carr, PhD, Helena Cronin, PhD, Allan Gibbard, PhD, Paul Gilbert, PhD, Ursula Goodenough, PhD, John Greden, MD, Annette Hollander, PhD, Gordon Kane, PhD, Lois Kane, Matthew Keller, BA, Kevin Kerber, MD, Timothy Ketelaar, PhD, Raymond Kloss, MD, Richard Lempert, PhD, David Lyons, MD, Jacquelyn Murphy, PhD, Margaret Nesse, MS,

Daphna Oyserman, PhD, Richard Price, PhD, Peter Railton, PhD, Barbara Smuts, PhD, Charles Webster, PhD, Brant Wenegrat, MD, and Elizabeth Young, MD, for comments on the ideas presented and on early drafts of this article. *Corresponding author: Randolph M. Nesse, MD, Institute for Social Research, University of Michigan, Room 5057, 426 Thompson St, Ann Arbor, MI 48106-1248 (e-mail: nesse@umich.edu).*

REFERENCES

1. Williams GW, Nesse RM. The dawn of Darwinian medicine. *Q Rev Biol.* 1991;66:1-22.
2. Nesse RM, Williams GC. *Why We Get Sick: The New Science of Darwinian Medicine.* New York, NY: Vintage Books; 1994.
3. DuPont HL, Hornick RB. Adverse effect of lomotil therapy in shigellosis. *JAMA.* 1973;226:1525-1528.
4. McGuire MT, Troisi A, Raleigh MM. Depression in evolutionary context. In: Baron-Cohen S, ed. *The Maladapted Mind.* Hillsdale, NJ: Lawrence A Erlbaum Associates; 1997:255-282.
5. Akiskal HS, McKinney WT Jr. Depressive disorders: toward a unified hypothesis. *Science.* 1973;182:20-29.
6. Shaver P, Schwartz J, Kirson D, O'Connor C. Emotion knowledge: further exploration of a prototype approach. *J Pers Soc Psychol.* 1987;52:1061-1086.
7. Watson D, Clark LA. Affects separable and inseparable: on the hierarchical arrangement of the negative affects. *J Pers Soc Psychol.* 1992;62:489-505.
8. Kessler RC, McGonagle KA, Swartz M, Blazer DG, Nelson CB. Sex and depression in the National Comorbidity Survey, I: lifetime prevalence, chronicity and recurrence. *J Affect Disord.* 1993;29:85-96.
9. Olfson M, Broadhead WE, Weissman MM, Leon AC, Farber L, Hoven C, Kathol R. Subthreshold psychiatric symptoms in a primary care group practice. *Arch Gen Psychiatry.* 1996;53:880-886.
10. Judd LL, Akiskal HS, Paulus MP. The role and clinical significance of subsyndromal depressive symptoms (SSD) in unipolar major depressive disorder. *J Affect Disord.* 1997;45:5-17.
11. Kendler KS, Gardner CO Jr. Boundaries of major depression: an evaluation of *DSM-IV* criteria. *Am J Psychiatry.* 1998;155:172-177.
12. Whybrow PC, Akiskal HS, McKinney WT. *Mood Disorders: Toward a New Psychobiology.* New York, NY: Plenum Publishing Corp; 1984.
13. Akiskal HS, Judd LL, Gillin JC, Lemmi H. Subthreshold depressions: clinical and polysomnographic validation of dysthymic, residual and masked forms. *J Affect Disord.* 1997;45:53-63.
14. Angst J, Merikangas KR, Presig M. Subthreshold syndromes of depression and anxiety in the community. *J Clin Psychiatry.* 1997;58:6-10.
15. Janzen DH. Evolutionary physiology of personal defense. In: Townsend CR, Calow P, eds. *Physiological Ecology: An Evolutionary Approach to Resource Use.* Cambridge, Mass: Blackwell Publishers; 1981:145-164.
16. Vander A, Sherman JH, Luciano DS. *Human Physiology: The Mechanisms of Body Function.* 5th ed. New York, NY: McGraw-Hill Book Co; 1985.
17. Mrosovsky N. *Rheostatis.* New York, NY: Oxford University Press; 1990.
18. Brown GW, Harris T. *Social Origins of Depression.* New York, NY: The Free Press; 1978.
19. Monroe SM, Simons AD. Diathesis-stress theories in the context of life stress research: implications for the depressive disorders. *Psychol Bull.* 1991;110:406-425.
20. Brown GW, Harris TO, Hepworth C. Loss, humiliation and entrapment among women developing depression: a patient and non-patient comparison. *Psychol Med.* 1995;25:7-21.
21. Monroe SM, Simons AD, Thase ME. Onset of depression and time to treatment entry: roles of life stress. *J Consult Clin Psychol.* 1991;59:566-573.
22. Frank E, Anderson B, Reynolds CF III, Ritenour A, Kupfer DJ. Life events and the research diagnostic criteria endogenous subtype: a confirmation of the distinction using the Bedford College methods. *Arch Gen Psychiatry.* 1994;51:519-524.
23. Johnson-Laird PN, Oatley K. The language of emotions: an analysis of a semantic field. *Cogn Emotion.* 1989;3:81-123.
24. Barr RG. The early crying paradox: a modest proposal. *Hum Nature.* 1990;1:355-389.
25. Lummaa V, Vuorisalo T, Barr RG, Lehtonen L. Why cry? adaptive significance of intensive crying in human infants. *Evolution Hum Behav.* 1998;19:193-202.
26. Rosenblum LA, Plimpton EH. The infant's effort to cope with separation. In: Lewis M, Rosenblum LA, eds. *The Uncommon Child.* New York, NY: Plenum Publishing Corp; 1981:225-257.
27. Lewis AJ. Melancholia: a clinical survey of depressive states. *J Mental Sci.* 1934;80:1-43.
28. Coyne JC, Kessler RC, Tal M, Turnbull J. Living with a depressed person. *J Consult Clin Psychol.* 1987;55:347-352.
29. Hagen EH. The functions of postpartum depression. *Evolution Hum Behav.* In press.
30. Watson PW, Andrews PW. An evolutionary theory of unipolar depression as an adaptation for overcoming constraints of the social niche. Presented at: Annual Meeting of the Human Behavior and Evolution Society; July 10, 1998; Davis, Calif.
31. Lief A, ed. *The Common Sense Psychiatry of Dr Adolf Meyer.* New York, NY: McGraw Hill Book Co; 1948.
32. Klerman GL. Depression and adaptation. In: Friedman RJ, Katz MM, eds. *The Psychology of Depression.* Washington DC: VH Winston & Sons; 1974:127-156.
33. Engel G, Schmale A. Conservation-withdrawal: a primary regulatory process for organismic homeostasis. In: Porter R, Night J, eds. *Physiology, Emotion, and Psychosomatic Illness.* Amsterdam, the Netherlands: Associated Scientific Publishers; 1972:57-85.
34. Schmale A, Engel GL. The role of conservation-withdrawal in depressive reactions. In: Benedek T, Anthony EJ, eds. *Depression and Human Existence.* Boston, Mass: Little Brown & Co; 1975:183-198.
35. Thierry B, Steru L, Chermat R, Simon P. Searching-waiting strategy: a candidate for an evolutionary model of depression? *Behav Neural Biol.* 1984;41:180-189.
36. Beck AT. Depression as an evolutionary strategy. Presented at: Annual Meeting of the Human Behavior and Evolution Society; June 27, 1996; Evanston, Ill.
37. Rosenthal NE, Sack DA, Gillin JC, Lewy AJ, Goodwin FK, Davenport Y, Mueller PS, Newsome DA, Wehr TA. Seasonal affective disorder: a description of the syndrome and preliminary findings with light therapy. *Arch Gen Psychiatry.* 1984;41:72-80.
38. Bowlby J. *Attachment and Loss.* New York, NY: Basic Books Inc Publishers; 1969.
39. Archer J. *The Nature of Grief.* New York, NY: Oxford University Press; 1999.
40. Nesse RM. Is grief really maladaptive? *Evolution Hum Behav.* In press.
41. Price JS. The dominance hierarchy and the evolution of mental illness. *Lancet.* 1967;2:243-246.
42. Price J, Sloman L, Gardner R Jr, Gilbert P, Rohde P. The social competition hypothesis of depression. *Br J Psychiatry.* 1994;164:309-315.
43. Sloman L, Price J, Gilbert P, Gardner R. Adaptive function of depression: psychotherapeutic implications. *Am J Psychother.* 1994;48:401-416.
44. Gardner R Jr. Mechanisms in manic-depressive disorder: an evolutionary model. *Arch Gen Psychiatry.* 1982;39:1436-1441.
45. Gilbert P. *Depression: The Evolution of Powerlessness.* New York, NY: Guilford Publications; 1992.
46. Hartung J. Deceiving down. In: Lockard JS, Paulhus D, eds. *Self-deception: An Adaptive Mechanism?* Englewood Cliffs, NJ: Prentice-Hall International Inc; 1988:170-185.
47. Bibring E. The mechanisms of depression. In: Greenacre P, ed. *Affective Disorders.* New York, NY: International Universities Press; 1953:13-48.
48. Davis DR. Depression as adaptation to crisis. *Br J Med Psychol.* 1970;43:109-116.
49. Gut E. *Productive and Unproductive Depression.* New York, NY: Basic Books Inc Publishers; 1989.
50. Baumeister RF. Suicide as escape from self. *Psychol Rev.* 1990;97:90-113.
51. Hamburg DA. Coping behavior in life-threatening circumstances. *Psychother Psychosom.* 1974;23:13-25.
52. Seligman MEP. *Helplessness: On Depression, Development, and Death.* San Francisco, Calif: WH Freeman & Co; 1975.
53. Wortman CB, Brehm JW. Responses to uncontrollable outcomes: an integration of reactance theory and the learned helplessness model. In: Berkowitz L, ed. *Advances in Experimental Social Psychology.* New York, NY: Academic Press Inc; 1975:277-336.
54. Peterson C, Maier SF, Seligman ME. *Learned Helplessness.* New York, NY: Oxford University Press; 1993.
55. Tiger L. *Optimism: The Biology of Hope.* New York, NY: Simon & Schuster; 1979.
56. Klinger E. Consequences of commitment to and disengagement from incentives. *Psychol Rev.* 1975;82:1-25.
57. Klinger E. *Meaning and Void: Inner Experience and the Incentives in People's Lives.* Minneapolis: University of Minnesota Press; 1977.
58. Janoff-Bulman R, Brickman P. Expectations and what people learn from failure. In: Feather NT, ed. *Expectations and Action.* Hillsdale, NJ: Lawrence A Erlbaum Associates; 1982.
59. Brickman P. *Commitment, Conflict, and Caring.* Englewood Cliffs, NJ: Prentice-Hall International Inc; 1987.
60. Carver CS, Scheier MF. *Attention and Self-regulation: A Control Theory Approach to Human Behavior.* New York, NY: Springer-Verlag; 1983.
61. Hyland ME. Control theory interpretation of psychological mechanisms of depression: compari-

son and integration of several theories. *Psychol Bull.* 1987;102:109-121.
62. Carver CS, Scheier MF. Origins and functions of positive and negative affect: a control-process view. *Psychol Rev.* 1990;97:19-35.
63. Higgins ET. Self-discrepacy: a theory relating self and affect. *Psychol Rev.* 1987;94:319-340.
64. Schwartz N. Feelings as information: informational and motivational functions of affective states. In: Higgins ET, Sorrentino R, eds. *Handbook of Motivation and Cognition.* New York, NY: Guilford Press; 1990:527-559.
65. Brunstein JC. Personal goals and subjective well-being. *J Pers Soc Psychol.* 1993;65:1061-1070.
66. Schwartz N, Clore GL. Feelings and phenomenal experiences. In: Higgens ET, Kruglanski AW, eds. *Social Psychology: Handbook of Basic Principles.* New York, NY: Guilford Publications; 1996: 433-465.
67. Alloy LB, Abramson L. Depressive realism: four theoretical perspectives. In: Alloy L, ed. *Cognitive Processes in Depression.* New York, NY: Guilford Press; 1988.
68. Taylor SE, Brown JD. Illusion and well-being: a social psychological perspective on mental health. *Psychol Bull.* 1988;103:193-210.
69. Martin LL, Tesser A, eds. *Striving and Feeling: Interactions Among Goals, Affect, and Self-regulation.* Hillsdale, NJ: Lawrence A Erlbaum Associates; 1996.
70. Nesse RM. Evolutionary explanations of emotions. *Hum Nature.* 1990;1:261-289.
71. Nesse RM. What is mood for? *Psycholoquy* [journal online]. 1991;2:9.2. Available at: ftp://ftp.princeton.edu/pub/harnad/Psycholoquy/1991.volume.2/psyc.91.mood.1.nesse. Accessed October 19, 1999.
72. Nesse RM. What good is feeling bad? *The Sciences.* November/December 1991:30-37.
73. Wender PH, Klein DF. *Mind, Mood and Medicine.* New York, NY: New American Library; 1982.
74. Tooby J, Cosmides L. The past explains the present: emotional adaptations and the structure of ancestral environments. *Ethol Sociobiol.* 1990; 11:375-424.
75. Oatley K, Jenkins JM. Human emotions: function and dysfunction. *Annu Rev Psychol.* 1992;43:55-85.
76. Ekman P, Davidson RJ, eds. *The Nature of Emotion: Fundamental Questions.* New York, NY: Oxford University Press; 1994:97-143.
77. Frijda NH. Varieties of affect: emotions and episodes, moods and sentiments. In: Ekman P, Davidson RJ, eds. *The Nature of Emotion: Fundamental Questions.* New York, NY: Oxford University Press; 1994:59-67.
78. Nesse RM, Berridge KC. Psychoactive drug use in evolutionary perspective. *Science.* 1997;278: 63-66.
79. Charnov EL. Optimal foraging: the marginal value theorem. *Theor Popul Biol.* 1976;9:129-136.
80. Stephens DW, Krebs JR. Foraging theory. In: Krebs JR, Clutton-Brock T, eds. *Monographs in Behavior and Ecology.* Princeton, NJ: Princeton University Press; 1986.
81. Ellsworth P. Some implications for cognitive appraisal theories of emotion. *Int Rev Stud Emotion.* 1991;1:143-161.
82. Lazarus RS. *Emotion and Adaptation.* New York, NY: Oxford University Press; 1991.
83. Cantor N. From thought to behavior: "having" and "doing" in the study of personality and cognition. *Am Psychol.* 1990;45:735-750.
84. Diener E, Fujita F. Resources, personal strivings, and subjective well-being: a nomothetic ideographic approach. *J Pers Soc Psychol.* 1995; 68:926-935.
85. Fleeson W, Cantor N. Goal relevance and the affective experience of daily life: ruling out situational explanations. *Motivation Emotion.* 1995; 19:25-57.
86. Gollwitzer PM. Action phases and mind-sets. In: Higgins ET, Sorrentine RM, eds. *Handbook of Motivation and Cognition.* New York, NY: Guilford Press; 1990:53-92.
87. de Waal FB. *Peacemaking Among Primates.* Cambridge, Mass: Harvard University Press; 1989.
88. Beck AT. *Depression: Clinical, Experimental, and Theoretical Aspects.* New York, NY: Hoeber Medical Division; 1967.
89. Teasdale JD. Negative thinking in depression: cause, effect, or reciprocal relationship? *Adv Behav Res Ther.* 1983;5:3-25.
90. Pyszczynski T, Greenberg J. Self-regulatory perseveration and the depressive self-focusing style: a self-awareness theory of reactive depression. *Psychol Bull.* 1987;102:122-138.
91. Nolen-Hoeksema S, Morrow J. Effects of rumination and distraction on naturally occurring depressed mood. *Cogn Emotion.* 1993;7:561-570.
92. Seligman ME. *Learned Optimism.* New York, NY: Random House Inc; 1991.
93. Vaillant GE. *Adaptation to Life.* Boston, Mass: Little Brown & Co; 1977.
94. Nesse RM. Testing evolutionary hypotheses about mental disorders. In: Stearns S, ed. *Evolution in Health and Disease.* New York, NY: Oxford University Press; 1999:260-266.
95. Nesse RM, Williams GC. Research designs that address evolutionary questions about medical disorders. In: Stearns S, ed. *Evolution in Health and Disease.* New York, NY: Oxford University Press; 1999:16-26.
96. Gilbert P, Allan S. The role of defeat and entrapment (arrested flight) in depression: an exploration of an evolutionary view. *Psychol Med.* 1998;28:585-598.
97. Gray JA. *Fear and Stress.* 2nd ed. Cambridge, England: Cambridge University Press; 1987.
98. Maser J, Cloninger R. *Comorbidity of Mood and Anxiety Disorders.* Washington, DC: American Psychiatric Press; 1990.
99. Little BR, Lecci L, Watkinson B. Personality and personal projects: linking big five and PAC units of analysis. *J Pers.* 1992;60:501-525.
100. Wenegrat B. *Illness and Power.* New York: New York University Press; 1995.
101. Palys TS, Little BR. Perceived life satisfaction and the organization of personal project systems. *J Pers Soc Psychol.* 1983;44:1221-1230.
102. Emmons RA. Abstract versus concrete goals: personal striving level, physical illness, and psychological well-being. *J Pers Soc Psychol.* 1992; 62:292-300.
103. Emmons RA, King LA. Conflict among personal strivings: immediate and long-term implications for psychological and physical well-being. *J Pers Soc Psychol.* 1988;54:1040-1048.
104. Kendler KS, Karkowski-Shuman L. Stressful life events and genetic liability to major depression: genetic control of exposure to the environment? *Psychol Med.* 1997;27:539-547.
105. Kendler KS. Major depression and the environment: a psychiatric genetic perspective. *Pharmacopsychiatry.* 1998;31:5-9.
106. Kahnemann D, Deiner E, Schwarz N. *Well-Being: Foundations of Hedonic Psychology.* New York, NY: Russell Sage Foundation; 1999.
107. Cross-National Collaborative Group. The changing rate of major depression: cross-national comparisons. *JAMA.* 1992;268:3098-3105.
108. Murray CJ, Lopez AD. *The Global Burden of Disease: A Comprehensive Assessment of Mortality and Disability From Diseases, Injuries, and Risk Factors in 1990 and Projected to 2020.* Cambridge, Mass: Harvard University Press; 1996.

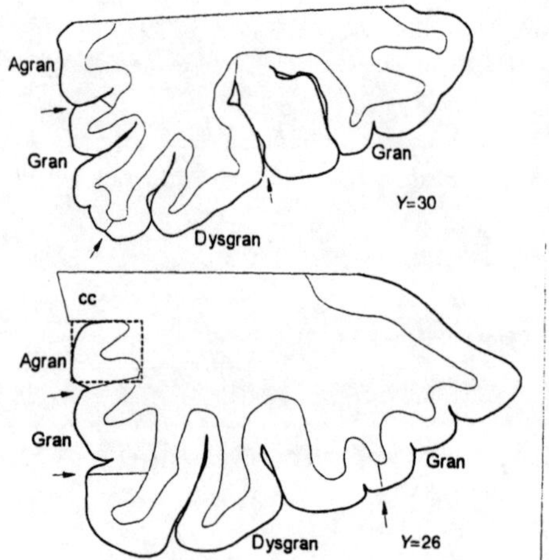

Figure 1 Drawings of coronal sections through the genu of the corpus callosum (CC) and subgenual and posterior orbital PFC of a human brain at levels 26 and 30 mm rostral to the anterior commissure. Agranular ('agran'), dysgranular ('dysgran') and granular ('gran') cortical regions are marked. The subgenual PFC consists of agranular cortex on the anterior cingulate gyrus immediately ventral to the genu of the corpus callosum[30]. Dashed line indicates the centre of the smaller ROI used for regional measures in the 953B images. This cylindrical ROI, 1 cm in diameter and spanning 1-9 mm ventral to the bicommissural plane, was placed[29] *a priori* in each subject's image over the coordinates of the peak $|t|$ value identified in the subgenual PFC in the t image from group A: $x = 5$, $y = 25$, $z = -6$ (in mm from the anterior commissure, with positive x as right, positive y as rostral, and negative z as ventral to the bicommissural plane[28]).

Subgenual prefrontal cortex abnormalities in mood disorders

Wayne C. Drevets*†‡§, Joseph L. Price‡, Joseph R. Simpson Jr†, Richard D. Todd*‖, Theodore Reich*‖, Michael Vannier†§ & Marcus E. Raichle†‡¶‖**

* *Department of Psychiatry,* † *Division of Radiological Sciences, Mallinckrodt Institute of Radiology,* ‡ *Department of Anatomy and Neurobiology,* ‖ *Department of Genetics,*
¶ *Department of Neurology and Neurological Surgery (Neurology),*
** *McDonnell Center for Studies of Higher Brain Function, Washington University School of Medicine, St Louis, Missouri 63110, USA*

Pathological disturbances of mood may follow a 'bipolar' course, in which normal moods alternate with both depression and mania, or a 'unipolar' course, in which only depression occurs[1–3]. Both bipolar and unipolar disorders can be heritable illnesses associated with neurochemical, neuroendocrine and autonomic abnormalities. The neurobiological basis for these abnormalities has not been established[2,3]. Using positron emission tomographic (PET) images of cerebral blood flow and rate of glucose metabolism to measure brain activity, we have now localized an area of abnormally decreased activity in the prefrontal cortex ventral to the genu of the corpus callosum in both familial bipolar depressives and familial unipolar depressives. This decrement in activity was at least partly explained by a corresponding reduction in cortical volume[4], as magnetic resonance imaging (MRI) demonstrated reductions in the mean grey matter volume in the same area of 39 and 48% in the bipolar and unipolar samples, respectively. This region has previously been implicated in the mediation of emotional and autonomic responses to socially significant or provocative stimuli, and in the modulation of the neurotransmitter systems targeted by antidepressant drugs[3,5–10].

Low-resolution PET images of cerebral blood flow (BF) (full width at half-maximum (FWHM, 17 mm) from unmedicated, bipolar depressives and from controls were divided into two groups (A and B) for hypothesis generation and subsequent testing (Table 1). Using the images from group A, a statistical image composed of unpaired t values (the difference between the mean values for each subject sample divided by the standard error of this difference) was computed by subtracting the mean blood flow for the controls from that of the depressives at every voxel (volume element) and then dividing the resulting differences by the local variance[11]. Regions-of-interest (ROI) were defined in this t-image, which highlighted areas where blood flow inherently differed between the bipolar-depressives and controls from group A (ref. 11). The ROI containing the largest absolute difference in mean flow between groups was defined in the subgenual prefrontal cortex, where flow was decreased by 7.7% in the depressives relative to the controls from group A (the proximity of this abnormality to the midline precluded laterality determinations from the PET image data; Fig. 2 legend). The hypothesis that blood flow was abnormal in bipolar depression in this ROI was confirmed by comparing regional measures from the independent subject group B, in which mean flow was decreased by 6.6% in the depressives relative to the controls ($t = -4.3$, corrected d.f. $= 16$, corrected P(1-tailed) < 0.01).

§ Present addresses: Departments of Psychiatry and Radiology, University of Pittsburgh Medical Center, 3811 O'Hara Street, Pittsburgh, Pennsylvania 15213-2593, USA (W.C.D.); Department of Radiology, University of Iowa, Iowa City, Iowa 52242, USA (M.V.).

Table 1 PET image comparison of regional BF and metabolic rates for bipolar depressed, unipolar depressed, bipolar manic and control patients

Hypothesis:	Generating		Testing		Testing and extending		Extending	Extending
Subject group:	A		B		C		FPDD	Manic
PET camera	PETT VI		PETT VI		Siemens CTI 953B		953B	953B
Measure	Relative BF		Relative BF		Relative BF and MRglu		Relative MRglu	Relative MRglu
Subsample:	BP-D	Control	BP-D	Control	BP-D	Control		
n	6	24	5	15	7	12	10	4
Mean age, yr (± s.d.)	29 ± 5.5	29 ± 7.1	27 ± 6.5	27 ± 8.5	37 ± 8.7	33 ± 11	39 ± 7.3	30 ± 11
Right-handed (%)	100	100	100	100	86	92	100	100
Conclusion, subgenal PFC activity:			BF is reduced in BP-D versus control		BF and MRglu are both reduced in BP-D versus control		MRglu is reduced in FPDD versus control	MRglu appears raised in manic versus control, BP-D and FPDD

For abbreviations, see Methods.

To localize this abnormality more precisely, glucose metabolism images were acquired in a third, independent set of unmedicated, bipolar depressives and controls (group C in Table 1) using a higher-resolution camera (Siemens/CTI 953B; reconstructed resolution, 5 mm FWHM). A smaller ROI was stereotaxically positioned in each group C image at the coordinates of the $|t|$ value identified in the subgenual prefrontal cortex in the t-image from group A (Fig. 1). Mean normalized metabolism was decreased 16.3% and mean blood flow was decreased 18.5% in this ROI in the bipolar depressives relative to the controls (mean ± one standard deviation for metabolism $= 0.87 \pm 0.15$ and 1.04 ± 0.15, respectively; $t = -2.3$, corrected d.f. = 12, P(1-tail) < 0.025; and for blood flow $= 1.01 \pm 0.15$ and 1.24 ± 0.17, respectively, $t = -3.0$, corrected d.f. = 13, P(1-tail) < 0.01). The greater magnitude and variance of the differences measured in this sample was probably accounted for by the higher spatial resolution of the images.

The same high-resolution PET methods were applied to unipolar depressives with familial pure depressive disease (FPDD; criteria that exclude depressives with a family history of mania[12]) and to bipolar subjects scanned in the manic phase[1]. The unipolar group ($n = 10$; 7 female) met criteria for recurrent, major depressive disorder[1] and FPDD[12], and their mean age, depression severity (mean Hamilton Depression Rating Scale (HDRS) score, 25.5 ± 5.4) and medication free period (>4 weeks) were similar to those of bipolar group C (Table 1). The mean subgenual prefrontal cortex metabolism in the unipolar depressives (0.91 ± 0.11) was decreased 12.2% relative to the controls ($t = -2.3$, d.f. = 20, P(1-tail) < 0.025) and did not significantly differ from that of the bipolar depressives. Previously, the only functional neuroimaging finding consistently identified in both bipolar and unipolar depressives was located in the dorsolateral prefrontal cortex where reduced activity is thought to correlate with the neuropsychological manifestations of depression (for example, slowing of thought speed)[13–20].

The manic subjects ($n = 4$) met criteria for bipolar disorder–manic phase[1] (mean Mania Rating Scale[21] score was 20 ± 4.4, one female, one medicated within 4 weeks). In contrast to the findings in the depressed groups, the mean metabolism in the manic group (1.15 ± 0.054) was increased relative to that of the control ($t = 2.2$, d.f. = 12, P(2-tail) < 0.05), bipolar-depressed ($t = 4.6$, $P < 0.01$) and unipolar-depressed groups ($t = 5.5$, $P < 0.01$). Consistent with these differences, in one subject scanned in both phases, normalized metabolism in the subgenual prefrontal cortex was 0.84 while depressed and 1.11 eight weeks later while manic. Although these preliminary observations in mania require replication in a larger sample, they suggest that subgenual prefrontal cortex metabolism is mood-state dependent.

Decreased blood flow and metabolism in the subgenual prefrontal cortex in depression could reflect a regional reduction in either synaptic activity[22] or tissue volume (because of the low spatial resolution of PET, reductions in tissue associated with atrophy or hypoplasia reduce the magnitude of local blood flow and metabolic measures from PET images, a phenomenon known as the partial volume averaging effect)[4]. The grey matter volume of the corresponding cortex was therefore measured in MRI images acquired in mood-disordered and control subjects (Figs 2, 3). MRI scans were not available for the subjects in groups A and B, so to improve the sensitivity for detecting intergroup differences (regional brain volume measures have greater variability than PET measures), the sample sizes were increased by adding MRI data from subjects not involved in the PET comparisons. The expanded bipolar group included the unmedicated, bipolar depressives from group C together with two medicated-depressed, four manic and eight remitted (six medicated) subjects with bipolar disorder[1] (total $n = 21$; age = 35 ± 8.2; 13 female; 20 right-handed; all had a parent or sibling with bipolar disorder). The expanded unipolar group combined the FPDD group with seven additional unipolar depressives who met criteria for recurrent, major depressive disorder[1], but not for FPDD[12] (total $n = 17$; mean age = 35 ± 9.4; 10 female, 16 right-handed). Additional controls were combined with those from group C (total $n = 21$; age = 34 ± 8.2; 11 female; 19 right-handed).

The left subgenual prefrontal cortex grey matter volume was reduced by 39% in the bipolar subjects and 48% in the unipolar depressives relative to the controls ($F = 9.8$; $P < 0.0002$, after covarying for age, gender and whole brain volume; Fig. 3), and did not significantly differ between the unipolar and bipolar groups. (Notably, post hoc tests showed that the volumetric differences identified in the expanded group of bipolar subjects were also significant when the controls were compared either to the seven bipolar subjects from group C ($P < 0.05$) or to the 14 bipolar subjects not included in group C ($P < 0.005$).) No significant differences in mean volume were found between the bipolar and control groups in other portions of the anterior cingulate gyrus, including the right subgenual prefrontal cortex (219 ± 95 and 209 ± 66 mm^3, respectively) or the dorsal anterior cingulate cortex (left: 418 ± 184 and 389 ± 211 mm^3, respectively, $t = 0.47$; right: 456 ± 134 and 406 ± 134 mm^3, respectively, $t = 1.2$). Post hoc analysis indicated that the volumetric difference in the subgenual prefrontal cortex is present irrespective of mood state in bipolar disorder (mean values for the symptomatic (manic or depressed) and remitted subsamples were 131 ± 72 and 146 ± 99 mm^3, respectively). The anatomical abnormality also persisted during antidepressant drug treatment in 15 of the unipolar depressives who were reimaged following a mean treatment period of 3.2 ± 3.5 months (the mean volume was 126 ± 66 mm^3 pre-treatment and 123 ± 61 mm^3 post-treatmnent). Thus, the reduction in the left subgenual prefrontal cortex grey matter volume in mood disorders, localized by synergistic use of PET and MRI image data, could reflect either an abnormality of brain development related to the tendency to develop mood episodes or a degenerative change resulting from recurrent illness.

In monkeys and other experimental animals, the subgenual prefrontal cortex has extensive connections with structures implicated in emotional behaviour and autonomic/neuroendocrine responses to stressors, including the amygdala, the lateral hypotha-

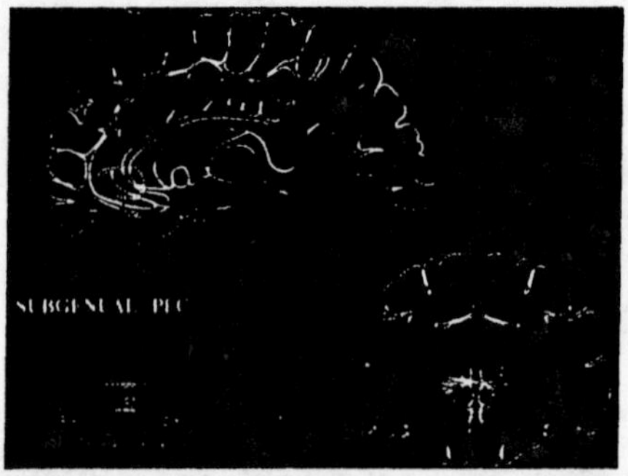

Figure 2 Coronal ($y = 31$ mm) and sagittal ($x = -3$ mm) sections showing negative voxel t values where metabolism is decreased in depressives relative to controls. This image, generated *post hoc* to provide optimal localization of the subgenual PFC abnormality, compares all unmedicated depressives scanned with the 953B (bipolar depressives from group C plus unipolar depressives with FPDD) with the group C controls. The stereotaxic centre-of-mass of this difference ($x = -2, y = 32, z = -2$) lay within one FWHM (17 mm for PET VI) from the peak BF difference in group A (Fig. 1) and from the centre-of-mass of the BF difference computed post hoc for the entire PET VI image set (groups A plus B): $x = 1, y = 25, z = -6$. All three coordinate sets localize to the agranular region of the anterior cingulate gyrus ventral to the CC (Fig. 1). The spatial resolution of PET precludes clear laterality distinctions. Anterior, or left, is to the left.

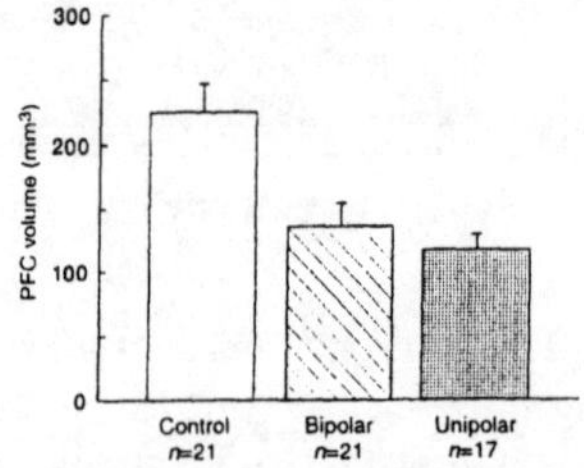

Figure 3 MRI-based volumes of the left subgenual prefrontal cortex (PFC) grey matter differed between the dipolar disordered, unipolar depressed and control groups (ANOVA, $F = 9.8$; $P < 0.0002$, co-varying for gender, age and whole brain volume). Post hoc tests (Tukey-Kramer) showed significant volumetric decreases in the bipolar and unipolar groups relative to the control group. Whole-brain MRI volume and skull X-ray measures (product of anterior-posterior distance between the inner tables of the skull at the estimated bicommissural segment[29] and perpendicular distance from the midpoint of the bicommissural segment to the vertex[29]) were slightly smaller in the unipolar group compared with the bipolar and control groups, and did not differ between the bipolar and control groups. The left subgenual PFC/whole brain volume ratio was also reduced in the bipolar and unipolar groups, being $1.8 \times 10^{-4} \pm 0.74 \times 10^{-4}$, $1.1 \times 10^{-4} \pm 0.64 \times 10^{-4}$, and $1.1 \times 10^{-4} \pm 0.51 \times 10^{-4}$ in the control, bipolar, and unipolar groups, respectively ($F = 8.4$; $P < 0.001$).

lamus, the nucleus accumbens, and the brainstem serotonergic, noradrenergic and dopaminergic nuclei (the function of these neurotransmitter systems appears to be blunted during depressive episodes and to be augmented by antidepressant drug treatments)[2,3,5–7]. Humans with lesions that include the subgenual prefrontal cortex demonstrate abnormal autonomic responses to emotional experiences, inability to experience emotion related to concepts that ordinarily evoke emotion, and impaired comprehension of the adverse consequences of pernicious social behaviours[8,9]. Based partly upon these observations, Damasio *et al.*[8,10] proposed that the ability to discern the outcome of social behaviour in terms of punishment and reward depends upon visceral feedback mediated through interactions between the ventromedial prefrontal cortex and autonomic centres. If so, disordered interactions between the subgenual prefrontal cortex and interconnected structures may be related to the pathological guilt or anxiety characterizing depression, or the rapid shifts between inappropriate euphoria and anger seen in mania[2,3]. The neural network formed by these structures may contain a disease process that is not confined to the subgenual prefrontal cortex, as reduced left amygdala volume[23] and third ventricle enlargement[18] (the subgenual prefrontal cortex shares substantial, predominantly ipsilateral connections with the amygdala and the medial thalamic nuclei surrounding the third ventricle[5]) have also been reported in bipolar disorder. Post-mortem histopathological assessments within this circuitry may elucidate the neurobiology of familial mood disorders. □

Methods

Subjects. Characteristics of subgroups appear in Table 1. The bipolar-depressed (BP-D) subjects met criteria for bipolar disorder, depressed phase[1], and had a parent or sibling with probable or definite bipolar disorder. Hamilton Depression Rating Scale (HDRS) scores (21 items)[24] were in the moderately-to-severely-depressed range (mean = 24.2 ± 3.5 (20–29) for groups A and B, and 23.4 ± 6.5 (16–35) for group C). Subjects had not received psychotropic or other drugs likely to alter blood flow (BF) or glucose metabolism for >4 weeks. Exclusion criteria included substance abuse within one year and major medical disorders.

Controls met the same exclusions and denied having had major psychiatric disorders. Group A controls consisted of 24 subjects involved in our previous study of unipolar depression[11], who also denied a family history of psychiatric disorders. This large, carefully screened control group was used to generate the composite normative image for the t-image computation. Group B controls were matched with bipolar subjects in group B (40% female in each) and group C controls with the bipolar subjects in group C (50 and 57% female, respectively) for age, handedness and gender.

Image acquisition. PET scans were acquired as subjects rested with eyes closed. For groups A and B, images were obtained using PETT VI and 60–80 mCi of $H_2{}^{15}O$ (ref. 25). Tissue radioactivity was measured, which over the range tested accurately reflects differences in regional BF[26].

For group C, images were acquired with a Siemens 953B tomograph (resolution was 5 mm FWHM, septa inserted). Glucose metabolism was measured using 5–10 mCi of $[^{18}F]$2-fluorodeoxyglucose, adaptions of the Sokoloff method,[27] and arterial blood sampling. A linear normalization was applied by dividing regional-by-global metabolic rate for glucose (MRglu; mean global values did not significantly differ across the control, bipolar-depressed, and unipolar-depressed (FPDD) groups, being 6.0 ± 0.95, 6.2 ± 1.2 and 5.7 ± 1.1 mg per 100 mg per min, respectively). The metabolic images were not filtered (that is, FWHM was 5 mm). Regional BF was also measured[25] and the reconstructed BF images were filtered to a 3-dimensional resolution of 14 mm FWHM. Technical problems precluded acquisition of the metabolic image for one bipolar depressive and the BF image for another.

Image analysis. To guide regional analyses, PET scans from group A were used to compute a composite statistical image highlighting differences between bipolar depressives and controls. After remapping primary images into a common, stereotaxic array[28,29], an image of unpaired t-values was computed, with each voxel representing the difference in mean BF between depressives and controls divided by the local variance[11]. The t image was searched for t values above a threshold $|t|$ that would correspond to $P < 0.05$ in a single test. ROI were defined to encompass the voxel containing the peak $|t|$ value and adjacent voxels with similar t values. The size of each ROI was optimized by computing regional t for progressively larger ROI, and the ROI for which the regional t was maximized was selected. Eleven ROI were defined, located in the following regions (per cent difference in mean normalized flow in depressives relative to controls appears in parentheses): subgenual prefrontal cortex (PFC) (− 7.7%), right (R) insula (− 7.5%), R and left (L) temporoparietal cortex (− 7.4 and − 6.7%, respectively), R and L lentiform nucleus (− 6.3 and − 5.7%, respectively), rostral thalamus (− 6.1%), posterior cingulate (− 5.6%), L hippocampus (− 5.2%), L frontal pole (4.4%) and R precuneate (4.5%).

The hypothesis that BF differed between depressives and controls in each ROI was tested by comparing the mean BF of the depressed and control samples from group B in one-tailed t-tests, corrected for multiple comparisons (Bonferroni), with degrees of freedom corrected for unequal variance (Satterthwaite). Thus, the ROI used to obtain the BF measures for both groups A and B were identical in size and location, having been generated from the t-image from group A, and stereotaxically placed in each subject's PET image[11,28,29]. The only mean BF difference between the depressives and controls from group B achieving significance after corrections from 11 tests was found in the subgenual PFC.

Because of the higher spatial resolution of the 953B images, regional measures in group C were obtained using the smaller ROI shown in Fig. 1. Thus, they were not guided by information regarding inherent differences between the depressives and controls from groups B or C.

Neuromorphometric measures. MR images acquired using a Siemens VISION 1.5T scanner and a 3D MPRAGE sequence (T1, 300 ms; TR, 9.7; TE, 4; flip angle, 12°; matrix, 256 × 256 × 128, 1 × 1 × 25 mm voxels) were resliced to 1 mm^3 voxels with coronal sections oriented perpendicular to the bicommissural line using ANALYZE. The grey matter was manually traced for the first full gyrus beneath the corpus callosum in all coronal slices between the anteriormost point of the callosum and the anteriormost plane where the internal capsule no longer divided the striatum. Segmentation was performed by one investigator (W.C.D.) blinded to diagnosis. Virtually identical mean intergroup differences were obtained by a second rater (J.R.S.) blinded to the measures of the first. Variance components estimates (intraclass correlation coefficients) showed that 1.0% of the total variability was due to interrater differences and 99% to inter-subject differences.

Received 12 September 1996; accepted 18 February 1997.

1. *Diagnostic and Statistical Manual of Mental Disorders (DSM-III-R)* (American Psychiatric Association, Washington, DC, 1987).
2. Goodwin, F. K. & Jamison, K. R. *Manic-depressive Illness* (Oxford University Press, New York, 1990).
3. Drevets, W. C. & Todd, R. D. in *Adult Psychiatry* (ed. Guze, S. B.) 99–142 (Mosby, St Louis, 1997).
4. Mazziotta, J. C., Phelps, M. E., Plummer, D. & Kuhl, D. E. Quantitation in positron emission computed tomography: 5. Physical-anatomical effects. *J. Comput. Assist. Tomogr.* **5**, 734–743 (1981).
5. Carmichael, S. T. & Price, J. L. Limbic connections of the orbital and medial prefrontal cortex in macaque monkeys. *J. Comp. Neurol.* **363**, 615–641 (1995).
6. Neafsey, E. J., Terreberry, R. R., Hurley, K. M., Ruit, K. G. & Frysztak, R. J. in *Neurobiology of Cingulate Cortex and Limbic Thalamus* (eds Vogt, B. A. & Gabriel, M.) 206–223 (Birkhauser, Boston, 1993).
7. Sesack, S. R., Deutch, A. Y., Roth, R. H. & Bunney, B. S. Topographic organization of the efferent projections of the medial prefrontal cortex in the rat: an anterograde tract-tracing study using *Phaseolus vulgaris* leucoagglutinin. *J. Comp. Neurol.* **290**, 213–242 (1989).
8. Damasio, A. R., Tranel, D. & Damasio, H. Individuals with sociopathic behavior caused by frontal damage fail to respond autonomically to social stimuli. *Behav. Brain Res.* **41**, 81–94 (1990).
9. Bechara, A., Tranel, D., Damasio, H. & Damasio, A. R. Failure to respond autonomically to anticipated future outcomes following damage to the prefrontal cortex. *Cerebr. Cort.* **6**, 215–225 (1996).
10. Damasio, A. R. *Descarte's Error: Emotion, Reason, and the Human Brain.* (Grosset/Putnam, New York, 1994; Picador MacMillan, London, 1995).
11. Drevets, W. C. *et al.* A functional anatomical study of unipolar depression. *J. Neurosci.* **12**, 3628–3641 (1992).
12. Winokur, G. The development and validity of familial subtypes in primary unipolar depression. *Pharmacopsychiatry* **15**, 142–146 (1982).
13. Baxter, L. R. *et al.* Cerebral metabolic rates for glucose in mood disorders. *Arch. Gen. Psychiat.* **42**, 441–447 (1985).
14. Baxter, L. R. *et al.* Reduction of prefrontal cortex glucose metabolism common to three types of depression. *Arch. Gen. Psychiat.* **46**, 243–250 (1989).
15. Buchsbaum, M. S. *et al.* Frontal cortex and basal ganglia metabolic rates assessed by positron emission tomography with $[^{18}F]$2-deoxyglucose in affective illness. *J. Affect. Dis.* **10**, 137–152 (1986).
16. Cohen, R. M. *et al.* Evidence for common alterations in cerebral glucose metabolism in major affective disorders and schizophrenia. *Nauropsychopharmacology* **2**, 241–254 (1989).
17. Dolan, R. J. *et al.* Dorsolateral prefrontal cortex dysfunction in the major psychoses: symptom or disease specificity? *J. Neurol. Neurosurg. Psychiat.* **56**, 1290–1294 (1993).
18. Drevets, W. C. & Botteron, K. in *Adult Psychiatry* (ed. Guze, S. B.) 53–82 (Mosby, St Louis, 1996).
19. Drevets, W. C. & Raichle, M. E. Reciprocal suppression of regional cerebral blood flow during emotional versus higher cognitive processes: implications for interactions between emotion and cognition. *Cognit. Emot.* (in the press).
20. Drevets, W. C., Spitznagel, E. L., MacLeod, A. K. & Raichle, M. E. Discriminatory capability of PET measurements of regional blood flow in familial pure depressive disease. *Abstr. Soc. Neurosci.* **18**, 1596 (1992).
21. Young, R. C., Biggs, J. T., Ziegler, V. E. & Meyer, D. A. A rating scale for mania: reliability, validity and sensitivity. *Brit. J. Psychiat.* **133**, 429–435 (1978).
22. DiRocco, R. J., Kageyama, G. H. & Wong-Riley, M. T. The relationship between CNS metabolism and cytoarchitecture: a review of ^{14}C-deoxyglucose studies with correlation to cytochrome oxidase histochemistry. *Comp. Med. Imag. Graph.* **13**, 81–92 (1989).
23. Pearlson, G. D. *et al.* Medial and superior temporal gyral volumes and cerebral asymmetry in schizophrenia versus bipolar disorder. *Biol. Psychiat.* **41**, 1–14 (1997).
24. Hamilton, M. A rating scale for depression. *J. Neurol. Neurosurg. Psychiat.* **23**, 56–62 (1960).
25. Raichle, M. E., Martin, W. R. W., Herscovitch, P., Mintun, M. A. & Markham, J. Brain blood flow measured with intravenous $H_2^{15}O$. II. Implementation and validation. *J. Nucl. Med.* **24**, 790–798 (1983).
26. Fox, P. T. & Mintun, M. A. Noninvasive functional brain mapping by change distribution analysis of averaged PET images of $H_2^{15}O$ tissue activity. *J. Nucl. Med.* **30**, 141–149 (1989).
27. Phelps, M. E. *et al.* Tomographic measurements of local cerebral glucose metabolic rate in humans with [F-18]2-fluoro-2-deoxy-D-glucose: validation of method. *Ann. Neurol.* **6**, 371–388 (1979).
28. Talairach, J. & Tournoux, P. in *Co-Planar Stereotaxic Atlas of the Human Brain* 1–122 (Theime, Stuttgart, 1988).
29. Fox, P. T., Perlmutter, J. S. & Raichle, M. E. A stereotactic method of anatomical localization for positron emission tomography. *J. Comput. Assist. Tomogr.* **9**, 141–153 (1985).
30. Carmichael, S. T. & Price, J. L. Architectonic subdivision of the orbital and medial prefrontal cortex in the macaque monkey. *J. Comp. Neurol.* **346**, 366–402 (1994).

Acknowledgements. This work was supported by the US NIH and the Charles A Dana Foundation. We thank T. Videen and J. Haller, for advice on image analysis. W. Powers for guidance on metabolic imaging, E. Spitznagel and T. Pilgram for assistance with statistical analysis, and L. Gardner for technical assistance.

Correspondence and requests for materials should be addressed to W.C.D.

A Molecular and Cellular Theory of Depression

Ronald S. Duman, PhD; George R. Heninger, MD; Eric J. Nestler, MD, PhD

Recent studies have begun to characterize the actions of stress and antidepressant treatments beyond the neurotransmitter and receptor level. This work has demonstrated that long-term antidepressant treatments result in the sustained activation of the cyclic adenosine 3′, 5′-monophosphate system in specific brain regions, including the increased function and expression of the transcription factor cyclic adenosine monophosphate response element-binding protein. The activated cyclic adenosine 3′, 5′-monophosphate system leads to the regulation of specific target genes, including the increased expression of brain-derived neurotrophic factor in certain populations of neurons in the hippocampus and cerebral cortex. The importance of these changes is highlighted by the discovery that stress can decrease the expression of brain-derived neurotrophic factor and lead to atrophy of these same populations of stress-vulnerable hippocampal neurons. The possibility that the decreased size and impaired function of these neurons may be involved in depression is supported by recent clinical imaging studies, which demonstrate a decreased volume of certain brain structures. These findings constitute the framework for an updated molecular and cellular hypothesis of depression, which posits that stress-induced vulnerability and the therapeutic action of antidepressant treatments occur via intracellular mechanisms that decrease or increase, respectively, neurotrophic factors necessary for the survival and function of particular neurons. This hypothesis also explains how stress and other types of neuronal insult can lead to depression in vulnerable individuals and it outlines novel targets for the rational design of fundamentally new therapeutic agents.

Arch Gen Psychiatry. 1997;54:597-606

Depression is thought to be a heterogenous illness that can result from the dysfunction of several neurotransmitter or

For editorial comment see page 607

metabolic systems. Basic and clinical studies have provided evidence that the serotonin and norepinephrine (NE) neurotransmitter systems are involved in the treatment of depression. These studies have led to a series of hypotheses concerning the mechanism of the action of anti- [illegible], as well as the pathophysiology of depression, that have focused on alterations in levels of these monoamines or their receptors. Although these models have guided research efforts in the field for 3 decades, they have not generated a compelling model of antidepressant action or the pathophysiology of depression. For example, studies to date have failed to identify a common action of antidepressant treatments at the level of monoamines or their receptors. This is not surprising given that different types of antidepressant treatments exert widely dif-

From the Laboratory of Molecular Psychiatry, Departments of Psychiatry and Pharmacology, Yale University School of Medicine, Connecticut Mental Health Center, New Haven.

ferent effects on the serotonin and NE systems. It is also possible that there is more than a single mechanism by which antidepressant treatments exert their therapeutic actions.

An updated hypothesis that builds on previous work suggests that the long-term, therapeutic action of antidepressant treatments is mediated by postreceptor intracellular targets. Advances in molecular and cellular biology have elucidated the intracellular machinery through which monoamines ultimately act to control the functioning of neurons. These advances have made it possible to begin the process of delineating the specific signal transduction pathways that mediate the short-term effects of different types of antidepressant treatments and that underlie the adaptations in neuronal function responsible for the long-term effects of these treatments.

We present a brief review of the basic and clinical work about the role of serotonin and NE systems in the treatment of depression. We also discuss, in greater detail, recent advances that demonstrate a role for intracellular signal transduction pathways and the regulation of specific target genes in antidepressant treatments. Specifically, we describe recent findings that demonstrate that the transcription factor cyclic adenosine 3′, 5′-monophosphate (cAMP) response element-binding protein (CREB) is one intracellular target of long-term antidepressant treatment and that brain-derived neurotrophic factor (BDNF) is one target gene of CREB. These studies support an emerging hypothesis of the mechanisms by which stress and other environmental insults may damage specific populations of neurons and, thereby, contribute to the pathophysiology of depression in vulnerable individuals. This provides a framework for future studies needed to test this potentially unifying hypothesis for antidepressant action and the pathophysiology of at least certain forms of depression.

MONOAMINES AND DEPRESSION

Early studies indicated that agents that deplete monoamines, such as reserpine, could lead to depression in a small percentage of individuals. This led to the theory that reduced availability of monoamine neurotransmitters, particularly NE and serotonin, could play a role in the formation of depression.[1-3] This hypothesis was supported by the discovery that prototypical antidepressant treatments, the tricyclics and monoamine oxidase inhibitors, cause a short-term increase in synaptic levels of monoamines. However, despite extensive research, it remains unclear whether long-term antidepressant treatments result in the increased or decreased function of the many monoamine pathways located throughout the brain.

The role of monoamines in depression has been further examined with the use of serotonin and NE depletion paradigms in normal and drug-remitted individuals with depression.[4-6] The results of these studies demonstrate that although the depletion of serotonin or NE does not lead to depressive symptoms in normal individuals, patients who experienced remission on either serotonin or NE selective reuptake inhibitors are vulnerable to relapse on depletion of the corresponding monoamine. This indicates that serotonin and NE are somehow involved in the maintenance of an antidepressant response, but cannot alone explain either the mechanism of action of antidepressant treatments or the pathophysiology of depression. This conclusion is also supported by the time required for the therapeutic action of antidepressant treatments (several weeks), even though levels of monoamines are increased rapidly by these treatments. Together, the results suggest that additional factors contribute to antidepressant responses and the onset of depression.

MONOAMINE RECEPTORS AND DEPRESSION

A consequence of antidepressant treatment and elevated levels of serotonin or NE is the activation of monoamine receptors. One possibility is that persistent activation of these receptors would lead to adaptations in the receptors that would then contribute to the delayed therapeutic action of antidepressant treatments.[7-9] Indeed, early studies demonstrated that long-term antidepressant treatments down-regulate the density of receptor sites for serotonin and NE. The best-characterized example is that the long-term, but not short-term, administration of many types of antidepressant treatments decreases levels of β-adrenergic receptor (βAR) ligand–binding sites in limbic brain regions, such as the cerebral cortex and the hippocampus.[10,11] The ability of βARs to stimulate the formation of cAMP is similarly decreased in these regions by long-term antidepressant treatments. Serotonin$_2$-receptor–binding sites were also found to be down-regulated by many antidepressant treatments.[12] These and other receptor studies led to various receptor sensitivity hypotheses—for example, that the action of antidepressant treatments is dependent on the down-regulation of βAR or serotonin$_2$ receptors and that enhanced sensitivity of these receptors may lead to depression.[7,8]

However, there are many problems with these hypotheses. First, not all antidepressant treatments effectively regulate the levels of βAR or serotonin$_2$-receptor sites.[9] This could mean that the action of different antidepressant treatments is mediated by different receptors or that other sites are more relevant. Second, the time course for down-regulation of βAR and serotonin$_2$ receptor–binding sites is more rapid than the therapeutic onset of these treatments.[9,13,14] Third, levels of serotonin$_2$ receptors are increased, not decreased, by long-term electroshock seizure treatment, one of the most effective therapies for depression.[9,14] Fourth, the reduction of βAR function by the administration of selective βAR receptor antagonists is not an effective treatment for depression and actually produces depression in some individuals.[15,16] In fact, the activation or facilitation of βAR function by the administration of thyroid hormone or a specific receptor agonist can have antidepressant efficacy in some patients.[17]

A serotonin$_{1A}$ receptor sensitivity hypothesis has also been put forth by Blier and de Montigny.[18] This hypothesis states that long-term antidepressant treatments increase the function of postsynaptic $serotonin_{1A}$ receptors in the hippocampus. Depending on the type of antidepressant treatment, they propose that this could occur by either the increased sensitivity of postsynaptic $serotonin_{1A}$ receptors or the desensitization of serotonin autoreceptors. One problem with this hypothesis is that direct-acting $serotonin_{1A}$ receptor agonists are not clearly effective antidepressant treatments, although the $serotonin_{1A}$ agonists tested (buspirone hydrochloride and gepirone) are thought to be partial agonists at postsynaptic $serotonin_{1A}$ receptors and may not adequately test the hypothesis. Another possibility is that increased $serotonin_{1A}$ neurotransmission is necessary, but insufficient, for antidepressant efficacy and that the activation of additional factors is required.

Several other monoamine receptor subtypes are reported to be regulated by antidepressant treatments.[8,9] However, as with the βAR, $serotonin_2$, and $serotonin_{1A}$ receptors, regulation of these other monoamine receptors alone cannot account for the mechanism of action of antidepressant treatments. Rather, alterations in the levels of these receptors or in their functional sensitivity probably represent adaptations to increased levels of monoamines. In fact, it can be argued that the observed receptor down-regulations are indicative of continued receptor activation secondary to continued elevations in monoamine levels after long-term antidepressant treatments. Indeed, levels of these receptors are decreased, and not completely eliminated, by long-term antidepressant treatments, raising the possibility that there could be sufficient levels of receptor remaining to respond to the elevated levels of serotonin and NE (**Figure 1**). If this is the case, the functional output of the monoamine receptors would be increased, not decreased, by long-term treatments, a possibility that was entertained in an early review.[19] This would suggest that long-term antidepressant treatments result in the sustained activation of the intracellular signal transduction cascades that mediate the actions of monoamine receptors. Such intracellular factors represent potential common targets for many different types of antidepressant treatments because they could be regulated by the activation of either the serotonin or NE receptor systems. This could include the activation of serotonin and NE receptor subtypes that are not themselves regulated by antidepressant treatments. It will be important in future studies to determine which serotonin and NE receptor subtypes mediate the relevant therapeutic actions of antidepressant treatments, although identification of the critical intracellular targets will likely facilitate this process.

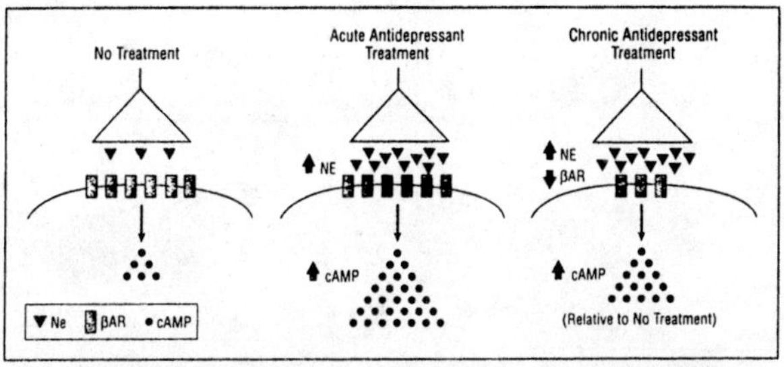

Figure 1. *A model demonstrating antidepressant regulation of the β-adrenergic receptor (βAR)–coupled cyclic adenosine 3', 5'-monophosphate (cAMP) system. When there is no treatment, basal levels of norepinephrine (NE) stimulate the βAR–coupled cAMP system. Short-term administration of certain types of antidepressants elevates levels of NE, increasing levels of βAR–stimulated cAMP formation. Long-term administration of many types of antidepressants causes down-regulation of the number of βAR-binding sites available to stimulate cAMP production. This in turn leads to a decrease in the maximal level of βAR–stimulated cAMP formation. However, with synaptic levels of NE still elevated as a result of continued antidepressant treatment, the level of cAMP formed remains elevated relative to the no-treatment condition. This possibility requires further testing to determine if levels of βAR–stimulated cAMP formation are indeed elevated. However, this model provides a mechanism to explain how long-term antidepressant treatments activate the cAMP pathway even though levels of βAR are decreased.*

INTRACELLULAR MESSENGERS, NEUROTROPHIC FACTORS, AND DEPRESSION

Advances in molecular and cellular biology have paved the way for studies to determine how antidepressant treatments ultimately regulate the function of target neurons in the brain. There are many comprehensive reviews on intracellular signal transduction pathways,[20-25] and this information will not be discussed in detail herein except as it pertains to antidepressant treatments. In general, these pathways can be divided into 2 broad categories. The first category includes those pathways that are controlled by receptor-coupled second messengers (eg, cAMP, inositol triphosphate, Ca^{2+}, and nitric oxide) and are usually regulated by classic neurotransmitters, such as the monoamines, amino acids, and neuropeptides (**Figure 2**). The second category includes those pathways that are controlled by receptors that contain, or interact with, protein tyrosine kinases and are usually regulated by neurotrophic factors and cytokines; activation of these receptors leads to the regulation of other intracellular cascades, such as the mitogen-activated protein kinase pathway (Figure 2). As the protein kinases and phosphatases, phosphoproteins, transcription factors, and target genes that make up these pathways are increasingly identified and characterized, it is becoming possible to examine how adaptations of these complex pathways are involved in the long-term actions of antidepressant treatments and other psychotropic drugs.

The ability to study these adaptations is a critical advance because these pathways control all aspects of neuronal function and ultimately underlie the ability of the brain to adapt and respond to pharmacological and environmental inputs. The functional consequences of such molecular adaptations can be determined at the cellular level by analysis of the electrophysiological and morpho-

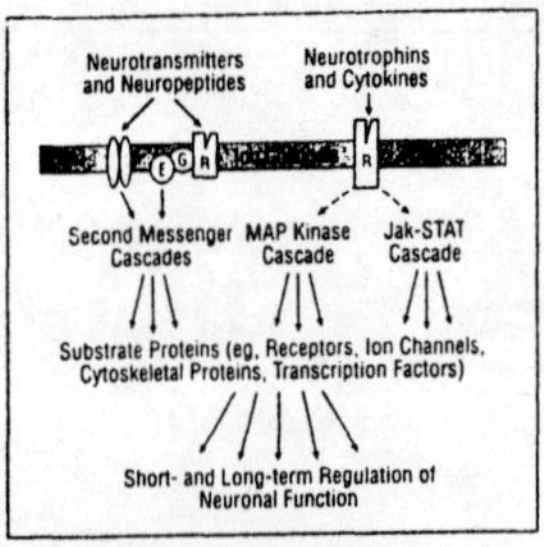

Figure 2. *A general model of receptor-coupled intracellular signal transduction pathways. Intracellular pathways can be subdivided into 2 general categories. Intracellular pathways in the first general category are the second messenger-regulated signaling cascades. These pathways are activated by neurotransmitter or neuropeptide receptors that couple to effector (E) proteins via G proteins. Examples of second messenger cascades include cyclic adenosine monophosphate, cyclic guanosine monophosphate, Ca^{2+}, inositol triphosphate, and nitric oxide. Neurotransmitter regulation of ion channels can also result in regulation of second messenger-dependent pathways. These second messengers lead to the regulation of second messenger-dependent protein serine–threonine kinases. Intracellular pathways in the second general category are the tyrosine kinase–mediated cascades. These pathways are regulated by neurotrophins and cytokines via the activation of receptors (R) that have intrinsic tyrosine kinase activity on the intracellular aspect of the receptors (eg, trkB) or interact with cytoplasmic tyrosine kinases. Activation of these kinases leads to association with other proteins that subsequently activate the mitogen-activated protein (MAP) kinase and Jak-STAT cascades. Regulation of these and the second messenger-dependent protein kinase cascades results in the short- and long-term regulation of neuronal function via the phosphorylation of specific substrate proteins.*

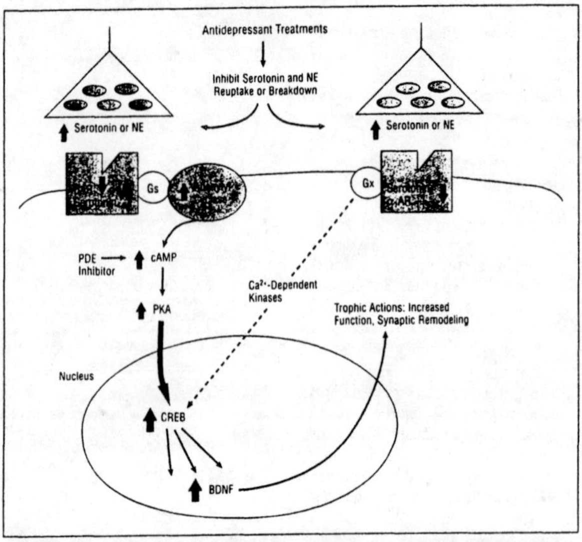

Figure 3. *A model for the molecular mechanism of action of long-term antidepressant treatments. Antidepressants cause a short-term increase in levels of serotonin and noreprinephrine (NE) by inhibiting the reuptake or breakdown of these monoamines. Long-term antidepressant administration decreases the function and expression of certain serotonin and NE receptors (eg, β-adrenergic receptor [βAR] and $serotonin_2$), but the cyclic adenosine 3', 5'-monophosphate (cAMP) signal transduction pathway is increased by long-term antidepressant treatments, including increased levels of adenylyl cyclase and cAMP-dependent protein kinase (PKA), as well as the translocation of PKA to the cell nucleus. Moreover, recent studies demonstrate that expression and function of the transcription factor cAMP response element–binding protein (CREB) is increased by different types of antidepressant treatments, suggesting that CREB is a common postreceptor target for antidepressants. Cyclic adenosine monophosphate response element–binding protein could be regulated by monoamine receptors that couple to the cAMP-PKA cascade ($serotonin_{4,6,7}$ and βAR) or via receptors that lead to the activation of Ca^{2+}-dependent kinases (eg, $serotonin_2$ and α_1-adrenergic receptor [α_1AR]). Increased activity of the cAMP signal transduction cascade indicates that the functional output of serotonin and NE are up-regulated at least in some brain regions, even though levels of certain serotonin and NE receptors are partially down-regulated. This conclusion is further supported by the finding that expression of brain-derived neurotrophic factor (BDNF) and trkB, 2 potential targets of CREB, is also increased by long-term antidepressant treatment. Up-regulation of BDNF and trkB could influence the function of hippocampal neurons or the neurons innervating this brain region, such as serotonin and NE neurons. This could include increased neuronal survival, function, and remodeling of synaptic or cellular architecture.*

logical properties of neurons. Examples of these types of adaptations are the enhanced or diminished synaptic efficacy that is observed in cellular models of learning and memory.[26-29] Morphological changes include atrophy or the sprouting of neurons in response to damaging or growth-promoting stimuli.[30-32]

These types of responses can be viewed as prototypical ways in which the brain adapts to repeated perturbations. Our hypothesis is that similar types of molecular and cellular adaptations occur in response to antidepressant treatments and are involved in the pathophysiology of depression. These types of adaptations are complicated and, in many cases, are difficult to identify, but recognition of their potential importance has stimulated studies that have investigated the role of intracellular pathways and their cellular adaptations in antidepressant action and in depression. Characterization of such adaptations is at a relatively early stage, but has already led to notable conceptual advances in the field.

ANTIDEPRESSANT TREATMENTS ACTIVATE THE cAMP SIGNAL TRANSDUCTION PATHWAY

There are many potential intracellular pathways that could mediate the action of antidepressant treatments. One such pathway that is regulated by the serotonin and NE systems is the cAMP signal transduction cascade (**Figure 3**). Receptor activation leads to the formation of cAMP by coupling to adenylyl cyclase via the stimulatory G protein subtype, Gs. Certain forms of adenylyl cyclase can be activated independent of Gs in response to elevated cellular Ca^{2+} levels.[24] The effects of cAMP are then mediated by the activation of cAMP-dependent protein kinase, which, in turn, leads to the regulation of cellular function by the phosphorylation of specific proteins. One of these is the transcription factor CREB, which mediates many of the actions of the cAMP system on gene expression.[33,34] In addition to its regula-

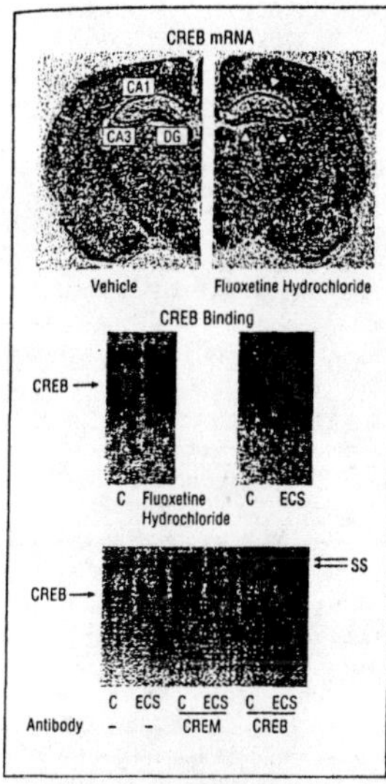

Figure 4. *Long-term antidepressant treatments increase levels of cyclic adenosine 3′, 5′-monophosphate (cAMP) response element–binding protein (CREB) messenger RNA (mRNA) and binding in the hippocampus. The finding that long-term antidepressant treatments increase the expression and function of CREB in the hippocampus is illustrated. The influence of long-term (21 days) fluoxetine hydrochloride administration on levels of CREB messenger RNA was determined by in situ hybridization analysis. Levels of CREB messenger RNA were increased in the major subfields of the hippocampus, including CA3 and CA1 pyramidal and dentate gyrus granule cell layers. Levels of CREB binding were also increased by long-term fluoxetine treatment, as well as electroshock seizures (ECS) (10 days). For this assay, homogenates of the hippocampus are incubated with a radiolabeled, synthetic fragment of DNA that contains a consensus cAMP response element. Binding of CREB shifts the migration of the radiolabeled DNA through the gel. The identity of CREB is confirmed in several ways. First, the CREB binding is reduced by competition with unlabeled DNA containing the cAMP response element, but not with DNA containing a mutated cAMP response element sequence (not shown). Second, supershift (SS) studies (bottom) demonstrate that a specific antibody to CREB, but not CREM (cAMP response element modulatory protein), alters the cAMP response element–binding band. For ss analysis, the homogenate is preincubated with antibody before the radiolabeled DNA is added. If the specific antibody binds to the protein-DNA complex, it either disrupts the complex or supershifts the migration of the complex through the gel.*[44]

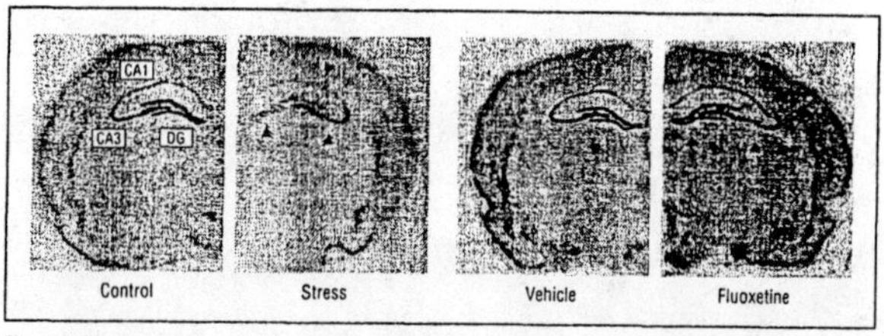

Figure 5. *Stress decreases and antidepressant treatments increase the expression of brain-derived neurotrophic factor in the hippocampus. The influence of acute restraint stress (90 minutes) or long-term fluoxetine hydrochloride administration (21 days) on levels of brain-derived neurotrophic factor messenger RNA were determined by in situ hybridization analysis. The CA3 and CA1 pyramidal and dentate gyrus granule cell layers of the hippocampus are indicated. Pretreatment with fluoxetine or other antidepressants also blocks the down-regulation of brain-derived neurotrophic factor in response to stress.*[52]

tion by phosphorylation, recent studies have demonstrated that expression of the total amount of CREB is another mechanism by which the function of CREB can be regulated.[35-37] The cAMP system is a potential common target for serotonin and NE because there are receptor subtypes for both monoamines that stimulate the formation of this second messenger (Figure 3). In addition to the βAR, there are 3 serotonin receptor subtypes that stimulate the cAMP system (serotonin$_{4,6,7}$), and one of these (serotonin$_7$) is reported to be regulated by long-term antidepressant treatments.[38] Moreover, CREB may represent a common intracellular target for antidepressant treatments because other serotonin or NE receptors (eg, serotonin$_{2A,C}$ and α_1-adrenergic receptors) could also activate CREB via the stimulation of Ca^{2+}-dependent protein kinases (**Figure 4**).[33,34]

Several studies have demonstrated that the postreceptor components of the cAMP system are regulated by long-term antidepressant treatments (Figure 3). Levels of guanine nucleotide–stimulated adenylyl cyclase and cAMP–dependent protein kinase enzyme activity are reported to be increased by long-term antidepressant treatments.[39-43] In addition, we have found that the levels of CREB messenger RNA and protein in the hippocampus are increased by long-term antidepressant treatments, including serotonin and NE selective reuptake inhibitors (Figure 4 and **Figure 5**).[44] The time course for the induction of CREB is consistent with that for the therapeutic actions of antidepressant treatments (ie, 10-21 days of treatment). To further test the hypothesis that CREB is involved in antidepressant actions, it will be important to determine whether the time course for the reversal of these effects is consistent with the offset of therapeutic actions. Increased expression of CREB could be mediated by the up-regulation of cAMP function discussed previously because CREB expression can be induced in cultured cells by the activation of the cAMP cascade.[35] These findings contrast to those of a recent study of CREB function in PC12 cells, an adrenal chromafin cell line.[45] However, in the latter study, the short-term incubation of PC12 cells with antidepressant treatments inhibited depolarization-induced activation of CREB, an effect owing to the blockade of Ca^{2+} channels. To our knowledge, such inhibition of CREB has not been demonstrated in vivo.

Increased function and expression of CREB provides direct support for the proposal that the cAMP signal transduction system is increased in the hippocampus by long-term antidepressant treatments. Induction of the intracellular components of the cAMP cascade may also explain the requirement for long-term antidepressant treatments, even though levels of cAMP may be elevated by short-term antidepressant treatments (Figure 1 and Figure 3). Our results also indicate the types of specific gene elements likely to be regulated by long-term antidepressant treatments; that is, those with functional cAMP response elements. However, not all genes with a cAMP response element would be expected to be activated by antidepressant treatments. First, up-regulation of the cAMP system and CREB is not observed in all brain regions (there is evidence for down-regulation of the cAMP system in the locus coeruleus[46]). Second, regulation of gene expression is dependent on the activity and interaction of several different promoter elements and transcription factors. Thus, activation of the cAMP system and CREB may lead to the regulation of a specific set of genes in the hippocampus that are involved in the action of antidepressant treatments. One goal of current studies is to identify these genes and to determine their relevance to the clinical responses to antidepressant treatments. Recent studies have identified BDNF and its receptor, trkB, as 2 potential target genes of interest.

ANTIDEPRESSANT TREATMENTS REGULATE NEUROTROPHINS

Brain-derived neurotrophic factor is a member of the nerve growth factor family, which also includes the prototype nerve growth factor as well as neurotrophin-3 and neurotrophin-4. These growth factors are involved in the differentiation and growth of many types of neurons in the developing brain as well as the maintenance and survival of neurons in the mature brain.[30-32,47] For example, the survival and growth of serotonin neurons in the adult brain is increased by BDNF and, to a lesser degree, by neurotrophin-3, but not by the nerve growth factor.[48] Also, neurotrophins can rapidly influence the function of neurons, as demonstrated by the finding that short-term exposure of hippocampal slices to BDNF increases the strength of certain synaptic connections.[28,29] These types of findings, along with an increasing appreciation of the neurotrophic actions of the monoamines,[49,50] highlight the large overlap between the roles played by neurotrophins and monoamines in the regulation of brain function. The actions of neurotrophins are mediated by binding to specific receptors, referred to as trkB receptors, which lead to the activation of protein tyrosine kinase activity located on the intracellular domain of the receptors.

Recent studies have provided support for the notion that neurotrophins and neuronal plasticity and survival may be involved in the treatment of depression. First, BDNF is reported to have antidepressant effects in 2 behavioral models of depression, the forced swim and learned helplessness paradigms.[51] Second, long-term, but not short-term, antidepressant administration, including serotonin and NE selective reuptake inhibitors, a monoamine oxidase inhibitor, an atypical antidepressant, as well as electroshock seizures, increases the expression of BDNF and trkB in the hippocampus (Figure 3 and Figure 5).[44,52] Third, BDNF is reported to enhance the growth of serotonin and NE neurons, as well as to protect these neurons from neurotoxic damage.[48,53] While these findings support a role for BDNF in the actions of antidepressant treatments, studies of additional antidepressant and nonantidepressant agents are required to further test this hypothesis. In addition, the role of other neurotrophic factors (eg, nerve growth factor, neurotrophin-3, and neurotrophin-4) should be examined.

The possibility that increased expression of BDNF results from the activation of CREB is supported by several lines of evidence. First, the time course for the up-regulation of CREB is similar to that of BDNF. Second, the regulation of CREB and BDNF is observed in the same populations of neurons in the hippocampus (Figure 4 and Figure 5). Third, studies in primary neuronal cultures have demonstrated that the stimulation of cAMP- or Ca^{2+}-activated protein kinases increases the expression of BDNF.[54,55] Finally, the reduction of CREB levels in the hippocampus by the administration of antisense oligonucleotides to CREB messenger RNA decreases basal levels of BDNF and blocks the induction of BDNF by antidepressant treatments.[49] Additional in vitro and in vivo studies are needed to demonstrate a direct link between CREB and the expression of BDNF.

A ROLE FOR NEUROTROPHINS IN DEPRESSION

There is also evidence of a neurotrophic element in the pathophysiology of certain forms of depression. First, immobilization stress causes a dramatic reduction in BDNF expression in the hippocampus of rats (Figure 5).[56] The relevance of this finding requires further examination. For example, do other types of stress (eg, psychosocial), which can precipitate or exacerbate depression, also decrease the expression of BDNF? Second, chronic stress of several types (ie, restraint or psychosocial) or glucocorticoid treatments are reported to cause atrophy, or even death, of vulnerable neurons in the hippocampus in rats and nonhuman primates.[57-63] The CA3 pyramidal neurons seem to be most vulnerable to stress, although other populations of neurons seem to be sensitive to stress, glucocorticoids, cytokines, and other types of neuronal insult, such as hypoxia-ischemia or hypoglycemia.[64] Third, the ability of the hippocampus to inhibit the hypothalamic–pituitary–adrenal axis is reduced in certain patients with depression, consistent with a deficit of hippocampal function in these individuals.[65] Fourth, there is a small decrease in hippocampal volume as determined by magnetic resonance imaging in patients with depression or posttraumatic stress disorder.[66-68] In addition, a recent review of the literature provides evidence to suggest that there may be a decrease in the size of certain brain structures in depression.[69] Down-regulation of BDNF may contribute to the atrophy of neurons in the hippocampus in response to stress. However, not all episodes of depression are associated with stress, and the model presented may be limited to certain subtypes of depression. Postmortem studies to demonstrate atrophy or neuronal death directly in the hippocampus of patients with depression are required to further test this hypothesis.

These studies form the basis of a molecular and cellular model of depression and antidepressant action (**Figure 6**). Depression, particularly stress-associated cases, may result from the atrophy or death of vulnerable pyramidal neurons in the CA3 region of the hippocampus. This could be a consequence, at least in part, of the decreased levels of BDNF available to these neurons. Elevated levels of glucocorticoids are also known to play a notable role in stress-induced damage of CA3 neurons.[57-63] Antidepressant treatments could reverse this atrophy by increasing BDNF expression and function. In fact, we have found that long-term antidepressant pretreatment blocks the down-regulation of BDNF in response to stress.[52] Normalization of glucocorticoid levels by antidepressant treatments in some individuals could be an additional mechanism for the prevention of further neuronal damage.[70] Further studies are required to determine whether antidepressant treatments have direct neuroprotective effects or neurotrophic actions on hippocampal neurons as suggested by early studies.[71,72] Recent studies are encouraging. We have found that long-term electroshock treatment causes sprouting of granule neurons in the hippocampus.[73] Unlike the sprouting observed in response to kindling or excitotoxin treatment, there was no obvious cell damage after long-term electroshock treatment. In addition, electroshock-induced sprouting was markedly attenuated in mutant knockout mice that express reduced levels of BDNF. These results indicate that electroshock induces sprouting of certain hippocampal neurons and that the response is mediated by the increased expression of BDNF in these neurons. The observation that antidepressant treatments can lead to the reinstatement of hippocampal control of the hypothalamic–pituitary–adrenal axis in some patients further supports the possibility that the function of these neurons, indeed, can be improved.[65]

One challenge in depression research is the difficulty of identifying specific anatomical substrates involved in the disorder. The hippocampus is involved in the control of emotion, learning and memory, and the regulation of the hypothalamic–pituitary–adrenal axis, as well as other vegetative processes. Changes in the structure or function of hippocampal neurons could be involved in the affective, neuroendocrine, cognitive, and vegetative abnormalities observed in depression. However, these abnormalities are also likely to be influenced by several other limbic brain structures and it is possible that stress alters the structure and function of neurons in these brain regions as well.

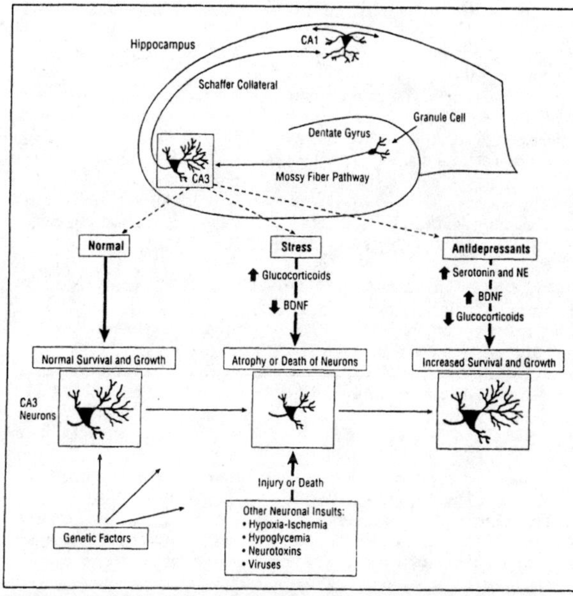

Figure 6. *A molecular and cellular model for the action of antidepressant treatments and the pathophysiology of stress-related disorders. This model of the hippocampus shows the major cell types in the hippocampus and how stress and antidepressant treatments may influence CA3 pyramidal cells. The 3 major subfields of the hippocampus (CA3 and CA1 pyramidal cells and dentate gyrus granule cells) are connected by the mossy fiber and Schaffer collateral pathways. Recent studies demonstrate that chronic stress decreases the expression of brain-derived neurotrophic factor (BDNF) in the hippocampus. This could contribute to the atrophy or death of neurons in the CA3 pyramidal cell layer of the hippocampus. Long-term elevation of glucocorticoid levels is also known to decrease the survival of these neurons. Other types of neuronal insult such as hypoxia-ischemia, hypoglycemia, neurotoxins, and viral infections could also cause atrophy or damage of neurons and could, thereby, make an individual vulnerable to subsequent insults. These types of interactions could underlie the observations of decreased function and volume of hippocampus in patients with affective disorders and could explain the selective vulnerability of certain individuals to become depressed. Long-term antidepressant treatments increase the expression of BDNF, as well as trkB, and prevent the down-regulation of BDNF elicited by stress. This could increase the growth or survival of neurons, or help repair or protect neurons from further damage. Increased expression of BDNF and trkB seems to be mediated by the sustained elevation of the serotonin and norepinephrine (NE) systems and the cyclic adenosine monophosphate cascade. Normalization of glucocorticoid levels by long-term antidepressant treatments could also contribute to the recovery of CA3 neurons.*

A HYPOTHESIS FOR GENETIC AND ENVIRONMENTAL VULNERABILITIES

It is widely believed that depression results from a combination of genetic and environmental factors. Yet, virtually nothing is known about the specific genes that may predispose certain individuals to depression and render others relatively resistant. Studies of the cAMP pathway, CREB, and BDNF, discussed previously, demonstrate the enormous number of genes that could be involved. Indeed, these studies highlight the naivete of candidate gene strategies to identify depression vulnerability genes, which remain focused on monoamine metabolic enzymes, receptors, and reuptake proteins. These studies indicate the need for more open-ended investigations of the genetic factors involved in depression.

However, it could be immediately informative to examine how

various types of environmental factors may predispose certain individuals to mood disorders based on our hypothesis. One possibility is that many individuals who become depressed may have had a prior exposure to stress that causes a small amount of neuronal damage, but not enough to precipitate a behavioral change. If additional damage occurs, either as a result of normal aging or further stressful stimuli, these effects may then be manifested in the symptoms of a mood disorder. These types of events could explain the decreased volume of specific brain structures in depression. This model could also explain how other types of neuronal insult predispose an individual to mood disorders. Insults such as hypoxia-ischemia, hypoglycemia, neurotoxins, or viral infections could cause direct neuronal damage or render neurons more vulnerable to psychosocial stress (Figure 6). Such changes could lead to depression at later times or, if severe enough, could immediately precipitate a depressive episode. For example, a high incidence of depression is well documented in patients who have had a stroke.[74-76] The possible involvement of myriad environmental factors implicates many additional sets of genes that could conceivably alter an individual's inherent responses to stress and establish a diathesis for depression. The possible role of a subtle neurodegenerative contribution to the pathophysiology of depression should be directly examined by analysis of postmortem tissue, as discussed previously.

RATIONAL DESIGN OF NOVEL THERAPEUTIC AGENTS

New information indicating a role for the cAMP pathway and CREB in the actions of antidepressant treatments suggests novel approaches to develop faster-acting and more effective agents. The development and testing of such agents will also help to further test our hypothesis. First, receptor agonists could be targeted at the specific serotonin or NE receptors that stimulate cAMP- or Ca^{2+}-activated protein kinases and mediate the antidepressant induction of BDNF. These receptor sites must first be identified, although the βAR and the $serotonin_{4,6,7}$ receptor sites are likely candidates. Second, identification of other neurotransmitter receptors that stimulate cAMP- or Ca^{2+}-activated protein kinases in the hippocampus could be additional targets. Third, agents that directly stimulate cAMP- or Ca^{2+}-activated kinases, or that directly activate CREB, could be developed. Fourth, the inhibition of cAMP breakdown would enhance the function of CREB and increase BDNF expression. Fifth, agents that activate the BDNF-trkB signaling pathway may be of some use. The first 2 possibilities have the potential for regulating the function of CREB and the expression of BDNF specifically in the hippocampus, depending on the distribution of the receptors targeted, but may not be much more effective than available treatments. Conversely, the last 3 possibilities may be less specific because they would be expected to influence many brain regions as well as peripheral tissues that express these intracellular targets, but may be more effective. There has been legitimate concern regarding the specificity and safety of such agents. However, it is impossible to predict the effects of such agents until prototypical compounds are available for evaluation. Moreover, some agents, such as lithium and nonsteroidal anti-inflammatory agents (which affect arachidonic acid metabolism), are enormously effective for their respective indications despite their generalized actions.

The possibility that the inhibition of cAMP breakdown increases BDNF expression has been examined. Long-term administration of inhibitors of phosphodiesterases, the enzymes that metabolize cAMP, increases the expression of CREB and BDNF in the hippocampus of rats.[44] Moreover, coadministration of a phosphodiesterase inhibitor with a tricyclic antidepressant results in a more rapid induction of CREB and BDNF.[44] These findings provide additional support for the hypothesis that the cAMP system regulates the expression of BDNF and suggest that the inhibition of cAMP metabolism may provide a mechanism for a more rapid treatment of depression. The notion that the inhibition of cAMP metabolism may have antidepressant effects was raised several years ago[77] and was supported by preliminary clinical studies with rolipram, a potent phosphodiesterase inhibitor.[78] The lack of further progress on the therapeutic potential of phosphodiesterase inhibitors raises questions about the efficacy of these agents in the treatment of depression. However, given the recent observations, it may be time to reevaluate the therapeutic potential of phosphodiesterase inhibitors. One potential application that has not been investigated is the use of phosphodiesterase inhibitors as augmenting agents with other antidepressant treatments that block the reuptake or metabolism of monoamines. This approach could allow the cAMP system to be augmented in specific brain regions that contain the appropriate serotonin and NE receptors.

COMMENT

Although the regulation of CREB and BDNF may be important in the actions of antidepressant treatments, it would be preliminary and naive to suggest that these are the sole targets of these treatments. There are many genes that are known to be regulated by the cAMP system and certain antidepressant treatments.[70,79-86] In addition, the cAMP cascade is just one of many intracellular pathways that could be regulated by serotonin and NE and could be important to the action of antidepressant treatments. One example is the regulation of the phosphatidylinositol system and protein kinase C by lithium.[87-91]

The findings discussed herein indicate that antidepressant action is not mediated by the simple up- or down-regulation of monoamines and their receptors. Elucidation of the role of the cAMP system and BDNF in the response to antidepressant treatments provides fundamentally new leads in understanding antidepressant action and the pathophysiology of depression. Although the studies discussed provide a framework for a unifying hypothesis, it requires further testing of its several components. However, the model incorporates the important role of the monoamines in these phenomena and begins to elaborate the many molecular and cellular mechanisms influenced by the monoamines that are more proximal to the complex adaptations in brain function that underlie depression and its treatment.

Accepted for publication June 18, 1996.

This study was supported by grants MH45481, MH53199, and 2 PO1 MH25642 from the National Institute of Mental Health, National Institutes of Health, Bethesda, Md; a Veterans Administration National Center Grant, Veterans Affairs Medical Center, West Haven, Conn; and the Abraham Ribicoff Research Facilities of the Connecticut Mental Health Center, State of Connecticut Department of Mental Health and Addiction Services, New Haven.

Corresponding author: Ronald S. Duman, PhD, Connecticut Mental Health Center, 34 Park St, New Haven, CT 06508.

REFERENCES

1. Schildkaut JJ. The catecholamine hypothesis of affective disorders: a review of supporting evidence. *Am J Psychiatry.* 1965;122:509-522.
2. Bunney WE, Davis J. Norepinephrine in depressive reactions: a review. *Arch Gen Psychiatry.* 1965;13:483-494.
3. Coppen A. The biochemistry of affective disorders. *Br J Psychiatry.* 1967;113:1237-1264.
4. Shopsin B, Gershon S, Goldstein M, Friedman E, Wilk S. Use of synthesis inhibitors in defining a role for biogenic amines during imipramine treatment in depressed patients. *Psychopharmacol Commun.* 1975;1:239-249.
5. Delgado PL, Price LH, Miller HL, Salomon RM, Aghajanian G, Heniner GR, Charney D. Serotonin and the neurobiology of depression. *Arch Gen Psychiatry.* 1994;51:865-874.
6. Miller HL, Delgado PL, Salomon RM, Berman R, Krystal JH, Heninger GR, Charney DS. Clinical and biochemical effects of catecholamine depletion on antidepressant-induced remission of depression. *Arch Gen Psychiatry.* 1996;53:117-128.
7. Sulser F, Vetulani J, Mobley P. Mode of action of antidepressant drugs. *Biochem Pharmacol.* 1978; 27:257-261.
8. Charney DS, Menkes DB, Heninger GR. Receptor sensitivity and the mechanism of action of antidepressant treatment: implications for the etiology and therapy of depression. *Arch Gen Psychiatry.* 1981;38:1160-1180.
9. Heninger GR, Charney DS. Mechanisms of action of antidepressant treatments: implications for the etiology and treatment of depressive disorders. In: Meltzer HY, ed. *Psychopharmacology: The Third Generation of Progress.* New York, NY: Raven Press; 1987:535-544.
10. Vetulani J, Sulser F. Action of various antidepressant treatments reduces reactivity of noradrenergic cAMP-generating system in limbic forebrain. *Nature.* 1975;257:495-496.
11. Banerjee SP, Kung LS, Riggi SJ, Chanda SK. Development of β-adrenergic receptor subsensitivity by antidepressants. *Nature.* 1977;268:455-456.
12. Peroutka SL, Snyder SH. Long-term antidepressant treatment decreases spiroperidol-labeled serotonin receptor binding. *Science.* 1980;210:88-90.
13. Riva MA, Creese I. Re-evaluation of the regulation of β-adrenergic receptor binding by desipramine treatment. *Mol Pharmacol.* 1989;36:211-218.
14. Butler MO, Morinobu S, Duman RS. Chronic electroconvulsive seizures increase the expression of serotonin$_2$ receptor mRNA in rat frontal cortex. *J Neurochem.* 1993;61:1270-1276.
15. Paykel ES, Fleminger R, Watson JP. Psychiatric side effects of antihypertensive drugs other than reserpine. *J Clin Psychopharmacol.* 1982;2:14-39.
16. Avorn J, Everitt DE, Weiss S. Increased antidepressant use in patients prescribed β-blockers. *JAMA.* 1986;255:357-360.
17. Goodwin FK, Prange AJ, Post RM, Muscettola G, Lipton MA. Potentiation of antidepressant effect by triiodothyronine in tricyclic nonresponders. *Am J Psychiatry.* 1982;139:34-38.
18. Blier P, de Montigny C. Current advances and trends in the treatment of depression. *Trends Pharmacol Sci.* 1994;15:220-226.
19. Stone EA. Problems with the current hypotheses of antidepressant agents: speculations leading to a new hypothesis. *Behav Brain Sci.* 1983;6:535-577.
20. Berridge MJ. Inositol triphosphate and calcium signaling. *Nature.* 1993;361:315-325.
21. Blenis J. Signal transduction via the MAP kinases: proceed at your own RSK. *Proc Natl Acad Sci U S A.* 1993;90:5889-5892.
22. Hudson CJ, Young LT, Li PP, Warsh JJ. CNS signal transduction in the pathophysiology and pharmacotherapy of affective disorders and schizophrenia. *Synapse.* 1993;13:278-293.
23. Darnell JE, Kerr IM, Stark GR. Jak-STAT pathways and transcriptional activation in response to IFNs and other extracellular signaling proteins. *Science.* 1994;264:1415-1421.
24. Nestler EJ, Duman RS. G proteins and cyclic nucleotides in the nervous system. In: Siegel G, Agranoff B, Albers RW, Molinoff P, eds. *Basic Neurochemistry.* 5th ed. New York, NY: Raven Press; 1994:429-448.
25. Duman RS, Nestler EJ. Signal transduction pathways for catecholamine receptors. In: Meltzer H, ed. *Psychopharmacology: The Fourth Generation of Progress.* New York, NY: Raven Press; 1995:303-320.
26. Madison DV, Malenka RC, Nicoll RA. Mechanisms underlying long-term potentiation of synaptic transmission. *Ann Rev Neurosci.* 1991;14: 379-397.
27. Bliss TVP, Collingridge G. A synaptic model of memory: long-term potentiation in the hippocampus. *Nature.* 1993;361:31-39.
28. Kang H, Schuman EM. Long-lasting neurotrophin-induced enhancement of synaptic transmission in the adult hippocampus. *Science.* 1995;267:1658-1662.
29. Levine ES, Dreyfus CF, Black IB, Plummer MR. Brain-derived neurotrophic factor rapidly enhances transmission in hippocampal neurons via postsynaptic tyrosine kinase receptors. *Proc Natl Acad Sci U S A.* 1995;92:8074-8077.
30. Lindsay RM, Wiegand SJ, Altar CA, Di Stefano PS. Neurotrophic factors: from molecule to man. *Trends Neurosci.* 1994;17:182-190.
31. Lindvall O, Kokaia Z, Bengzon J, Elmer E, Kokaia M. Neurotrophins and brain insults. *Trends Neurosci.* 1994;17:490-496.
32. Thoenen H. Neurotrophins and neuronal plasticity. *Science.* 1995;270:593-598.
33. Meyer TE, Habener JF. Cyclic adenosine 3',5'-monophosphate response element-binding protein (CREB) and related transcription-activating deoxyribonucleic acid-binding proteins. *Endocr Rev.* 1993;14:269-290.
34. Ghosh A, Greenberg ME. Calcium signaling in neurons: molecular mechanisms and cellular consequences. *Science.* 1995;268:239-247.
35. Walker WH, Fucci L, Habener JF. Expression of the gene encoding transcription factor cyclic adenosine 3',5'-monophosphate (cAMP) response element-binding protein (CREB): regulation by follicle-stimulating hormone-induced cAMP signalling in primary rat Sertoli cells. *Endocrinology.* 1995; 136:3534-3545.
36. Widnell KL, Russell DS, Nestler EJ. Regulation of expression of cAMP response element-binding protein in the locus coeruleus in vivo and in a locus coeruleus-like cell line in vitro. *Proc Natl Acad Sci U S A.* 1994;91:10947-10951.
37. Widnell KL, Self DW, Lane SB, Russell DS, Vaidya VA, Miserendino MJD, Rubin CR, Duman RS, Nestler EJ. Regulation of CREB expression: in vivo evidence for a functional role in morphine action in the nucleus accumbens. *J Pharmacol Exp Ther.* 1996;276:306-315.
38. Sleight AJ, Carolo C, Petit N, Zwingelstein C, Bourson A. Identification of 5-hydroxytryptamine$_7$ receptor binding sites in rat hypothalamus: sensitivity to chronic antidepressant treatments. *Mol Pharmacol.* 1995;47:99-103.
39. Menkes DB, Rasenick MM, Wheeler MA, Bitensky MW. Guanosine triphosphate activation of brain adenylate cyclase: enhancement by long-term antidepressant treatment. *Science.* 1983; 129:65-67.
40. Ozawa H, Rasenick MM. Chronic electroconvulsive treatment augments coupling of the GTP-binding protein Gs to the catalytic moiety of adenylyl cyclase in a manner similar to that seen with chronic antidepressant drugs. *J Neurochem.* 1991; 56:330-338.
41. Colin SF, Chang HC, Mollner S, Pfeuffer T, Reed RR, Duman RS, Nestler EJ. Chronic lithium regulates the expression of adenylate cyclase and Gi-protein alpha in rat cerebral cortex. *Proc Natl Acad Sci U S A.* 1991;88:10634-10637.
42. Nestler EJ, Terwilliger RZ, Duman RS. Chronic antidepressant administration alters the subcellular distribution of cyclic AMP-dependent protein kinase in rat frontal cortex. *J Neurochem.* 1989; 53:1644-1647.
43. Perez J, Tinelli D, Brunello N, Racagni G. cAMP-dependent phosphorylation of soluble and crude microtubule fractions of rat cerebral cortex after prolonged desmethylimipramine treatment. *Eur J Pharmacol.* 1989;172:305-316.
44. Nibuya M, Nestler EJ, Duman RS. Chronic antidepressant administration increases the expression of cAMP response element-binding protein (CREB) in rat hippocampus. *J Neurosci.* 1996;16: 2365-2372.
45. Schwaninger M, Schoel C, Blume R, Rossig L, Knepel W. Inhibition by antidepressant drugs of cyclic AMP response element-binding protein/ cyclic AMP response element-directed gene transcription. *Mol Pharmacol.* 1995;47:1112-1118.

46. Melia KR, Rasmussen K, Haycock J, Terwilliger RZ, Nestler EJ, Duman RS. Coordinate regulation of firing rate, tyrosine hydroxylase, and the cyclic AMP system in rat locus coeruleus: effects of chronic stress and norepinephrine depleting agents. *J Neurochem.* 1992;58:494-502.
47. Lo DC. Neurotrophic factors and synaptic plasticity. *Neuron.* 1995;15:979-981.
48. Mamounas LA, Blue ME, Siuciak JA, Altar CA. BDNF promotes the survival and sprouting of serotonergic axons in the rat brain. *J Neurosci.* 1995;15:7929-7939.
49. Duman RS, Vaidya VA, Nibuya M, Morinobu S, Rydelek-Fitzgerald L. Stress, antidepressant treatments, and neurotrophic factors: molecular and cellular mechanisms. *Neuroscientist.* 1995;1:351-360.
50. Azmitia EC, Rubenstein VJ, Strafaci JA, Rios JC, Whitaker-Azmitia PM. 5-HT_{1A} agonist and dexamethasone reversal of para-chloroamphetamine-induced loss of MAP-2 and synaptophysin immunoreactivity in adult rat brain. *Brain Res.* 1995;677:181-192.
51. Siuciak JA, Lewis D, Wiegand SJ, Lindsay RM. Antidepressant-like effect of brain-derived neurotrophic factor. *Pharmacol Biochem Behav.* 1996;56:131-137.
52. Nibuya M, Morinobu S, Duman RS. Regulation of BDNF and trkB mRNA in rat brain by chronic electroconvulsive seizure and antidepressant drug treatments. *J Neurosci.* 1995;15:7539-7547.
53. Sklair-Tavron L, Nestler EJ. Opposing effects of morphine and the neurotrophins NT-3, NT-4, and BDNF, on locus coeruleus neurons in vitro. *Brain Res.* 1995;702:117-125.
54. Ghosh A, Carnahan J, Greenberg ME. Requirement for BDNF in activity-dependent survival of cortical neurons. *Science.* 1994;263:1618-1623.
55. Condorelli DF, Dell'Albani P, Mudo G, Timmusk T, Belluardo N. Expression of neurotrophins and their receptors in primary astroglial cultures: induction by cAMP-elevating agents. *J Neurochem.* 1994;63:509-516.
56. Smith MA, Makino S, Kvetnansky R, Post RM. Stress alters the expression of brain-derived neurotrophic factor and neurotrophin-3 mRNAs in the hippocampus. *J Neurosci.* 1995;15:1768-1777.
57. Sapolsky RM, Krey LC, McEwen BS. Prolonged glucocorticoid exposure reduces hippocampal neuron number: implications for aging. *J Neurosci.* 1985;5:1222-1227.
58. Uno H, Tarara R, Else JG, Suleman MA, Sapolsky RM. Hippocampal damage associated with prolonged and fatal stress in primates. *J Neurosci.* 1989;9:1705-1711.
59. Sapolsky RM, Uno H, Robert CS, Finsh CE. Hippocampal damage associated with prolonged glucocorticoid exposure in primates. *J Neurosci.* 1990;10:2897-2902.
60. Wooley CS, Gould E, McEwen BS. Exposure to excess glucocorticoids alters dendritic morphology of adult hippocampal pyramidal neurons. *Brain Res.* 1990;531:225-231.
61. Watanabe Y, Gould E, McEwen BS. Stress induces atrophy of apical dendrites of hippocampal CA3 pyramidal neurons. *Brain Res.* 1982;588:341-345.
62. Stein-Behrens B, Mattson MP, Chang I, Yeh M, Sapolsky R. Stress exacerbates neuron loss and cytoskeletal pathology in the hippocampus. *J Neurosci.* 1994;14:5373-5380.
63. Magarinos AM, McEwen BS, Flugge G, Fuchs E. Chronic psychosocial stress causes apical dendritic atrophy of hippocampal CA3 pyramidal neurons in subordinate tree shrews. *J Neurosci.* 1996;16:3534-3540.
64. Sapolsky R. Glucocorticoids, hippocampus, and the glutamatergic synapse. *Prog Brain Res.* 1990;86:13-23.
65. Young EA, Haskett RF, Murphy-Weinberg V, Watson SJ, Akil H. Loss of glucocorticoid fast feedback in depression. *Arch Gen Psychiatry.* 1991;48:693-699.
66. Sheline YI, Wany P, Gado MH, Csernansky JG, Vannier MW. Hippocampal atrophy in recurrent major depression. *Proc Natl Acad Sci U S A.* 1996;93:3908-3913.
67. Sapolsky RM. Glucocorticoids and atrophy of the human hippocampus. *Science.* 1996;273:749-775.
68. Bremner JD, Randall P, Scott TM, Bronen RA, Seibyl JP, Southwick SM, Delaney RC, McCarthy G, Charney DS, Innis RB. MRI-based measurement of hippocampal volume in patients with combat-related posttraumatic stress disorder. *Am J Psychiatry.* 1995;152:973-981.
69. Elkis H, Friedman L, Wise A, Meltzer HY. Meta-analysis of studies of ventricular enlargement and cortical sulcal prominence in mood disorders. *Arch Gen Psychiatry.* 1995;52:735-746.
70. Barden N, Reul JMH, Holsboer F. Do antidepressants stabilize mood through actions on the hypothalamic-pituitary-adrenocortical system? *Trends Neurosci.* 1995;18:6-11.
71. Nakamura S. Antidepressants induce regeneration of catecholaminergic axon terminals in the rat cerebral cortex. *Neurosci Lett.* 1990;111:64-68.
72. Watanabe Y, Gould E, Daniels DC, Cameron H, McEwen BS. Tianeptine attenuates stress-induced morphological changes in the hippocampus. *Eur J Pharmacol.* 1992;222:157-162.
73. Vaidya VA, Duman RS. Chronic ECS induces mossy fiber sprouting. *Soc Neurosci.* 1996;22:181.
74. Reding MJ, Orto LA, Winter SW, Firtuna IM, Di Ponte P, McDowell FH. Antidepressant therapy after stroke: a double-blind trial. *Arch Neurol.* 1986;43:763-765.
75. Stern RA, Bachmann DL. Depressive symptoms following stroke. *Am J Psychiatry.* 1991;148:351-356.
76. Fedoroff J, Starkstein S, Forrester A, et al. Depression in patients with acute traumatic brain injury. *Am J Psychiatry.* 1992;149:918-923.
77. Wachtel H. Potential antidepressant activity of rolipram and other selective cyclic adenosine 3',5'-monophosphate phosphodiesterase inhibitors. *Neuropharmacology.* 1983;22:267-272.
78. Horowski R, Sastre-Y-Hernandez M. Clinical effects of the neurotrophic selective cAMP phosphodiesterase inhibitor rolipram in depressed patients: global evaluation of the preliminary reports. *Curr Ther Res.* 1985;38:23-29.
79. Duman RS, Heninger GR, Nestler EJ. Adaptations of receptor-coupled signal transduction pathways underlying stress- and drug-induced neural plasticity. *J Nerv Ment Disease.* 1994;182:692-700.
80. Hosoda K, Duman RS. Regulation of β-adrenergic receptor mRNA and ligand binding by antidepressant treatments and norepinepnrine depletion in rat frontal cortex. *J Neurochem.* 1993;60:1335-1343.
81. Hosoda K, Feussner GK, Rydelek-Fitzgerald L, Fishman PH, Duman RS. Agonist and cyclic AMP-mediated regulation of β_1-adrenergic receptor mRNA and gene transcription in rat C6 glioma cells. *J Neurochem.* 1994;63:1635-1645.
82. Li PP, Tam YK, Young T, Warsh JJ. Lithium decreases Gs, Gi-1 and Gi-2α-subunit mRNA levels in rat cortex. *Eur J Pharm.* 1991;206:165-166.
83. Winston SM, Hayward MD, Nestler EJ, Duman RS. Chronic electroconvulsive seizures down-regulate expression of the immediate-early genes c-fos and c-jun proto-oncogenes in rat cerebral cortex. *J Neurochem.* 1990;54:1920-1925.
84. Duncan GE, Johnson KB, Breese GR. Topographic patterns of brain activity in response to swim stress: assessment by 2-deoxyglucose uptake and expression of fos-like immunoreactivity. *J Neurosci.* 1993;13:3932-3934.
85. Hope BT, Kelz M, Duman RS, Nestler EJ. Chronic electroconvulsive seizure (ECS) treatment results in expression of a long-lasting AP-1 complex in brain with altered composition and characteristics. *J Neurosci.* 1994;14:4318-4328.
86. Morinobu S, Nibuya M, Duman RS. Chronic antidepressant treatment down-regulates the induction of c-fos mRNA in response to acute stress in rat frontal cortex. *Neuropsychopharmacology.* 1995;12:221-228.
87. Casebolt TL, Jope RS. Effects of chronic lithium treatment on protein kinase C and cyclic AMP-dependent protein phosphorylation. *Biol Psychiatry.* 1991;29:233-243.
88. Lenox RH, Watson DG, Patel J, Ellis J. Chronic lithium administration alters a prominent PKC substrate in rat hippocampus. *Brain Res.* 1992;570:333-340.
89. Li PP, Sibony D, Green MA, Warsh JJ. Lithium modulation of phosphoinositide signaling system in rat cortex: selective effect on phorbol ester binding. *J Neurochem.* 1993;61:1722-1730.
90. Manji HK, Etcheberrigaray R, Chen G, Olds JL. Lithium decreases membrane-associated protein kinase C in hippocampus: selectivity for the a isozyme. *J Neurochem.* 1993;61:2303-2310.
91. Manji HK, Potter WZ, Lenox RH. Signal transduction pathways: molecular targets for lithium's actions. *Arch Gen Psychiatry.* 1995;52:531-543.

The Impact of Early Adverse Experiences on Brain Systems Involved in the Pathophysiology of Anxiety and Affective Disorders

Christine Heim and Charles B. Nemeroff

The relative contribution of genetic and environmental factors to the development of the major psychiatric disorders has long been debated. Recently, considerable attention has been given to the observations that adverse experiences early in life predispose individuals to the development of affective and anxiety disorders in adulthood. Corticotropin-releasing factor (CRF) is the central coordinator of the endocrinologic, autonomic, immunologic, and behavioral stress responses. When centrally administered, CRF produces many physiologic and behavioral changes reminiscent of both acute stress and depression. Moreover, CRF has also been implicated in the pathogenesis of a variety of anxiety disorders, mainly through CRF neurocircuits connecting the amygdala and the locus ceruleus. Clinical studies have provided convincing evidence for central CRF hypersecretion in depression, and, to a lesser extent, in some anxiety disorders. Evidence mainly from preclinical studies suggests that stress early in life results in persistent central CRF hyperactivity and increased stress reactivity in adulthood. Thus, genetic disposition coupled with early stress in critical phases of development may result in a phenotype that is neurobiologically vulnerable to stress and may lower an individual's threshold for developing depression and anxiety upon further stress exposure. This pathophysiologic model may provide novel approaches to the prevention and treatment of psychopathology associated with stress early in life. Biol Psychiatry 1999;46:1509–1522 © *1999 Society of Biological Psychiatry*

Key Words: Anxiety, depression, development, stress, corticotropin-releasing factor

Are neuroses exogenous or endogenous illnesses? Are they the inevitable result of a particular constitution or the product of certain detrimental (traumatic) experiences in life? (Freud 1895)

From the Department of Psychiatry and Behavioral Sciences, Emory University School of Medicine, Atlanta, Georgia.

Address reprint requests to Charles B. Nemeroff, Department of Psychiatry and Behavioral Sciences, Emory University School of Medicine, 1639 Pierce Drive, WMRB, Suite 4000, Atlanta, GA 30322.

Received April 6, 1999; revised August 3, 1999; accepted August 10, 1999.

Introduction

From the past to present times, the relative contribution of disposition and experience to the pathogenesis of mental disorders has been explored in numerous studies. Evidence from these studies suggests a strong genetic contribution to the development of the major psychiatric disorders. In addition, a preeminent role of stressful life events has been documented for several disorders, especially mood and anxiety disorders, but schizophrenia as well. A number of studies have shown that the onset of depression is often preceded by stressful life events, and there is evidence that concomitant chronic stress enhances the effects of major life events on depression (Kessler 1997). Likewise, stressful life events along with recent minor difficulties have been identified as predictors of an episode of depression in a monozygotic female twin study (Kendler and Magee 1993). Moreover, genetically vulnerable individuals are more likely to develop major depression in response to stress than individuals without genetic loading (Kendler et al 1995).

The strong impact of untoward life events in childhood on the development of mood and anxiety disorders in adulthood has been well documented in recent years. One study comprising almost 2000 women revealed that women with a history of childhood sexual or physical abuse exhibited more symptoms of depression and anxiety and had more frequently attempted suicide than women without a history of childhood abuse (McCauley et al 1997). Another recent study reported that women who had been abused in childhood were four times more likely to develop major depression in adulthood than women who had not been abused (Mullen et al 1996). The magnitude of childhood abuse is correlated to the severity of depression in adulthood. Moreover, child abuse is associated with the early onset of depression and a greater likelihood for chronic depression (Young et al 1997; Zlotnick et al 1995).

Childhood abuse also has been shown to predispose for the development of several anxiety disorders in adulthood, including panic disorder and generalized anxiety disorder

0006-3223/99/$20.00
PII S0006-3223(99)00224-3

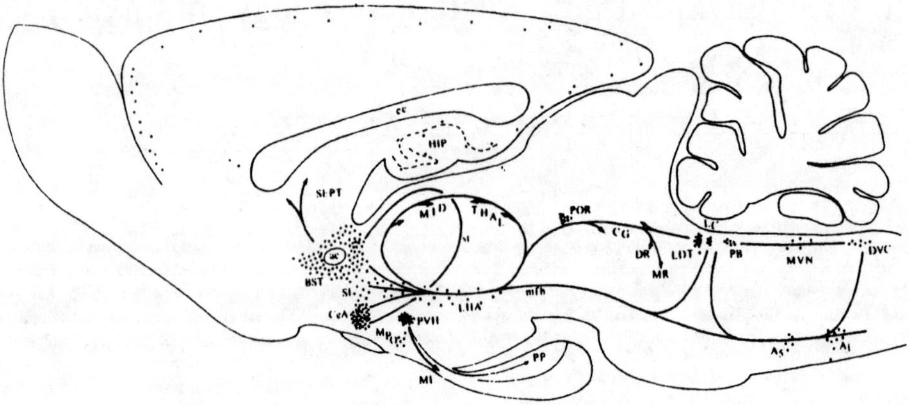

Figure 1. Major CRF-stained cell groups (dots) and fiber systems in the rat brain. cc, corpus callosum; HIP, hippocampus; SEPT, septal region; AC, anterior commissure; BST, bed nucleus of the stria terminalis; SI, substantia innominata; CeA, central nucleus of the amygdala; MPO, medial preoptic area; PVH, paraventricular nucleus of the hypothalamus; ME, median eminence; PP, posterior pituitary; LHA, lateral hypothalamic area; mfb, medial forebrain bundle; MID THAL, midline thalamic nuclei; st, stria terminalis; POR, perioculomotor nucleus; CG, central gray; DR, dorsal raphe; MR, median raphe, LDT, laterodorsal tegmental nucleus; LC, locus ceruleus; PB, parabrachial nucleus; MVN, medial vestibular nucleus; DVC, dorsal vagal complex; A_5, A_1, noradrenergic cell groups. (Reproduced with permission from Swanson et al 1983.)

(Portegijs et al 1996; Stein et al 1996). Moreover, post-traumatic stress disorder (PTSD), an anxiety disorder consisting of symptoms of intrusion, avoidance, and increased arousal related to the experience of a traumatic event, has also been related to childhood adversities; PTSD may be a direct consequence of the experience of childhood abuse. Childhood abuse, however, appears to increase an individual's risk to develop PTSD in response to extreme stressors in adulthood (Bremner et al 1993; Browne and Finkelhor 1986; Zaidi and Foy 1993).

In addition to childhood physical and sexual abuse, parental loss and other childhood adversities have also been related to the development of depression and anxiety disorders, including PTSD, in adulthood (Kendler et al 1993; Kessler and Magee 1993; McCranie et al 1992). Several studies have shown that depression and anxiety disorders are often comorbid in individuals with a history of childhood adversities, whereas there is little specificity regarding the consequences of different kinds of experiences (Mullen et al 1996; Saunders et al 1992).

Based on these observations, we assume that genetic predisposition coupled with early adverse experiences in critical phases of development induce a persistent vulnerability to the effects of stress later in life and, thus, increase vulnerability of an individual to develop mood and anxiety disorders. This stress vulnerability was posited to be mediated by persistent changes in stress-responsive neurobiological systems involved in both mood and anxiety disorders.

Corticotropin-Releasing Factor

It is likely that persistent changes in central nervous system (CNS) corticotropin-releasing factor (CRF) systems mediate the association between stressful experiences and the development of mood and anxiety disorders. The 41–amino acid sequence of CRF was isolated and characterized by Vale et al (1981). Subsequent immunohistochemical and radioimmunoassay mapping suggested a heterogeneous distribution of CRF neurons throughout the CNS (see Owens and Nemeroff 1991 for review; Figure 1). Cell bodies that contain CRF are found in high densities in the medial parvocellular region of the hypothalamic paraventricular nucleus (PVN). These neurons project mainly to the median eminence, where CRF is released from nerve terminals into the portal vascular system connecting the hypothalamus and the pituitary gland (Antoni et al 1983). The parvocellular CRF neurons of the hypothalamic PVN, thus, form the central constituent of the neuroendocrine stress-response system. Outside the hypothalamus, an abundant presence of CRF-containing neurons is found in cortical regions. These CRF neurons may be involved in the mediation of behavioral stress responses as well as the cognitive appraisal of stressful situations. A high density of CRF neurons is also found in the central nucleus of the amygdala (CeA), a limbic brain region involved in the processing of emotions. The presence of CRF in the CeA suggests a role for CRF in the modulation of affective stress responses. Amygdaloid CRF neurons project directly to the parvocellular division of the PVN and to brain stem regions. There are also indirect projections to these regions passing to (and through) the bed nucleus of the stria terminalis (BNST). These projections likely mediate endocrine and autonomic nervous system function (Gray et al 1989). Finally, CRF immunoreactivity has been measured in brain stem nuclei, which comprise the source of the major noradrenergic and serotonergic projections to the forebrain. These include the locus ceruleus, the parabrachial nucleus, and the raphe nuclei. These findings plausibly infer a role of CRF in modulating monoaminergic neurotransmitter systems, long believed to be involved in the pathophysiology of mood and anxiety disorders.

An equally widespread distribution of CRF messenger ribonucleic acid (mRNA) in those brain regions that also contain CRF has been described (Beyer et al 1988). Two subtypes of CRF receptors have further been identified, both G-protein–linked receptors (Chalmers et al 1996). The CRF_1 receptors are found in high density in the anterior pituitary gland, but are also found in a variety of subcortical and cortical brain regions. The CRF_2 receptors are expressed mostly in peripheral tissues, e.g., heart, testes, and in some brain areas, including the septum, hypothalamus, and the dorsal raphe nuclei. Only recently, urocortin has been identified, which shows partial sequence homology with CRF and binds to both CRF receptors. It has been posited to be the endogenous ligand for the CRF_2-receptor subtype. The functional significance and relevance of urocortin for neuropsychiatric disorders is currently unknown (Arborelius et al 1999). Thus, CRF appears to function not only as a releasing factor, but also as a neurotransmitter that functions as primary CNS mediator of the endocrine, autonomic, immune, and behavioral responses to stress.

CRF and the Stress Responses

Endocrinologically, the stress response is largely characterized by activation of the hypothalamic–pituitary–adrenal (HPA) axis. Stress-activated neurotransmitter systems are believed to stimulate both the synthesis and secretion of CRF into the hypothalamo–hypophysial portal circulation. The CRF binds to receptors of the adenohypophysial corticotrophs and thereby stimulates the production and release of the pro-opiomelanocortin (POMC) derivatives derivatives, adrenocorticotropin (ACTH) and β-endorphin. In turn, ACTH, stimulates the synthesis and secretion of glucocorticoids from the adrenal cortex. The metabolic and immune-modulating effects of glucocorticoids (cortisol in primates and corticosterone in most rodents) maintain homeostatic balance during stress. Circulating glucocorticoids control the activity of the HPA axis by negative-feedback inhibition (Dallman et al 1987). There are two types of adrenal steroid receptors, the mineralocorticoid (MR) and the glucocorticoid receptors (GR). High-affinity MR are located in the hippocampus and are believed to be involved in the circadian regulation of the HPA axis. Low-affinity GR, in contrast, are widely distributed throughout the CNS and in the pituitary and are thought to regulate HPA axis reactivity to stress in concert with MR (DeKloet et al 1991). During the feedback process, glucocorticoids bind to the cytoplasmic receptor, which then undergoes a conformational change (activation) and translocates to the nucleus of the cell to alter levels of gene expression. The ability of these receptors to dampen HPA-axis responses to stress is critical to the adaptation of an organism. Interestingly, there is a positive feed-forward cascade between glucocorticoids and extrahypothalamic CRF, in which stress-induced increases in glucocorticoid secretion may further enhance CRF neuronal activity in circuits involved in behavioral responses to stress.

As noted previously, an extensive literature has provided evidence that CRF mediates autonomic, immune, and behavioral stress responses beyond its role as a hypothalamic hypophysiotropic hormone (see Figure 2). Direct CNS administration of CRF to laboratory animals results in many physiologic and behavioral changes that closely parallel signs of stress (Dunn and Berridge 1990). These changes include activation of the autonomic nervous system and subsequent elevations of peripheral catecholamines, increases in heart rate and mean arterial pressure, and changes in gastrointestinal activity. Behavioral effects of central CRF administration include decreased reproductive behavior, decreased food intake and feeding behavior, disruption of slow-wave sleep, increased grooming behavior, and increased locomotor activity in a familiar environment. In nonhuman primates, CRF application results in a behavioral despair syndrome, characterized by inactivity, frequent vocalizations, reclining, and huddling (Kalin 1990). Many of these CRF-induced changes are reminiscent of the symptoms of depression, including loss of libido and appetite, sleep disturbances, changes in motor activity, and loss of interest.

Centrally administered CRF also produces many behavioral changes that are indicative of anxiety. These include suppression of exploratory behavior in a novel environment, potentiation of acoustic startle responses, facilitation of fear conditioning, and enhancement of shock-induced freezing and fighting behavior (Dunn and Berridge 1990;

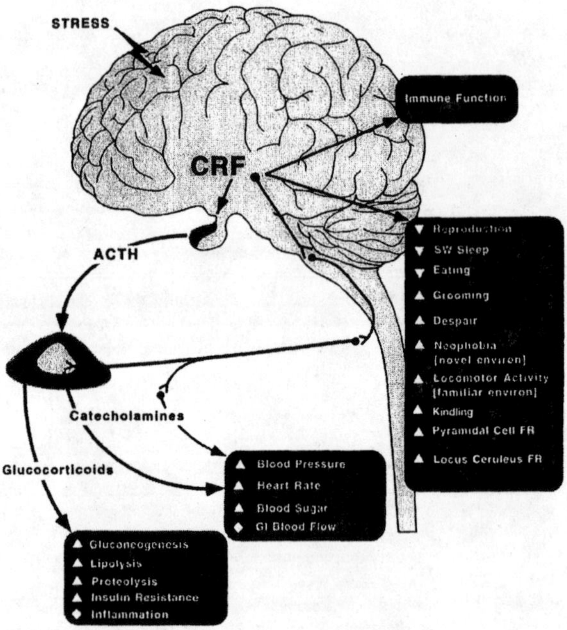

Figure 2. Effects of central corticotropin-releasing factor (CRF). Triangles, increase; inverted triangles, decrease; diamonds, bidirectional changes; ACTH, adrenocorticotropin; GI, gastrointestinal; FR, firing rate; SW, slow wave.

Koob et al 1994; Owens and Nemeroff 1991). The behavioral effects of CRF can be blocked by central administration of CRF-receptor antagonists or a CRF antisense oligo-deoxynucleotide (Dunn and Berridge 1990; Skutella et al 1994). Findings of an attenuating effect of CRF receptor antagonists on stress-induced behavior and findings of increased or decreased anxiety in transgenic mice overexpressing CRF or lacking CRF_1 receptors, respectively, substantiate a role for endogenous CRF in the mediation of anxiety (Arborelius et al 1999).

There is increasing evidence that the CRF neuronal system connecting the amygdala with the noradrenergic neurons of the locus ceruleus is involved in the mediation of the anxiogenic effects of the peptide. The amygdala has long been implicated in the regulation of emotions (LeDoux 1994). Stress increases CRF concentrations in the amygdala (Pich et al 1993). Microinjection of CRF directly into the amygdala suppresses exploratory behavior in an open-field test and facilitates fear conditioning (Liang and Lee 1988). Corticotropin-releasing factor–receptor antagonists locally administered into the amygdala attenuate shock-induced freezing behavior. Furthermore, lesions of the amygdala completely abolish CRF-induced potentiation of startle responses as well as conditioned emotional responses, suggesting a role for CRF in the encoding of emotional memories (Hitchcock and Davis 1996; LeDoux 1994).

Originating from the amygdala, CRF neurons project to the locus ceruleus and synapse onto noradrenergic neurons (van Bockstaele et al 1996). The locus ceruleus has also been implicated in the mediation of anxiety (Schulkin et al 1994). Acute and chronic stress increase CRF concentrations in the locus ceruleus (Chappell et al 1986). Microinjection of CRF directly into the locus ceruleus increases neuronal firing rates and the release of excitatory amino acids (Singewald et al 1996; Valentino et al 1983). The presence of CRF in the locus ceruleus appears to increase tyrosine hydroxylase activity, the rate-limiting step in norepinephrine synthesis (Melia and Duman 1991). Along with these modulatory effects of CRF on the locus ceruleus, CRF may be involved in the regulation of arousal and vigilance. Microinjections of CRF into the locus ceruleus and into the neighboring parabrachial nucleus also induce anxiety-like behavior, including decreased exploratory behavior in a novel environment and increased conflict behavior (Butler et al 1990; Weiss et al 1994). The CRF-induced increases in defensive withdrawal behavior can be reversed by infusion of CRF-receptor antagonists

Table 1. Comparison of Neurobiological Correlates of Major Depression and Anxiety Disorders

	Major depression	Anxiety disorders
Basal cortisol levels	↑	→PD, ↓PTSD
Cortisol suppression by dexamethasone	↓	↓GAD, ↓OCD, →PD, ↑PTSD, →SP
GR binding in PBMC	↓	↑PTSD
ACTH response to CRF challenge	↓	↑/↓PD, ↓PTSD
Cortisol response to CRF challenge	→	→PD, →PTSD
ACTH response to DEX/CRF challenge	↑	↑PD
Cerebrospinal fluid CRF levels	↑	→PD, ↑PTSD, ↑OCD
Hippocampal volume	↓	↓PTSD

ACTH, adrenocorticotropic hormone; CRF, corticotropin-releasing factor; DEX, dexamethasone; GAD, generalized anxiety disorder; GR, glucocorticoid receptor; OCD, obsessive–compulsive disorder; PBMC, peripheral blood mononuclear cells; PD, panic disorder, PTSD, posttraumatic stress disorder; SP, social phobia.

into the locus ceruleus (Smagin et al 1996). Benzodiazepines have been shown to attenuate several of the anxiogenic effects of CRF, and this anxiolytic effect may, in part, depend on a reduction of CRF concentrations in the locus ceruleus (Owens et al 1989). Thus, extrahypothalamic CRF pathways projecting from the amygdala to the locus ceruleus may serve as the major neurotransmitter system mediating various anxiety states. By these pathways, enhanced CRF activity may explain many symptoms of anxiety disorders, including PTSD, such as imprinted emotional memories, symptoms of avoidance, and increased vigilance, along with enhanced startle reactivity. A comparable dysregulation of CNS CRF systems may be the biological basis for the high symptom overlap and frequent comorbidity between depression and anxiety disorders.

Clinical Findings in Depression

Increased HPA-axis activity in major depression is one of the most robust findings in the history of biological psychiatry (see Table 1). Board et al (1957) reported increased adrenocortical activity in depressed patients, and this finding has now been replicated in numerous studies (Holsboer 1991). After the intake of a standard dose of dexamethasone, a synthetic glucocorticoid that suppresses pituitary–adrenal activity through negative-feedback inhibition in healthy subjects, the majority of depressed patients exhibit nonsuppression of ACTH, β-endorphin, and cortisol (Carroll et al 1981). Nonsuppression in the dexamethasone suppression test (DST) is more prevalent among patients with severe forms of depression, such as depression with psychotic features. Consistent with impaired feedback inhibition, decreased glucocorticoid-receptor binding and function has been measured in peripheral mononuclear cells of depressed patients (see Pariante et al 1995). All of these features are state rather than trait dependent and reverse with clinical remission.

When administered exogenous CRF intravenously, which stimulates pituitary ACTH release, depressed patients exhibit a reduced ACTH response when compared with normal control subjects (Gold et al 1984; Holsboer et al 1985). Cortisol responses to CRF in depressed patients are normal, and this suggests an increased adrenocortical reactivity to endogenously secreted ACTH. Indeed, increased cortisol responses in depressed patients after exogenously administered $ACTH_{1\text{-}24}$, a biologically active fraction of ACTH, has been reported (Amsterdam et al 1983). Potential mechanisms underlying the blunted ACTH response to CRF in depressed patients include down-regulation of pituitary CRF receptors in response to chronic hypersecretion of hypothalamic CRF and/or increased feedback inhibition of the corticotrophs to the basal hypercortisolemia. Similar to other HPA-axis alterations in depression, the blunted ACTH response to CRF is state dependent and normalizes upon clinical recovery (Amsterdam et al 1988). When pretreated with dexamethasone and subsequently administered CRF intravenously, depressed patients exhibit "escape" from dexamethasone suppression that cannot be observed in healthy subjects (von Bardeleben and Holsboer 1989). This finding strongly suggests that increased hypothalamic CRF release mediates the development of DST nonsuppression observed in depressed patients. The combined DST/CRF stimulation test appears to be a highly sensitive diagnostic test for depression, which also detects trait vulnerability, because of its relative persistence after recovery and its documented alterations in asymptomatic first-degree relatives of depressed patients (Heuser et al 1994).

In direct support of the hypothesis of CNS CRF hypersecretion in depression is the well-documented increase in CRF concentrations in lumbar cerebrospinal fluid (CSF) of depressed patients compared with healthy control subjects and patients with other psychiatric disorders in a series of studies (Bánki et al 1987, 1992a; Nemeroff et al 1984; Widerlöv et al 1988). Increased CRF concentrations were also observed in cisternal CSF of suicide victims, most of whom presumably suffered from depression (Arató et al 1989). Other studies failed to find elevated CRF levels in CSF of patients with major depression (Kling et al 1991), although these findings appear to be explained by the inclusion of patients with atypical depression. Indeed, a recent study has provided evidence for decreased rather than increased CSF CRF concentrations in eucortisolemic depressed patients with at least one atypical symptom (Geracioti et al 1997).

Because CSF measures likely reflect overall peptide release from several brain areas, it is difficult to infer conclusions on increases in CRF neuronal activity in specific regions, such as the hypothalamus or the cortex. Postmortem studies can, however, provide such information. Thus, increased CRF concentrations, as well as increased CRF mRNA expression, has been observed in hypothalamic tissue obtained from depressed patients compared with control subjects (Raadsheer et al 1994, 1995). Moreover, decreased CRF-receptor binding in the frontal cortex of suicide victims, likely due to chronic CRF hypersecretion, has been reported (Nemeroff et al 1988) and confirmed in a second study (Owens and Nemeroff, unpublished observations).

Consistent with findings from animal studies (Brady et al 1992), several classes of antidepressant drugs have been shown to reduce central CRF activity in humans. Antidepressant treatment and symptom remission appear to be associated with normalization of central CRF activity. Twenty-four hours after a regimen of electroconvulsive therapy, depressed patients exhibited a decrease in CSF CRF levels (Nemeroff et al 1992). Short-term treatment with desipramine reduces CSF CRF concentrations in normal volunteers (Veith et al 1993). Chronic treatment of depressed patients with fluoxetine results in a decrease in CSF CRF concentrations that is associated with clinical recovery (DeBellis et al 1993). Patients who remain depression-free during a 6-month antidepressant treatment period exhibit reduced CSF CRF concentrations, whereas patients with persistently elevated CSF CRF concentrations did not exhibit remission (Bánki et al 1992b). Thus, central CRF hyperactivity is a state, rather than a trait marker of depression. Reduction of CNS CRF activity appears to be one final common pathway of antidepressant action.

Consistent with the neuroendocrine findings are the radiologically demonstrable increases in pituitary and adrenal gland volumes in depressed patients that have been reported (Krishnan et al 1991; Nemeroff et al 1993). Research from laboratory animal studies provides evidence that chronic ACTH stimulation of the adrenal gland results in increased adrenal gland volumes (Orth et al 1992). In a recent study, chronic intracerebroventricular infusion of CRF induced adrenal gland hyperplasia (Buwalda et al 1997). Sustained hypercortisolemia in depression may contribute to the development of hippocampal atrophy due to the direct neurotoxic effects of corticosteroids. Although we failed to find atrophy of the hippocampus in depressed patients in an early study (Axelson et al 1993), a higher-resolution magnetic resonance imaging study detected significant reductions in hippocampal volume in women with a history of recurrent depression (Sheline et al 1996). Moreover, there was a correlation between the total duration of depressive episodes and the extent of atrophy. Because of the seminal role of the hippocampus in inhibiting paraventricular nucleus CRF activity, alterations in hippocampal function may initiate a feed-forward cascade, whereby increasing damage to the hippocampus would lead to further disinhibition of CRF secretion, leading to further increases in cortisol secretion, which in turn further damage the hippocampus.

Finally, concordant with the notion that CNS CRF regulates outflow pathways of the sympathetic nervous system (vide supra), significant positive correlations between plasma cortisol and epinephrine levels have been reported in depressed patients (Rosenbaum et al 1983; Stokes et al 1981).

Clinical Findings in Anxiety Disorders

Stress early in life appears to predispose to the development not only of depression, but to several anxiety disorders as well. Findings from basic research provide compelling evidence for a role for CRF in mediating states of anxiety (vide supra). Clinical studies in patients with several anxiety disorders, including panic disorder, generalized anxiety disorder, and obsessive–compulsive disorder (OCD), are less conclusive than the findings reviewed previously in depression (see Table 1). Patients with panic disorder exhibit normal basal plasma cortisol concentrations; hypercortisolemia is present only if these patients suffer from comorbid depression (Holsboer et al 1987; Roy-Byrne et al 1986). A standard DST results in normal suppression of cortisol in patients with either panic disorder or social phobia (Goldstein et al 1987; Roy-Byrne et al 1985; Tancer 1993). Patients with generalized anxiety disorder and patients with OCD, however, have been reported to exhibit DST nonsuppression, which is not related to comorbid depression (Insel et al 1982; Schweizer et al 1986). As in depressed patients, the more sensitive DST/CRF stimulation test induces an escape from cortisol suppression in patients with panic disorder, providing evidence for a hyperactive HPA axis (Schreiber et al 1996). Thus, patients with panic disorder have been shown to demonstrate a blunted ACTH response in a standard CRF stimulation test (Holsboer et al 1987; Roy-Byrne et al 1986). Because blunted ACTH responses were also observed in the presence of basal eucortisolemia, these findings support pituitary CRF-receptor downregulation secondary to hypothalamic CRF hypersecretion as underlying this endocrine abnormality in panic disorder; however, in a recent report, increased ACTH responses to CRF were observed in patients with panic disorder, and treatment with alprazolam, reported to decrease hypothalamic CRF activity (Owens et al 1989), normalized pituitary responsiveness (Curtis et al 1997). A possible explanation for these discrepant findings may be differences in the HPA axis in panic disorder, depending on when, in the longitudinal course of the illness, the patients are studied. Thus, an initial CRF sensitization may evolve into CRF receptor down-regulation upon long-term CRF hypersecretion. Although these findings would suggest an involvement of CRF systems in panic disorder, CSF CRF concentrations are unaltered in these patients (Jolkkonen et al 1993). Patients with OCD, in contrast, have been reported to exhibit increased CSF CRF concentrations which normalize upon clinical recovery (Altemus et al 1992, 1994).

A considerable number of studies in recent years have focused on HPA-axis alterations in patients with PTSD, an anxiety disorder that also is increased in prevalence by stress early in life (vide supra). Several studies provide evidence for abnormally low, rather than high, adrenocortical activity in PTSD patients, as evidenced by decreased urinary cortisol excretion and low cortisol concentrations in single plasma or saliva samples (see Yehuda 1997). In a chronobiological study, Vietnam veterans with PTSD demonstrated a decreased nadir and an increased peak of cortisol release when compared with healthy normal control subjects and depressed patients (Yehuda et al 1996a). Increased GR binding in peripheral mononuclear cells of Vietnam veterans with PTSD compared with healthy control subjects and other psychiatric patients has been reported (Yehuda et al 1991, 1993a). Although no alterations in feedback sensitivity could be detected in the standard DST, patients with PTSD were shown to exhibit an exaggerated suppression of cortisol in response to a low dose of dexamethasone (Yehuda et al 1993b, 1995). Moreover, dexamethasone induces a more pronounced decrease in GR binding in patients with PTSD than in control subjects, possibly reflecting increased translocation of the activated GR from the cytoplasm to the nucleus of the cell. Together, these findings suggest that decreased adrenocortical activity and increased negative-feedback sensitivity occur in PTSD. This neuroendocrine pattern has been observed in PTSD patients, even in those with comorbid depression.

Interestingly, patients with PTSD demonstrate increased ACTH responses to blockade of endogenous cortisol production with the β-hydroxylase inhibitor, metyrapone (Yehuda et al 1996b). This finding not only supports the hypothesis of increased feedback inhibition of the HPA axis in PTSD, but also implies a pronounced increase in CRF secretion in these patients. Our group has observed blunted ACTH responses to CRF in Vietnam veterans with PTSD; both baseline and CRF-stimulated cortisol concentrations did not differ from control subjects. One half of the PTSD patients had comorbid major depression (Smith et al 1989). This finding is concordant with down-regulation of adenohypophysial CRF receptors secondary to chronically increased CRF secretion, although enhanced feedback sensitivity of the pituitary gland may contribute to this finding. Indeed, CSF CRF concentrations are increased in Vietnam veterans with PTSD, lending support to hyperactivity of CRF neuronal systems in this disorder (Bremner et al 1997). Thus, whereas depression and PTSD are discordant at peripheral HPA axis loci, both disorders share hypersecretion of CRF in the CNS.

As has been reported in depression, hippocampal atrophy has also been observed in combat veterans with PTSD (Bremner et al 1995; Gurvits et al 1996), despite the reported hypocortisolism. This hippocampal atrophy may reflect a preexisting risk factor for the development of stress-related neuropathology; alternatively, it may be due to toxic effects of high cortisol levels at the time of trauma associated with increased vulnerability of the hippocampus because of increased GR function. Patients with PTSD also demonstrate elevated plasma catecholamine concentrations and behavioral sensitization to the selective α_2-receptor antagonist, yohimbine, which stimulates the central noradrenergic system by blockade of presynaptic feedback (Kosten et al 1987; Southwick et al 1993). This hyperreactivity of the central noradrenergic system may be due, at least in part, to increased CRF release in the locus ceruleus.

Indices of CRF hypersecretion have been obtained in patients with certain anxiety disorders. It would appear that in several anxiety disorders some form of peripheral adaptation occurs in response to increased central CRF activity, resulting in normal or decreased adrenocortical activity.

Preclinical and Clinical Findings in Early Life Stress

Given the relationship between severe childhood adversity and the development of mood and anxiety disorders, for which a neurobiological substrate has been posited, preclinical and clinical studies of the neurobiological effects of early adverse experiences would appear to provide the best opportunity to elucidate the precise pathogenesis (see Table 2). Among rodent models of early life stress are repeated brief removals of rat pups from their mothers during the neonatal period. Whereas the mild stress of early handling produces a phenotype that is less sensitive to stress and, thus, better adapted, the more severe stress of prolonged maternal separation results in heightened stress vulnerability in adulthood (Plotsky and Meaney 1993). Thus, adult rats who were repeatedly separated from their mothers for 180 min per day on postnatal days 2–14 demonstrate increased ACTH and corticosterone responses to a variety of stressors in adulthood (Plotsky and

Table 2. Summary of Long-Term Neuroendocrine Changes in Selected Models of Early Life Stress

Model	Species	Timing	Neuroendocrine changes	
Maternal separation	Rats	180 min/day pnd 2–14	ACTH after psychological stress	↑
			CORT after psychological stress	↑
			CRF in ME and LC	↑
			CRF–receptor binding in LC	↑
			CRF mRNA in ME, CeA, BNST	↑
		4–6 h/day pnd 2–14	ACTH basal and after stress	↑
			CORT basal and after stress	→
			CRF in ME and PB	↑
			Pituitary CRF–receptor binding	↓
			CRF–receptor binding in NR	↑
	Nonhuman primates	Separated after birth and peer reared	ACTH after stress	↑
			CORT after stress	↑
Variable foraging demand	Nonhuman primates	12 weeks (beginning at ~17 weeks of age)	CSF CRF	↑
			CSF CORT	↓
Childhood abuse	Humans	Before the onset of puberty	ACTH after psychosocial stress	↑ [a,b]
			CORT after psychosocial stress	→ [a], ↑ [b]
			ACTH after CRF challenge	↑ [a], ↓ [b]

[a] Without current major depression.
[b] With current major depression.
ACTH, adrenocorticotropic hormone; BNST, bed nucleus of the stria terminalis; CORT, corticosterone or cortisol; CeA, central nucleus of the amygdala; CRF, corticotropin-releasing factor; LC, locus coruleus; ME, median eminence; mRNA, CRF messenger ribonucleic acid; NR, nucleus raphe; PB, parabrachial nucleus; pnd, postnatal day.

Meaney 1993). Maternal separation of 4 hours per day on postnatal days 2–5 and 6 hours per day on postnatal days 6–20 also results in increased ACTH concentrations in adulthood (postnatal day 108), both basally and in response to stress, although corticosterone responses appear to be normal (Ladd et al 1996). Interestingly, prolonged maternal separation over 24 hours at postnatal days 3–4 produces normal ACTH and increased corticosterone responses to stress at postnatal day 20, whereas prolonged maternal separation at postnatal day 11–12 produces blunted ACTH and normal corticosterone responses to stress at postnatal day 20 (Workel et al 1997; van Oers et al 1998). Although these findings contribute only indirectly to our knowledge of the long-term neurobiological consequences of early stress, they suggest that there are critical time windows for the effects of early stress on neurobiological systems. Moreover, with prolonged maternal separation, adrenocortical responsiveness may dissociate from pituitary responsiveness.

Enhanced pituitary responsiveness seems to be mediated by persistent changes in hypothalamic CRF neurons, because increased CRF concentrations in the median eminence, along with reduced pituitary CRF receptors (as well as increased CRF mRNA expression in the hypothalamic PVN), have been repeatedly demonstrated in maternally separated rats under resting conditions (Ladd et al 1996; Plotsky and Meaney 1993). Increased CRF mRNA expression in the PVN after stress exposure has also been observed in these rats relative to rats that had been reared under normal animal-facility conditions. Remarkably, the heightened stress responses at all levels of the HPA axis are reversed by treatment of the maternally separated rats with the selective serotonin reuptake inhibitor, paroxetine, as well as with the selective norepinephrine reuptake inhibitor, reboxetine (Plotsky et al, in press).

Increased sensitivity of the HPA axis seems to be limited to psychological stress (i.e., air puff startle, restraint stress, or novel environment), and is not observed after physical stress (i.e., hemorrhage, cold, nitroprusside-induced hypotension; Ladd et al, in press). These findings suggest the involvement of corticolimbic pathways in the mediation of the heightened stress response. Interesting in this regard are findings of changes in extrahypothalamic CRF systems as a result of maternal separation in rats. Indeed, increased CRF concentrations were also measured in the parabrachial nucleus after maternal separation (Ladd et al 1996). Moreover, increased CRF mRNA expression was observed in the CeA and in the BNST, through which polysynaptic CRF neurons from the amygdala project to the hypothalamus (Plotsky et al, in press). In addition, increased CRF concentrations, along with increased CRF-receptor binding, were observed in the locus ceruleus (Plotsky et al, in press), which receives projections from the amygdala and sends projections to the hypothalamus. Both of these pathways may be involved in the modulation of the HPA-axis response to psychological stress. Accordingly, increased norepinephrine levels in the PVN of the hypothalamus were measured in maternally separated rats after exposure to restraint stress (Liu et al, in press). In the study by Ladd et al (1996), increased CRF-receptor binding was observed in the raphe nuclei (the major origin of forebrain serotonergic pathways), which has been implicated in the pathophysiology of depression and also PTSD (Connor and Davidson 1998; Owens and Nemeroff 1994).

Concordant with increased extrahypothalamic CRF activity, maternally separated rats exhibit marked behavioral abnormalities. These include anhedonia, i.e., reduced consumption of sweetened solution and changes in food intake. Moreover, these rats exhibit increased anxiety-like behavior, such as suppressed exploration of a novel environment, increased freezing in an open field, and increased startle responses (Caldji et al, in press). Many of these behavioral changes resemble symptoms of depression and anxiety disorders. It appears that both endocrine and behavioral long-term consequences of maternal separation in rats are mediated through changes in maternal behavior, because cross-fostering of handled and maternally separated rats results in reversed changes (Huot et al 1997; Ladd et al, in press).

The effects of early life stress have also been studied in nonhuman primates. Similar to findings in rodents, young adult nonhuman primates who have been maternally deprived and reared with peers during infancy exhibit increased pituitary–adrenal activation as well as increased levels of distress vocalizations and passive behavior in response to separation from peers as compared with primates who have been reared by their mothers for the first 6 months of life (Suomi 1991). Another paradigm, which more closely resembles stress experiences of human infants, consists of exposure of infant nonhuman primates to differential rearing conditions, in which the mothers are confronted with different foraging demands. Mothers with constantly low foraging demand (LVD) can obtain food without any effort, whereas mothers with constantly high foraging demand (HVD) have to complete a daily task to obtain their food. In a variable foraging demand (VFD) condition, mothers are exposed to unpredictable conditions with respect to food access, resulting in a diminished perception of security in terms of maternal attachment in the infants (Rosenblum and Paully 1984). Adult (2–4 years) bonnet macaques that have been exposed to VFD over a 12-week period during infancy, beginning at approximately 17 weeks of age, demonstrate significantly elevated CSF CRF concentrations when compared with primates reared under LVD or HVD conditions. Cerebrospinal fluid CRF concentrations did not correlate with CSF cortisol concentrations. Indeed, CSF cortisol concentrations were actually lower in the animals exposed to the variable foraging demand (Coplan et al 1996). The dissociation between increased central CRF activity and decreased adrenal activity parallels our findings in PTSD. Moreover, VFD-reared nonhuman primates exhibit stable traits of anxiety along with exaggerated anxiety-like responses to the administration of the selective α_2-receptor antagonist, yohimbine (Rosenblum and Paully 1984; Rosenblum et al 1994).

Whereas a number of studies have characterized the behavioral and neurobiological consequences of early life stress in rodents and nonhuman primates, only a small number of studies have focused on human subjects. Sexually abused girls, many of whom suffered from dysthymia, exhibit blunted ACTH responses to CRF (DeBellis et al 1994). In another study, abused children who still lived under conditions of ongoing stress and suffered from comorbid PTSD and depression showed increased ACTH responses to CRF, whereas cortisol responses were normal (Kaufman et al 1997), paralleling findings in rats exposed to prolonged maternal separation (Ladd et al 1996).

Our group has obtained preliminary findings on stress responsiveness in adult survivors of childhood abuse with and without major depression. Upon exposure to standardized psychosocial laboratory stress, women with a history of childhood abuse, with and without current major depression, demonstrated markedly increased ACTH responses as compared with healthy control subjects without a history of early life stress (Heim et al 1998a). The mean ACTH response was highest in women with a history of childhood abuse and current major depression. Moreover, women with a history of childhood abuse and current major depression also showed significantly increased cortisol responses to psychosocial stress as compared with control subjects and abused women without depression. Net ACTH and cortisol responses were positively correlated with the degree of childhood abuse and the severity of depression and PTSD. Women with a history of childhood abuse, with and without depression, also demonstrated higher and more persistent heart rate responses to psychosocial stress relative to control subjects. Women with a history of childhood abuse and current depression suffered more often from comorbid PTSD and had been exposed to more recent life stress when compared with women with a history of childhood abuse without depression (Heim et al 1998a). Corticotropin-releasing factor stimulation tests were also obtained in these women. Interestingly, women with a history of childhood abuse without current major depression exhibited increased ACTH responses along with normal to decreased cortisol responses (C. Heim et al, unpublished data, 1999). This finding parallels findings in maternally deprived rats and abused children (Kaufman et al 1997; Ladd et al 1996). In contrast, women with a history of childhood abuse with comorbid major depression exhibited blunted ACTH responses, likely due to chronic overexposure of the pituitary to CRF. Together, these findings suggest that there may be an initial sensitization of the stress hormone system, representing a biological vulnerability for the

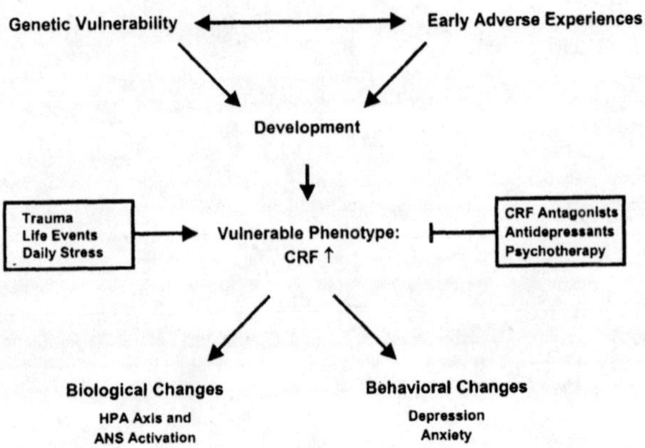

Figure 3. The relationship between early life stress, sensitization of corticotropin-releasing factor (CRF) neuronal systems, and the development of depression and anxiety. HPA, hypothalamic–pituitary–adrenal; ANS, autonomic nervous system.

development of depression and anxiety disorders. This vulnerability may result in relatively high CRF secretion whenever these women are stressed, which may then lead to pituitary receptor down-regulation. The increased ACTH response to laboratory stress in depressed women with a history of childhood abuse may reflect the involvement of corticolimbic pathways as well as enhanced PVN CRF activity, overriding the receptor down-regulation. Interestingly, there are several studies suggesting hippocampal atrophy in adult survivors of childhood abuse (Bremner et al 1997; Stein et al 1997), and an impaired hippocampus may contribute to the development of an enhanced HPA-axis response to stress as a consequence of childhood abuse.

Summary and Future Directions

An interaction of genetic and environmental factors has long been postulated to determine an individual's vulnerability to developing affective and anxiety disorders. A strong relationship between early adverse experiences and the development of these disorders in adulthood appears well documented. Both endocrine and behavioral responses to stress are predominantly controlled by CNS CRF systems. Corticotropin-releasing factor neurons in limbic and brain stem regions appear to mediate, at least in part, anxiety. There is evidence for increased CRF activity in both patients with depression and patients with anxiety disorders. Preclinical studies suggest that stress during development may result in persistently increased activity of one or more CNS CRF systems and a sensitization of the HPA axis to stress. Our group has suggested that stress early in life results in a persistent sensitization of these CRF circuits to even mild stress in adulthood, forming the basis for the development of mood and anxiety disorders (see Figure 3). This hypothesis is supported by our recent clinical study of adult survivors of childhood abuse.

These findings have multiple implications for future research. First, genetic factors and the effects of early stress experiences on neurobiological systems should now be coupled in animal models or human twin studies. Second, central mechanisms underlying increased stress reactivity in human survivors of childhood adversities should be evaluated, particularly with respect to CRF-neuronal systems and functional properties of the amygdala and the hippocampus. Third, the reversibility of this stress vulnerability should be investigated. Potential candidates for facilitating this reversal are antidepressants, which have been shown to reverse neuroendocrine consequences of maternal separation in rats. It would also be of interest to explore whether various forms of psychotherapy may prevent or reverse neurobiological consequences of early life stress. If CRF hyperactivity remains, blockade of central CRF effects using selective CRF_1-receptor antagonists may provide an important tool for the prevention and treatment of depression and anxiety disorders. Finally, preclinical and clinical studies have found that severe early trauma may result in decreased adrenocortical activity. This abnormality has been observed in several anxiety disorders, even in the case of comorbidity with depression. One may thus assume that there is a specific traumatic type of mixed anxiety and depression, which is associated with low adrenocortical activity, but central CRF hyperactivity. Similar patterns have been reported for patients with trauma-related bodily disorders (Heim et al 1998b), and thus reduced pituitary–adrenal activity may have important implications for the physical adaptation of the organism to stress (McEwen 1998). Future studies focusing on these issues may have important potential in increasing our knowledge of the pathogenesis of stress-related disorders and may provide novel approaches in the prevention and treatment of such disorders.

The authors are supported by NIH MH-42088, NIH MH-50113, and DFG He2561/2-1.

This work was presented at the scientific satellite conference, "The Role of Biological and Psychological Factors on Early Development and Their Impact on Adult Life," that preceded the Anxiety Disorders Association of America (ADAA) annual meeting, San Diego, March 1999. The conference was jointly sponsored by the ADAA and the National Institute of Mental Health through an unrestricted educational grant provided by Wyeth-Ayerst Laboratories.

References

Altemus M, Pigott T, Kalogeras KT, Demitrack M, Dubbert B, Murphy DL, et al (1992): Abnormalities in the regulation of vaspressin and corticotropin-releasing factor secretion in obsessive-compulsive disorder. *Arch Gen Psychiatry* 49:9–20.

Altemus M, Swedo SE, Leonard HL, Richter D, Rubinow DR, Potter WZ, et al (1994): Changes in cerebrospinal fluid neurochemistry during treatment of obsessive-compulsive disorder with clomipramine. *Arch Gen Psychiatry* 51:794–803.

Amsterdam JD, Winokur A, Abelman E, Lucki I, Rickels K (1983): Cosyntropin (ACTH alpha 1-24) stimulation test in depressed patients and healthy subjects. *Am J Psychiatry* 140:907–908.

Amsterdam JD, Maislin G, Winoku A, Berwish N, Kling M, Gold P (1988): The oCRH test before and after clinical recovery from depression. *J Affect Disord* 14:213–222.

Antoni FA, Palkovits T, Makara GB, Linton EA, Lowry PJ, Kiss JZ (1983): Immunoreactive corticotropin-releasing hormone in the hypothalamoinfundibular tract. *Neuroendocrinology* 36:415–423.

Arató M, Bánki CM, Bisette G, Nemeroff CB (1989): Elevated CSF CRF in suicide victims. *Biol Psychiatry* 25:355–359.

Arborelius L, Owens MJ, Plotsky PM, Nemeroff CB (1999): The role of corticotropin-releasing factor in depression and anxiety disorders. *J Endocrinol* 160:1–12.

Axelson DA, Doraiswamy MP, McDonald WM, Boyko OB, Tupier LA, Patterson LJ, et al (1993): Hypercortisolemia and hippocampal changes in depression. *Psychiatry Res* 47:163–173.

Bánki CM, Bissette G, Arató M, O'Connor L, Nemeroff CB (1987): Cerebrospinal fluid corticotropin-releasing factor-like immunoreactivity in depression and schizophrenia. *Am J Psychiatry* 144:873–877.

Bánki CM, Karmaksi L, Bissette G, Nemeroff CB (1992a): Cerebrospinal fluid neuropeptides in mood disorder and dementia. *J Affect Disord* 25:39–46.

Bánki CM, Karmaksi L, Bissette G, Nemeroff CB (1992b): CSF corticotropin-releasing hormone and somatostatin in major depression: response to antidepressant treatment and relapse. *Eur Neuropharmacol* 2:107–113.

Beyer HS, Matta SG, Sharp BM (1988): Regulation of the messenger ribonucleic acid for corticotropin-releasing factor in the paraventricular nucleus and other brain sites of the rat. *Endocrinology* 123:2117–2123.

Board F, Wadeson R, Persky H (1957): Depressive affect and endocrine function: Blood levels of adrenal cortex and thyroid hormones in patients suffering from depressive reactions. *Arch Neurol Psychiatry* 78:612–620.

Brady LS, Gold P, Herkenham M, Lynn A, Whitfield HJ (1992): The antidepressants fluoxetine, idazoxan, and phenelzine alter corticotropin-releasing hormone and tyrosine hydroxylase mRNA levels in rat brain: Therapeutic inplications. *Brain Res* 572:117–125.

Bremner JD, Southwick SM, Johnson DR, Yehuda R, Charney DS (1993): Childhood physical abuse and combat-related posttraumatic stress disorder in Vietnam veterans. *Am J Psychiatry* 150:235–239.

Bremner JD, Randall P, Scott TM, Bronen RA, Seibyl JP, Southwick SM, et al (1995): Magnetic resonance imaging-based measurement of hippocampal volume in patients with combat-related posttraumatic stress disorder. *Am J Psychiatry* 152:973–981.

Bremner JD, Licino J, Darnell A, Krystal JH, Owens MJ, Southwick SM, et al (1997): Elevated CSF corticotropin-releasing factor concentrations in PTSD. *Am J Psychiatry* 154:624–629.

Browne A, Finkelhor D (1986): Impact of childhood sexual abuse. *Psychol Bull* 99:66–77.

Butler PD, Weiss JM, Stout JC, Nemeroff CB (1990): Corticotropin-releasing factor produces fear-enhancing and behavioral activating effects following infusion into the locus coeruleus. *J Neurosci* 10:176–183.

Buwalda B, de Boer SF, van Kalkeren AA, Koolhaas JM (1997): Physiological and behavioral effects of of chronic intracerebroventricular infusion of corticotropin-releasing factor in the rat. *Psychoneuroendocrinology* 22:297–309.

Caldji C, Francis D, Sharma S, Plotsky PM, Meaney MJ (in press): The effects of early rearing environment on the development of $GABA_A$ and central benzodiazepine receptor levels and novelty-induced fearfulness in the rat. *J Neurosci.*

Carroll BJ, Feinberg M, Greden JF, Tarika J, Albala AA, Haskett RF, et al (1981): A specific laboratory test for the diagnosis of melancholia. *Arch Gen Psychiatry* 38:15–22.

Chalmers DT, Lovenberg TW, Grigoriadis DE, Behan DP, De Souza EB (1996): Corticotropin-releasing factor receptors: From molecualr biology to drug design. *Trends Pharmacol Sci* 17:166–172.

Chappell PB, Smith MA, Kilts CD, Bissette G, Ritchie JC, Andersen C, et al (1986): Alterations in corticotropin-releasing factor-like immunoreactivity in discrete brain regions after acute and chronic stress. *J Neurosci* 6:2908–2914.

Connor KM, Davidson JRT (1998): The role of serotonin in posttraumatic stress disorder. *CNS Spectrums* 3:43–51.

Coplan JD, Andrews MW, Rosenblum LA, Owens MJ, Friedman S, Gorman JM, et al (1996): Persistent elevations of cerebrospinal fluid concentrations of corticotropin-releasing factor in adult nonhuman primates exposed to early life stressors: Implications for the pathophysiology of mood and anxiety disorders. *Proc Natl Acad Sci U S A* 93:1619–1623.

Curtis GC, Abelson JL, Gold PW (1997): Adrenocorticotropic and hormone and cortisol responses to corticotropin-releasing hormone: Changes in panic disorder and effects of alprazolam treatment. *Biol Psychiatry* 41:76–85.

Dallman MF, Akana S, Cascio CS, Darlington DN, Jacobson L, Levin N, et al (1987): Regulation of ACTH secretion: Variations on a theme of B. *Rec Prog Horm Res* 43:113–173.

DeBellis MD, Gold P, Geracioti TD, Listwak SJ, Kling MA (1993): Association of fluoxetine treatment with reductions in CSF concentrations of corticotropin-releasing hormone and arginine vasopression in patients with major depression. *Am J Psychiatry* 150:656–657.

DeBellis MD, Chrousos GP, Dorn LD, Burke L, Helmers K, Kling MA, et al (1994): Hypothalamic pituitary adrenal dysregulation in sexually abused girls. *J Clin Endocrinol Metab* 78:249–255.

DeKloet ER, Vreugdenhil E, Oitzl MS, Joels M (1991): Brain corticosteroid receptor balance in health and disease. *Endocr Rev* 19:269–301.

Dunn AJ, Berridge CW (1990): Physiological and behavioral responses to corticotropin-releasing factor administration: Is CRF a mediator of anxiety or stress responses? *Brain Res Rev* 15:71–100.

Freud S (1895): General theory on neuroses. In: Freud A, editor. *The Standard Edition of the Complete Psychological Works of Sigmund Freud*. London: Hogarth.

Geracioti TD, Loosen PT, Orth DN (1997): Low cerebrospinal fluid corticotropin-releasing hormone concentrations in eucortisolemic depression. *Biol Psychiatry* 42:166–174.

Gold PW, Chrousos G, Kellner C, Post R, Roy A, Augerinos P, et al (1984): Psychiatric implications of basic and clinical studies with corticotropin-releasing factor. *Am J Psychiatry* 141:619–627.

Goldstein S, Halbreich U, Asnis G, Endicott J, Alvir J (1987): The hypothalamic-pituitary-adrenal system in panic disorder. *Am J Psychiatry* 144:1320–1323.

Gray TS, Carney ME, Magnuson DJ (1989): Direct projections from the central amygdaloid nucleus to the hypothalamic paraventricular nucleus: Possible role in stress-induced adrenocorticotropin release. *Neuroendocrinology* 50:433–446.

Gurvits TG, Shenton MR, Hokama H, Ohta H, Lasko NB, Gilberson MW, et al (1996): Magnetic resonance imaging study of hippocampal volume in chronic, combat-related posttraumatic stress disorder. *Biol Psychiatry* 40:193–199.

Heim C, Graham YP, Heit SC, Bonsall R, Miller AH, Nemeroff CB (1998a): Increased sensitivity of the hypothalamic-pituitary-adrenal axis to psychosocial stress in adult survivors of childhood abuse. *Soc Neurosci Abst* 28:201.12.

Heim C, Ehlert U, Hanker JP, Hellhammer DH (1998b): Abuse-related posttraumatic stress disorder and alterations of the hypothalamic-pituitary-adrenal axis in women with chronic pelvic pain. *Psychosom Med* 60:309–318.

Heuser I, Yassouridis A, Holsboer F (1994): The combined dexamethasone/CRF test: A refined laboratory test for psychiatric disorders. *J Psychiatr Res* 28:341–356.

Hitchcock J, Davis M (1996): Lesions of the amygdala, but not of the cerebellum block conditioned fear measured with the potentiated startle paradigm. *Behav Neurosci* 100:11–22.

Holsboer F (1991): The hypothalamic-pituitary-adrenocortical system. In: Paykel ES, editor. *Handbook of Affective Disorders*. Livingston: Churchill, 267–287.

Holsboer F, Gerken A, Stalla GK, Mueller OA (1985): ACTH, cortisol and corticosterone output after ovine corticotropin-releasing factor challenge during depression and after recovery. *Biol Psychiatry* 20:276–286.

Holsboer F, von Bardeleben U, Buller R, Heuser I, Steiger A (1987): Stimulation response to corticotropin-releasing hormone (CRH) in patients with depression, alcoholism and panic disorder. *Horm Metab Res* 16:80–88.

Huot RL, Smith M, Plotsky PM (1997, July): Alterations of maternal-infant interaction as a result of maternal separation in Long Evans rats and its behavioral and neuroendocrine consequences. Presented at the 28th Congress of the International Society for Psychoneuroendocrinology, San Francisco.

Insel TR, Kalin NH, Guttmacher LB, Cohen RM, Murphy DL (1982): The dexamethasone suppression test in patients with primary obsessive compulsive disorder. *Psychiatry Res* 6:153–160.

Jolkkonen J, Lepola U, Bissette G, Nemeroff CB, Riekkinen (1993): CSF corticotropin-releasing factor is not affected in panic disorder. *Biol Psychiatry* 33:136–138.

Kalin NH (1990): Behavioral and endocrine studies of corticotropin-releasing hormone in primates. In: De Souza EB, Nemeroff CB, editors. *Corticotropin-Releasing Factor: Band and Clinical Studies of a Neuropeptide*. Boca Raton, FL: CRC Press, 275–289.

Kaufman J, Birmaher B, Perel J, Dahl RE, Moreci P, Nelson B, et al (1997): The corticotropin-releasing hormone challenge in depressed abused, depressed nonabused, and normal control children. *Biol Psychiatry* 42:669–679.

Kendler KS, Kessler RC, Neale MC, Heath AC, Eaves LJ (1993): The prediction of major depression in women: Toward an integrated model. *Am J Psychiatry* 150:1139–1148.

Kendler KS, Kessler RC, Walters EE, MacLean C, Neale MC, Heath AC, et al (1995): Stressful life events, genetic liability and onset of an episode of major depression. *Am J Psychiatry* 152:833–842.

Kessler RC (1997): The effects of stressful life events on depression. *Annu Rev Psychol* 48:191–214.

Kessler RC, Magee WJ (1993): Childhood adversities and adult depression: Basic patterns of association in a US national survey. *Psychol Med* 23:679–690.

Kling MA, Roy A, Doran AR, Calabrese JR, Rubinow DR, Whitfield HJ, et al (1991): Cerebrospinal fluid immunoreactive corticotropin-releasing hormone and adrenocorticotropin secretion in Cushing's disease and major depression: Potential clinical implications. *J Clin Endocrinol Metab* 71:260–271.

Koob GF, Heinrichs SC, Menzaghi F, Pich EM, Britton KT (1994): Corticotropin-releasing factor, stress and behavior. *Semin Neurosci* 6:221–229.

Kosten TR, Mason JW, Giller EL, Harkness L (1987): Sustained urinary norepinephrine and epinephrine elevation in posttraumatic stress disorder. *Psychoneuroendocrinology* 12:13–20.

Krishnan RR, Doraiswamy PM, Lurie SM, Figiel GS, Husain MM, Boyko OB, et al (1991): Pituitary size in depression. *J Clin Endocrinol Metab* 72:256–259.

Ladd CO, Owens MJ, Nemeroff CB (1996): Persistent changes in corticotropin-releasing factor neuronal systems induced by maternal deprivation. *Endocrinology* 137:1212–1218.

Ladd CO, Huot RL, Thrivikraman KV, Nemeroff CB, Meaney MJ, Plotsky PM (in press): Long-term behavioral and neuroendocrine adaptations to adverse early experience. In: Mayer E, Saper C, editors. *Progress in Brain Research: The Biological Basis for Mind Body Interactions.* Amsterdam: Elsevier.

LeDoux JE (1994): The amygdala: Contributions to fear and stress. *Semin Neurosci* 6:231–237.

Liang KC, Lee EHY (1988): Intra-amygdala injections of corticotropin-releasing factor facilitate inhibitory avoidance learning and reduce exploratory behavior in rats. *Psychopharmacology (Berl)* 96:232–236.

Liu D, Caldji C, Sharma S, Plotsky PM, Meaney MJ (in press): Influence of neonatal rearing condition on stress-induced hypothalamic-pituitary-adrenal responses and norepinephrine release in the hypothalamic paraventricular nucleus. *J Neurosci.*

McCauley J, Kern DE, Kolodner K, Dill L, Schroeder AF, DeChant, et al (1997): Clinical characteristics of women with a history of childhood abuse. *JAMA* 277:1362–1368.

McCranie EW, Hyer LA, Boudewyns PA, Woods MG (1992): Negative parenting behavior, combat exposure and PTSD symptom severity: Test of a person-event interaction model. *J Nerv Ment Dis* 180:431–438.

McEwen BS (1998): Protective and damaging effects of stress mediators. *N Engl J Med* 338:171–179.

Melia KR, Duman RS (1991): Involvement of corticotropin-releasing factor in chronic stress regulation of the brain noradrenergic system. *Proc Natl Acad Sci U S A* 88:8382–8386.

Mullen PE, Martin JL, Anderson JC, Romans SE, Herbison GP (1996): The long-term impact of the physical, emotional, and sexual abuse of children: A community study. *Child Abuse Negl* 20:7–21.

Nemeroff CB, Widerlöv E, Bisette G, Walleus H, Karlsson L, Eklund K, et al (1984): Elevated concentrations of CSF corticotropin releasing factor like immunoreactivity in depressed patients. *Science* 226:1342–1344.

Nemeroff CB, Owens MJ, Bisette G, Andorn AC, Stanley M (1988): Reduced corticotropin-releasing factor (CRF) binding sites in the frontal cortex of suicide victims. *Arch Gen Psychiatry* 45:577–579.

Nemeroff CB, Bissette G, Akil H, Fink M (1992): Neuropeptide concentrations in the cerebrospinal fluid of depressed patients treated with electroconvulsive therapy. *Br J Psychiatry* 158: 59–63.

Nemeroff CB, Krishnan RR, Reed D, Leder R, Beam C, Dunnick NR (1993): Adrenal gland enlargement in major depression. *Arch Gen Psychiatry* 49:384–387.

Orth DN, Kovacs WJ, deBold CR (1992): The adrenal cortex. In: Wilson JD, Foster DW, editors. *Williams Textbook of Endocrinology.* Philadelphia: Saunders, 489–619.

Owens MJ, Nemeroff CB (1991): Physiology and pharmacology of corticotropin-releasing factor. *Pharmacol Rev* 43:425–473.

Owens MJ, Nemeroff CB (1994): Role of serotonin in the pathophysiology of depression: Focus on the serotonin transporter. *Clin Chem* 40:288–295.

Owens MJ, Bissette G, Nemeroff CB (1989): Acute effects of alprazolam on the concentrations of corticotropin-releasing factor in the rat brain. *Synapse* 4:196–202.

Pariante CM, Nemeroff CB, Miller AH (1995): Glucocorticoid receptors in depression. *Isr J Med Sci* 31:705–712.

Pich EM, Koob OF, Sattler SC, Menzaghi F, Heilig M, Heinrichs SC, et al (1993): Stress-induced release of corticotropin-releasing factor in the maygdala measured by in vivo microdialysis. *Neurosci Abstr* 18:535.

Plotsky PM, Meaney MJ (1993): Early, postnatal experience alters hypothalamic corticotropin-releasing factor (CRF) mRNA, median eminence CRF content and stress-induced release in adult rats. *Mol Brain Res* 18:195–200.

Plotsky PM, Thrivikraman KV, Caldji C, Sharma S, Meaney MJ (in press): The effects of neonatal rearing environment on CRF mRNA and CRF receptor levels in adult rat brain. *J Neurosci.*

Portegijs PJM, Jeuken FMH, van der Horst FG, Kraan HF, Knottnerus JA (1996): A troubled youth: Relations with somatization, depression and anxiety in adulthood. *Fam Pract* 13:1–11.

Raadsheer FC, Hoogendijk WJ, Stam FC, Tilders FJ, Swaab DF (1994): Increased numbers of corticotropin-releasing hormone expressing neurons in the hypothalamic paraventricular nucleus of depressed patients. *Neuroendocrinology* 60:436–444.

Raadsheer FC, van Heerikhuize JJ, Lucassen PJ, Tilders FJ, Swaab DF (1995): Corticotropin-releasing hormone mRNA levels in the paraventricular nucleus of patients with Alzheimer's disease and depression. *Am J Psychiatry* 152:1372–1376.

Rosenbaum AH, Maruta T, Schatzberg AF, Orsulak PJ, Jiang NS, Cole JO, et al (1983): Toward a biochemical classification of depressive disorders, VII: Urinary free cortisol and urinary MHPG in depression. *Am J Psychiatry* 140:314–318.

Rosenblum SA, Paully GS (1984): The effects of varying environmental demands on maternal and infant behavior. *Child Dev* 55:305–314.

Rosenblum LA, Coplan JD, Friedman S, Gorman JM, Andrews MW (1994): Adverse early experiences affect noradrenergic and serotonergic functioning in adult primates. *Biol Psychiatry* 35:221–227.

Roy-Byrne PP, Bierer LM, Uhde TW (1985): The dexamethasone suppression test in panic disorder: Comparison with normal control. *Biol Psychiatry* 20:1237–1240.

Roy-Byrne PP, Uhde TW, Post RM, Gallucci W, Chrousos GP, Gold PW (1986): The corticotropin-releasing hormone stimulation test in patients with panic disorder. *Am J Psychiatry* 143:896–899.

Saunders BE, Villoponteaux LA, Lipovsky JA (1992): Child sexual assault as a risk factor for mental disorders among women: A community survey. *J Interpers Violence* 7:189–204.

Schreiber W, Lauer CJ, Krumrey K, Holsboer F, Krieg JC (1996): Dysregulation of the hypothalamic-pituitary-adrenal system in panic disorder. *Neuropsychopharmacology* 15:7–15.

Schulkin J, McEwen BS, Gold PW (1994): Allostasis, the amygdala and anticipatory angst. *Neurosci Biobeh Rev* 18:1–12.

Schweizer EE, Swenson CM, Winokur A, Rickels K, Maislin G (1986): The dexamethasone suppression test in generalized anxiety disorder. *Br J Psychiatry* 149:320–322.

Sheline YI, Wang PW, Gado MH, Csernansky JG, Vannier MW (1996): Hippocampal atrophy in recurrent major depression. *Proc Natl Acad Sci U S A* 93:3908–3913.

Singewald N, Zhou GY, Chen F, Philippu A (1996): Corticotropin-releasing factor modulates basal and stress-induced excitatory amino acid release in the locus coeruleus of conscious rats. *Neurosci Lett* 204:45–48.

Skutella T, Montkowski A, Stohr T, Probst JC, Landgraf R, Holsboer F, et al (1994): Corticotropin-releasing hormone (CRH) antisense oligodeoxynucleotide treatment attenuates social-defeat induced anxiety in rats. *Cell Mol Neurobiol* 14:579–588.

Smagin GN, Harris RBS, Ryan DH (1996): Corticotropin-releasing factor antagonist infused into the locus coeruleus attenuates immobilization stress-induced defensive withdrawal in rats. *Neurosci Lett* 220:167–170.

Smith MA, Davidson MA, Ritchie JC, Kudler H, Lipper S, Chappell P, et al (1989): The corticotropin-releasing hormone test in patients with posttraumatic stress disorder. *Biol Psychiatry* 26:349–355.

Southwick SM, Krystal JH, Johnson DR, Nagy LM, Nicolau A, Heninger GR, et al (1993): Abnormal noradrenergic function in posttraumatic stress disorder. *Arch Gen Psychiatry* 50: 266–274.

Stein MB, Walker JR, Anderson G, Hazen AL, Ross CA, Eldridge G, et al (1996): Childhood physical and sexual abuse in patients with anxiety disorders in a community sample. *Am J Psychiatry* 153:275–277.

Stein MB, Koverola C, Hanna C, Torchia MG, McClarty B (1997): Hippocampal volume in women victimized by childhood sexual abuse. *Psychol Med* 27:951–959.

Stokes PE, Frazer A, Casper R (1981): Unexpected neuroendocrine transmitter relationships. *Psychopharmacol Bull* 17:72–75.

Suomi SJ (1991): Early stress and adult emotional reactivity in rhesus monkeys. *Ciba Found Symp* 156:171–183.

Swanson LW, Sawchenko PE, Rivier J, Vale WW (1983): Organization of ovine corticotropin-releasing factor immunoreactive cells and fibers in the rat brain: An immunohistochemical study. *Neuroendocrinology* 36:165–186.

Tancer ME (1993): Neurobiology of social phobia. *J Clin Psychiatry* 54:26–30.

Vale W, Spiess J, Rivier C, Rivier J (1981): Characterization of a 41-residue ovine hypothalamic peptide that stimulates secretion of corticotropin and beta-endorphin. *Science* 213: 1394–1397.

Valentino RJ, Foote SL, Aston-Jones G (1983): Corticotropin-releasing factor activates noradrenergic neurons of the locus coeruleus. *Brain Res* 270:363–367.

van Bockstaele EJ, Colago EEO, Valentino RJ (1996): Corticotropin-releasing factor-containing axon terminals synapse onto catecholamine dendrites and may presynaptically modulate other afferents in the rostral pole of the nucleus locus coeruleus in the rat brain. *J Comp Neurol* 364:523–534.

van Oers HJ, DeKloet ER, Levine S (1998): Early versus late maternal deprivation differentially alters the endocrine and hypothalamic responses to stress. *Brain Res* 111:245–252.

Veith RC, Lewis N, Langohr JI, Murburg MM, Ashleigh EA, Castillo S, et al (1993): Effect of desipramine on cerebrospinal fluid concentrations of corticotropin-releasing factor in human subjects. *Psychiatry Res* 46:1–8.

von Bardeleben U, Holsboer F (1989): Cortisol response to a combined dexamethasone-human corticotrophin-releasing hormone challenge in patients with depression. *J Neuroendocrinol* 1:485–488.

Weiss JM, Stout JC, Aaron M, Owens MJ, Nemeroff CB (1994): Experimental studies of anxiety and depression: Locus coeruleus and corticotropin-releasing factor. *Brain Res Bull* 35: 561–572.

Widerlöv E, Bissette G, Nemeroff CB (1988): Monoamine metabolites, corticotropin-releasing factor and somatostatin as CSF markers in depressed patients. *J Affect Disord* 14:99–107.

Workel JO, Oitzl MS, Ledeboer A, DeKloet ER (1997): The Brown Norway rat displays enhanced stress-induced ACTH reactivity at day 18 after 24 h maternal deprivation at day 3. *Brain Res* 103:199–203.

Yehuda R (1997): Sensitization of the hypothalamic-pituitary-adrenal axis in posttraumatic stress disorder. *Ann N Y Acad Sci* 821:57–75.

Yehuda R, Lowy MT, Southwick SM, Shaffer D, Giller EL (1991): Increased number of glucocorticoid receptor in posttraumatic stress disorder. *Am J Psychiatry* 148:499–504.

Yehuda R, Boisoneau D, Mason J, Giller EL (1993a): Glucocorticoid receptor number and cortisol excretion in mood, anxiety, and psychotic disorders. *Biol Psychiatry* 34:18–25.

Yehuda R, Southwick SM, Krystal JH, Bremner DJ, Charney DS, Mason JW (1993b): Enhanced suppression of cortisol following dexamethasone administration in posttraumatic stress disorder. *Am J Psychiatry* 150:83–86.

Yehuda R, Boisoneau D, Lowy MT, Giller EL (1995): Dose-response changes in plasma cortisol and lymphocyte glucocorticoid receptors following dexamethasone administration in combat veterans with and without posttraumatic stress disorder. *Arch Gen Psychiatry* 52:538–593.

Yehuda R, Levengood RA, Schmeidler J, Wilson S, Guo LS, Gerber D (1996a): Increased pituitary activation following metyrapone administration in post-traumatic stress disorder. *Psychoneuroendocrinology* 21:1–16.

Yehuda R, Teicher RL, Trestman R, Siever LJ (1996b): Cortisol regulation in posttraumatic stress disorder and major depression: A chronobiological analysis. *Biol Psychiatry* 40:79–88.

Young EA, Abelson JL, Curtis GC, Nesse RM (1997): Childhood adversity and vulnerability to mood and anxiety disorders. *Depression Anx* 5:66–72.

Zaidi LY, Foy DW (1993): Childhood abuse experiences and combat related PTSD. *J Traum Stress* 7:33–42.

Zlotnick C, Ryan CE, Miller IW, Keitner GI (1995): Childhood abuse and recovery from major depression. *Child Abuse Negl* 19:1513–1516.

ELSEVIER

PERSPECTIVES

The Corticosteroid Receptor Hypothesis of Depression

Florian Holsboer, M.D., Ph.D.

Signs and symptoms that are characteristic for depression include changes in the setpoint of the hypothalamic-pituitary-adrenocortical (HPA) system, which in the majority of these patients result in altered regulation of corticotropin (ACTH) and cortisol secretory activity. More refined analysis of the HPA system revealed that corticosteroid receptor (CR) signaling is impaired in major depression, resulting among other changes, in increased production and secretion of corticotropin-releasing hormone (CRH, also frequently abbreviated CRF) in various brain regions postulated to be involved in the causality of depression. This article summarizes the clinical and preclinical data, supporting the concept that impaired CR signaling is a key mechanism in the pathogenesis of depression. Mouse genetics, allowing for selective inactivation of genes relevant for HPA regulation and molecular pharmacology, dissecting the intracellular cascade of CR signaling, are the most promising future research fields, suited for identifying genes predisposing to depression. Focusing on these two research lines may also allow to gain insight into understanding how current antidepressants work and further, how more specific targets for future antidepressant drugs can be identified. **[Neuropsychopharmacology 23:477-501, 2000]** *© 2000 American College of Neuropsychopharmacology. Published by Elsevier Science Inc.*

KEY WORDS: *Corticosteriod receptors; CRH; HPA; Stress; Depression; Antidepressants*

FUNCTIONAL IMPAIRMENT OF CENTRAL CORTICOSTEROID RECEPTORS

Clinical Evidence

Until now, the serendipitous discovery of antidepressants in the 1950s has profoundly inspired hypotheses of the pathogenesis of depression. The well-known pharmacological effects of antidepressants on presynaptic uptake transporters and degradating enzymes (i.e., MAO) of serotonin and norepinephrine has focused research on causality and treatment of depression on the metabolism of functional biogenic amines and the capacity of their respective receptors to alter intracellular signaling pathways that ultimately induce changes in gene activity. Elevated circulating levels of stress hormones among depressives were recognized even before antidepressants were discovered, but these changes were seen as epiphenomena, reflecting the stressful experience of depression, although M. Bleuler (1919) already demonstrated that hormones have diverse psychotropic effects and suggested hormone treatments as potential antidepressants. A vast amount of evidence has accumulated, that reject the view that altered stress hormone secretions in depression are epiphenomenal.

During the past decade, several research groups formulated a hypothesis relating aberrant stress hormone dysregulation to causality of depression and submitted that antidepressants may act through normalisation of these HPA changes (review: Holsboer and Barden

From the Max Planck Institute of Psychiatry, Munich, Germany.

Address correspondence to: Florian Holsboer, M.D., Ph.D., Max Planck Institute of Psychiatry, Kraepelinstr. 2–10, D-80804 Munich, Germany.

Received February 28, 2000; revised June 22, 2000; accepted June 23, 2000.

NEUROPSYCHOPHARMACOLOGY 2000–VOL. 23, NO. 5

Published by Elsevier Science Inc.
655 Avenue of the Americas, New York, NY 10010

0893-133X/00/$–see front matter
PII S0893-133X(00)00159-7

1996). This hypothesis was derived from the following clinical observations in depressives: 1) the number of ACTH and cortisol secretory pulses is increased which is also reflected in elevated urinary cortisol production rates (Rubin et al. 1987); 2) levels of CRH in the CSF are elevated (Nemeroff et al. 1984); 3) the number of CRH secreting neurons in limbic brain regions is increased (Raadsheer et al. 1994); and 4) the number of CRH binding sites in the frontal cortex is reduced secondary to increased CRH concentration (Nemeroff et al. 1988). These studies were complemented by many neuroendocrine function tests including the suppressibility of ACTH and corticosteroids by the synthetic glucocorticoid dexamethasone (dexamethasone suppression test, DST). The DST showed that a high proportion of patients with various affective disorders have elevated cortisol levels (Carroll 1982), thus escaping the suppressive effect of dexamethasone. After CRH was discovered and characterized by Vale and coworkers (1981) initial studies employing ovine or human CRH in depressives showed that the ACTH response after injection of this neuropeptide was decreased, suggesting desensitized pituitary CRH receptors due to homologous downregulation by hypersecreted CRH (Gold et al. 1986; Holsboer et al. 1986).

The most sensitive neuroendocrine function test to detect HPA dysregulation combines the DST and the CRH stimulation test (dex/CRH test) (von Bardeleben and Holsboer 1989, 1991; Heuser et al. 1994; Rybakowski and Twardowska 1999). In this test, patients are pretreated with a single low dose (1.5 mg) of dexamethasone at 23:00 h and receive intravenously 100 μg CRH at 15:00 h the following day. The amount of ACTH and cortisol subsequently released is much higher among depressives. In fact, Heuser and coworkers (1994) concluded from their studies that the sensitivity of this test (i.e., likelihood to differentiate between normal and pathological states) is above 80%, depending on age and gender. Whereas CRH-elicited ACTH response is blunted in depressives, dexamethasone pretreatment produces the opposite effect and paradoxically enhances ACTH release following CRH. Similarly, CRH-induced cortisol release is much higher in dexamethasone-pretreated patients than following a challenge with CRH alone. The interpretation of the above findings is as follows: dexamethasone, due to its low binding to corticosteroid binding globulin and its decreased access to the brain (Meijer et al. 1998), acts primarily at the pituitary to suppress ACTH. The subsequent decrease of cortisol and the failure of dexamethasone to compensate for the decreased cortisol levels in the nervous tissue creates a situation that is sensed by central regulatory elements of the HPA system as a partial and transient adrenalectomy. In response to this situation, the secretion of central neuropeptides which are capable of activating ACTH secretion—mainly CRH and vasopressin—is increased. Vasopressin is known to synergize with CRH, overriding dexamethasone suppression at human corticotrophs: When vasopressin is infused at a low rate into dexamethasone pretreated controls, concurrent infusion with CRH induces an ACTH and cortisol response which is similar to the hormone secretory profile of depressives receiving the combined dex/CRH-test but without simultaneous vasopressin treatment (von Bardeleben et al. 1985). This finding led us to postulate that hypothalamic vasopressin is increased in depressives (von Bardeleben and Holsboer 1989). A more recent study by Purba and coworkers (1996) reporting increased numbers of vasopressin-expressing neurons in the parvocellular part of the hypothalamic paraventricular nucleus of depressives ultimately confirmed this view.

All three tests (DST, CRH test, and dex/CRH test) have been frequently administered to depressed patients by several research groups. Serial DSTs during a variety of antidepressant drug treatment revealed that whenever cortisol suppression was inappropriate, i.e., above a certain threshold, normalization of the neuroendocrine dysregulation was necessary for clinical remission to become manifest. In addition, if post-dexamethasone plasma cortisol levels increased over time or remained elevated the likelihood for an unfavorable clinical course or nonresponse to treatment was high (Holsboer et al. 1982; Greden et al. 1983).

Blunted ACTH response to CRH and the normalization of elevated CRH in the CSF after antidepressant-induced clinical remission has also been reported; these findings confirm a close association between HPA dysregulation and depressive psychopathology (de Bellis et al. 1993). The combined dex/CRH test proved particularly useful as a predictor of increased risk for relapse (Holsboer et al. 1987; Holsboer-Trachsler et al. 1994; Heuser et al. 1996; Zobel et al. 1999).

In those patients where the neuroendocrine abnormality persisted, the risk of relapse or resistance to treatment was much higher. Together, all studies reported so far indicate that reinstatement of a "normal" HPA setpoint is an important prerequisite for clinical improvement and furthermore, if HPA abnormalities persist or become more pronounced during drug treatment the respective individual is at increased risk for relapse.

A study that administered different doses of dexamethasone prior to CRH showed that ACTH and cortisol suppression occurs at higher dexamethasone dosages in the depressives than in matched controls. This shift of the dose response curve to higher dexamethasone dosages corroborates the view that negative feedback mechanisms through glucocorticoid receptors (GR), to which dexamethasone binds, are impaired in depressives (Modell et al. 1997).

The consequences of impaired regulation of cortisol secretion are manifold, ranging from untoward effects in peripheral tissues (e.g., osteoporosis) to changes in the central nervous system. The latter are believed to comprise effects on morphology as well as on cognitive function. Studies by Sheline et al. (1996, 1998, 1999) and Bremner et al. (2000) suggested that recurrent major depression is associated with hippocampal volume loss and that the degree of this change is determined by the duration of the illness. Considering the findings that depressed patients are frequently hypercortisolemic and that the degree of hippocampal atrophy in aged humans correlates with the degree of plasma cortisol increase over time and the current basal cortisol levels (Lupien et al. 1998), it has been proposed that the neuroendocrine changes in depression may account for the changes in hippocampal size seen in this disease. Importantly, these reductions in hippocampal volume which are also seen in patients with schizophrenia—a disease not particularly associated with enduring hypercortisolemia—do not necessarily reflect cell death (Nelson et al. 1998). Moreover, in post-traumatic stress disorder, decreased hippocampal volume is associated with normal or even reduced plasma and urine glucocorticoid contents (Bremner et al. 1999).

Studies in rats and tree shrews showed that psychological stressors may also induce atrophy in hippocampal CA3 pyramidal neurons which involves reversible remodeling of apical dendrites, a process where elevated excitatory amino acids are believed to be a primary cause, possibly amplified by increased glucocorticoids (Watanabe et al. 1992; Gould et al. 1997; Magariños et al. 1996, 1997). That factors—other than glucocorticoids—account for stress-induced reversible or permanent morphological changes in the hippocampus has also been underscored by a study in nonhuman primates (Leverenz et al. 1999). Based on works by Landfield et al. (1981), Kerr et al. (1991), and Sapolsky (1992), the study by Leverenz et al. (1999) administered high doses of glucocorticoids to aged macaques for 12 months, however, no evidence for decreased hippocampal volume, subfield volumes, subfield neuronal density, and subfield total neuronal number emerged. This finding is in accordance with a report by Müller and coworkers (1998), who studied postmortem brains of patients with depression and of patients treated with various synthetic corticosteroids and failed to observe morphological changes and signs of cell death under these clinical conditions. In this context, it is important to note that there is evidence that primates, unlike rats, have a relative paucity in GR, but a high density in mineralocorticoid (MR) in the hippocampus (Sánchez et al. 2000). Since, unlike cortisol, synthetic corticosteroids bind only poorly to MRs, studies using synthetic glucocorticoids, e.g., dexamethasone, in humans produce a situation where MRs remain unliganded in this brain formation. If it holds true that also in humans MRs are predominating over GR in hippocampus, dexamethasone pretreatment would deprive this brain region from CR signaling.

As reviewed by McEwen and coworkers (1992), adrenal steroids can exert a manifold of effects sometimes opposing on the rat hippocampus, i.e., they can be protective as well as deleterious. In line with this view, studies by Hassan et al. (1996, 1999) and Almeida et al. (2000) showed that corticosterone and dexamethasone given at low dosages can exert opposite effects on hippocampal cell viability. It is yet unclear whether these opposing effects are due to differences in penetration of these two corticosteroids through the blood brain barrier or whether they are due to differences in relative occupation of GR and MR. It also seems important to recognize in future studies that neurochemical and neuroanatomical effects of stress hormones can only be studied to a limited extent by exogenous administration of corticosteroids. Producing stress-like plasma cortisol concentrations results in a variety of central changes including altered expression of CRH and neurotrophins, which in turn may exert neuroprotective and other behavioral effects (Behl et al. 1997).

Another issue that deserves attention in future clinical and preclinical studies relates to the difference in the effects mediated by GR and MR (reviews: Trapp and Holsboer 1996a; de Kloet et al. 1998). To dissect their respective effects on cognition, studies similar to that of Newcomer et al. (1999), but using selective MR and GR agonists and antagonists, are needed. This is of particular importance if the provocative study of Sánchez and coworkers (2000) that reported a relative absence of GR in the primate hippocampus is corroborated. Based on measurements of GR and MR mRNA, Seckl et al. (1991) showed that in human hippocampus both receptors are highly expressed, but also confirmed that differences between species exist regarding the subfield distribution of GR and MR.

In the past, much emphasis had been put on the possibility that neurochemical and neuroendocrine changes associated with depression account for the morphological changes observed in the CNS of these patients. A recent study by Rajkowska et al. (1999) found reductions in density and size of neurons and glial cells in the dorsolateral prefrontal cortex of depressed patients and raised the question whether the observed specific histopathological changes in major depression may be due to a genetic predisposition for cortical cell changes. Studies that help to resolve this question are awaited and they need to include studies on gene networks that are involved in early brain development.

Genetic Studies

The patient population which would be ideally suited to study shifted HPA setpoints are subjects with inherited glucocorticoid resistance. These patients may either have a polymorphism in the GR gene or other alterations in genes, whose products are involved in glucocorticoid signaling. As a consequence of the ubiquitous GR resistance, elevated ACTH and cortisol secretion occurs without leading to symptoms of Cushing's syndrome. Nonetheless, other disturbances emerge that are mediated by those elevated adrenocortical hormones that bind to other steroid receptors, such as MR or androgen receptors. Thus, subjects with detected familial GR resistance were diagnosed to have hypertension, and among females hirsutism, menstrual irregularities, and acne were prevalent (Lamberts et al. 1992, 1996). Because such symptoms are not apparent in depression and because of the episodic course of this disease, it seems unlikely at first sight that the pathology underlying depression involves a major GR gene mutation.

Recent data, however, suggest that relative glucocorticoid resistance caused by GR mutations may not be as infrequent as previously thought (Koper et al. 1997). Thus, it seems pertinent to study whether psychiatric syndromes are more prevalent in patients with GR resistance and also whether such mutations may occur among psychiatric patients with dysregulation of the HPA system. It is of note that the presence of polymorphisms or mutations in the GR cannot be automatically inferred from glucocorticoid resistance because structure or assembly of cellular components, such as chaperones or other transcription factors involved in hormone signaling, may also be defective. On the other hand, the episodic nature of depression does not reject the possibility of GR gene polymorphism since compensatory mechanisms, which help to maintain stress hormone homeostasis most of the time, may be present. One such mechanism may include interaction of polymorphic GR with chaperones, which are responsible for individual GR-binding properties and in cooperation with other transcription factors can determine the activation or repression of gene expression through ligand-activated GRs (see Section III). The capacity of the chaperone/transcription factor assembly to compensate for functional deficits due to allelic GR variants may fluctuate and become less effective whenever other counteracting non-genetic factors (e.g., intracellular signals induced by environmental stressors) are activated.

Munich Vulnerability Study. In this light, the data from the Munich Vulnerability Study are of interest as they show that subjects who never suffered from a psychiatric disorder, but belong to families with a high genetic load for depression may display abnormal responses to the dex/CRH test (see Figure 1). These abnormalities were found to be constant over time and

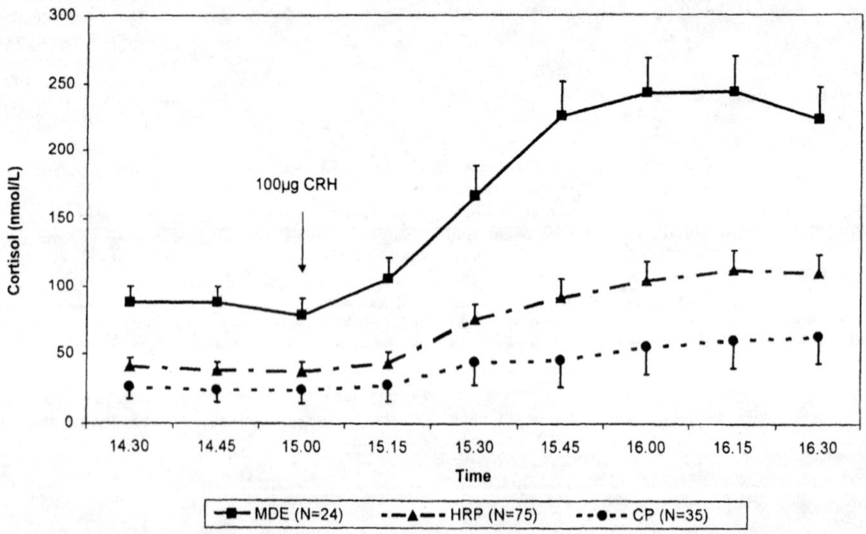

Figure 1. Munich Vulnerability Study. Seventy-five healthy probands selected from families with a high genetic load for depression (high risk probands, HRP) received 100 µg human CRH (i.v.) at 15:00 h after pretreatment with an oral dose of 1.5 mg dexamethasone at 23:00 h the day before. The plasma cortisol response (adjusted means ± SEM; adjusted by age and sex) of the HRPs, matched patients with major depressive episode (MDE) and matched healthy controls (CP) from families without history for psychiatric morbidity were found to be significantly ($F_{2,129} = 16.36$, $p < .001$) different. (Adapted from Holsboer et al. 1995 and additional data).

those subjects showing these depression-like HPA changes were considered to be at risk for developing depression (Holsboer et al. 1995; Modell et al. 1998). The possibility that these HPA disturbances are acquired and rather reflect the stressful experience of having a family member suffering from a mood disorder than a genetic risk can be rejected, as only a fraction of about 20% of the probands show these alterations. Interestingly, this figure corresponds well with the calculated risk for developing depression in later life of high risk probands (Lauer et al. 1998). Whether it proves true that these individuals are indeed prone to develop depression is currently under investigation in longitudinal follow-up studies.

While it may well be that some of the individuals showing impaired corticosteroid receptor function and increased risk for depression do have a GR mutation, e.g., a single amino acid substitution in the ligand binding domain leading to reduced corticosteroid sensitivity, most genetic studies reported so far reject the GR gene as a possible locus of inherited pathology (Detera-Wadleigh et al. 1992; Morissette et al. 1999). It would not be surprising, however, if genetic studies of large kindreds would reveal that GR-regulated genes or genes whose products are involved in stress hormone signaling are contributing to genetic susceptibility for depression.

Preclinical Studies

The CR hypothesis implies that intracellular signaling of adrenocortical steroids is impaired in specific areas of the brain, resulting in a number of changes in gene activity and neurotransmitter production involved in causality of depression. Particular emphasis is put on the interaction of hormone-activated GR and the effects on CRH, which is believed to be a key neuropeptide in the pathogenesis of depression and other stress-related disorders (reviews: Owens and Nemeroff 1991; Holsboer et al. 1992).

There is no uniform relationship, however, between activated GRs and CRH secretion, as CRH is differentially regulated by GR in different regions of the brain. In most parts of the hypothalamic paraventricular nuclei (PVN), glucocorticoids suppress CRH and vasopressin as they suppress proopiomelanocortin, the precursor of ACTH of the anterior pituitary (Erkut et al. 1998). In some brain areas that include the central amygdala expression (Schulkin et al. 1998) and those nuclei of the PVN that project to the spinal cord accounting for CRH content in the cerebrospinal fluid (Swanson and Simmons 1989), corticosteroids upregulate CRH gene expression. Positive feedback of glucocorticoids on CRH synthesis and secretion in many brain areas is life-sustaining as it keeps the organism responsive to acute stressors under conditions of chronic stress. Elevated CRH in the amygdala, for example, is pertinent to maintaining appropriate emotional responsivity, particularly if stress exposure endures (review: Gray and Bingaman 1996).

The effects of CRH are mediated through specific receptors of which two different subtypes (CRH-R1 and CRH-R2) have yet been identified (Chalmers et al. 1995). Their neuroanatomical distributions suggest that they mediate different effects. Recent studies using antisense probes directed against CRH-R1 and CRH-R2 mRNA supported this notion as they showed that only reduced CRH-R1 levels produce anxiolytic effects in stressed rats (Liebsch et al. 1999). Reports on mouse mutants where one of these receptors was genetically inactivated confirmed that CRH-R1 mediates anxiety-like behavior (Timpl et al. 1998; Smith et al. 1998). In contrast, two out of three studies where the CRH-R2 was invalidated noted increased anxiety-like behavior (Bale et al. 2000; Kishimoto et al. 2000; Coste et al. 2000) (see also Section II)

GRs are present in all rodent brain areas and are most abundant in the hypothalamus where they repress CRH and vasopressin gene activity. Most MRs in the brain are located in the hippocampus where they may be co-expressed with GR by many, but not all neurons. Hippocampal MRs are not selective for the prototypic mineralocorticoid aldosterone, but bind the glucocorticoid corticosterone (or cortisol in primates) with approximately tenfold higher affinity than GRs. This "nonselectivity" of brain MRs is determined by the fact that unlike in peripheral cells, the enzyme 11β-hydroxysteroid dehydrogenase (11βHSD) does not effectively exclude corticosterone or cortisol from MR-targets in the hippocampus. For example, in epithelial cells of the human kidney containing MR, this enzyme converts cortisol into cortisone, which binds only poorly to MR, allowing electrolyte homeostasis through aldosterone alone. In the hippocampus, a different 11βHSD isoform is present, which does not provide such selectivity (van Haarst et al. 1996a; Seckl 1997).

Because of the about tenfold higher affinity of "non selective" hippocampal MRs for corticosterone, these receptors are already almost completely occupied at basal levels of corticosteroid secretion. On the other hand, hippocampal GRs are only occupied when corticosteroid levels increase under stress conditions or at the peak of the circadian rhythm of corticosteroid secretion. The coexistence of MRs activated at low corticosteroid concentrations, and of GRs activated only at high concentrations, allows the brain to differentially respond to the wide range of concentrations over which corticosteroids are secreted. These responses are extremely diverse and include steroid effects on cell membranes. At low concentrations, corticosterone maintains neuronal excitability which is a predominantly MR-governed effect, whereas at higher hormone concentrations this is opposed by increasing GR activation (Joëls and de Kloet 1992). Specifically, under basal conditions where most of the MRs, but only a fraction of GRs are occupied, Ca^{++} inward currents are small in hippocampal neurons; this results in a stable firing rate, thus contributing to the "proactive" role of corticosterone in maintaining homeostasis (review: de Kloet et al. 1998). Under stress, more GRs are activated and there is an associated increase in Ca^{++} influx and responsivity to serotonin (5-HT), for example, increases. This condition is referred to as the "reactive" mode by which corticosteroids protect neurons through GR and MR by reinstating homeostasis (de Kloet et al. 1998). Thus, it is the ratio of activated MR and GR, which determines not only the effects of corticosteroids on hippocampal neurons themselves but also in their projection areas, e.g., the amygdala.

The effects of the predominant amino acid transmitters in the brain, glutamate and γ-aminobutyric acid (GABA), which mediate excitatory and inhibitory effects on synaptic transmission respectively, are also controlled by the relative occupancy and activation of MR and GR. This is demonstrated by the modulatory effects of these two receptors on long-term potentiation (LTP), a phenomenon that refers to strengthening of synaptic contacts by repeated stimulation. When glutamatergic afferents to the hippocampus, particularly the CA1 area, are repeatedly stimulated, prolonged enhancement of synaptic responsivity is observed as a consequence. It has been suggested that changes in LTP correlate with the capacity to learn and retrieve memorized material. The induction of LTP has been found to be critically determined by the level of corticosteroids. As recently argued by de Kloet and coworkers (1998, 1999), this effect can be best explained by appreciating the specific roles of MRs and GRs and the ratio of ligand activated MR/GR on neuronal activity in the hippocampus. Under resting conditions, when corticosteroid levels are in the normal range, LTP is most pronounced and the MR/GR ratio is high because MRs but not GRs are fully occupied. This condition is associated with a facilitated adaptation to stressful situations where MR activation accounts for behavioral reactivity to acute stressors. Under chronic stress, a reduced MR/GR ratio results from increased GR occupation under increased corticosteroid levels and a gradual desensitization of MRs which precedes GR desensitization; the latter changes are associated with reduced LTP. It seems likely that such changes in synaptic efficiency represent the neural correlate of memory impairment associated with hypercortisolism. These cognitive deficits not only include disruption of memory consolidation but also impaired memory retrieval (de Quervain et al. 1998). In this context, it is important to note that such effects do not solely result from altered corticosteroid effects in the hippocampus. For example, GR-mediated memory consolidation is also influenced by β-adrenoceptor stimulation in the amygdala (Roozendaal et al. 1999).

The interaction between hippocampal GR and MR also plays a role in HPA regulation of rat. Studies using MR antagonists or MR antisense probes under trough (morning) or stress conditions resulted in exaggerated HPA activity (Oitzl et al. 1994; Reul et al. 1997). Interestingly, the GR antagonist mifepristone (RU 486, also blocking progesterone receptors) when injected intracerebroventricularly (icv) has no effect on basal trough levels because of low GR occupancy during early daytime hours. Administration of the same drug in the early evening, when corticosteroid levels are rising, leads to further HPA activity increase. However, if RU 486 is injected directly into the hippocampus, this results in a decrease of ACTH and corticosterone secretion (van Haarst et al. 1996b), indicating that hippocampal GRs, when activated by corticosterone binding, are opposing the inhibitory effects of MRs. In other words, MRs mediate an inhibitory tone on the HPA system which is opposed by activated hippocampal GR. Following icv administration, the excitatory effect of GR antagonism at the hypothalamus overrides the inhibitory effect of GR antagonism at the hippocampus. If the balance between MR and GR is intact, then hypothalamic and pituitary GR capacity is sufficient to maintain adequate feedback upon CRH neurons and corticotrophic cells. However, if corticosteroid signaling is defunct, stress-elicited HPA activity is gradually shifted towards operating at higher setpoints, resulting in continuous HPA hyperdrive with accompanying behavioral effects due to CRH and vasopressin disinhibition as well as the many other sequelae of MR/GRdysbalance.

The Nature-Nurture Conundrum

The risk of developing depression or other major affective disorders is determined by a complex interplay between genetic susceptibility, environmental exposures, and aging. These influences also account for long-term changes in the regulation of the stress hormone system. This is particularly well illustrated by animal studies in which stressors were administered pre- or postnatally, followed by evaluations of HPA function and emotionality during later life. From these experiments, it was concluded that context and timing are critical determinants for predicting whether early stress exposure results in hypo- or hyperactive HPA-status. For example, Reul and coworkers (1994) stressed pregnant female rats with immunostimulants and observed that their pups had increased activity throughout adulthood.

Since the original report by Levine and Mullins (1966), it has been repeatedly demonstrated that the effect of postnatal "handling", i.e., a very brief daily separation of mother and pup results in reduction of both, emotionality and corticosterone secretion. Similarly, rats that had received normal maternal care (licking, grooming) during the first 10 days of their life had reduced plasma ACTH and corticosterone response to stress increased hippocampal GR and MR mRNA levels and decreased CRH mRNA when examined as adults. However, opposite effects were found, when these rats were severely traumatized postnatally by long mother-pup separations alone or in combination with mild foot shocks (Ladd et al. 1996). These rats showed increased CRH concentrations in the median eminence, decreased number of CRH receptors and pituitary ACTH-secreting cells, and hypercorticoidism, thus bearing resemblance to the neuroendocrine state found in depressives. Of special importance is the observation that rats that were postnatally traumatized perform poorly in learning and memory tests, as opposed to rats that had received optimal maternal care (Plotsky and Meaney 1993). These findings, which were also confirmed in experiments with non-human primates (Coplan et al. 1996), suggest that early trauma may persistently weaken corticosteroid signaling, leading to disinhibited release of hypothalamic CRH, ACTH, and corticosterone which, in turn, may have behavioral sequelae that are related to a number of depressive symptoms. These data might even be extrapolated to the human situation, explaining why individuals who were abused during childhood may be more likely to develop depression in later life (Heim et al. 2000).

A number of different experiments, however, demonstrates that early trauma does not necessarily result in HPA disinhibition and cognitive impairment. Oitzl et al. (unpublished results, cited in de Kloet et al., 1998) used a different strain of rats than the previous investigators and showed that in Brown Norway rats, which are known for their long and healthy life spans, early trauma (i.e., long mother-pup separation) resulted in a bimodal distribution of cognitive performance in later life. Among animals that were traumatized as pups, these investigators identified good as well as poor learners but only a few intermediate learners. In the control group, however, the majority of rats were intermediate learners and only few good or poor learners were observed. The maternally-deprived rats had decreased GR expression in the hypothalamus and in the hippocampus. Among these traumatized rats, the good performers had lower plasma ACTH and corticosterone concentrations as compared to the poor performers. These experiments point to strain-dependent effects and suggest that it is the individual genotype that determines the consequences of early trauma on the HPA-system and related behaviors. In view of this, the studies by Kendler and coworkers (1999) are important and have introduced an additional level of complexity as they show that the genetic endowment interacts with the environment; individuals with a high genetic risk for depression are more susceptible to the depressive episode-triggering effect of an adverse life event. In addition, genetic factors influence not only the sensitivity to potentially depressogenic life events, but also influence the likelihood to expose oneself to such an event. Hypothetically then, individuals with an inherited genetic trait that weakens stress hormone regulation through impaired corticosteroid receptor function may be more vulnerable to stressors and in addition they may select themselves into adversive situations which then trigger the onset of a depressive episode.

MOUSE GENETICS AS A TOOL TO PROBE THE CR HYPOTHESIS

Knock-out or Transgenic Manipulation of CRH and Corticosteroid Signaling

Mouse mutants with manipulations of the genes encoding either CRH or its receptors or CRs have been generated. As predicted from studies where CRH was injected into rodent brains, overexpression of CRH in mice results in an enhancement of anxiety-like behavior (Stenzel-Poore et al. 1994). Mice with deletions of the CRH gene exhibit normal stress-induced behavior, confirming that CRH may not be the only physiologically active ligand of CRH receptors. If CRH is absent, other neuropeptides such as urocortin or other yet-to-be identified molecules acting at CRH1 or CRH2 receptors (and possibly CRH receptors yet-to-be discovered) can serve as anxiogenic or depressogenic signals (Weninger et al. 1999).

Studies by Liebsch et al. (1995, 1999), Heinrichs et al. (1997), and Skutella et al. (1998), who used antisense probes directed against the mRNA-encoding CRH-R1 and CRH-R2 in rats, and also studies involving mouse mutants lacking CRH-R1, suggested that CRH-R1 mediates anxiety-like behavior (Timpl et al. 1998; Smith et al. 1998) (Figure 2). In contrast, CRH-R2 deficiency was shown to increase anxiety-like behavior in some (Bale et al. 2000; Kishimoto et al. 2000) but not all (Coste et al. 2000) studies, raising the possibility that the two so far identified CRH receptors mediate opposite effects on anxiety-like behavior. Recently, Radulovic and coworkers (1999) confirmed that the role of CRH in enhancing learning and precipitating anxiety-like behavior is brain area- and receptor type-dependent and that previous stressful experience can also modulate the CRH-mediated behaviors. CRH signaling through CRH receptors is further complicated because CRH is bound to CRH-binding protein (CRH-BP) which has an affinity for CRH that is equal to or greater than the respective CRH receptors (Potter et al. 1991). This 37-kDA protein binds 40–90% of total CRH and is present in most human brain regions at tenfold higher concentrations than total CRH, which points to a major role of CRH-BP as regulator of CRH, "buffering" its actions under conditions of excessive release (Behan et al. 1995).

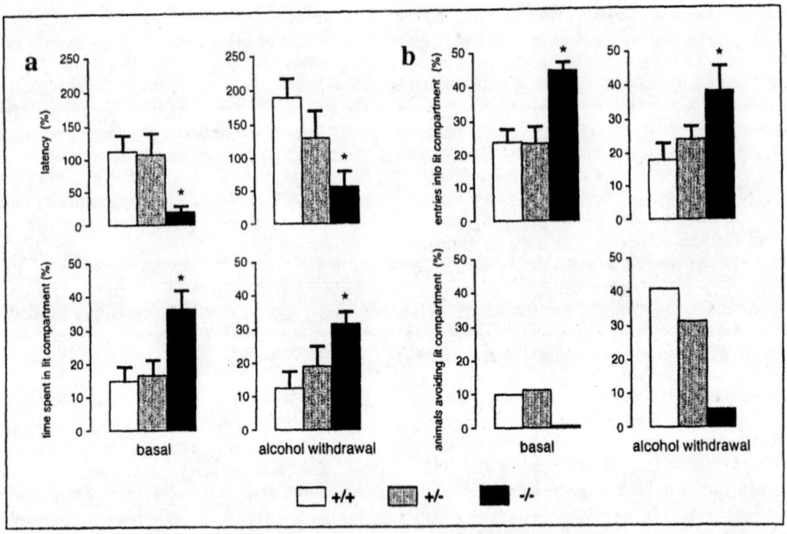

Figure 2. CRH_1 Receptor Knockout Mouse. A mouse mutant lacking a functional CRH_1 receptor by using homologous recombination in embryonic stem cells was generated where the coding sequences of the transmembrane regions V, VI, and VII, including the G-coupling protein domain and the intracellular cytoplasmatic trial were deleted. Analysis of their behavioral phenotype employing the light-dark box revealed that these mice showed less anxiety-like behavior at basal and stress (alcohol withdrawal) conditions. **(a)** Latency to enter the lit compartment was increased during withdrawal from comparison of 20 wild-type, 18 heterozygous, and 19 null mutants under basal and 22 wild-type, 22 heterozygous, and 20 null mutants under stress conditions, significant ($F_{1,115} = 8.4$, $p < .005$) treatment effects emerged. **(b)** A similar effect of withdrawal stress was observed for animals avoiding the lit compartment. For latency, percent of time spent in the lit compartment and percent of entries into the lit compartment (genotype at $F_{2,115} > 12.1$, $p < .0001$). All these and data from Smith et al. (1998) are consistent with reduced anxiety-like behavior in the full or partial absence of CRH_1 receptors. (From Timpl et al. 1998).

Compounds that displace CRH from this carrier in the brain produce anxiety-like and anorectic behavior, which is similar to the behavioral phenotype of mice where the gene for CRH-BP had been deleted (Karolyi et al. 1999). The loss of appetite seen in these animals is plausibly explained by the increased "free" CRH and urocortin levels since both of these peptides exert anorectic effects through CRH-R1 and/or CRH-R2. The behavioral role of urocortin still needs to be clarified. This neuropeptide binds with higher affinity to both CRH receptors and this may explain why anxiety-like responses to stressors in CRH null mutant mice are indistinguishable from wild-type mice (Weninger et al. 1999). In the absence of CRH, urocortin may bind to CRH-R1 compensating the loss of CRH. Consistent with the notion that CRH and CRH receptors are involved in depression, anxiety and other stress-related conditions, transgenic mice which overexpress CRH-BP show decreased anxiety-like behavior and enhanced locomotor activity (Burrows et al. 1998).

The above mentioned studies confirmed the central role of CRH and its receptors in mediating stress-related hormonal and behavioral responses and are complemented by recent studies in mice with targeted mutations of corticosteroid receptors. In order to gain further insight into the causality of HPA aberrancies, the GR gene was disrupted, which resulted in a phenotype with 90–95% lethality (Cole 1996). Survivors had excessive ACTH and corticosterone levels and almost absent adrenal medullas. In these mutants, Meijer and coworkers (1997) showed that the GR deficit results in impaired processing of spatial information. Because this behavior had previously been attributed to MR, these authors suggested that MR effects in the hippocampus require intact GR function which is consistent with a role for GR/MR heterodimers in mediating these effects (Trapp et al. 1994). The fact that only a minor fraction of litters survives the disruption of GR suggests that these animals were the few that could successfully compensate GR deficiency, which has profound peripheral effects.

The true nature of these complex compensatory mechanisms is not clear and it will be difficult to identify their specific involvement in the observed behavioral phenotype. Therefore, the recently developed mouse mutants where the GR knockout was restricted to neural tissue using the Cre/LoxP-recombination system should be more promising for studies of the effects of GR disruption in the brain (Tronche et al. 1999). In these mice, exon 3, encoding the first zinc-finger GR DNA binding domain, was flanked by LoxP sites. Crossing these mice with mice that express the nestin-Cre transgene resulted in animals where GR protein was absent only in neurons and glia cells. In these mice, CRH was elevated in the hypothalamus and ACTH and corticosterone were hypersecreted indicating that ligand-activated pituitary GRs (which remained intact) are unable to fully compensate for effects of hypersecreted CRH through suppression of POMC gene expression. These mice also showed signs of reduced anxiety and impaired stress response suggesting that loss of corticosteroid signaling through GR in the brain has direct consequences for emotional behavior (Tronche et al. 1999).

These initial studies did not address whether GR deletion leads to reduced CRH gene expression in the central amygdala. In this brain region, CRH is believed to be enhanced by activated GR and the absence of neuronal GR function could plausibly result in decreased anxiety-like behavior (Schulkin et al. 1998). Notably, even cell-specific gene disruption does not resolve the issue of compensatory mechanisms which are perhaps also reflected in the surprising dissociation of ACTH and corticosterone secretion in these mice. Given the specific role of hippocampal MR in behavior and neuroendocrine regulation, it would be of great interest to study a mouse mutant where the MR gene deletion is restricted to the hippocampus. The MR knockout mice obtained by gene targeting that is not tissue specific, died between postnatal day 8 and day 13 due to massive sodium loss and subsequent electrolyte disturbance (Berger et al. 1998). Studies using techniques to inactivate MR selectively in the hippocampal formation are now warranted to better understand the role of this receptor, which in non-human primates is believed to be the predominant corticosteroid receptor in this brain region (Sánchez et al. 2000).

Transgenic Mice Expressing GR Antisense

Pepin and coworkers (1992) generated a transgenic mouse in which an 1815 base pair fragment of the 3′ non-coding region of the GRcDNA, downstream from a 2.3 kb Eco R1/Hind III human neurofilament promoter element, was inserted into the mouse genome. This resulted in a mouse expressing GR antisense mainly in neuronal tissue and this mutant was expected to be a well-suited animal model of depression associated with impaired GR function (Pepin et al. 1992). This transgenic mouse was extensively studied and the main findings that emerged were the following: 1) these mice needed higher dexamethasone dosages than control mice in order to display corticosterone suppression under basal conditions or following CRH (Stec et al. 1994); 2) CRH-elicited ACTH was higher in transgenic mice but corticosterone was lower in comparison to controls (Barden et al. 1997); 3) these mice showed decreased corticosterone response to exogenous ACTH (Barden et al. 1997); 4) when stressed, these mice showed increased ACTH levels, whereas corticosterone levels remain unchanged (Karanth et al. 1997); 5) Dijkstra et al. (1998) showed reduced activity of CRH neurons in the PVN of these mice and decreased sensitivity of pituitary CRH-R1 mRNA to stimulus-induced desensitisation; 6) these mice displayed an enhanced locomotor-stimulating effect to morphine, a response that is reflected by an enhanced dopaminergic activity within the mesolimbic system (Spanagel et al. 1996); 7) in these mice, responses to endotoxin were aberrant as noted by Linthorst and coworkers (1999), confirming that immune function is critically determined by appropriate GR function; 8) several studies (e.g., Montkowski et al. 1995; Rousse et al. 1997; Rochford et al. 1997; Ströhle et al. 1998) showed that these mice have impairments in learning and memory paradigms which are also influenced by age; 9) Steckler et al. (1999) concluded that allocentric spatial navigation is impaired whereas egocentric navigation is unimpaired. The latter authors suggested that the observed effects were due to hippocampal dysfunction secondary to GR deficiency and possible compensatory changes. From their study follows that the observed deficit is related to a general impairment in storage or retrieval of information; 10) Steckler and coworkers (2000a) further concluded that the behavioral phenotype of GR-impaired transgenic mice is characterized by altered motivation and enhanced impulsive responding rather than from mnemonic deficiency; 11) Linthorst et al. (2000) studied putative disturbances at the synaptic level in these mice employing an *in vivo* microdialysis probe. In transgenic mice, serotonin release was higher than in control mice when exposed to rats, usually perceived as a profound stressor by mice. Paradoxically, transgenic mice did not show typical stress-like behaviors (e.g., freezing), but exhibited arousal behavior (e.g., exploration and approach toward a rat). The exaggerated serotonin release in these mice perhaps reflects the reciprocal interaction between CRH and raphe-hippocampal serotonin activity. Chronically elevated levels of central CRH have been shown to cause hyporesponsiveness of hippocampal serotonin following an acute stressful stimulus (Linthorst et al. 1997). In these transgenic mice, hypothalamic release of CRH is low, possibly explaining the enhanced serotonin release (Dijkstra et al. 1998).

Critical appreciation of the herein referred to studies using mouse mutants allows one to conclude that manipulations of the expression of CRH and its receptors have largely confirmed what was expected from pharmacological experiments. Alteration of GR gene expression (knockout or antisense expression) has led to several unexpected findings, e.g., reduced anxiety-like behavior in mice with GR gene disruption in the CNS and decreased CRH expression in hypothalami of mice expressing GR antisense. It is of note that none of the mouse mutants generated so far, can be viewed as animal model of a specific psychiatric disease defined by common diagnostic procedures. However, as discussed below these mouse mutants seem to be of great value to study several selected symptoms such as anxiety, abnormal stress response, cognition, withdrawal from drugs of abuse, appetite, reproductive behavior, sleep, etc., that are associated with HPA disturbances.

MOLECULAR MECHANISMS OF CORTICOSTEROID SIGNALING

Cytosolic Activities

The translation of the corticosteroid signal into a cellular response can be dissected into three steps: 1) entry of corticosteroids into the cell which occurs by passive transmembrane passage; 2) binding to corticosteroid receptors whose binding capacity is determined by chaperone-assisted folding; 3) trafficking to the nucleus that involves dissociation of chaperones and cooperative actions of transporters; and 4) nuclear actions of ligand-activated receptors either through DNA binding at specific response elements (GRE) or through protein-protein interaction with other transcription factors.

The first step in corticosteroid signaling, its passage through the cell membrane, is regarded as a passive process due to the lipophilic nature of steroid molecules. Because the affinity of steroid molecules for intracellular receptors is higher than for extracellular transport proteins (corticosteroid-binding globulin), there is enrichment of corticosteroid molecules within target cells. Only recently, specific interactions of corticosteroids with molecules residing within the cell membrane have been identified. From studies with ion channels composed of $GABA_A$ receptor subunits, evidence emerged that so-called neuroactive steroids (usually reduced at the ring A of the steroid molecule) interact by modulating chloride ion conductance (reviews: Paul and Purdy 1992; Rupprecht and Holsboer 1999).

In non-mammalian cells, Orchinik and coworkers (1991) found preliminary evidence for a corticosterone receptor-like structure in synaptic membranes and others (Alléra and Wildt 1992; Lackner et al. 1998) suggested the existence of a glucocorticoid carrier within the membrane of rat liver cells. It is yet unresolved whether such mechanisms also exist in neurons. These studies need to be substantiated in various tissues before the possibility of membrane-mediated actions can be recognised as crucial step in steroid signaling. That the access of corticosteroids to nerve cells can also be limited by an active process has recently been shown by Schinkel et al. (1995). Uptake of moderate amounts of dexamethasone was found to be limited by a multidrug resistance gene product, a P-glycoprotein extrusion pump that actively exports synthetic corticosteroids, but not naturally occurring hormones out of the cell. Mice lacking this gene have a higher central uptake of some synthetic neuroactive compounds (Uhr et al. 2000) including dexamethasone (Meijer et al. 1998).

When entering the cell, the corticosteroid molecule binds to MR or GR which are part of a dynamic multiprotein complex, composed of the steroid receptor and an array of chaperones which include heat shock proteins. Chaperones function as assembly systems for steroid receptors as well as other protein molecules involved in corticosteroid signal transduction. The basic assembly system (termed "foldosome") has been reconstituted *in vitro* and was shown to require hsp90, hsp70, p60/hop (hsp70-organizing protein) and hsp40 (Pratt and Dittmar 1998). The foldosome initially associates with the nonsteroid binding state of the receptor. Under *in vivo* conditions the foldosome may require additional proteins, e.g., hip (hsp70-interacting protein). In the final heterocomplex, hop is replaced by immunophilins, e.g., FKBP 51 (also termed FKBP 59) or FKBP 52 (also termed FKBP 59, p59, or hsp56). This heterocomplex is further stabilized by p23, a protein that binds directly to hsp90 and maintains the corticosteroid receptor in a conformation that facilitates hormone binding. It is of note that the stepwise assembly and conformational maturation of the heterocomplex requires energy input through ATP. Both chaperones, hsp90 and hsp70, are ATP-binding and -hydrolyzing proteins. The role for hsp90 and the importance of ATP to maintain receptor conformation has been studied using the benzoquinone geldanamycin, which occupies the nucleotide binding site on hsp90 and prevents the switch to its ATP-bound conformation. Through this inhibition, the corticosteroid receptor is prevented from being assembled into the heterocomplex and is kept in a low affinity state for its ligands and steroid receptor-induced transactivation is therefore abolished.

Another example how chaperoning determines CR signaling is that the ratio between hsp70 and a protein that binds hsp70 as a co-chaperone, termed BAG-1 (Bcl-2-associated gene product-1) modulates the glucocorticoid-binding activity of the GR hsp90 heterocomplex, as increasing BAG-1 inhibits GR folding and thus decreases corticosteroid signaling (Kanelakis et al. 1999; Nollen et al. 2000). From these findings, it can be concluded that changes in the chaperone assembly can have a manifold of effects on activation and repression of GRE-regulated genes. The relevance of stoichiometric changes in chaperone expression has been demonstrated in the squirrel monkey, a species with excessively high cortisol levels, but no signs of Cushing's syndrome (Chrousos et al. 1982). This discrepancy is currently best explained by a markedly decreased binding affinity of GR, due to an overexpression of immunophilin FKBP 51 in squirrel monkey (Reynolds et al. 1999).

Once the steroid is bound, it induces a conformational change in the receptor and subsequently heat shock proteins and immunophilins dissociate, allowing for nuclear actions of activated MRs and GRs. This dissociation equilibrium is a dynamic process and GR and MR can be recycled by reassociating with chaperones. There is increasing evidence that (co)chaperones are not only important for GR activity in the cytosol, but also in the nucleus. For example, hsp90 may participate in the nuclear-cytoplasmic shuttling of GR (Kang et al. 1999) and it may also facilitate chromatin recycling of GR (Liu and DeFranco 1999). More recently, the cochaperone RAP 46 (also known as HAP 46 or BAG-IL) which can associate with hsp90 and GR has been identified as a non-specific DNA-binding protein which may act as a general transcriptional activator (Zeiner et al. 1999), on the other hand, Schneikert and coworkers (1999) reported that RAP 46 downregulates GR-mediated transactivation, but not transrepression. Altogether, it becomes clear from these few selected examples that future research linking HPA function with causality of depression and course of treatment needs to include studies on the role of chaperones in GR signaling.

Nuclear Activities

Ligand-activated GRs and MRs can either activate or deactivate expression of target genes. Activation occurs through formation of GR-GR and MR-MR homodimers or GR-MR heterodimers, which bind to short palindromic DNA sequences called glucocorticoid response elements (GRE, see above) in the promoter region of corticosteroid-responsive target genes. Whether the response elements to which receptor homodimers or heterodimers can bind are all identical is not yet known. The role of activated GR and MR functioning as nuclear transcription factors is to recruit various factors that are able to remodel the chromatin structure at the promoter of the target gene and to recruit and maintain a transcriptional pre-initiation complex. A fine-tuned mechanism orchestrates gene activation through GRE and only a few aspects highlighting possible causes of impaired GR and MR function at this level and consequences for potential targets are briefly discussed (reviews: Beato et al. 1995; Mangelsdorf et al. 1995; Shibata et al. 1997; Freedman 1999) (see Figure 3).

When bound to DNA, the steroid receptor associates with coactivators, such as steroid receptor coactivator 1 (SRC-1, member of the p160 family). If SRC-1 is coexpressed in an assay system analysing GRE-regulated gene expression (such as the mouse mammary tumor virus, MMTV) then the transcriptional efficacy of GRs is strongly enhanced. The situation is even more complex as the enhancement of GR by the coactivator SRC-1 is amplified by CBP, a protein that binds CREB (cyclo AMP response element binding protein). This synergy may function through more efficient recruitment of basic ("general") transcription factors (GTF) and stabilization of the preinitiation complex, thus enhancing mRNA synthesis by polymerase II. SRC-1 and CBP are only two of the many recently discovered coactivators of GR-mediated transcriptional activity and the mechanism by which they drive transcription is only poorly understood. One such mechanism is the acetylation of histones by SRC-1 which results in localized chromatin remodelling and assembly of the basal transcription machinery into a stable preinitiation complex (Spencer et al. 1997). While all coactivators identified so far are proteins, a recent study by Lanz and coworkers (1999) identified an RNA molecule that fulfills all characteristics of a coactivator of SRC-1. This RNA transcript called SRA (steroid receptor RNA activator), if coexpressed in assays of steroid receptor-mediated transactivation, can induce a tenfold enhancement of receptor gene activity, which can be abolished when SRA antisense oligodeoxynucleotides are added to the cells. It is not clear whether modulation of GR mediated transactivation by RNA molecules is a physiologically relevant mechanism. This theoretical possibility, however, opens up many new opportunities to interfere with glucocorticoid actions in the nucleus.

Reduction of gene expression by glucocorticoid receptors can be achieved through DNA-bound GRs as well as by interference of GRs with those nuclear transcription factors, that otherwise enhance gene activity. The physiological role of response elements, which reduce transcription when GR dimers are bound, is still debated. Only in a few cases, for example, the negative GRE-mediated regulation of the proopiomelanocortin gene expression, a mechanism requiring DNA-binding receptor dimers, seems to be effective (Drouin et al. 1993). Another example is that of the recently localized cis-acting site of the human CRH promoter that mediates negative regulation by ligand-activated GR (CRHnGRE) (Malkoski et al. 1997). Under the experimental conditions used (transient expression in mouse corticotroph-derived AtT-20 cells), the CRHnGRE, however, can be activated by cAMP or CREB (Malkoski and Dorin 1999).

To further appreciate these findings in the context of the CR hypothesis, it would be desirable to reproduce these findings under conditions that allow extrapolations on the *in vivo* condition. Still another possibility of GR-induced reduction of gene activity is that some molecules associated with GRE bound receptors act as corepressors (see Figure 3). Such a functional interaction be-

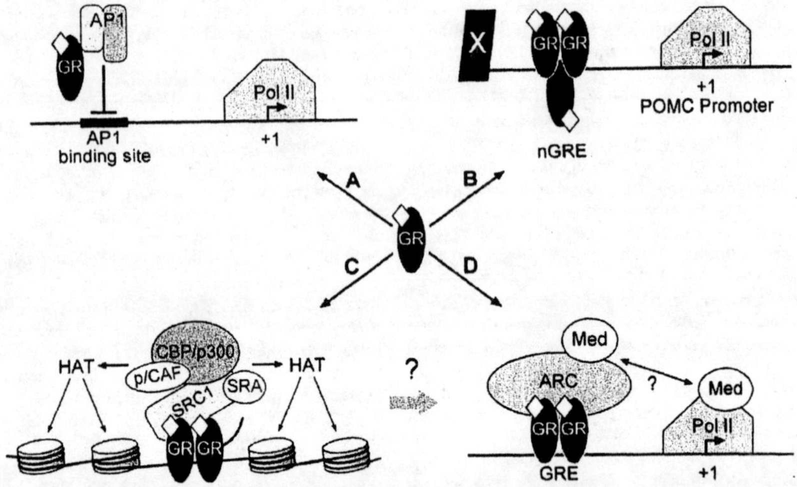

Figure 3. Positive and Negative Regulation of Gene Transcription by GR. **(A)** *Transrepression.* Ligand-activated GR interacts with transcription factors like AP1 or NF-κβ by direct protein-protein contacts, thereby preventing them from binding to their cognate DNA sites and from activating the RNA polymerase II initiation complex. **(B)** *nGREs.* Negative regulation of gene transcription by ligand-activated GR in the POMC promoter involves binding of a GR trimer to a negative GRE (nGRE), thereby presumably intervening with upstream activating factors (X). Negative regulation at other nGREs, e.g., in the gene promoters of CRH, GnRH, prolactin, IL-1β, and osteocalcin involves the interplay with other transcription factors, e.g., AP-1, Pbx, and Oct-1. **(C)** *Chromatin Remodeling.* Coactivators of the p160 family such as SRC-1 (= NCoA-1), RAC3, GRIP1 (= TIF2 = NCoA-2), p/CIP (= ACTR), AIB1, and TRAM-1 bridge the DNA-bound GR dimer with a complex consisting of CBP or its homologue p300 and p/CAF. In addition, a ribonucleoprotein complex containing SRA (steroid receptor RNA activator) . RNA probably stabilizes the interaction of p160 proteins (e.g., SRC-1) with GR. Since the p160 family members, CBP/p300 and p/CAF all possess HAT (histone acetyl transferase) activity, this complex would result in remodeling the chromatin structure, thereby opening promoter regions. Moreover, CBP has the capability to directly bind to components of the basal transcription machinery. **(D)** *Transactivation.* DNA-bound GR dimer recruits the activation complex DRIP (probably identical to ARC and TRAP) which leads to activation of the RNA polymerase II complex. Mammalian homologues of the mediator/SRB proteins have been found both as components of the DRIP complex and associated with the CTD of RNA polymerase II, a functional interaction between these two protein complexes. Whether the chromatin remodeling complex **(C)** and the transactivating complex **(D)** function subsequently or concomitantly is not clear yet. *Abbreviations:* ACTR, activator of the thyroid and retinoic acid receptors; AIB1, amplified in breast cancer 1; ARC, activator-recruited cofactor; CBP, CRE binding protein; CRH, corticotropin-releasing hormone, DRIP, vitamin D receptor-interacting protein; GnRH, gonadotropin releasing hormone; GRE, glucocorticoid responsive element; GRIP1, glucocorticoid receptor interacting protein; HAT, histone acetyl transferase; Med, Mediator; NCoA, nuclear receptor coactivator; p/CAF, p300/CBP-associated factor; p/CIP, p300/CBP-cointegrator associated protein; POMC, pro-opiomelanocortin; RAC3, receptor-associated coactivator; SRA, steroid receptor RNA activator; SRC-1, steroid receptor coactivator 1; SRB, suppressor of RNA polymerase B mutations; TIF2, transcriptional intermediary factor; TRAM-1, Thyroid hormone receptor activator molecule 1; TRAP, thyroid receptor-associated protein.

tween a latent transcription factor called Stat5 (signal transducer and activator of transcription) and the GR has been shown (Stoecklin et al. 1996). The GR can form a physical complex with Stat5, which decreases its DNA binding and thus GR-driven transactivation. This effect, first demonstrated in the mouse mammary tumor virus (MMTV) promoter (which contains four copies of the GRE), required phosphorylation and dimerisation of Stat5. The MR is similarly affected by Stat5, however, at a lower rate (Stoecklin et al. 1997).

The best studied example of how corticosteroid receptors negatively regulate gene transcription through protein-protein binding is a group of negatively GR-regulated genes that contain an AP-1 (activating protein 1) binding site in the promoter. AP-1 is a dimer composed of Jun and Fos (review: Pfahl 1993). If GR is ligand-activated it interacts as a monomer with the Jun/Fos dimer resulting in decreased AP-1 driven transcription (Figure 3). An example where both mechanisms (transactivation through genomic action and transrepression through protein-protein interaction) occur simultaneously is the effect of ligand-activated GR on the activity of NFκB (nuclear factor κB), a factor which is induced by many stimuli, predominantly those related to inflammation. In its inactive form NFκB (composed of a p50-p65 heterodimer, although other members of the RelA family can also constitute this transcription factor) is complexed by the inhibitory IκB subunit. When activated by corticosteroids, GRs can activate IκB expression through a GRE in the IκB gene promoter (Auphan et al. 1995). Furthermore, activated GRs interact with p65 and may therefore prevent p50-p65 binding to κB sites in the promoters of cytokines or cell adhesion factors which mediate inflammatory response (Caldenhoven et al. 1995). This dual action of corticosteroids through GR-protein interaction and gene activation works concurrently to suppress clinical symptoms associated with inflammation (Wissink et al. 1998; van der Burg et al. 1997).

Another mechanism which may reduce the efficiency of GR induced gene activation is altered splicing of GR pre-mRNA, resulting in overexpression of the GRβ variant that is devoid of transactivity. Heterodimerisation of GRβ with the transactive GRα results in diminished GRE regulated gene activity (Bamberger et al. 1995). A nuclear orphan receptor has also been identified that represses GR mediated transcriptional activity (Trapp and Holsboer 1996b). Other orphan nuclear receptors that interfere with GR and are directly involved in HPA activity belong to the nurr1/nur77 subfamily. These molecules do not require ligand binding and can confer transcriptional activity through specific response elements without ligand activation (Drouin et al. 1998; Murphy and Conneely 1997). Nur77, which transactivates either as a monomer or as a dimer through specific response elements, is of particular importance for the maintenance of basal ACTH secretion. Only during stress, when CRH is released from the hypothalamus reaching the anterior pituitary through portal vessels, CRH-R1 receptor-mediated enhancement of proopiomelanocortin gene expression and subsequent increased secretion of ACTH from corticotrophs occurs.

While most experiments elucidating cellular effects of ligand-activated corticosteroid receptors have been conducted in artificial cell systems, some of the conclusions drawn so far have been corroborated in a mouse mutant where a specific point mutation was introduced into the GR (Reichardt et al. 1998). These authors mutated the GR gene by exchanging alanine and threonine, in position 458. This was based on a study by Heck and coworkers (1994) who observed that this mutation, which is located in the second zinc-finger in the DNA binding domain of the GR, abolishes receptor dimerisation and thus DNA binding. In mice homozygous for this point mutation, CRH expression was unimpaired, whereas POMCmRNA and ACTH were elevated. This finding is consistent with a negative regulation of the CRH gene through GR monomers that do not bind to DNA but transrepress through protein-protein interaction. Alternatively, the activation of a negative GRE in the CRH promoter may not require GR dimerisation (Malkoski and Dorin 1999). In contrast, pituitary corticotrophs require GR dimerisation which is in accord with DNA binding at a negative response element or interaction as a dimer with nur77 (Philips et al. 1997).

The examples referred to in this section show that a great number of possibilities exist for changing the setpoint of an individuals HPA activity. It is important to note that such setpoints are variable across individuals, but fairly stable intra-individually (Huizenga et al. 1998). This is even true among individuals with an increased genetic risk for depression where alterations of this setpoint are believed to be causally related to pathogenesis (Modell et al. 1998).

CONSEQUENCES FOR FUTURE DRUG TREATMENT OF DEPRESSION

Current Antidepressants

Antidepressants are clinically effective not only in depression and panic disorder, but also in generalized anxiety and social phobia, and constitute one of the most successful treatment modalities in medicine. In contrast to this clinical situation, elucidation of the mechanisms of action of these drugs has been less successful. The hypothesis that has dominated the psychopharmacology of depression for decades is based on the assumption that a biogenic amine-deficiency underlies mood disorders and that this can be remedied by inhibition of presynaptic reuptake transporters of serotonin (synthesized and released from dosal raphe nucleus) and/or norepinephrine (originating from the locus coeruleus), thus increasing the transmitter concentration at postsynaptic sites. This hypothesis does not explain why it takes many weeks, often months, before antidepressants become effective, whereas reuptake inhibition occurs immediately.

A refinement of the monoamine hypothesis was forwarded by studies that depleted central serotonin and norepinephrine bioavailability. These studies found that normal individuals do not develop depressive symptoms when serotonin or norepinephrine is depleted through specific diets (Delgado et al. 1990). It was found, however, that patients having previously responded to a selective serotonin reuptake inhibitor (SSRI) worsen clinically when experimentally deprived from serotonin, but not from norepinephrine. In turn, those patients having responded to a norepinephrine reuptake inhibitor had increased depressive symptomatology when norepinephrine depletion was induced through diet with methyl para-tyrosine (Delgado et al. 1992). It was concluded from these studies that antidepressants rather than acting through a specific pharmacological mechanism may trigger a long cascade of events which then converge to act through a final common pathway. The view that the primary effect of antidepressant-induced changes on uptake transporters is remote from the therapeutically-relevant action is also fueled by a recent study that failed to find a difference in the clinical efficacy of the selective serotonin reuptake inhibitor paroxetine when compared to tianeptine, which enhances serotonin reuptake (Nickel et al., unpublished results), which is in accord with results of a study that compared tianeptine with fluoxetine (Lôo et al. 1999).

Two new hypotheses, which are complementary rather than mutually exclusive, have been forwarded to explain how antidepressants work at the neurobiological level. One hypothesis, developed by Duman et al. (1997), focusses on the effects of activation of the cAMP cascade through cell membrane receptors, followed by enhanced induction of CREB and hippocampal brain derived neurotrophic factor (BDNF). The other hypothesis, which is the fundament of this treatise, submits that antidepressants act through improving CR function. In the CNS, these modulations also affect brain regions not or only indirectly connected to the peripheral HPA system, which regularly stabilizes under the influence of antidepressants.

Studies supporting the cAMP/CREB/BDNF-hypothesis documented that the expression of CREB is enhanced by antidepressants and electroconvulsive treatments. In addition, the stress-induced decrease of BDNF is blocked by antidepressants. Because the BDNF gene contains a cAMP response element (CRE) to which phosphorylated CREB (P-CREB) binds and enhances transcription, it is assumed that activating cAMP through increased amine binding at G protein-coupled cell membrane receptors will ultimately result in increased expression of BDNF. This neurotrophic factor, when injected centrally in high dosages to rats produces changes in behavior that are reminiscent of changes induced by antidepressants (Siuciak et al. 1996). The antidepressant-induced expression of BDNF would also explain the beneficial effect of these drugs upon neuronal survival and growth of hippocampal neurons which are believed to be potentially endangered as a consequence of the neuroendocrine changes during a depressive episode (see Section I).

As the authors of this hypothesis point out themselves, CREB and BDNF regulation are not the sole targets of antidepressants (review: Duman et al. 1997). Their hypothesis rather exemplifies a new approach in exploring how antidepressants may exert their therapeutic of action beyond the receptor level. More specifically, studies related to the cAMP/CREB/BDNF-hypothesis will prove whether the absolute amount of CREB, increased by antidepressants is relevant for transactivation of CRE-regulated genes. In the future, the degree of phosphorylation of CREB (P-CREB) following acute and long-term treatments with antidepressants needs to be analysed, because only P-CREB can bind to DNA, thereby accounting for CRE-induced transactivation. Such studies are pertinent since Rossby and coworkers (1999) examined the long-term effects of venlafaxine, which inhibits both, the serotonin and the norepinephrine reuptake transporter. These authors reported that CREB expression was unchanged by venlafaxine, whereas the transcriptionally active phosphorylated P-CREB was reduced in the cortex of rats. Because neither endogenous nor cAMP-stimulated protein kinase A (PKA) activity was changed by venlafaxine, the decrease of P-CREB was not attributed to decreased cAMP. If this venlafaxine-induced decrease in CREB phosphorylation is also effective in the hippocampus, BDNF expression would be expected to be decreased by this drug in this brain area. This would be not consistent with a general enhancement of BDNF expression by effective antidepressants.

The important information obtained from these studies is that antidepressants exert nuclear effects that are not necessarily mediated by the well-characterized signaling pathways. This seems particularly true when one tries to unify the CR hypothesis and the cAMP/CREB/BDNF hypothesis. First, there is substantial cross-talk between CR signaling and CREB phosphorylation. GR does not prevent CREB binding at DNA but physically associates with CREB and thus decreases phosphorylation of CREB. Provided that the observation of Rossby and coworkers (1999) is not limited to the specific effects of venlafaxine in the cortex, then decreased P-CREB should result in decreased expression of CRH, which contains a CRE in its promoter (Seasholtz et al. 1988; Spengler et al. 1992). Legradi and coworkers (1997) observed that glucocorticoids can abolish CREB phosphorylation in CRH neurons. Thus, if GR signaling is impaired, CRH expression through P-CREB is enhanced and this effect is counteracted by venlafaxine (and perhaps also by other antidepressants) which reduces P-CREB (Rossby et al. 1999). Still, other impairments in cAMP-PKA pathways may possibly exist in depression (Shelton et al. 1999), including impaired CRE-regulated gene expression which can be restored by antidepressants. Since cross-talk between cAMP-PKA pathways and corticosteroid signaling is well documented, impaired corticosteroid receptor function could not only result from altered cAMP-PKA activity but may in turn account for disturbances in cAMP-PKA-elicited activation of CRE.

The second observation that allows both hypothesis to converge is that postreceptor effects of antidepressants do not necessarily implicate cell membrane receptor G protein cAMP-PKA pathways or ion channel-mediated activation of kinases. Inasmuch as BDNF can be regulated by other mechanisms than cAMP-CREB, corticosteroids can also be functionally regulated by antidepressants in the absence of adrenoceptors. Pepin and coworkers (1992) have demonstrated increased GR promoter activity in fibroblast cells that are devoid of aminergic receptors, and other studies (Rossby et al. 1995; Eiring and Sulser 1997) found that increased hippocampal GR mRNA expression is independent of increased adrenoceptor stimulation and, in general, independent of norepinephrine bioavailability. In this context, another interesting aspect that has been introduced by Pariante et al. (1997), is that GR trafficking can be induced by antidepressants independently of ligand binding and receptor activation, thus pointing to an interaction of antidepressants with chaperones, and an interference with the energy supply (ATP) necessary to maintain corticosteroid receptors in a hormone-binding mode through energy-requiring activities of chaperones.

In vivo experiments showed that rats, when treated for five weeks with different antidepressants (MAO inhibitors, SSRIs, norepinephrine reuptake inhibitors, serotonin reuptake enhancer), displayed decreased baseline and stress-induced levels of plasma ACTH and corticosterone. Upon analyzing the capacity of MR and GR in the hippocampus of these rats, it was found that the first change was seen in MR binding, which increased after one week of treatment (Reul et al. 1993, 1994, and unpublished results). In the light of the inhibitory effect of MRs on HPA activity which is reflected by studies employing MR antagonists in rats (Spencer et al. 1998) and humans (Dodt et al. 1993; Young et al. 1998) or MR antisense in rats (Reul et al. 1997), the observed upregulation of MR capacity seems to be a first step necessary for the inhibition of hypothalamic CRH neurons. This effect on MR is followed by increased GR capacity (Brady et al. 1991; Seckl and Fink 1992; Reul et al. 1993, 1994).

The physiological significance of MR function is further underscored by studies that showed that acute stress in the hippocampus is associated with increased hippocampal (CA1) MR density and function, an effect that is mediated by CRH and associated with an increased inhibitory tone on HPA activity (Gesing et al., unpublished results). The MR-upregulating effect of antidepressants and the subsequent reduction of HPA overactivity in depressed patients points toward the importance of appropriate MR function. This is further supported by a clinical trial in which antidepressant response to amitriptyline in major depression was impaired by coadministration of spironolactone, an MR antagonist (Hundt et al., unpublished results, cited in Holsboer 1999).

The effects of antidepressants on GR function have been studied using the transgenic mouse that expresses GR antisense (see Section III). After long-term treatment with moclobemide, a reversible inhibitor of MAO A, these mutated mice not only showed normalized HPA activity but also changes in several tests of anxiety and memory (Montkowski et al. 1995). Some of these behavioral alterations may be explained by the recent electrophysiological observation that in these animals the threshold for induction of hippocampal LTP is shifted towards low stimulation frequencies by long-term treatment with moclobemide (Steckler et al. 2000b).

Because long-term administration of moclobemide suppresses HPA activity and activates cAMP-mediated CREB phosphorylation via PKA, the expression of BDNF may be enhanced and followed by a profound alteration in synaptic efficiency (Korte et al. 1995, 1996; Chen et al. 1999; Kafitz et al. 1999). Furthermore, in these transgenic mice, morphine-induced mesolimbic release of serotonin and dopamine as well as the psychomotor-stimulant effects of morphine were enhanced. This is in accordance with the well-established modulation of these neurotransmitters by GR and their modulation of responses to drugs of abuse. After long-term treatment with moclobemide, these neurochemical and behavioral abnormalities disappeared (Sillaber et al. 1998). In addition, tranylcypromin, an irreversible nonselective MAO-inhibitor, was found to induce the AP-1 complex, probably indicating stimulation of a large number of genes by antidepressants (Hope et al. 1994). As outlined above, AP-1 is negatively modulated by GR, whose function is most likely enhanced by this antidepressant drug. These findings support the notion that antidepressants act by improving the negative feedback capacity of the HPA system at various levels and that the setpoint of the HPA system activity is modified in a way that "buffers" the hormonal response to stressors. This may represent one mechanism by which patients who have recovered from a depressive episode may be protected by long-term antidepressant treatment against further stress-triggered relapses.

CRH Receptor Antagonists

If one assumes that normalization of an altered HPA setpoint is an essential mechanism for antidepressant drug action, the question arises as to how this goal is achieved. One explanation involves the well founded β-adrenoceptor desensitization and decrease in cAMP-mediated phosphorylation of transcription factors including CREB, following antidepressant treatment. If this effect of antidepressants, which to date has only been demonstrated *in vivo* for venlafaxin (Rossby et al. 1999), *in vitro*, however, for several other antidepressants (Schwaninger et al. 1995), is a general phenomenon of antidepressants, then this decreased activation of CREB would result in decreased CRH expression via CRE (see above). An alternative treatment approach would, therefore, be to either suppress the behavioral symptoms of enhanced CRH by CRH receptor antagonist or to block the many untoward effects excessive corticosteroid secretion may have by administration of GR antagonists.

One recently developed pyrazolopyrimidine, R121919, is a compound with high affinity for CRH-R1 that is now clinically tested and appears to not suppress stress-induced HPA response: patients and controls treated with varying dosages of R121919 did not have an impaired CRH-elicited ACTH and cortisol release (Zobel et al. 2000). This is consistent with the selectivity of such compounds for CRH-R1, leaving pituitary CRH-R2 still responsive to CRH challenges, which in conjunction with other ACTH secretagogues such as vasopressin may override the CRH-R1 blockade at corticotrophs. This is in accord with a report by Sánchez et al. (1999), who found that CRH2-R exist at primate corticotrophs. In addition, the possibility exists that the doses used in human studies still leaves sufficient CRH-R1 available for CRH-elicited ACTH response.

The first open label trial with a CRH1-R antagonist observed significant reductions in depression and anxiety scores using both clinician and patient ratings, suggesting that this type of compound may have considerable therapeutical potential. The question of whether CRH-R1 antagonists resolve the entire depressive syndrome or only several stress-related symptoms, such as pathological anxiety, loss of appetite and sexual drive, sleep disturbance, psychomotor and cardiovascular changes, etc. as found in animal experiments, remains to be validated in controlled clinical studies. Another important aspect are the consequences of CRH-R1 antagonist withdrawal. Long-term CRH-R1 antagonist treatment may result in receptor upregulation and enhanced CRH secretion in a similar way as was seen in CRH-R1 knockout mice where CRH accumulation occurs in all areas in which CRH-R1 is normally expressed, e.g., in the amygdala. After cessation of long-term treatment, patients with depression may have upregulated CRH_1 receptors and accumulated ligand (CRH), which together may increase liability for relapse, possibly making tapering of the drug necessary (Zobel et al. 2000).

Cortisol Synthesis Inhibitors

The other alternative focusses on reduction of cortisol either by cortisol synthesis inhibitors or by blocking their action by antagonizing their effects at receptors and has only been investigated in a small number of studies. Administration of metyrapone results in an inhibition of hydroxylation at position C11 of the steroid molecule, thus preventing synthesis of cortisol and corticosterone. Metyrapone treatment has produced antidepressant-like behavioral changes in two frequently used rodent models for screening antidepressive compounds, the forced swim-test and the olfactory-bulbectomized rat (Healy et al. 1999).

Metyrapone and the antidepressant desimipramine produced similar effects in these models, in agreement with a clinical study by O'Dwyer and coworkers (O'Dwyer et al. 1995), who confirmed the antidepressant potential of metyrapone in a placebo-controlled trial already suggested in numerous exploratory studies. This clinical effect seems to contradict the notion that decreased cortisol-mediated feedback may elicit increased CRH in all those brain areas where CRH gene expression is negatively controlled by GR. It was hypothesized that such an increase in CRH may either directly or indirectly precipitate some of the cardinal symptoms of depression. However, as discovered in a series of studies by Patchev et al. (1994, 1996, 1997), the additional bioavailability of non C11-hydroxylated adrenal steroids increases the pool of so-called neuroactive steroids (such as tetrahydro11-deoxy-cortisol or tetrahydro11-deoxycorticosterone) which can exert a number of neuroendocrine and behavioral symptoms such as reduction of anxiety-like behavior and suppression of CRH expression. These results indicate that neuroactive steroids may be able to compensate for the loss of corticosterone (or cortisol in humans) following metyrapone. In this context it is of interest that these neuroactive steroids may exert both genomic and nongenomic effects (Rupprecht et al. 1993) and that the concentration of these steroids is modulated by antidepressants in animals and humans (Romeo et al. 1998; Uzunova et al. 1998; Ströhle et al. 2000).

Other strategies comprise treatments with aminoglutethimide, which is a less selective inhibitor of cortisol biosynthesis, and with ketokonazole. Aminogluthetimide blocks 3β-steroiddehydrogenase and 11β-hydroxylase. Ketokonazole, in addition to blocking adrenal steroid synthesis, inhibits cytochrome P450-dependent enzymes (11-hydroxylase, 17-hydroxylase, C17,20 lyase) similar to aminogluthetimide and has direct inhibitory effects on other anterior pituitary cells than corticotrophs (Stalla et al. 1989) thus, for example, affecting gonadal steroid secretion. Consistent with predictions from open label studies (e.g., Murphy 1991; Thakore and Dinan 1995), a recent double blind placebo-controlled study suggested that ketokonazole is superior to placebo among hypercortisolemic depressed patients (Wolkowitz et al. 1999). Here again, it is difficult to dissociate the effects of ketokonazole from the effects of other adrenal steroids which are produced at much higher rates because of the enzyme blockade. Interestingly, in the study by Wolkowitz and coworkers (1999) pregnenolone sulfate which is a negative allosteric modulator of the $GABA_A$ receptor is increased eightfold by ketokonazole. Thus, ketokonazole may exert psychotropic effects through increased pregnenolone which has been reported to improve cognitive impairment in animals (Flood et al. 1995).

Appreciation of studies examining the effects of corticosteroid synthesis inhibitors thus requires recognition of the very complex changes in steroid metabolism which may be induced by the applied drugs; these changes can result in a manifold of different psychotropic effects. Controlled studies evaluating the potential benefits of metyrapone either given alone or in combination with standard antidepressants in depression are warranted.

Corticosteroid Receptor Antagonists

Blockade of corticosteroid receptors as a treatment strategy has been poorly studied due to the lack of specific antagonists. Preliminary results from Murphy et al. (1993) suggested that mifepristone (RU 486) may be a useful treatment approach in major depression. Theoretically, mifepristone may be particularly effective in psychotic depression where the HPA system is most frequently hyperactive and where cortisol induced inhibition of dopamine metabolism may be involved in the pathogenesis of this subtype of depression (Schatzberg et al. 1985). In fact, trimipramin, an effective antidepressant monotherapy of psychotic depression, suppresses hypersecretion of cortisol very effectively (Holsboer-Trachsler et al. 1994; Sonntag et al. 1996).

In contrast to GR antagonism, more substantial data are available for the MR antagonist spironolactone, which if coadministered with the antidepressant amitriptyline impairs antidepressant drug response (Hundt et al., unpublished, cited in Holsboer 1999). The explanation for this finding is related to the studies discussed above, supporting the notion that the first neuroendocrine response to antidepressants is an increase in hippocampal MR, which apparently is required to initiate the cascade that ultimately leads to clinical response (Reul et al. 1993, 1994). Notably, MR agonists enhance hypothalamic CRH release through their hippocampal action. Selective GR antagonists most likely enhance CRH secretion from the hypothalamus which is in line with data from Tronche and coworkers (1999) where a neuron-specific deletion of the GR led to an increase in CRH and PVN of these mice. In other brain areas, e.g., in those where CRH is activated by GR, treatment with GR antagonists may repress CRH gene activity. Clinical trials are therefore needed to clarify the therapeutic potential of GR antagonists in depression and related disorders.

It is not fully clear, however, how disturbed corticosteroid receptor signaling can be influenced therapeutically. Conservatively, administration of a CRH-R1 antagonist is expected to shorten the onset of coadministered antidepressants. Such drugs may also act as antidepressants when administered as monotherapy. Similarly, GR antagonists might not be effective enough as a monotherapy, but they may be a worthwhile adjunct to antidepressants. Whether corticosteroid synthesis inhibitors have therapeutic potential is an open question, since these drugs induce many other psychotropic steroid metabolites. Some studies, however, suggest that metyrapone may taper untoward effects of stress under experimental conditions in rats (Calvo et al. 1998) as well as in patients with cancer (Deguchi et al. 1998).

OUTLOOK

The examples discussed in this article support the hypothesis that impaired central stress hormone regulation is causally involved in the development and course of depression. In addition, experimental evidence is provided, suggesting that the mechanism of action of antidepressants includes normalization of HPA activity. This hypothesis can now be tested clinically as well as in basic laboratories. While clinical studies are needed to test whether specific intervention at various levels of stress hormone regulation, i.e., CRH-R1 or GR antagonists are equal or superior to current antidepressants, basic studies need to elaborate intracellular signaling and DNA effects of antidepressants and how stress hormones interfere.

The advent of the detailed human genome map in the near future combined with the use of the techniques that allow gene expression profiling on a large scale in a short time offers the possibility to discover novel candidate drug targets. Once identified, the possible relevance of such candidate genes can be verified by generating mouse mutants where the corresponding gene had been inactivated. Only if a relevant phenotype emerges from behavioral screening, a more detailed analysis and the search for molecules that modulate expression of the respective gene or its nuclear effects is warranted.

Techniques that allow large scale analysis of the proteom, and in particular transcription factor activation by phosphorylation in a similar way to that presently used for profiling of gene activation by DNA microarrays still need to be developed. The clinical observations pointing to stress hormone dysregulation causing depression on the one hand and the manifold cellular and nuclear effects of hormone-activated GR and MR on the other, predicts that CR-regulated genes and derived proteins may ultimately be identified as optimal drug targets for depression and possibly other stress-related disorders. Drugs that will emerge from new strategies in biomedicine are likely to be more selectively targeted to specific elements of the HPA system than standard antidepressants. These new drugs promise to act much faster, however only in cases where the central stress hormone system is defunct.

Because these changes in stress-related neuropeptide and corticosteroid secretion are not uniform in the CNS, but subjected to a neuroanatomical microheterogeneity, i.e., may not affect all brain areas in the same way, it seems important to keep in mind that peripheral measures of the pituitary-adrenocortical activity do not necessarily reflect alterations in the release of CR-regulated neuropeptides such as CRH, e.g., in the central amygdala, locus coeruleus, or prefrontal cortex. Therefore, the challenge for clinical research is to develop laboratory tests that allow to specifically identify those patients who may potentially benefit from a therapeutic strategy that specifically targets the central stress hormone system.

REFERENCES

Alléra A, Wildt L (1992): Glucocorticoid-recognizing and -effector sites in rat liver plasma membrane. Kinetics of corticosterone uptake by isolated membrane vesicles. I. Binding and transport. J Steroid Biochem Mol Biol 42:737–756

Almeida OF, Conde GL, Crochemore C, Demeneix BA, Fischer D, Hassan AH, Meyer M, Holsboer F, Michaelidis TM (2000): Subtle shifts in the ratio between pro- and antiapoptotic molecules after activation of corticosteroid receptors decide neuronal fate. FASEB J 14:779–790

Auphan N, Didonato JA, Rosette C, Helmberg A, Karin M (1995): Immunosuppression by glucocorticoids: Inhibition of NF-κB activity through induction of IκB synthesis. Science 270:286–290

Bale TI, Gontarino A, Smith GW, Chan R, Gold LH, Sawchenko PE, Koob GF, Vale WW, Lee K-F (2000): Mice deficient for corticotropin-releasing hormone receptor-2 display anxiety-like behaviour and are hypersensitive to stress. Nature Genet 24:410–414

Bamberger CM, Bamberger AM, DeCastro M, Chrousos GP (1995): Glucocorticoid receptor beta, a potential endogenous inhibitor of glucocorticoid action in humans. J Clin Invest 95:2435–2441

Barden N, Stec I, Montkowski A, Holsboer F, Reul JMHM (1997): Endocrine profile and neuroendocrine challenge tests in transgenic mice expressing antisense RNA against the glucocorticoid receptor. Neuroendocrinology 66:212–220

Beato M, Herrlich P, Schütz G (1995): Steroid hormone receptors: Many actors in search of a plot. Cell 83:851–857

Behan DJP, Heinrichs SC, Troncoso JC, Liu XJ, Kawas CH, Ling N, De Souza EB (1995): Displacement of corticotropin releasing factor from its binding protein as a possible treatment for Alzheimer's disease. Nature 378:284–287

Behl C, Lezoualc'h F, Trapp T, Widmann M, Skutella T, Holsboer F (1997): Glucocorticoids enhance oxidative stress-induced cell death in hippocampal neurons *in vitro*. Endocrinology 138:101–106

Berger S, Bleich M, Schmid W, Cole TJ, Peters J, Watanabe HWK, Warth R, Greger R, Schütz G (1998): Mineralocorticoid receptor knockout mice: Pathophysiology of sodium metabolism. Proc Natl Acad Sci USA 95:9424–9429

Bleuler M (1919): The Internal Secretions and the Nervous System. (Nervous and Mental Disease Monograph Series, No. 30.) New York, Nervous and Mental Disease Publ Comp

Brady LS, Whitfield HJ Jr, Fox RJ, Gold PW, Herkenham M (1991): Long-term antidepressant administration alters corticotropin-releasing hormone, tyrosine hydroxylase, and mineralocorticoid receptor gene expression in rat brain. Therapeutic implications. J Clin Invest 87:831–837

Bremner J, Southwick S, Charney D (1999): The neurobiology of post-traumatic stress disorder: An integration of animal and human research. In Saigh P, Bremner J (eds), Post-traumatic Stress Disorder: A Comprehensive Text. Needham Heights, MA, Allyn & Cacon, pp 103–143

Bremner JD, Narayan M, Anderson ER, Staib LH, Miller HL, Charney DS (2000): Hippocampal volume reduction in major depression. Am J Psychiatry 157:115–117

Burrows HL, Nakajima M, Lesh JS, Goosens KA, Samuelson LC, Inui A, Camper SA, Seasholtz AF (1998): Excess corticotropin-releasing hormone-binding protein in the hypothalamic-pituitary-adrenal axis in transgenic mice. J Clin Invest 101:1439–1447

Caldenhoven E, Liden J, Wissink S, Van de Stolpe A, Raaijmakers J, Okret S, Gustafsson J-A, Van der Saag PT (1995): Negative crosstalk between RelA and the glucocorticoid receptor: A possible mechanism for the anti-inflammatory action of glucocorticoids. Mol Endocrinol 9:401–412

Calvo N, Martijena ID, Molina VA, Volosin M (1998): Metyrapone pretreatment prevents the behavioral and neurochemical sequelae induced by stress. Brain Res 800:227–235

Carroll J (1982): Clinical applications of the dexamethasone suppression test for endogenous depression. Pharmacopsychiatry 15:19–24

Chalmers DT, Lovenberg TW, De Souza EB (1995): Localization of novel corticotropin-releasing factor receptor (CRF2) mRNA expression to specific subcortical nuclei in rat brain: Comparison with CRF1 receptor mRNA expression. J Neurosci 15:6340–6350

Chen G, Kolbeck R, Barde Y-A, Bonhoeffer T, Kossel A (1999): Relative contribution of endogenous neurotrophins in hippocampal long-term potentiation. J Neurosci 19:7983–7990

Chrousos GP, Renquist D, Brandon D, Eil C, Pugeat M, Vigersky R, Cutler GB Jr, Loriaux DL, Lipsett MB (1982): Glucocorticoid hormone resistance during primate evolution: receptor-mediated mechanisms. Proc Natl Acad Sci USA 79:2036–2040

Cole TJ (1996): Steroid receptor knockouts. Curr Opin Endocrinol Diabet 3:363–368

Coplan JD, Andrews MW, Rosenblum LA, Owens MJ, Friedman S, Gorman JM, Nemeroff CB (1996): Persistent elevations of cerebrospinal fluid concentrations of corticotropin-releasing factor in adult non-human primates exposed to early-life stressors: Implications for the pathophysiology of mood and anxiety disorders. Proc Natl Acad Sci USA 93:1619–1623

Coste SC, Kesterson RA, Heldwein KA, Stevens SL, Heard AD, Hollis JH, Murray SE, Hill JK, Pantely GA, Hohimer AR, Hatton DC, Phillips TJ, Finn DA, Low MJ, Rittenberg MB, Stenzel P, Stenzel-Poore MP (2000): Abnormal adaptations to stress and impaired cardiovascular function in mice lacking corticotropin-releasing hormone receptor-2. Nature Genet 24:403–409 de Bellis MD, Gold, PW, Geracioti TD Jr, Listwak SJ, Kling MA (1993): Association of fluoxetine treatment with reductions in CSF concentrations of corticotropin-releasing hormone and arginine vasopressin in patients with major depression. Am J Psychiatry 150:656–657

de Kloet ER, Vreugdenhil E, Oitzl MS, Joëls M (1998): Brain corticosteroid receptor balance in health and disease. Endocrinol Rev 19:269–301

de Kloet ER, Oitzl MS, Joëls M (1999): Stress and cognition: Are corticosteroids good or bad guys? Trends Neurosci 22:422–426

de Quervain DJ-F, Roozendaal B, McGaugh JL (1998): Stress and glucocorticoids impair retrieval of long-term spatial memory. Nature 394:787–790

Deguchi M, Yoshiaki I, Matsukawa S, Yamaguchi A, Nakagawara G (1998): Useful of metyrapone treatment to suppress cancer metastasis facilitated by surgical stress. Surgery 123:440–449

Delgado PL, Charney DS, Price LH, Aghajanian GK, Landis H, Heninger GR (1990): Serotonin function and the mechanism of antidepressant action: Reversal of antidepressant-induced remission by rapid depletion of plasma tryptophan. Arch Gen Psychiatry 47:411–418

Delgado PL, Price LH, Heninger GR, Charney DS (1992): Neurochemistry of affective disorders. In Paykel ES (ed), Handbook of Affective Disorders. New York, NY, Churchill Livingstone, pp 219–253

Detera-Wadleigh SD, Berrettini WH, Goldin LR, Martinez M, Hsieh WT, Hoehe MR, Encio IJ, Coffman D, Rollins DY, Muniec D (1992): A systematic search for a bipolar predisposing locus on chromosome 5. Neuropsychopharmacology 6:219–229

Dijkstra I, Tilders FJH, Aguilera G, Kiss A, Rabandan-Diehl C, Barden N, Karanth S, Holsboer F, Reul JMHM (1998): Reduced activity of hypothalamic corticotropin-releasing hormone neurons in transgenic mice with impaired glucocorticoid receptor function. J Neurosci 18:3909–3918

Dodt C, Kern W, Fehm HL, Born J (1993): Antimineralocorticoid canrenoate enhances secretory activity of the hypothalamus-pituitary-adrenocortical (HPA) axis in humans. Neuroendocrinology 58:570–574

Drouin J, Sun YL, Chamberland M, Gauthier Y, De Lean A, Nemer M, Schmidt TJ (1993): Novel glucocorticoid receptor complex with DNA element of the hormone-repressed POMC gene. EMBO J 12:145–156

Drouin J, Maira M, Philips A (1998): Novel mechanism of action for Nur77 and antagonism by glucocorticoids: A convergent mechanism for CRH activation and glucocorticoid repression of POMC gene transcription. J Steroid Biochem Mol Biol 65:59–63

Duman RS, Heninger GR, Nestler EJ (1997): A molecular and cellular theory of depression. Arch Gen Psychiatry 54:597–606

Eiring A, Sulser F (1997): An increased synaptic availability of norepinephrine is *not* essential for antidepressant induced increases in hippocampal GR mRNA. J Neural Transm 104:1255–1258

Erkut ZA, Pool C, Swaab DF (1998): Glucocorticoids suppress corticotropin-releasing hormone and vasopessin expression in human hypothalamic neurons. J Clin Endocrinol Metab 83:2066–2073

Flood JF, Morley JE, Roberts E (1995): Pregnenolone sulfate enhances post-training memory processes when injected in very low doses into limbic system structures; the amygdala is by far the most sensitive. Proc Natl Acad Sci USA 92:10806–10810

Freedman LP (1999): Increasing the complexity of coactivation in nuclear receptor signaling. Cell 97:5–8

Gold PW, Loriaux DL, Roy A, Kling MA, Calabrese JR, Kellner CH, Nieman LK, Post RM, Pickar D, Gallucci W, Avgerinos P, Paul S, Oldfield EH, Cutler GB Jr, Chrousos GP (1986): Responses to corticotropin-releasing hormone in the hypoercortisolism of depression and Cushing's disease. N Engl J Med 314:1329–1335

Gould E, McEwen BS, Tanapat P, Galea LAM, Fuchs E (1997): Neurogenesis in the dentate gyrus of the adult tree shrew is regulated by psychosocial stress and NMDA receptor activation. J Neurosci 17:2492–2498

Gray TS, Bingaman EW (1996): The amygdala: Corticotropin-releasing factor, steroids, and stress. Critical Rev Neurobiol 10:155–168

Greden F, Gardner R, King D, Grunhaus L, Carroll J, Kronfol Z (1983): Dexamethasone suppression test in antidepressant treatment of melancholia. Arch Gen Psychiatry 40:493–500

Hassan AHS, von Rosenstiel P, Patchev VK, Holsboer F, Almeida OFX (1996): Exacerbation of apoptosis in the dentate gyrus of the aged rat by dexamethasone and the protective role of corticosterone. Exp Neurol 140:43–52

Hassan AHS, Patchev VK, von Rosenstiel P, Holsboer F, Almeida OFX (1999): Plasticity of hippocampal corticosteroid receptors during aging in the rat. FASEB J 13:115–122

Healy DG, Harkin A, Cryan JF, Kelly JP, Leonard BE (1999): Metyrapone displays antidepressant-like properties in preclinical paradigms. Psychopharmacology 145:303–308

Heck S, Kullmann M, Gast A, Ponta H, Rahmsdorf HJ, Herrlich P, Cato ACB (1994): A distinct modulating domain in glucocorticoid receptor monomers in the repression of activity of the transcription factor AP-1. EMBO J 13:4087–4095

Heim C, Newport DJ, Heit S, Graham YP, Wilcox M, Bonsall R, Miller AH, Nemeroff CB (2000): Increased pituitary-adrenal and autonomic responses to stress in adult women after sexual and physical abuse in childhood. JAMA, In press

Heinrichs SC, Lapsansky J, Lovenberg TW, De Souza EB, Chalmers DT (1997): Corticotropin-releasing factor CRF1, but not CRF2 receptors mediate anxiogenic-like behavior. Regul Peptides 71:15–21

Heuser I, Yassouridis A, Holsboer F (1994): The combined dexamethasone/CRH test: A refined laboratory test for psychiatric disorders. J Psychiatric Res 28:341–356

Heuser IJE, Schweiger U, Gotthardt U, Schmider J, Lammers CH, Dettling M, Yassouridis A, Holsboer F (1996): Pituitary-adrenal-system regulation and psychopathology during amitriptyline treatment in elderly depressed patients and in normal comparison subjects. Am J Psychiatry 153:93–99

Holsboer F (1999): The rationale for corticotropin-releasing hormone receptor (CRH-R) antagonists to treat depression and anxiety. J Psychiatric Res 33:181–214

Holsboer F, Barden N (1996): Antidepressants and HPA regulation. Endocrinol Rev 17:187–203

Holsboer F, Liebl R, Hofschuster E (1982): Repeated dexamethasone suppression test during depressive illness. Normalization of test result compared with clinical improvement. J Affect Disord 4:93–101

Holsboer F, Gerken A, Von Bardeleben U, Grimm W, Beyer H, Müller OA, Stalla GK (1986): Human corticotropin-releasing hormone (CRH) in patients with depression, alcoholism and panic disorder. Biol Psychiatry 21:601–611

Holsboer F, Von Bardeleben U, Wiedemann K, Müller OA, Stalla GK (1987): Serial assessment of corticotropin-releasing hormone response after dexamethasone in depression—implications for pathophysiology of DST nonsuppression. Biol Psychiatry 22:228–234

Holsboer F, Spengler D, Heuser I (1992): The role of corticotropin-releasing hormone in the pathogenesis of Cushing's disease, anorexia nervosa, alcoholism, affective disorders and dementia. Prog Brain Res 93:385–417

Holsboer F, Lauer CJ, Schreiber W, Krieg J-C. (1995): Altered hypothalamic-pituitary-adrenocortical regulation in healthy subjects at high familial risk for affective disorders. Neuroendocrinology 62:340–347

Holsboer-Trachsler E, Hemmeter U, Hatzinger M, Seifritz E, Gerhard U, Hobi V (1994): Sleep deprivation and bright light as potential augmenters of antidepressant drug treatment—neurobiological and psychometric assessment of course. J Psychiatric Res 28:381–399

Hope BT, Nye HE, Kelz MB, Self DW, Iadarola MJ, Nakabeppu Y, Duman RS, Nestler EJ (1994): Induction of a long-lasting AP-1 complex composed of altered Fos-like proteins in brain by chronic cocaine and other chronic treatments. Neuron 13:1235–1244

Huizenga NATM, Koper JW, de Lange P, Pols HAP, de Jong FH, Stolk RP, Grobbee DE, Lamberts SWJ (1998): Interperson variability, but intraperson reproducibililty of baseline cortisol concentrations and its relation to the feedback sensitivity of the hypothalamo-pituitary-adrenal axis to low dose dexamethasone. J Clin Endocrinol Metab 83:47–54

Joëls M, de Kloet ER (1992): Control of neuronal excitability by corticosteroid hormones. Trends Neurosci 15:25–30

Kafitz KW, Rose CR, Thoenen H, Konnerth A (1999): Neurotrophin-evoked rapid excitation through TrkB receptors. Nature 401:918–921

Kanelakis KC, Morishima Y, Dittmar KD, Galigniana MD, Takayama S, Reed JC, Pratt WB (1999): Differential effects of the hsp70-binding protein BAG-1 on glucocorticoid receptor folding by the hsp90-based chaperone machinery. J Biol Chem 274:34134–34140

Kang KI, Meng X, Devin-Leclerc J, Bouhouche I, Chadli A, Cadepond F, Baulieu E-E, Catelli M-G (1999): The molecular chaperone hsp90 can negatively regulate the activity of a glucocorticosteroid-dependent promoter. Proc Natl Acad Sci USA 96:1439–1444

Karanth S, Linthorst ACE, Stalla GK, Barden N, Holsboer F, Reul JMHM (1997): Hypothalamic-pituitary-adrenocortical axis changes in a transgenic mouse with impaired glucocorticoid receptor function. Endocrinology 138:3476–3485

Karolyi IJ, Burrows HL, Ramesh TM, Nakajima M, Lesh JS, Seong E, Camper SA, Seasholtz AF (1999): Altered anxiety and weight gain in corticotropin-releasing hormone-binding protein-deficient mice. Proc Natl Acad Sci USA 96:11595–11600

Kendler KS, Karkowski LM, Prescott CA (1999): Causal relationship between stressful life events and the onset of major depression. Am J Psychiatry 156:837–841

Kerr DS, Campell LW, Applegate MD, Brodish A, Landfield PW (1991): Chronic stress-induced acceleration of electrophysiologic and morphometric biomarkers of hippocampal aging. J Neurosci 11:1316–1324

Kishimoto T, Radulovic J, Radulovic M, Lin CR, Schrick C, Hooshmand F, Hermanson O, Rosenfeld MG, Spiess J (2000): Deletion of *Crhr2* reveals an anxiolytic role for corticotropin-releasing hormone receptor-2. Nature Genet 24:415–419

Koper JW, Stolk RP, de Lange P, Huizenga NATM, Molijn G-J, Pols HAP, Grobbee DE, Karl M, de Jong FH, Brinkmann AO, Lamberts SWJ (1997): Lack of association between five polymorphisms in the human glucocorticoid receptor gene and glucocorticoid resistance. Human Genet 99:663–668

Korte M, Carroll P, Wolff E, Brem G, Thoenen H, Bonhoeffer T (1995): Hippocampal long-term potentiation is impaired in mice lacking brain-derived neurotrophic factor. Proc Natl Acad Sci USA 92:8856–8860

Korte M, Griesbeck O, Gravel C, Carroll P, Staiger V, Thoenen H, Bonhoeffer T (1996): Virus-mediated gene transfer into hippocampal CA1 region restores long-term potentiation in brain-derived neurotrophic factor mutant mice. Proc Natl Acad Sci USA 93:12547–12552

Lackner C, Daufeldt S, Wildt L, Alléra A (1998): Glucocorticoid-recognizing and -effector sites in rat liver plasma membrane. Kinetics of corticosterone uptake by isolated membrane vesicles. III. Specificity and stereospecificity. J Steroid Biochem Mol Biol 64:69–82

Ladd CO, Owens MJ, Nemeroff CB (1996): Persistent changes in corticotropin-releasing factor neuronal systems induced by maternal deprivation. Endocrinology 137:1212–1218

Lamberts SWJ, Koper JW, Biemond P, den Holder FH, de Jong FH (1992): Cortisol receptor resistance: The variability of its clinical presentation and response to treatment. J Clin Endocrinol Metab 74:313–321

Lamberts SWJ, Huizenga ATM, de Lange P, de Jong FH, Koper JW (1996): Clinical aspects of glucocorticoid sensitivity. Steroids 61:157–160

Landfield PW, Baskin RK, Pitler TA (1981): Brain aging correlates: Retardation by hormonal-pharmacological treatments. Science 214:581–584

Lanz RB, McKenna NJ, Onate SA, Albrecht U, Wong J, Tsai SY, Tsai M-J, O'Malley BW (1999): A steroid receptor coactivator, SRA, functions as an RNA and is present in an SRC-1 complex. Cell 97:17–274

Lauer CJ, Schreiber W, Modell S, Holsboer F, Krieg J-C (1998): The Munich vulnerability study of affective disorders. J Psychiatric Res 32:393–401

Legradi G, Holzer D, Kapcala LP, Lechan RM (1997): Glucocorticoids inhibit stress-induced phosphorylation of CREB in corticotropin-releasing hormone neurons of the hypothalamic paraventricular nucleus. Neuroendocrinology 66:86–97

Leverenz JB, Wilkinson CW, Wamble M, Corbin S, Grabber JE, Raskind MA, Peskind ER (1999): Effect of chronic high-dose exogenous cortisol on hippocampal neuronal number in aged nonhuman primates. J Neurosci 19:2356–2361

Levine S, Mullins RF (1966): Hormonal influences on brain organization in infant rats. Science 152:1585–1592

Liebsch G, Landgraf R, Gerstberger R, Probst JC, Wotjak CT, Engelmann M, Holsboer F, Montkowski A (1995): Chronic infusion of a CRH_1 receptor antisense oligodeoxynucleotide into the central nucleus of the amygdala reduced anxiety-related behavior in socially defeated rats. Regul Peptides 59:229–239

Liebsch G, Landgraf R, Engelmann M, Lörscher P, Holsboer F (1999): Differential behavioural effects of chronic infusion of CRH_1 and CRH_2 receptor antisense oligodeoxynucleotides into the rat brain. J Psychiatric Res 33:153–163

Linthorst ACE, Flachskamm C, Hopkins SJ, Hoadley ME, Labeur MS, Holsboer F, Reul JMHM (1997): Long-term intracerebroventricular infusion of corticotropin-releasing hormone alters neuroendocrine, neurochemical, autonomic, behavioral, and cytokine responses to a systemic inflammatory challenge. J. Neurosci 17:4448–4460

Linthorst ACE, Karanth S, Barden N, Holsboer F, Reul JMHM (1999): Impaired glucocorticoid receptor function evolves in aberrant physiological responses to bacterial endotoxin. Eur J Neurosci 11:178–186

Linthorst ACE, Flachskamm C, Barden N, Holsboer F, Reul JMHM (2000): Glucocorticoid receptor impairment alters CNS responses to a psychological stressor: An *in vitro* microdialysis study in transgenic mice. Eur J Neurosci 12:283–291

Liu J, DeFranco DB (1999): Chromatin recycling of glucocorticoid receptors: Implications for multiple roles of heat shock protein 90. Mol Endocrinol 13:355–365

Lôo H, Saiz-Ruiz J, Costa e Silva JA, Ansseau M, Herrington R, Vaz-Serra A, Dilling H, de Risio S (1999): Efficacy and safety of tianeptine in the treatment of depressive disorders in comparison with fluoxetine. J Affect Disord 56:109–118

Lupien SJ, de Leon M, de Santi S, Convit A, Tarshish C, Nair NPV, Thakur M, McEwen BS, Hauger RL, Meaney MJ (1998): Cortisol levels during human aging predict hippocampal atrophy and memory deficits. Nature Neurosci 1:69–73

Magariños AM, McEwen BS, Flügge G, Fuchs E (1996): Chronic psychosocial stress causes apical dendritic atrophy of hippocampal CA3 pyramidal neurons in subordinate tree shrews. J Neurosci 16:3534–3540

Magariños AM, Verdugo JM, McEwen BS (1997): Chronic stress alters synaptic terminal structure in hippocampus. Proc Natl Acad Sci USA 94:14002–14008

Malkoski SM, Handanos CM, Dron RI (1997): Localization of a negative glucocorticoid response element of the human corticotropin releasing hormone gene. Mol Cell Endocrinol 127:189–199

Malkoski SP, Dorin RI (1999): Composite glucocorticoid regulation at a functionally defined negative glucocorticoid response element of the human corticotropin-releasing hormone gene. Mol Endocrinol 13:1629–1644

Mangelsdorf DJ, Thummel C, Beato M, Herrlich P, Schütz G, Umesono K, Blumberg B, Kastner P, Mark M, Chambon P, Evans RM (1995): The nuclear receptor superfamily: The second decade. Cell 83:835–839

McEwen BS, Angulo J, Cameron H, Chao HM, Daniels D, Gannon MN, Gould E, Mendelson S, Sakai R, Spencer R, Woolley C (1992): Paradoxical effects of adrenal steroids on the brain: Protection versus degeneration. Biol Psychiatry 31:177–199

Meijer OC, Cole TJ, Schmid W, Schütz G, Joëls M, De Kloet ER (1997): Regulation of hippocampal 5-HT1A receptor mRNA and binding in transgenic mice with a targeted disruption of the glucocorticoid receptor. Mol Brain Res 46:290–296

Meijer OC, de Lange ECM, Breimer DD, de Boer AG, Workel JO, De Kloet ER (1998): Penetration of dexamethasone into brain glucocorticoid targets is enhanced in mdr1AP-glycoprotein knockout mice. Endocrinology 139:1789–1793

Modell S, Yassouridis A, Huber J, Holsboer F (1997): Corticosteroid receptor function is decreased in depressed patients. Neuroendocrinology 65:216–222

Modell S, Lauer CJ, Schreiber W, Huber J, Krieg J-C, Holsboer F (1998): Hormonal response pattern in the combined DEX-CRH test is stable over time in subjects at high familial risk for affective disorders. Neuropsychopharmacology 18:253–262

Montkowski A, Barden N, Wotjak C, Stec I, Ganster J, Meaney M, Engelmann M, Reul JMHM, Landgraf R, Holsboer F (1995): Long-term antidepressant treatment reduces behavioural deficits in transgenic mice with impaired glucocorticoid receptor function. J Neuroendocrinol 7:841–845

Morissette J, Villeneuve A, Lordeleau L, Rochette D, Laberge C, Gagné B, Laprise C, Bouchard G, Plante M, Gobeil L, Shink E, Weissenbach J, Barden N (1999): Genome-wide search for linkage of bipolar affective disorders in a very large pedigree derived from a homogeneous population in Quebec points to a locus of major effect on chromosome 12q23–q24. Am J Med Genet 88:567–587

Müller MB, Lucassen PJ, Yassouridis A, Hoogendijk WJG, Holsboer F, Swaab DE (1998): The human hippocampus in major depression or following administration of glucocorticoids: No evidence for major structural alterations. Soc Neurosci Abstr 24:990

Murphy BEP (1991): Treatment of major depression with steroid suppressive drugs. J Steroid Biochem Mol Biol 39:239–244

Murphy BEP, Filipini D, Ghadirian AM (1993): Possible use of glucocorticoid receptor antagonists in the treatment of major depression: Preliminary results using RU 486. J Psychiatry Neurosci 18:209–213

Murphy EP, Conneely OM (1997): Neuroendocrine regulation of the hypothalamic pituitary adrenal axis by the nurr1/nur77 subfamily of nuclear receptors. Mol Endocrinology 11:39–47

Nelson MD, Saykin AJ, Flashman LA, Riordan HJ (1998): Hippocampal volume reduction in schizophrenia as assessed by magnetic resonance imaging. A meta-analytic study. Arch Gen Psychiatry 55:433–440

Nemeroff CB, Widerlov E, Bissette G, Walleus H, Karlsson I, Eklund K, Kilts DC, Loosen PT, Vale W (1984): Elevated concentrations of CSF corticotropin-releasing factor-like immunoreactivity in depressed patients. Science 226:1342–1344

Nemeroff CB, Owens MJ, Bissette G, Andorn AC, Stanley M (1988): Reduced corticotropin releasing factor binding sites in the frontal cortex of suicide victims. Arch Gen Psychiatry 45:377–379

Newcomer JW, Selke G, Melson AK, Hershey T, Craft S, Richards K, Alderson AL (1999): Decreased memory performance in healthy humans induced by stress-level cortisol treatment. Arch Gen Psychiatry 56:527–533

Nollen EAA, Brunsting JF, Song J, Kampinga HH, Morimoto RI (2000): Bag1 functions in vivo as a negative regulator of hsp70 chaperone activity. Mol Cell Biol 20:1083–1088

O'Dwyer AM, Lightman SL, Marks M, Checkley SA (1995): Treatment of major depression with metyrapone and hydrocortisone. J Affect Disord 33:123–128

Oitzl MS, Fluttert M, De Kloet ER (1994): The effect of corticosterone on reacitivity to spatial novelty is mediated by central mineralocorticosteroid receptors. Eur J Neurosci 6:1072–1079

Orchinik M, Murrey TF, Moore FL (1991): A corticosteroid receptor in neuronal membranes. Science 252:1848–1851

Owens MJ, Nemeroff CB (1991): Physiology and pharmacology of corticotropin-releasing factor. Pharmacol Rev 43:425–473

Pariante CM, Pearce BD, Pisell TL, Owens MJ, Miller AH (1997): Steroid-independent translocation of the glucocorticoid receptor by the antidepressant desipramine. Mol Pharmacol 52:571–581

Patchev VK, Shoaib M, Holsboer F, Almeida OFX (1994): The neurosteroid tetrahydroprogesterone counteracts corticotropin-releasing hormone-induced anxiety and alters the release and gene expression of corticotropin-releasing hormone in the rat hypothalamus. Neuroscience 62:265–271

Patchev VK, Hassan AHS, Holsboer F, Almeida OFX (1996): The neurosteroid tetrahydroprogesterone attenuates the endocrine response to stress and exerts glucocorticoid-like effects on vasopressin gene transcription in the rat hypothalamus. Neuropsychopharmacology 15:533–540

Patchev VK, Montkowski A, Rouskova D, Koranyi L, Holsboer F, Almeida OFX (1997): Neonatal treatment of rats with the neuroactive steroid tetrahydrodeoxycorticosterone (THDOC) abolishes the behavioral and neuroendocrine consequences of adverse early life events. J Clin Invest 99:962–966

Paul SM, Purdy RH (1992): Neuroactive steroids. FASEB J 6:2311–2322

Pepin MC, Pothier F, Barden N (1992): Impaired type II glucocorticoid-receptor function in mice bearing antisense RNA transgene. Nature 355:725–728

Pfahl M (1993): Nuclear receptor/AP-1 interaction. Endocrinol Rev 14:651–658

Philips A, Maira M, Mullick A, Chamberland M, Lesage S, Hugo P, Drouin J (1997): Antagonism between Nur77 and glucocorticoid receptor for control of transcription. Mol Cell Biol 17:5952–5959

Plotsky P, Meaney M (1993): Early, postnatal experience alters hypothalamic corticotropin-releasing factor (CRF) mRNA, median eminence CRF-content and stress-induced release in adult rats. Mol Brain Res 18:195–200

Potter E, Behan DP, Fischer WH, Linton EA, Lowry PJ, Vale WW (1991): Cloning and characterization of the cDNAs for human and rat corticotropin releasing factor-binding proteins. Nature 349:423–426

Pratt WB, Dittmar KD (1998): Studies with purified chaperones advance the understanding of the mechanism of glucocorticoid receptor-hsp90 heterocomplex assembly. TEM 9:244–252

Purba JS, Hoogendijk WJG, Hofman MA, Swaab DF (1996): Increased number of vasopressin- and oxytocin-expressing neurons in the paraventricular nucleus of the hypothalamus in depression. Arch Gen Psychiatry 53:137–143

Raadsheer FC, Hoogendijk WJG, Stam FC, Tilders FHJ, Swaab DF (1994): Increased numbers of corticotropin-releasing hormone expressing neurons in the hypothalamic paraventricular nucleus of depressed patients. Neuroendocrinology 60:433–436

Radulovic J, Rühmann A, Liepold T, Spiess J (1999): Modulation of learning and anxiety by corticotropin-releasing factor (CRF) and stress: Differential roles of CRF receptors 1 and 2. J Neurosci 19:5016–5025

Rajkowska G, Miguel-Hidalgo JJ, Wei J, Dilley G, Pittman SD, Meltzer HY, Overholser JC, Roth BL, Stockmeier CA (1999): Morphometric evidence for neuronal and glial prefrontal cell pathology in major depression. Biol Psychiatry 45:1085–1098

Reichardt HM, Kaestner KH, Tuckermann J, Kretz O, Wessely O, Bock R, Gass P, Schmid W, Herrlich P, Angel P, Schütz G (1998): DNA binding of the glucocorticoid receptor is not essential for survival. Cell 93:531–541

Reynolds PD, Ruan Y, Smith DF, Scammell JG (1999): Glucocorticoid resistance in the squirrel monkeys is associated with overexpression of the immunophilin FKBP51. J Clin Endocrinol Metab 84:663–669

Reul JMHM, Stec I, Söder M, Holsboer F (1993): Chronic treatment of rats with the antidepressant amitriptyline attenuates the activity of the hypothalamic-pituitary-adrenocortical system. Endocrinology 133:312–320

Reul JMHM, Labeur MS, Grigoriadis DE, De Souza EB, Holsboer F (1994): Hypothalamic-pituitary-adrenocortical axis changes in the rat after long-term treatment with the reversible monoamine oxidase-A inhibitor moclobemide. Neuroendocrinology 60:509–519

Reul JMHM, Probst JC, Skutella T, Hirschmann M, Stec IS, Montkowski A, Landgraf R, Holsboer F (1997): Increased stress-induced adrenocorticotropin response after long-term intracerebroventricular treatment of rats with antisense mineralocorticoid receptor oligodeoxynucleotides. Neuroendocrinology 65:189–199

Rochford J, Beaulieu S, Rousse I, Glowa J, Barden N (1997): Behavioral reactivity to aversive stimuli in a transgenic mouse model of impaired glucocorticoid (type II) receptor function: Effects of diazepam and FG-7142. Psychopharmacology 132:145–152

Romeo E, Ströhle A, Spalletta G, di Michele F, Hermann B, Holsboer F, Pasini A, Rupprecht R (1998): Effects of antidepressant treatment on neuroactive steroids in major depression. Am J Psychiatry 155:910–913

Roozendaal B, Nguyen BT, Power AE, McGaugh JL (1999): Basolateral amygdala noradrenergic influence enables enhancement of memory consolidation induced by hippocampal glucocorticoid receptor activation. Proc Natl Acad Sci USA 96:11642–11647

Rossby SP, Nalepa I, Huang M, Burt A, Perrin C, Schmidt DE, Sulser F (1995): Norepinephrine-independent regulation of GRII mRNA *in vivo* by a tricyclic antidepressant. Brain Res 687:79–82

Rossby SP, Manier DH, Liang S, Nalepa I, Sulser F (1999): Pharmacological actions of the antidepressant venlafaxine beyond aminergic receptors. Intl J Neuropsychopharmacol 2:1–8

Rousse I, Beaulieu S, Rowe W, Meaney MJ, Barden N, Rochford J (1997): Spatial memory in transgenic mice with impaired glucocorticoid receptor function. NeuroReport 8:841–845

Rubin RT, Poland RE, Lesser IM, Winston RA, Blodgett ALN (1987): Neuroendocrine aspects of primary endogenous depression. Arch Gen Psychiatry 44:328–336

Rupprecht R, Holsboer F (1999): Neuroactive steroids: Mechanisms of action and neuropsychopharmacological perspectives. Trends Neurosci 22:410–416

Rupprecht R, Reul JMHM, Trapp T, van Steensel B, Wetzel C, Zieglgänsberger W, Damm K, Holsboer F (1993): Progesterone receptor mediated effects of neuroactive steroids. Neuron 11:523–530

Rybakowski JK, Twardowska K (1999): The dexamethasone/corticotropin-releasing hormone test in depression in bipolar and unipolar affective illness. J Psychiatric Res 33:363–370

Sánchez MM, Young LJ, Plotsky PM, Insel TR (1999): Autoradiographic and *in situ* hybridization localization of corticotropin-releasing factor 1 and 2 receptors in non-human primate brain. J Comp Neurol 408:365–377

Sánchez MM, Young LJ, Plotsky PM, Insel TR (2000): Distribution of corticosteroid receptors in the rhesus brain: Relative absence of glucocorticoid receptors in the hippocampal formation. J Neuroscience 20:4657–4668

Sapolsky RM (1992): Stress, the Aging Brain and the Mechanism of Neuron Death. London, MIT Press

Schatzberg AF, Rothschild AJ, Langlais PJ, Bird ED, Cole JO (1985): A corticosteroid/dopamine hypothesis for psychotic depression and related states. J Psychiatric Res 19:57–64

Schinkel AH, Wagenaar E, Van Deemter L, Mol CAAM, Borst P (1995): Absence of the mdr1a P-glycoprotein in mice affects tissue distribution and pharmacokinetics of dexamethasone, digoxin, and cyclosporin A. J Clin Invest 96:1698–1705

Schneikert J, Hübner S, Martin E, Cato ACB (1999): A nuclear action of the eukaryotic cochaperone RAP46 in downregulation of glucocorticoid receptor activity. J Cell Biol 146:929–940

Schulkin J, Gold PW, McEwen BS (1998): Induction of corticotropin-releasing hormone gene expression by glucocorticoids: Implication for understanding the states of fear and anxiety and allostatic load. Psychoneuroendocrinology 23:219–243

Schwaninger M, Schoel C, Blume R, Rossig L, Knepel W (1995): Inhibition by antidepressant drugs of cyclic AMP response element-binding protein/cyclic AMP response element-directed gene transcription. Mol Pharmacol 47:1112–1118

Seasholtz AF, Thompson RC, Douglass JO (1988): Identification of a cyclic adenosine monophosphate-responsive element in the rat *corticotropin-releasing hormone* gene. Mol Endocrinol 2:1311–1319

Seckl JR (1997): 11β-Hydroxysteroid dehydrogenase in the brain: A neural regulator of glucocorticoid action? Front Neuroendocrinol 18:49–99

Seckl JR, Fink G (1992): Antidepressants increase glucocorticoid and mineralocorticoid receptor mRNA expression in rat hippocampus *in vivo.* Neuroendocrinology 55:621–626

Seckl JR, Dickson KL, Yates C, Fink G (1991): Distribution of glucocorticoid and mineralocorticoid receptor messenger RNA expression in human postmortem hippocampus. Brain Res 561:332–337

Sheline YI, Wang PW, Gado MH, Hsernansky JG, Vannier MW (1996): Hippocampal atrophy in recurrent major depression. Proc Natl Acad Sci USA 93:3908–3913

Sheline YI, Gado M, Price JL (1998): Amygdala core nuclei volumes are decreased in recurrent major depression. NeuroReport 9:2023–2028

Sheline YI, Sanghavi M, Mintun MA, Gado MH (1999): Depression duration but not age predicts hippocampal volume loss in medically healthy women with recurrent major depression. J Neurosci 19:5034–5043

Shelton RC, Manier DH, Peterson CS, Truitt CE, Sulser F (1999): Cyclic AMP-dependent protein kinase in subtypes of major depression and normal volunteers. Intl J Neuropsychopharmacol 2:187–192

Shibata H, Spencer TE, Onate SA, Jenster G, Tsai SY, Tsai M-J, O'Malley BW (1997): Role of co-activators and co-repressors in the mechanism of steroid/thyroid receptor action. Rec Progr Hormone Res 52:141–163

Sillaber I, Montkowski A, Landgraf R, Barden N, Holsboer F, Spanagel R (1998): Enhanced morphine-induced behavioural effects and dopamine release in the nucleus accumbens in a transgenic mouse model of impaired glucocorticoid (type II) receptor function: Influence of long-term treatment with the antidepressant moclobemide. Neuroscience 85:415–425

Siuciak JA, Lewis D, Wiegand SJ, Lindsay RM (1996): Antidepressant-like effect of brain-derived neurotrophic factor. Pharmacol Biochem Behav 56:131–137

Skutella T, Probst JC, Renner R, Holsboer F, Behl C (1998): Corticotropin-releasing hormone receptor (type I) antisense targeting reduces anxiety. Neuroscience 85:795–805

Smith GW, Aubry J-M, Dellu F, Contarino A, Bilezikjian LM, Gold LH, Hauser C, Bentley CA, Sawchenko PE, Koob GF, Vale W, Lee K-F (1998): Corticotropin-releasing factor receptor 1-deficient mice display decreased anxiety, impaired stress response, and aberrant neuroendocrine development. Neuron 20:1093–1103

Sonntag A, Rothe B, Guldner J, Yassouridis A, Holsboer F,

Steiger A (1996): Trimipramine and imipramine exert different effects on the sleep EEG and on nocturnal hormone secretion during treatment of major depression. Depression 4:1–13

Spanagel R, Stöhr T, Barden N, Holsboer F (1996): Morphine-induced locomotor and neurochemical stimulation is enhanced in transgenic mice with impaired glucocorticoid receptor function. J Neuroendocrinol 8:93–97

Spencer RL, Kim PJ, Kalman BA, Cole MA (1998): Evidence for mineralocorticoid receptor facilitation of glucocorticoid receptor-dependent regulation of hypothalamic-pituitary-adrenal axis activity. Endocrinology 139:2718–2726

Spencer TE, Jenster G, Burcin MM, Allis CD, Zhou J, Mizzen CA, McKenna NJ, Onate SA, Tsai SY, Tsai M-J, O'Malley BW (1997): Steroid receptor coactivator-1 is a histone acetyltransferase. Nature 389:194–198

Spengler D, Rupprecht R, Phi Van L, Holsboer F (1992): Identification and characterization of a 3',5'-cyclic adenosine monophosphate-responsive element in the human corticotropin-releasing hormone gene promoter. Mol Endocrinol 6:1931–1941

Stalla GK, Stalla J, von Werder K (1989): Nitroimidazole derivates inhibit anterior pituitary cell function apparently by a direct effect on the catalytic subunit of the adenylate cyclase holoenzyme. Endocrinology 155:699–706

Stec I, Barden N, Reul JMHM, Holsboer F (1994): Dexamethasone nonsuppression in transgenic mice expressing antisense RNA to the glucocorticoid receptor. J Psychiatric Res 28:1–5

Steckler T, Weis C, Sauvage M, Mederer A, Holsboer F (1999): Disrupted allocentric but preserved egocentric spatial learning in transgenic mice with impaired glucocorticoid receptor function. Behav Brain Res 100:77–89

Steckler T, Sauvage M; Holsboer F (2000a): Glucocorticoid receptor impairment enhances impulsive responding in transgenic mice performing on a simultaneous visual discrimination task. Eur J Neuroscience, In press

Steckler T, Rammes G, Sauvage M, van Gaalen MM, Weis C, Zieglgänsberger W, Holsboer F (2000b): Effects of the monoamine oxidase A inhibitor moclobemide on hippocampal plasticity in GR-impaired transgenic mice. J Psychiatric Res, In press

Stenzel-Poore MP, Heinrichs SC, Rivest S, Koob GF, Vale WW (1994): Overproduction of corticotropin-releasing factor in transgenic mice: A genetic model of anxiogenic behavior. J Neurosci 14:2579–2584

Stoecklin E, Wissler M, Gouilleux F, Groner B (1996): Functional interactions between Stat5 and the glucocorticoid receptor. Nature 383:726–728

Stoecklin E, Wissler M, Moriggl R, Groner B (1997): Specific DNA binding of Stat5, but not of glucocorticoid receptor, is required for their functional co-operation in the regulation of gene transcription. Mol Cell Biol 17:6708–6716

Ströhle A, Poettig M, Barden N, Holsboer F, Montkowski A (1998): Age- and stimulus-dependent changes in anxiety-related behaviour of transgenic mice with GR dysfunction. NeuroReport 9:2099–2102

Ströhle A, Pasini A, Romeo E, Hermann B, Spalletta G, di Michele F, Holsboer F, Rupprecht R (2000): Fluoxetine decreases concentrations of 3α,5α-tetrahydrodeoxycorticosterone (THDOC) in major depression. J Psychiatric Res 34:183–186

Swanson LW, Simmons DM (1989): Differential steroid hormones and neural influences on peptide mRNA levels in CRH cells of the paraventricular nucleus: A hybridization histochemical study in the rat. J Comp Neurol 285:413–435

Thakore JH, Dinan TG (1995): Cortisol synthesis inhibition: A new treatment strategy for the clinical and endocrine manifestations of depression. Biol Psychiatry 37:364–368

Timpl P, Spanagel R, Sillaber I, Kresse A, Reul JMHM, Stalla GK, Blanquet V, Steckler T, Holsboer F, Wurst W (1998): Impaired stress response and reduced anxiety in mice lacking a functional corticotropin-releasing hormone receptor 1. Nature Genet 19:162–166

Trapp T, Rupprecht R, Castrèn M, Reul JMHM, Holsboer F (1994): Heterodimerization between mineralocorticoid and glucocorticoid receptor: A new principle of glucocorticoid action in the CNS. Neuron 13:1457–1462

Trapp T, Holsboer F (1996a): Heterodimerization between mineralocorticoid and glucocorticoid receptor increases the functional diversity of corticosteroid action. Trends in Pharmacol Sci 17:145–149

Trapp T, Holsboer F (1996b): Nuclear orphan receptor as a repressor of glucocorticoid receptor transcriptional activity. J Biol Chem 271:9879–9882

Tronche R, Kellendonk C, Kretz O, Gass P, Anlag K, Orban PC, Bock R, Klein R, Schütz G (1999): Disruption of the glucocorticoid receptor gene in the nervous system results in reduced anxiety. Nature Genet 23:99–103

Uhr M, Steckler T, Yassouridis A, Holsboer F (2000): Penetration of amitriptyline, but not fluoxetine, into brain is enhanced in mice with blood-brain barrier deficiency due to mdr1a P-glycoprotein gene disruption. Neuropsychopharmacology 22:380–387

Uzunova V, Sheline Y, Davis JM, Rasmusson A, Uzunov DP, Costa E, Guidotti A (1998): Increase in the cerebrospinal fluid content of neurosteroids in patients with unipolar major depression who are receiving fluoxetine or fluvoxamine. Proc Natl Acad Sci USA 95:3239–3244

Vale W, Spiess J, Rivier C, Rivier J (1981): Characterization of a 41-residue ovine hypothalamic peptide that stimulates secretion of corticotropin and β-endorphin. Science 213:1394–1397

van der Burg B, Liden J, Okret S, Delaunay F, Wissink S, van der Saag PT, Gustafsson J-A (1997): Nuclear factor-κB repression in antiinflammation and immunosuppression by glucocorticoids. Trends Endocrinol Metab 8:152–157

van Haarst AD, Welberg LAM, Sutanto W, Oitzl MS, De Kloet ER (1996a): 11β-Hydroxysteroid dehydroxygenase activity in the hippocampus: Implications for *in vivo* corticosterone receptor binding and cell nuclear retention. J Neuroendocrinol 8:595–600

van Haarst AD, Oitzl MS, Workel JO, De Kloet ER (1996b): Chronic brain glucocorticoid receptor blockade enhances the rise in circadian and stress-induced pituitary-adrenal activity. Endocrinology 137:4935–4943

von Bardeleben U, Holsboer F (1989): Cortisol response to a combined dexamethasone-hCRH challenge in patients with depression. J Neuroendocrinol 1:485–488 von Bardeleben U, Holsboer F (1991): Effect of age upon the cortisol response to human CRH in depressed patients pretreated with dexamethasone. Biol Psychiatry 29: 1042–1050

von Bardeleben U, Holsboer F, Stalla GK, Müller OA (1985): Combined administration of human corticotropin-releasing factor and lysine vasopressin induces cortisol escape from dexamethasone suppression in healthy subjects. Life Sci 37:1613–1619

Watanabe Y, Gould E, McEwen BS (1992): Stress induces atrophy of spatial dendrites of hippocampal CA3 pyramidal neurons. Brain Res 588:341–345

Weninger SC, Dunn AJ, Muglia LJ, Dikkes P, Miczek KA, Swiergiel AH, Berridge CW, Majzoub JA (1999): Stress-induced behaviors require the corticotropin-releasing hormone (CRH) receptor, but not CRH. Proc Natl Acad Sci USA 96:8283–8288

Wissink S, van Heerde EC, van der Burg B, van der Saag PT (1998): A dual mechanism mediates repression of NF-κB activity by glucocorticoids. Mol Endocrinol 12:355–363

Wolkowitz OM, Reus VI, Chan T, Manfredi F, Raum W, Johnson R, Canick J (1999): Antiglucocorticoid treatment of depression: Double-blind ketoconazole. Biol Psychiatry 45:1070–1074

Young EA, Lopez JF, Murphy-Weinberg V, Watson SJ, Akil H (1998): The role of mineralocorticoid receptors in hypothalamic-pituitary-adrenal axis regulation in humans. J Clin Endocrinol Metab 83:3339–3345

Zeiner M, Niyaz Y, Gehring U (1999): The hsp70-associating protein Hap46 binds to DNA and stimulates transcription. Proc Natl Acad Sci USA 96:10194–10199

Zobel AW, Yassouridis A, Frieboes R-M, Holsboer F (1999): Cortisol response to the combined dexamethasone-CRH test predicts medium-term outcome in patients with remitted depression. Am J Psychiatry 156:949–951

Zobel AW, Nickel T, Künzel HE, Ackl N, Sonntag A, Ising M, Holsboer F (2000): Effects of the high-affinity corticotropin-releasing hormone receptor 1 antagonist R121919 in major depression: The first 20 patients treated. J Psychiatric Res, 34:171–181

Regular Articles

Reciprocal Limbic-Cortical Function and Negative Mood: Converging PET Findings in Depression and Normal Sadness

Helen S. Mayberg, M.D., Mario Liotti, M.D., Ph.D., Stephen K. Brannan, M.D., Scott McGinnis, B.S., Roderick K. Mahurin, Ph.D., Paul A. Jerabek, Ph.D., J. Arturo Silva, M.D., Janet L. Tekell, M.D., Charles C. Martin, Ph.D., Jack L. Lancaster, Ph.D., and Peter T. Fox, M.D.

Objective: Theories of human behavior from Plato to Freud have repeatedly emphasized links between emotion and reason, a relationship now commonly attributed to pathways connecting phylogenetically "old" and "new" brain regions. Expanding on this theory, this study examined functional interactions between specific limbic and neocortical regions accompanying normal and disease-associated shifts in negative mood state. **Method:** Regions of concordant functional change accompanying provocation of transient sadness in healthy volunteers and resolution of chronic dysphoric symptoms in depressed patients were examined with two positron emission tomography techniques: [^{15}O]water and [^{18}F]fluorodeoxyglucose, respectively. **Results:** With sadness, increases in limbic-paralimbic blood flow (subgenual cingulate, anterior insula) and decreases in neocortical regions (right dorsolateral prefrontal, inferior parietal) were identified. With recovery from depression, the reverse pattern, involving the same regions, was seen—limbic metabolic decreases and neocortical increases. A significant inverse correlation between subgenual cingulate and right dorsolateral prefrontal activity was also demonstrated in both conditions. **Conclusions:** Reciprocal changes involving subgenual cingulate and right prefrontal cortex occur with both transient and chronic changes in negative mood. The presence and maintenance of functional reciprocity between these regions with shifts in mood in either direction suggests that these regional interactions are obligatory and probably mediate the well-recognized relationships between mood and attention seen in both normal and pathological conditions. The bidirectional nature of this limbic-cortical reciprocity provides additional evidence of potential mechanisms mediating cognitive ("top-down"), pharmacological (mixed), and surgical ("bottom-up") treatments of mood disorders such as depression.

(Am J Psychiatry 1999; 156:675–682)

The development of functional connections between limbic structures and neocortex has long been considered critical to the evolution of complex emotional behaviors, although conclusive experimental evidence from studies of humans is relatively sparse (1–6). Clinical observation and personal experience none-

Presented in part at the Third International Conference on Functional Mapping of the Human Brain, Copenhagen, May 19–23, 1997. Received May 5, 1998; revision received Sept. 25, 1998; accepted Oct. 10, 1998. From the Research Imaging Center and the Departments of Psychiatry, Neurology, and Radiology, University of Texas Health Science Center at San Antonio. Address reprint requests to Dr. Mayberg, Rotman Research Institute, Baycrest Centre, 3560 Bathurst St., Toronto, Ont. M6A 2E1, Canada; hmayberg@rotman-baycrest.on.ca (e-mail).

Supported by NIMH grant MH-49553, the National Alliance for Research on Schizophrenia and Depression, the Charles A. Dana Foundation, and Eli Lilly and Co.

The authors thank Stanley Mayberg, M.D., Lawrence Parsons, Ph.D., James Redmond, M.D., and Marty Woldorff, Ph.D., for comments and criticisms.

theless confirm the inseparable and often intrusive effects of transient changes in mood state on attention span, decisiveness, and other cognitive abilities, be it the fleeting sadness one feels on hearing a tragic news event or the more sustained feelings of melancholia and impaired concentration that accompany intense grief. The chronic and more insidious disruption of attentional processing observed in depressive illness (7, 8)—an extreme instance of a sustained altered mood state—further suggests common neural pathways mediating both the normal and pathological interactions of these behaviors.

Comparative anatomical studies provide material support for these hypotheses. Reciprocal pathways linking midline limbic structures (cingulate, hypothalamus, hippocampus, amygdala) with widely distributed brainstem, striatal, paralimbic, and neocortical sites are now well-defined (9, 10), and clear associations with specific motivational, affective, and emotional behaviors in animals have been demonstrated (3, 4, 11). By extrapolation, these regions are also assumed to be the neural substrates responsible for the systematic integration of exteroceptive and interoceptive inputs required for the combined sensory, cognitive, and autonomic processing at the core of normal and abnormal human emotional experience.

Previous human experiments have generally approached the brain localization of mood and attention in isolation and have rarely addressed mechanisms underlying their interaction (12, 13). With the use of complementary lesion-deficit and physiological studies (14–18), components of attention have been localized to right prefrontal, parietal, and dorsal anterior cingulate regions in both humans and primates. Mood has been mapped to predominantly limbic and paralimbic areas (cingulate, insula) and prefrontal cortex, but with considerable variability (19–24). Focal limbic (anterior cingulate), paralimbic (ventral frontal, anterior insula), and neocortical (prefrontal, parietal) abnormalities have also been identified in depression (25–29). However, correlations of these regional changes with specific symptoms or relationships between regions have not been fully explored (30).

To clarify mechanisms mediating these known mood-attention relationships, this study targeted interregional interactions and regional reciprocity in functional brain activity present during both transient and sustained changes in affective state. Using positron emission tomography (PET), we investigated two experimental manipulations of mood: transient sadness provoked in healthy volunteers and treatment-induced resolution of sustained dysphoria in clinically depressed patients. On the basis of the location and direction of changes in neural activity seen in these studies, we propose that the well-recognized concurrence of negative mood and impaired attentional processing in both normal and pathological conditions is mediated by reciprocal interactions between specific limbic and neocortical sites.

METHOD

For experiment 1, healthy subjects were recruited by advertisement and word of mouth. Potential participants were asked to prepare scripts describing two recent sad personal experiences, and these were reviewed with the investigators during the screening interviews. The potential subjects were screened for the presence of medical, neurological, and psychiatric conditions, personal or family history of major affective disorder, and medication use, any of which precluded participation in the study. Semistructured interviews confirmed the absence of major or minor depressive symptoms and evidence of other previously unrecognized psychiatric syndromes or complaints. Potential subjects were then tested on their emotional reactions to their prepared scripts. Of 13 potential subjects so screened, eight right-handed euthymic women (mean age=36 years, SD=6; mean Beck Depression Inventory score=1.75, SD=1 [asymptomatic range=0–9]) were selected for participation on the basis of their ability to predictably provoke an intense sad mood state under laboratory conditions.

For experiment 2, patients who had responded in a 6-week inpatient, placebo-controlled, double-blind PET study of fluoxetine treatment in depression (20 mg/day fixed dose) were identified. All patients met the DSM-IV criteria for a major depressive episode, unipolar type, as diagnosed by two independent psychiatrists (J.A.S. and J.L.T.) and confirmed by means of a structured psychiatric interview (Structured Clinical Interview for DSM-IV [31]). Patients with cerebrovascular risk factors or a previous stroke, documented head trauma, neurodegenerative disorders, other axis I psychiatric diagnoses, or evidence of global cognitive impairment were excluded, as were patients with psychotic symptoms, alcohol or substance abuse, or previous ECT. Responders were defined as patients who had a minimum 50% decrease in Hamilton Depression Rating Scale score, independent of treatment group (i.e., fluoxetine or placebo). Eight of 15 participating male patients met these criteria (mean age=44 years, SD=8; initial 17-item Hamilton depression scale score=22, SD=3; 6-week score=11, SD=2.5). Four responders received fluoxetine, and four received placebo. Written informed consent was obtained from all subjects, and the experiment was conducted as approved by the University of Texas Health Science Center's institutional review board.

Experiment 1

Regional cerebral blood flow (rCBF) was measured with the use of [^{15}O]water and PET in two mood states: sad and neutral (euthymic). For each subject there were two trials in the sad condition and four neutral trials (three during rest with eyes closed and one with a neutral-emotion script) in a randomized design. Rehearsed autobiographical scripts were used to provoke the sad (or neutral) mood state. On the basis of prescan practice trials with each subject, the protocol allowed 8–10 minutes to achieve the maximum target mood. Mood state was then maintained, without active rumination on the script, for approximately 2 minutes before tracer injection. Scans were acquired during this state with the subject's eyes closed. While monitoring of one's internal mood state (whether sad or neutral) was required for all conditions, the intent of the protocol was to minimize participation of brain regions mediating the cognitive processes involved in generating the emotional state. Subjects were debriefed after completion of each 90-second scan, and mood was allowed to return to a baseline euthymic state before initiation of the next condition, generally after about 5 minutes. Mood state was rated every 2 minutes throughout the session with a visual analog scale and the subject's self-report. Rest or neutral mood conditions required a score of 6 of a maximum 7 on the calmness scale and a mandatory 0 of 7 on the sadness scale to initiate scan acquisition; sad mood conditions required a minimum score of 6 of 7 on the sadness scale.

Experiment 2

Changes in regional glucose metabolism associated with remission of both dysphoric mood and other syndromal features were measured by means of [^{18}F]fluorodeoxyglucose (FDG) and PET in the selected subset of unipolar depressed patients. Scans were performed before and after 6 weeks of treatment as described above.

TABLE 1. Location of Concordant and Reciprocal Regional Changes With Transient Sadness in Eight Healthy Volunteers and With Recovery From Depression in Eight Patients

Zone and Region	Brodmann Area	Side	Healthy Volunteers[a] Coordinate[c] x	y	z	z Score[d]	Extent (mm^3)	% Change	Depressed Patients[b] Coordinate[c] x	y	z	z Score[d]	Extent (mm^3)	% Change
Ventral														
Subgenual cingulate	25	Bilateral	0	22	–2	3.7	1,096	13	–2	6	–6	–3.0	296	–17
Ventral-anterior insula		Right	32	24	–2	2.7	336	5	30	18	–8	–2.3	16	–8
		Left	–28	32	–4	2.6	392	9	–16	18	–16	–2.6	150	–11
Mid-anterior insula		Right	34	10	10	2.5	1,008	7	30	–2	8	–2.3	16	–9
		Left	–30	2	10	4.3	2,400	11	–26	–4	8	–2.2	16	–10
Posterior insula		Right	32	–22	20	3.2	608	9	38	–18	20	–3.8	616	–18
		Left	–36	–16	18	3.0	800	9	–34	–14	20	–2.6	40	–15
Dorsal														
Lateral prefrontal	46	Right	42	12	20	–2.9	936	–5	42	14	20	3.3	488	12
	9	Right	30	12	38	–3.6	1,160	–7	28	12	38	3.1	224	15
Inferior parietal	40	Right	44	–50	32	–3.0	1,520	–5	42	–34	34	3.3	536	16
		Left	–46	–38	34	–3.2	400	–8	–40	–46	34	2.2	16	10
Posterior cingulate	23		0	–28	23	–2.8	536	–7	4	–28	22	4.4	840	20
	31		–12	–38	32	–3.0	480	–8	14	–42	28	2.6	80	15
Anterior cingulate	24/32	Left	–14	38	22	–2.6	48	–4	–10	24	24	2.1	112	11

[a] Change in regional blood flow measured with [^{15}O]water (value during sadness condition minus value during rest).
[b] Change in regional glucose metabolism measured with FDG (value after 6 weeks of treatment minus baseline value).
[c] Millimeters relative to anterior commissure (35): x=right (+)/left (–); y=anterior (+)/posterior (–); z=superior (+)/inferior (–).
[d] For z values >1.96, p<0.05; for z values ≥2.6, p<0.01; for z values ≥3.3, p<0.001.

Scans were acquired with the patients in the resting state, with eyes closed and ears uncovered. The patients were specifically instructed to relax, stay awake, and avoid rumination on any one topic. They were not explicitly instructed to monitor internal mood state. This approach aimed to examine regional effects associated with a sustained shift in overall mood state accompanying remission of illness without any overt acute manipulation of either affective or cognitive state.

General PET Method

All PET scans were acquired on a General Electric Scanditronix 4096 camera (15 parallel slices; 6.5-mm center-to-center interslice distance) with measured attenuation correction (68Ge/68Ga transmission scans) and were reconstructed to a final in-plane resolution of 7.0 mm full width at half maximum. In experiment 1, CBF was measured with a conventional bolus [^{15}O]water technique (60–65 mCi [^{15}O]water dose per scan; scan duration=90 seconds) (32). Glucose metabolism was measured in the resting state with FDG (5 mCi FDG dose; scan duration=20 minutes) following a standard 40-minute FDG uptake period (33). An anatomical magnetic resonance imaging (MRI) scan of each subject was also acquired for the purposes of spatial transformation of the PET data and parametric image display (Elscint Gyrex 2T-DLX, Haifa, Israel) (three-dimensional gradient/recall acquisition in the steady state sequence: TR=33 msec; TE=12 msec; flip angle=60°; 256×256×127 volume; spatial resolution of 1 mm^3).

PET Data Analysis

All analyses were performed with in-house software and validated methods. Following spatial transformation of PET and MR images into proportional bicommissural coordinate space (34) relative to the 1988 stereotaxic atlas of Talairach and Tournoux (35), voxel-wise tissue activity of either [^{15}O]water or FDG was first value-normalized to mean whole brain activity and then scaled to an arbitrary mean of 1000 (32). Value- and spatially normalized images were then trilinearly interpolated, resampled (60 slices; 8-mm^3 voxels), and Gaussian-filtered to a final resolution of 9.9 mm (full width at half maximum) before statistical analysis.

State-related changes in rCBF (experiment 1) and metabolism (experiment 2) were detected in the following manner. A pixel-by-pixel subtraction of the condition pairs was first performed for each trial in each individual. Within-subject differences were then averaged across subjects, creating a grand-mean difference image for each experiment (value for sad memory minus value for rest in healthy subjects; value with treatment minus baseline value in depressed patients). A beta-2 statistic measuring kurtosis of the histogram of the difference image (change distribution curve) was used as an omnibus test to assess overall significance (36). The beta-2 test was implemented in the MIPS software (Research Imaging Center, San Antonio) in a manner similar to the use of the gamma-2 statistic (37). The beta-2 improves on the gamma-2 by using a better estimate of the degrees of freedom (i.e., "number of resyls" in the PET images) (38). The omnibus test was followed by a maxima and minima search to identify local extrema within a search volume measuring 125 mm^3 (39). To facilitate reporting and visualization of these maxima and minima, group mean subtraction images were converted post hoc to statistical parametric images of z scores based on the variance of all local changes within the subtraction images. Locations of concordant focal maxima and minima exceeding a z score magnitude of 1.96 ($p \leq 0.05$, two-tailed) are listed in table 1, with the peak voxel of each area described in x, y, and z coordinates in millimeters relative to the anterior commissure. Concordance was defined as a common Brodmann area identifier for the coordinates of the maxima or minima locations in both experiment 1 and experiment 2 (40), as well as evidence of anatomical overlap in the extent of significant activations or deactivations seen with the use of a logical contrast of the two z score maps (figure 1, bottom) (41).

RESULTS

Experiment 1

Intense sadness was experienced by all subjects (sadness score=6.85, SD=0.55; resting score=0, SD=0). On average, a sad state (minimum sadness score of 4 or 5 of the maximum 7) was achieved within 5–7 minutes of initiation of the trial. The approximate duration of sustained sadness (score of 6 or 7) was 5 minutes. During the debriefing interview, the subjects confirmed that

FIGURE 1. Reciprocal Changes in Cortical and Paralimbic Function With Shifts in Negative Mood State[a]

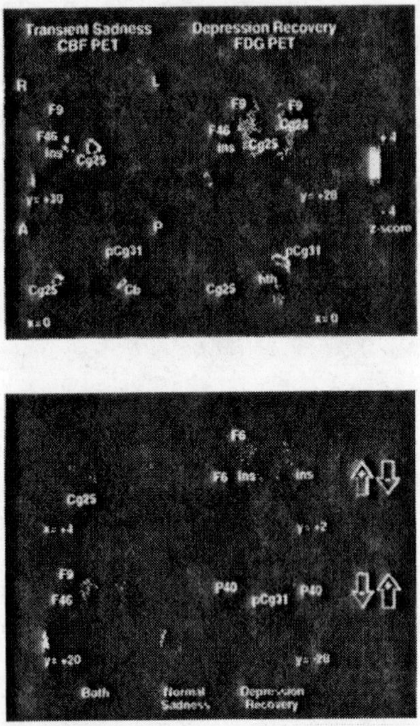

[a] Top: Left images: changes in regional cerebral blood flow (CBF) (with [^{15}O]water PET) associated with transient sadness in eight healthy volunteers. Right images: changes in regional glucose metabolism (with FDG PET) after 6 weeks of treatment in eight unipolar depressed patients. Coronal (top row) and sagittal (bottom row) views. Sadness is associated with increases in ventral paralimbic regions and decreases in dorsal frontal regions. With recovery from depression, the reverse is seen: ventral decreases and dorsal cortical increases. Slice locations are in millimeters relative to the anterior commissure. Numbers are Brodmann area designations. R=right; L=left; A=anterior; P=posterior; F=prefrontal; ins=anterior insula; Cg24=dorsal anterior cingulate; Cg25=subgenual cingulate; pCg=posterior cingulate; Cb=cerebellum; hth=hypothalamus. Color scale: red indicates increases and green indicates decreases in flow or metabolism.
Bottom: Logical images showing anatomical overlap of significant changes common to both experiments. Top row: concordant areas with increased flow during sadness and decreased metabolism during remission. Bottom row: areas with decreased flow during sadness and increased metabolism during remission. Numbers are Brodmann area designations. F=premotor; p=parietal. Red indicates changes unique to sadness; dark blue indicates changes unique to remission of depression; lighter blue indicates changes common to both. Arrows signify direction of change associated with each condition.

they had been able to comply with the instructions, and six of the eight described being tearful. All subjects also described being less aware of the scanning environment while intensely sad. Resting state debriefing identified no consistent repetitive thoughts in any subject.

Sadness compared with rest was associated with both increases and decreases in rCBF (omnibus: beta-2=3.216, df=1972, p=0.001, two-tailed) (figure 1, left). Increases were seen in ventral limbic and paralimbic sites (subgenual cingulate [Brodmann area 25] and ventral, mid-, and posterior insula); decreases were predominantly in dorsal cortical regions (right dorsal prefrontal [Brodmann area 46/9], inferior parietal [Brodmann area 40], dorsal anterior cingulate [Brodmann area 24b], and posterior cingulate [Brodmann area 23/31]) (table 1). Areas of significant change not seen in experiment 2 included decreases in the right temporal cortex (Brodmann area 37) and bilateral inferior frontal cortex (Brodmann area 10/47), as well as increases in the cerebellar vermis and right premotor cortex (Brodmann area 6).

Experiment 2

Posttreatment metabolism relative to pretreatment metabolism was associated with both increases and decreases in specific limbic-paralimbic and neocortical sites, but in a pattern inverse to that seen with provoked sadness (beta-2=3.178, df=1972, p=0.001, two-tailed) (figure 1, right). These regionally similar effects were obtained despite differences in gender, time course of mood-state change (sustained versus transient), and type of PET radiotracer used in the two experiments (FDG versus [^{15}O]water); they were seen with both active fluoxetine and placebo treatment, although the magnitude of changes in limbic regions was more robust with the active drug (data not shown).

Remission of depression was characterized by metabolic increases in dorsal cortical regions (right dorsolateral prefrontal [Brodmann area 46/9], inferior parietal [Brodmann area 40], dorsal anterior cingulate [Brodmann area 24b], and posterior cingulate [Brodmann area 23/31]) and concomitant decreases in ventral limbic and paralimbic sites (subgenual cingulate [Brodmann area 25] and ventral, mid-, and posterior insula) (table 1). The anatomical overlap of findings in the two experiments is presented in figure 1, bottom. Additional changes seen uniquely with recovery from depression included increases in the pons and left prefrontal cortex as well as decreases in the hippocampus and hypothalamus.

DISCUSSION

This study, using two separate subject populations and two different functional imaging approaches, independently demonstrated reciprocal changes involving nearly identical limbic-paralimbic and neocortical regions with both acute and chronic changes in negative mood state.

In the first and more direct assessment of brain regions mediating negative mood, the induction of transient normal sadness revealed most significantly increases in subgenual cingulate (Brodmann area 25) and decreases in right prefrontal cortex (Brodmann area 9). The increases in subgenual cingulate closely replicate previously reported findings in transient sadness with the use of a variety of provocation methods (12, 20). In contrast, the observed right prefrontal decreases (as well as the less significant decreases in inferior parietal and dorsal anterior cingulate) are the exact inverse of those seen in published studies where scanning occurred during overt processing of the sad stimuli (19, 20, 24). Such decreases are nonetheless comparable to those repeatedly described in resting-state studies of patients with clinical depression (26, 42). Furthermore, these decreases localize to areas previously implicated in both imaging and behavioral studies of attention (14, 18). In other words, the experience of sadness, as studied here, resulted not only in limbic activation but also in the simultaneous deactivation of cortical regions known to mediate attentional processing, independent of mood state. This observed reciprocal relationship between limbic increases and cortical decreases also appears consistent with changes in environmental awareness described by the subjects in the debriefing interview, as well as the large body of experimental evidence associating negative mood with impaired attention (8). While performance on attentional tasks was not explicitly monitored during or following the scanning period, performance deficits have been demonstrated in a separate event-related-potential study in which the identical sadness provocation method was used in a different group of subjects (43).

These reciprocal limbic-cortical and mood-attention relationships were confirmed, although more indirectly, in the second experiment, where resolution of chronic negative mood symptoms accompanying recovery from a chronic depressive episode was examined. The observed right dorsolateral prefrontal increases (also, increases in left prefrontal and dorsal anterior cingulate) are the normalization of a pretreatment frontal hypometabolic pattern characteristic of unipolar depression (relative regional glucose metabolism expressed as value-normalized tissue counts: pretreatment=1185, SD=108; posttreatment=1285, SD=25; healthy subjects=1236, SD=151). These pretreatment abnormalities have been linked to both severity of depression and impairments in psychomotor speed and cognition (26, 30, 42) and are consistent with the direction of cortical changes seen during acute sadness in experiment 1. The cortical increases accompanying remission generally replicate previous reports of antidepressant treatment effects (26, 44–46). In addition, resolution of mood symptoms in the present study was mirrored by significantly improved attentional performance. Simple reaction times were inversely correlated with right prefrontal cortex metabolism ($r=-0.47$, $N=16$, $p=0.05$), consistent with the initial hypothesis that changes in mood and attention are behaviorally linked.

In contrast to the normalization of pretreatment abnormalities seen in cortical regions, the decrease in the ventral limbic region (subgenual cingulate) was not the normalization of an existing abnormality. Rather, this change was suppression of activity below the expected normal level (relative regional glucose metabolism: healthy subjects=1115, SD=100; pretreatment=1119, SD=89; posttreatment=940, SD=126). This decrease in subgenual activity has not been previously described with pharmacological treatment of depression but has been suggested by changes reported with ECT (47), although anatomical localization of changes with ECT are less precise than those reported here. This relative subgenual cingulate suppression is also consistent with resting state decreases seen in remitted depressed patients on maintenance antidepressant therapy (48). These pretreatment and remission-related findings—normal subgenual cingulate (Brodmann area 25) metabolism when depressed; subnormal metabolism when well—would appear to contradict a recent report of subgenual cingulate/medial prefrontal hypometabolism and atrophy in acutely depressed unipolar and bipolar patients (49). This apparent contradiction can be reconciled if the reported hypometabolism is corrected for the described regional atrophy, which would likely result in a metabolic pattern similar to those reported here (i.e., normal or slightly increased) (50).

A potential confounding factor in considering the interpretation of these data, despite the regional convergence across the two experiments, is the contribution of the neutral control conditions. It has been proposed that task-associated decreases can be caused by suspension of activity present during a passive task or resting state (51, 52). This does not appear to apply here, since in the transient mood-induction experiment, comparable decreases were seen during both a resting state and a neutral memory condition (i.e., one that more precisely matched the cognitive activity present during the sadness trial) (53). This theory also would not explain the cortical increases seen in experiment 2. While the debriefing interviews revealed no specific repetitive cognitive thoughts in any of the patients nor subjective differences between the two scans, one might have expected, on the basis of previous reports targeting random episodic thinking, increased uncontrollable intrusive thoughts in the acutely depressed state (scan 1), resulting in a decrease rather than an increase in prefrontal and parietal metabolism with remission of illness (52).

A second potential confounding element was the presence of tearfulness in six of the eight subjects in experiment 1. While there was inadequate power to assess these effects independently, inspection of single-subject subtractions revealed similar patterns of limbic increases and cortical decreases in subjects who did and did not become tearful. In addition, changes in these same areas were observed with the resolution of negative mood symptoms in the second experiment,

FIGURE 2. Schematic Model Illustrating Relationships Among Regions Mediating Shifts in Negative Mood State[a]

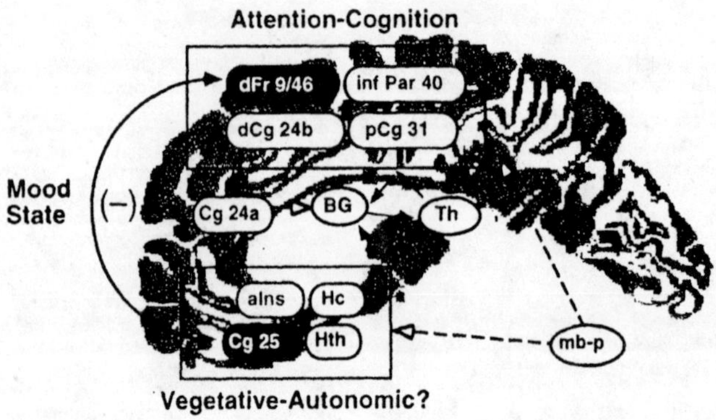

[a] Regions with known anatomical connections that also show synchronized changes (with PET) with both provocation and resolution of negative mood are grouped into two compartments: dorsal (blue) and ventral (red). The dorsal-ventral segregation also defines the brain regions where an inverse relationship is seen across the two PET paradigms (table 1, figure 1). Curved black arrows and color-filled regions further emphasize the significant inverse correlation between right dorsal prefrontal cortex (dFr 9/46, in blue) and subgenual cingulate (Cg 25, in red) seen with both transient sadness in healthy volunteers (Fr decreases, Cg increases) and mood symptom resolution in depressed patients (Fr increases, Cg decreases). Noncolored regions delineate brain areas potentially critical to the schematic model but where changes were not identified in both experiments. Short black arrows indicate known subcortical pathways. Numbers are Brodmann area designations. Abbreviations: in blue: dFr=dorsolateral prefrontal; inf Par=inferior parietal; dCg=dorsal anterior cingulate; pCg=posterior cingulate; in red: Cg25=subgenual cingulate; aIns=anterior insula; in black: Cg 24a=rostral anterior cingulate; BG=basal ganglia; Th=thalamus; Hc=hippocampus; Hth=hypothalamus; mb-p=midbrain-pons.

even though tearfulness was not observed in any of the patients during either scan.

To recapitulate, concordant changes in nearly identical dorsal cortical and ventral limbic regions were demonstrated in both experiments (figure 1, top and bottom). The two areas demonstrating the greatest magnitude of change, subgenual cingulate (Brodmann area 25) and right prefrontal cortex (Brodmann area 9), were also strongly intercorrelated. Using regions of interest (216 mm^3) centered on the maximal pixel identified in the two subtraction analyses, we found an inverse correlation between the activity in these two regions in both studies (sadness computed for all sadness and resting trials: r=–0.52, N=30, p=0.003; remission computed at baseline, 1 week, and 6 weeks: r=–0.46, N=24, p=0.02). These findings suggest that a reciprocal relationship between ventral limbic and dorsal cortical compartments is maintained through the interaction of these two nodes as mood shifts in either direction (figure 2). This statistical relationship further suggests that the negative influence of depressed mood on attention is probably attributable to functional connections between these two brain regions rather than concurrent changes in both sites independently.

The theory that these two regions are functionally linked and mutually inhibitory is supported by a large preclinical animal literature. Direct projections from subgenual cingulate to targets in dorsolateral prefrontal cortex have been delineated, as have bidirectional indirect pathways through multiple limbic and paralimbic nodes, including posterior cingulate, hippocampus, and anterior insula (4, 9, 10, 54).

The reciprocal nature of the changes observed in these two experiments suggests that treatments for depression targeting either "old" or "new" brain areas in this local circuit should be equally effective—a hypothesis supported by empirical clinical experience and by the finding of comparable regional changes in both drug and placebo responders. Mood symptoms can be ameliorated with cognitive therapy, which implies a "top-down" cortical influence on limbic pathways (55). Pharmacological treatments are more classically viewed as acting "bottom-up" (or combined bottom-up and top-down), since brainstem nuclei—most notably locus ceruleus and dorsal raphe—are major sites of action of most antidepressants, with secondary effects mediated in remote cortical sites through afferent projections and postsynaptic receptor mechanisms (56, 57). A more pure bottom-up effect is implicated by the surgical destruction of the subgenual cingulate region and surrounding white matter (the so-called limbic leukotomy or subcaudate tractotomy) (58), used to treat the most severely treatment-resistant depressed patients, suggesting that the critical change mediating clinical improvement is limbic suppression with secondary cortical release or disinhibition. These clinical observations might indicate that the requisite regional perturbation necessary for remission of disease is neither limbic nor cortical but a reconfiguration of their mutual interactions, whether initiated through top-down (cortical-limbic) or bottom-up (limbic-cortical) interventional strategies (42). If one assumes that these two approaches are equally viable, the related question of whether 1) suppression of ventral limbic regions allows normalization of dorsal cortical hypometabolism or 2) normalization of cortical activity causes a decrease in ventral limbic regions becomes moot. Clearly, this hypothesis requires examination of additional groups of patients of both genders as well as the focused evaluation of antidepressant medications that are not selective serotonin reuptake inhibitors. Further studies are also needed to delineate the specific behavioral correlates of the other identified regional changes, as well as to clarify how these results may be incorporated into other current theories of depression and mood regulation (5, 6, 59). Nonetheless, taken together, these data suggest that pathways connecting subgenual cingulate and dorsolateral prefrontal cortex are fundamental to the mediation of mood-attention interactions necessary for maintenance of emotional homeostasis in health and disease.

REFERENCES

1. James W: What is an emotion? Mind 1884; 9:188–205
2. Papez JW: A proposed mechanism of emotion. Arch Neurol Psychiatry 1927; 38:725–743
3. MacLean PD: Psychosomatic disease and the visceral brain: recent developments bearing on the Papex theory of emotion. Psychosom Med 1949; 11:338–353
4. Rolls ET: A theory of emotion, and its application to understanding the neural basis of emotion. Cognition & Emotion 1990; 4:161–190
5. Tucker DM, Luu P, Pribram KH: Social and emotional self-regulation. Ann NY Acad Sci 1995; 769:213–239
6. Damasio AR: The somatic marker hypothesis and the possible functions of the prefrontal cortex. Philos Trans R Soc Lond B Biol Sci 1996; 351:1413–1420
7. Weingartner H, Cohen RM, Murphy DL, Martello J, Gerdt C: Cognitive processes in depression. Arch Gen Psychiatry 1981; 38:42–47
8. Liotti M, Sava D, Rizzolatti G, Caffarra P: Differential hemispheric asymmetries in depression and anxiety: a reaction-time study. Biol Psychiatry 1991; 29:887–899
9. Carmichael ST, Price JL: Limbic connections of the orbital and medial prefrontal cortex in macaque monkeys. J Comp Neurol 1995; 363:615–641
10. Pandya DN, Yeterian EH: Comparison of prefrontal architecture and connections. Philos Trans R Soc Lond B Biol Sci 1996; 351:1423–1432
11. Dias R, Robbins TW, Roberts AC: Dissociation in prefrontal cortex of affective and attentional shifts. Nature 1996; 380:69–72
12. Baker SC, Frith CD, Dolan RJ: The interaction between mood and cognitive function studied with PET. Psychol Med 1997; 27:565–578
13. George MS, Ketter TA, Parekh PI, Rosinsky N, Ring HA, Pazzaglia PJ, Marangell LB, Callahan AM, Post RM: Blunted left cingulate activation in mood disorder subjects during a response interference task (the Stroop). J Neuropsychiatry Clin Neurosci 1997; 9:55–63
14. Pardo JV, Raichle ME, Fox PT: Localization of a human system for sustained attention by positron emission tomography. Nature 1991; 349:61–63
15. Corbetta M, Miezin FM, Shulman GL, Petersen SE: A PET study of visuospatial attention. J Neurosci 1993; 13:1202–1226
16. Pardo JV, Pardo PJ, Janer KW, Raichle ME: The anterior cingulate cortex mediates processing selection in the Stroop attentional conflict paradigm. Proc Natl Acad Sci USA 1990; 87: 256–259
17. Morecraft RJ, Geula C, Mesulam MM: Architecture of connectivity within a cingulo-fronto-parietal neurocognitive network for directed attention. Arch Neurol 1993; 50:279–284
18. Mesulam MM: Large-scale neurocognitive networks and distributed processing for attention, language and memory. Ann Neurol 1990; 28:597–613
19. Pardo JV, Pardo PJ, Raichle ME: Neural correlates of self-induced dysphoria. Am J Psychiatry 1993; 150:713–719
20. George MS, Ketter TA, Parekh PI, Horwitz B, Herscovitch P, Post RM: Brain activity during transient sadness and happiness in healthy women. Am J Psychiatry 1995; 152:341–351
21. Schneider F, Gur RE, Mozley LH, Smith RJ, Mozley PD, Censits DM, Alavi A, Gur RC: Mood effects on limbic blood flow correlate with emotional self-rating: a PET study with O-15 labeled water. Psychiatry Res 1995; 61:265–283
22. Gemar MC, Kapur S, Segal ZV, Brown GM, Houle S: Effects of self-generated sad mood on regional cerebral activity: a PET study in normal subjects. Depression 1996; 4:81–88
23. Paradiso S, Robinson RG, Andreasen NC, Downhill JE, Davidson RJ, Kirchner PT, Watkins GL, Boles Ponto LL, Hichwa RD: Emotional activation of limbic circuitry in elderly normal subjects in a PET study. Am J Psychiatry 1997; 154: 384–389
24. Lane RD, Reiman EM, Ahern GL, Schwartz GE, Davidson RJ: Neuroanatomical correlates of happiness, sadness, and disgust. Am J Psychiatry 1997; 154:926–933
25. Robinson RG, Kubos KL, Starr LB, Rao K, Price TR: Mood disorders in stroke patients: importance of location of lesion. Brain 1984; 107:81–93
26. Baxter LR Jr, Schwartz JM, Phelps ME, Mazziotta JC, Guze BH, Selin CE, Gerner RH, Sumida RM: Reduction of prefrontal cortex glucose metabolism common to three types of depression. Arch Gen Psychiatry 1989; 46:243–250
27. Mayberg HS: Frontal lobe dysfunction in secondary depression. J Neuropsychiatry Clin Neurosci 1994; 6:428–442
28. Bench CJ, Friston KJ, Brown RG, Scott LC, Frackowiak RS, Dolan RJ: The anatomy of melancholia—focal abnormalities of cerebral blood flow in major depression. Psychol Med 1992; 22:607–615
29. Mayberg HS, Brannan SK, Mahurin RK, Jerabek PA, Brickman JS, Tekell JL, Silva JA, McGinnis S, Glass TG, Martin CC, Fox PT: Cingulate function in depression: a potential predictor of treatment response. Neuroreport 1997; 8:1057–1061
30. Bench CJ, Friston KJ, Brown RG, Frackowiak RS, Dolan RJ: Regional cerebral blood flow in depression measured by positron emission tomography: the relationship with clinical dimensions. Psychol Med 1993; 23:579–590
31. First MB, Spitzer RL, Gibbon M, Williams JBW: Structured Clinical Interview for DSM-IV Axis I Disorders (SCID), Clinician Version: User's Guide. Washington, DC, American Psychiatric Press, 1996
32. Raichle ME, Martin WR, Herscovitch P, Mintun MA, Markham J: Brain blood flow measured with intravenous H2(15)O, II: implementation and validation. J Nucl Med 1983; 24:790–798
33. Phelps ME, Huang SC, Hoffman EH, Selin C, Sokoloff L, Kuhl DE: Tomographic measurement of local cerebral glucose metabolic rate in humans with (F-18)2-fluoro-2-deoxy-d-glucose: validation of method. Ann Neurol 1979; 6:371–388
34. Lancaster JL, Glass TH, Lankipalli BR, Downs H, Mayberg HS, Fox PT: A modality-independent approach to spatial normalization of tomographic images of the human brain. Human Brain Mapping 1995; 3:209–223

35. Talairach J, Tournoux P: Co-Planar Stereotaxic Atlas of the Human Brain. New York, Thieme Medical, 1988
36. D'Agostino RB, Belanger A, D'Agostino RB Jr: A suggestion for using powerful and informative tests of normality. Am Statistician 1990; 44:316–321
37. Fox PT, Mintun MA: Noninvasive functional brain mapping by change-distribution analysis of averaged PET images of $H_2{}^{15}O$ tissue activity. J Nucl Med 1989; 30:141–149
38. Worsley KJ, Evans AC, Marrett S, Neelin A: Three-dimensional statistical analysis for CBF activation studies in human brain. J Cereb Blood Flow Metab 1992; 12:900–918
39. Mintun MA, Fox PT, Raichle ME: A highly accurate method of localizing regions of neuronal activation in the human brain with positron emission tomography. J Cereb Blood Flow Metab 1989; 9:96–103
40. Lancaster JL, Rainey LH, Summerlin JL, Freitas CS, Fox PT, Evans AC, Toga AW, Mazziotta JC: Automated labeling of the human brain: a preliminary report on the development and evaluation of a forward-transform method. Human Brain Mapping 1997; 5:238–242
41. Fox PT, Ingham RJ, Ingham JC, Hirsch TB, Downs JH, Martin C, Jerabek P, Glass T, Lancaster JL: A PET study of the neural systems of stuttering. Nature 1996; 382:158–161
42. Mayberg HS: Limbic-cortical dysregulation: a proposed model of depression. J Neuropsychiatry Clin Neurosci 1997; 9:471–481
43. Liotti M, Mayberg HS, Ryder K, Brannan SK, Woldorff MG: An ERP study of mood provocation in remitted depression. Abstracts of the Society for Neuroscience 1996; 23:1657
44. Martinot J-L, Hardy P, Feline A, Huret J-D, Mazoyer B, Attar-Levy D, Pappata S, Syrota A: Left prefrontal glucose hypometabolism in the depressed state: a confirmation. Am J Psychiatry 1990; 147:1313–1317
45. Bench CJ, Frackowiak RSJ, Dolan RJ: Changes in regional cerebral blood flow on recovery from depression. Psychol Med 1995; 25:247–251
46. Buchsbaum MS, Wu J, Siegel BV, Hackett E, Trenary M, Abel L, Reynolds C: Effect of sertraline on regional metabolic rate in patients with affective disorder. Biol Psychiatry 1997; 41:15–22
47. Nobler MS, Sackeim HA, Prohovnik I, Moeller JR, Mukherjee S, Schnur DB, Prudic J, Devanand DP: Regional cerebral blood flow in mood disorders, III: treatment and clinical response. Arch Gen Psychiatry 1994; 51:884–897
48. Liotti M, Mayberg HS, Brannan SK, McGinnis S, Jerabek PA, Martin CC, Fox PT: Mood challenge in remitted depression: a ^{15}O-water PET study. NeuroImage 1997; 5:S114
49. Drevets WC, Price JL, Simpson JR Jr, Todd RD, Reich T, Vannier M, Raichle ME: Subgenual prefrontal cortex abnormalities in mood disorders. Nature 1997; 386:824–827
50. Meltzer CC, Zubieta JK, Brandt J, Tune LE, Mayberg HS, Frost JJ: Regional hypometabolism in Alzheimer's disease as measured by positron emission tomography after correction for effects of partial volume averaging. Neurology 1996; 47:454–461
51. Shulman GL, Fiez JA, Corbetta M, Buckner RL, Miezin FM, Raichle ME, Petersen SE: Common blood flow changes across visual tasks, II: decreases in cerebral cortex. J Cognitive Neuroscience 1997; 9:647–662
52. Andreasen NC, O'Leary DS, Cizadlo T, Arndt S, Rezai K, Watkins GL, Boles Ponto LL, Hichwa RD: Remembering the past: two facets of episodic memory explored with positron emission tomography. Am J Psychiatry 1995; 152:1576–1585
53. Mayberg HS, Liotti M, Jerabek PA, Martin CC, Fox PT: Induced sadness: a PET model of depression. Human Brain Mapping 1995; 1(suppl):396
54. Vogt BA, Pandya DN: Cingulate cortex of the rhesus monkey, II: cortical afferents. J Comp Neurol 1987; 262:271–289
55. Beck AT, Rush JA, Shaw BS, Emery G: Cognitive Therapy of Depression. New York, Guilford Press, 1979
56. Chaput Y, deMontigny C, Blier P: Presynaptic and postsynaptic modifications of the serotonin system by long-term administration of antidepressant treatments: an in vitro electrophysiologic study in the rat. Neuropsychopharmacology 1991; 5:219–229
57. Hyman SE, Nestler EJ: Initiation and adaptation: a paradigm for understanding psychotropic drug action. Am J Psychiatry 1996; 153:151–162
58. Cosgrove GR, Rausch SL: Psychosurgery. Neurosurg Clin North Am 1995; 6:167–176
59. Henriques JB, Glowacki JM, Davidson RJ: Reward fails to alter response bias in depression. J Abnorm Psychol 1994; 103:460–466

The Journal of Neuroscience, June 15, 1999, 19(12):5034–5043

Depression Duration But Not Age Predicts Hippocampal Volume Loss in Medically Healthy Women with Recurrent Major Depression

Yvette I. Sheline,[1,2,3] Milan Sanghavi,[1] Mark A. Mintun,[1,2,3] and Mokhtar H. Gado[2,3]

Departments of [1]Psychiatry and [2]Radiology 2 and the [3]Mallinckrodt Institute of Radiology, Washington University School of Medicine, St. Louis, Missouri 63110

This study takes advantage of continuing advances in the precision of magnetic resonance imaging (MRI) to quantify hippocampal volumes in a series of human subjects with a history of depression compared with controls. We sought to test the hypothesis that both age and duration of past depression would be inversely and independently correlated with hippocampal volume. A sample of 24 women ranging in age from 23 to 86 years with a history of recurrent major depression, but no medical comorbidity, and 24 case-matched controls underwent MRI scanning. Subjects with a history of depression (post-depressed) had smaller hippocampal volumes bilaterally than controls. Post-depressives also had smaller amygdala core nuclei volumes, and these volumes correlated with hippocampal volumes. In addition, post-depressives scored lower in verbal memory, a neuropsychological measure of hippocampal function, suggesting that the volume loss was related to an aspect of cognitive functioning. In contrast, there was no difference in overall brain size or general intellectual performance. Contrary to our initial hypothesis, there was no significant correlation between hippocampal volume and age in either post-depressive or control subjects, whereas there was a significant correlation with total lifetime duration of depression. This suggests that repeated stress during recurrent depressive episodes may result in cumulative hippocampal injury as reflected in volume loss.

Key words: hippocampus; depression; age; amygdala; magnetic resonance imaging; MRI; glucocorticoids; neurotoxicity; stereology

Hippocampal volume loss in humans has been associated with depression (Sheline et al., 1996) and aging (Jernigan et al., 1991). One explanation for volume loss in depression might be increased neuronal cell death secondary to glucocorticoid (GC) neurotoxicity (Sapolsky et al., 1986; McEwen, 1992). The pathophysiology of major depression involves impairment in negative feedback control of the hypothalamic–pituitary–adrenal (HPA) axis (Young et al., 1991), resulting in elevated cortisol levels during depressive episodes (Carroll et al., 1981). Prolonged exposure to elevated levels of glucocorticoids reduces hippocampal cell number (Sapolsky et al., 1985) and can induce cultured neurons to undergo apoptosis (Reagan and McEwen, 1997). This same effect has been shown in intact animals. Chronic stress or chronic administration of glucocorticoids to rodents (Watanabe et al., 1992) or nonhuman primates (Sapolsky et al., 1990) results in the degeneration of vulnerable hippocampal neurons, especially CA3 pyramidal cells. Animals exposed to high physiological levels of corticosterone (CORT) exhibited a persistent depletion of hippocampal CORT receptors and evidence of an impaired HPA axis (Sapolsky et al., 1983). Furthermore, a recent study (Lupien et al., 1998) has shown that in human aging, higher cortisol levels correlated longitudinally with greater hippocampal volume loss. In addition to direct neurotoxicity, glucocorticoid exposure may also enhance neuronal vulnerability to other insults, including hypoxia/ischemia (Tombaugh and Sapolsky, 1992), superoxide radical generators (McIntosh and Sapolsky, 1996), and hypoglycemia (Lawrence and Sapolsky, 1994).

Some studies in rodents have found age-related hippocampal neuronal loss based on neuron density studies (Landfield et al., 1981; Meaney et al., 1988; Issa et al., 1990). However, studies using unbiased stereological techniques have not found age-related loss of neurons in the CA1–CA3 hippocampal regions in humans, monkeys, or rodents (West, 1993; Rapp and Gallagher, 1996; Rasmussen et al., 1996). Differences in sampling procedures and counting methods could possibly account for some of the discrepancies between studies. Aged animals have decreases in hippocampal CORT receptors and evidence of an impaired HPA axis (Sapolsky et al., 1983) similar to animals exposed to high physiological levels of CORT. Although both aging and neurotoxic exposure produce loss of vulnerable hippocampal neurons, the combination of neurotoxic exposure and aging may have a synergistic effect through enhanced vulnerability to cell damage (Sapolsky, 1992). The analogy between aging and glucocorticoid exposure-induced neuronal vulnerability raises the question of the nature of the interaction between glucocorticoids and age. Because neuropathological studies of cell loss in Alzheimer's disease have been associated with volume loss in magnetic resonance imaging (MRI) studies, observable volume loss in MRI studies of depression may also result from cell loss. The present study was intended to use advances in the precision of MRI of the brain to quantify hippocampal volumes in a series of normal and depressed human subjects in mid and late life. We sought to test the hypothesis that both increasing age and increasing duration of depression would be independently associated with reductions in hippocampal volume. In addition we tested whether there would

Received Dec. 3, 1998; revised March 9, 1999; accepted April 6, 1999.

This work was supported by National Institutes of Health Grants MH K07 1370 (Y.I.S.), MH 58444 (Y.I.S.), and MH 54731 (M.A.M), and by the Washington University General Clinical Research Center National Institutes of Health Grant 5M01 RR00036. We thank Dr. Rosalind Neuman for helpful statistical advice.

Correspondence should be addressed to Dr. Yvette I. Sheline, Department of Psychiatry, Box 8134, Washington University School of Medicine, 4940 Childrens Place, St. Louis, MO 63110.

be an interaction between the two variables to produce synergistic effects in reducing hippocampal volume.

MATERIALS AND METHODS

Subjects. Depressed subjects were recruited to the outpatient psychiatry service at Washington University School of Medicine (WUSM), primarily from referrals from other psychiatrists who knew the inclusionary and exclusionary criteria (17/24 subjects) and also from advertisements to the general public (7/24 subjects). Control subjects were recruited primarily from the Aging and Development Project maintained by the Psychology Department at Washington University (13/24 subjects) and also from notices posted at the medical center (11/24 subjects). Subjects were recruited over a 4 year period. Subjects ranged in age from 23 to 86 years (mean = 54; median = 56). Inclusionary criteria were a history of recurrent major depression, with at least one previous episode requiring psychiatric treatment, female gender, right-handedness, and no medical illness potentially affecting the CNS. No subjects with current acute depression were included in the study to eliminate potential confounds in MRI volumetric measurements related to state-dependent changes such as hypercortisolemia. None of the subjects had been acutely depressed within the past 4 months. Only women were selected to decrease the incidence of occult cardiovascular disease and to minimize gender-based brain differences (Aboitiz et al., 1992). A case-control design was used to match patients with a history of depression (post-depressed) for age and educational level within 2 years. Groups were matched *post hoc* for height, a predictor of general brain size (Andreason et al., 1994). Potential subjects were screened by one of us (Y.I.S.) using a questionnaire, medical history, review of medical records, and physical exam to exclude those with medical problems potentially affecting the CNS. Exclusionary conditions included a current or past neurological disorder, head trauma, uncontrolled hypertension, myocardial infarction or ischemia, diabetes, Cushing's disease, steroid use, and drug/alcohol abuse. All subjects had documented normotension. In addition, subjects who had received more than three courses of electroconvulsive therapy (ECT) were excluded. Subjects gave written informed consent before inclusion in the study.

Clinical assessment was conducted by a psychiatrist (Y.I.S.) experienced in the use of the Diagnostic Interview for Genetic Studies (DIGS). The DIGS is a structured interview with high reliability (Nurnberger et al., 1993) that was used to make the diagnosis of past episodes of recurrent major depression by Diagnostic and Statistical Manual of Mental Disorders-IV criteria and to exclude other psychiatric diagnoses. The DIGS was used to assess both depressed and control subjects. Current antidepressant status and dosage were determined. To determine the presence and severity of any current depressive symptoms, all patients and controls were assessed using the Hamilton Rating Scale for Depression (HAMD).

Estimation of total time depressed. The number of symptoms and duration (days) of each episode were determined using the DIGS, as described above to define episodes of major depression. This was conducted using the Post Life Charting Method (Post et al., 1988) to anchor each episode. The total cumulative duration of depression was then calculated, summing over all episodes. Rigorous diagnostic criteria were used to establish each episode, and whenever possible, corroborating information was obtained from family members or treating psychiatrists, because in depressed populations, self-reporting may underestimate the duration of earlier episodes. Patients with more severe histories of depression, such as those in the current study, have been shown to have greater stability of diagnosis (Rice et al., 1987).

Neuropsychological testing. To determine the functional significance of brain volumetric changes, neuropsychological testing was performed. Subjects were administered the following tests: Wechsler Memory Scale-Revised (WMS-R), Logical Memory I (LMI) and II (LMII) subtests (Wechsler, 1987); Auditory Verbal Learning Test (AVLT) (Rey, 1964); Trail Making Test, parts A and B; and Weschler Adult Intelligence Scale-Revised (WAIS-R), Information and Block Design subtests (Wechsler, 1981). All tests were administered before administration of the dexamethasone suppression test (see below).

The Logical Memory subtest was administered according to the standardized protocol outlined in the WMS-R Manual (1987). Two stories were read aloud to the subject by the examiner. The subject was asked to repeat the story using as many of the same words as they could recall from memory after each story. One point was given for each verbatim or accepted alternate response phrase. After a 30 min delay the subject was asked to recall each story again. Subjects' responses were recorded on audiotape and transcribed to ensure accurate scoring. Scores were tabulated for each story as well as the total score for the immediate (LMI) and delayed (LMII) trials.

The AVLT was administered using a standard protocol (Lezak, 1995) to present a 12-word list five times followed each time by recall of as many words as possible, then a second 12-word list with recall. After a 30 min delay subjects were asked to recall the first list again. One point was given for each recalled word during each presentation. The sum of the total number of words recalled in presentations one through five was also calculated.

Trails A and B were administered in two parts according to a standard protocol (Lezak, 1995). On part A, subjects were asked to draw a line to connect consecutively numbered circles as quickly as possible, with time necessary to complete the task recorded in seconds. On part B, subjects were asked to draw a line connecting consecutively numbered and lettered circles as quickly as possible, alternating between numbers and letters (1 to A, A to 2, 2 to B, etc). Time to completion was recorded in seconds.

WAIS-R Information was administered according to the WAIS-R Manual (1981). Twenty-nine questions arranged in order of increasing difficulty were read directly from the manual, and the subjects' responses were recorded. The test was discontinued after five consecutive failures. One point was scored for each correctly answered question. WAIS-R Block Design also was administered according to the WAIS-R Manual (1981). Subjects were presented with designs requiring assembly of four blocks (first five designs) or nine blocks (last four designs). For each design the subject was shown a card with a picture of the design. There was a 1 min time limit on the first five designs and a 2 min time limit on the last four designs. The test was discontinued after two consecutive failed design constructions. Subjects were given points according to time needed for completion of each correctly assembled design, and the total earned points was calculated.

Magnetic resonance imaging. MRI scans were obtained using a Magnetom SP-4000 1.5T imaging system (Siemens Medical Systems, Iselin, NJ), and a standard Siemens 30 cm circularly polarized radio frequency (rf) head coil. Anatomic images consisted of 128 contiguous 1.25-mm-thick sagittal slices and were acquired using magnetization-prepared rapid gradient echo (MPRAGE) acquisition. No sedation was used during scanning. Specific MPRAGE scanning parameters were as follows: TR = 10 msec, TE = 4 msec, inversion time = 300 msec, flip angle = 8, matrix = 256 × 256 pixels, voxel size = 1 × 1 × 1.25 mm, slice thickness = 1.25 mm.

Image preprocessing. A graphics workstation (Sun Sparcstation 20, Sun Microsystems, Mountain View, CA) was used for initial image processing using ANALYZE software (Biomedical Imaging Resource, Mayo Foundation) (Robb, 1990). Images were interpolated to 0.5 mm sections. They were then reoriented to the anterior-posterior commissure plane for standard alignment. To minimize inter-scan variations, MR images underwent gray-scale normalization. Cylindrical regions-of-interest subvolumes inclusive of the amygdala and hippocampus were generated to aid in tissue classification. These subvolumes were analyzed using PeakFit software (Jandel Scientific, San Rafael CA), by the Marquardt-Levenberg algorithm for nonlinear curve fitting (Donald and Marquardt, 1963). The images were then scaled to create high contrast between gray and white matter in an eight-bit format.

Stereological method and reliability. Two raters (Y.I.S., M.S.) measured unilateral hippocampal gray matter volumes after training and assessment standardization with a neuroradiologist (M.H.G.) expert in hippocampal neuroanatomy. Stereological estimation methods, which have been used with precision in microscopy and MR volume determination (Mayhew, 1992) were used to estimate all hippocampal, amygdala, and whole brain volumes. Sampling parameters and grid size were set to yield at least 150 "hits" per measurement, a number that has previously been determined to yield reliable measurements in brain volume determination (Gundersen, 1988). From three-dimensional MRI cubical subvolumes composed of 0.5 × 0.5 × 0.5 mm voxels, coronal slices were sampled every 1.5 mm for hippocampus, every 1.0 mm for total amygdala, and every 0.5 mm for amygdala core nuclei. A rigid grid of points was then superimposed on the images. Grid points falling within the hippocampal, total amygdala, or amygdala core nuclei gray matter (see definitions below) were counted. Measurements were made using MEASURE (courtesy of P. Barta, Johns Hopkins University) in the coronal orientation, but the program displays grid points simultaneously in three orthogonal perspectives: sagittal, axial, and coronal (Fig. 1) to aid in anatomic localization. Volume estimates were calculated by MEASURE based on the number of selected grid points. Raters were blind to subject

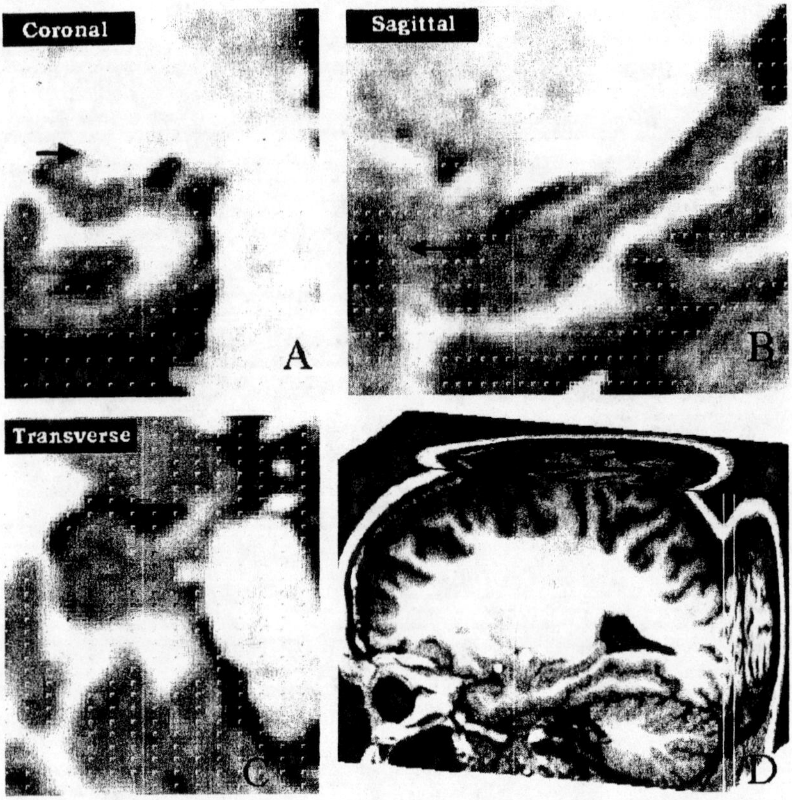

Figure 1. Hippocampal volume measurement using stereology. *A*, Coronal section through the hippocampus. Points within the hippocampus highlighted in *red* were selected from a randomly placed 5 × 5 mm^2 grid overlying the hippocampus and are simultaneously displayed in (*A*) coronal, (*B*) sagittal, and (*C*) horizontal views. *Arrow* indicates the caudate (*A*), and ↔ indicates the amygdala 171 (*B*). *D*, Cubic volumes containing the hippocampus were sectioned out from the total brain volume.

identity and measured left and right volumes separately. Mean volumes were determined from an average of four measurements of each volume, two measurements each by two independent raters for hippocampal, amygdala core nuclei, and total cerebral volumes. Means for total amygdala volumes, left and right, were determined from an average of two independent measures by the same rater. Intra-rater and inter-rater reliability were determined using the intraclass R. Intra-rater correlation coefficients were calculated for total (0.94 and 0.95), left (0.90 and 0.95), and right (0.95 and 0.98) hippocampal volumes, total (0.97 and 0.96), left (0.94 and 0.93), and right (0.92 and 0.90) amygdala core nuclei volumes, total (0.90), left (0.86), and right (0.88) whole amygdala volumes, and whole brain volumes (0.93 and 0.93). Inter-rater correlation coefficients were calculated for total (0.95), left (0.90), and right (0.95) hippocampal volumes, total (0.89), left (0.90), and right (0.82) amygdala core nuclei volumes, and whole brain volumes (0.92). For hippocampus, 48 pairs of intra-rater measurements and 48 pairs of inter-rater comparisons were made. For amygdala, 48 pairs of intra-rater and inter-rater core amygdala measurements were made, and 48 pairs of intra-rater measurements were made for whole amygdala by one rater. For whole brain, 48 pairs of intra-rater reliability measurements were made, and 28 pairs of inter-rater reliability measurements were made.

Anatomic definition of the hippocampus. Anatomical boundaries were defined by specific rules (Duvernoy, 1988; Bartzokis et al., 1993) as follows: every third coronal slice was assessed, beginning with the posterior-most slice in which the hippocampus was visualized. Orthogonal views were consulted in cases of anatomic uncertainty, although the coronal view retained priority. Posteriorly, the tail of the hippocampus continues as the indusium griseum, a thin strip of gray matter overlying the surface of the corpus callosum. For purposes of measurement, the posterior-most slice for inclusion was defined as the slice where the hippocampus first appeared adjacent to the trigone of the lateral ventricle. Included tissues were an elongated gray matter complex bordered superiorly by the fornix-fimbria white matter junction, inferiorly by parahippocampal gyrus white matter, medially by the subarachnoid spaces of various cisterns (e.g., ambient cistern), and laterally by the CSF-filled lateral ventricle. The gray matter complex included the cornu ammonis (CA), dentate gyrus, and subiculum, (i.e., the head and body of the hippocampus were included). The vertical digitation of the head of the hippocampus, which curves up and medial to the amygdala in coronal sections, was included. Excluded tissues were the fornix-fimbria white matter complex; the alveus, the intraventricular white matter covering of the hippocampus; the white matter of the parahippocampal gyrus; vari-

Table 1. Demographic and clinical characteristics of subjects with a history of major depression and matched controls

Variable	Depressed subjects (n = 24)		Matched controls (n = 24)		Paired t test	
	Mean	SD	Mean	SD	t	p
Age (year)	52.8	18.4	52.8	17.8	0.0001	0.99
Education (year)	16.3	3.5	16.3	4.1	−0.08	0.94
Height (cm)	162.1	5.4	163.8	6.9	−1.2	0.24
Cortisol (μg/l)						
Baseline	21.86[a]	11.70	21.37[b]	10.13	−0.51[c]	0.62[c]
DST	1.99[a]	1.26	1.99[b]	1.13	−0.98[c]	0.35[c]
HAMD	5.9	4.8	1.3	1.5	4.7	0.0001
Days depressed	1058	1032				

[a]Cortisol levels based on n = 17.

[b]Cortisol levels based on n = 17.

[c]Calculated from 14 matched pairs.

ous fluid-filled spaces including ventricles, subarachnoid spaces, and sporadic fluid-density spaces in the hippocampus complex; and the amygdala proper and the white matter border with it, a thin white matter line, discernible in high resolution MR images, which separated the hippocampus from the amygdala.

The subiculum extends medially from the cornu ammonis. The superior component of the CA does not extend medially far enough to aid in demarcating the border of the hippocampus, and the inferior component of the CA is in direct continuity with the subiculum. Because no clear gross anatomic separation exists between the hippocampus, subiculum, presubiculum, or parasubiculum, we adopted a previous procedure to include the subiculum in the measured volume of the hippocampus (Bartzokis et al., 1993).

Anatomic definition of the amygdala core nuclei. As described (Sheline et al., 1998), these structures were defined by the white matter tracts (longitudinal association bundles) surrounding them. Included were the basal nucleus, accessory basal nucleus, and the lateral nucleus (medial portions). Excluded structures were the periamygdaloid areas, the medial nucleus, and the central nucleus.

Anatomic definition of the noncore amygdala. The amygdala was visualized in three planes simultaneously during measurement, and some boundaries were better visualized in one plane than in another. The noncore amygdala was defined by measuring the total amygdala and subtracting the core amygdala. The anterior boundary of the amygdala, visualized in coronal section, was the first section in which the temporal stalk connected to the white matter of the insula. Dorsally, visualized in coronal section, the border was defined in anterior sections by the endorhinal sulcus between the basal forebrain and temporal lobe, and posteriorly in sagittal sections by a horizontal to the posteroinferior edge of the temporal stem with the temporal horn of the lateral ventricle. Ventrally, visualized in sagittal section, the amygdala was bounded by a horizontal line connecting to the ventral/anterior edge of the hippocampus. Posteriorly, seen in sagittal section, the amygdala was bounded by its border with the hippocampus. Medially, seen in coronal section, the amygdala was bounded by subarachnoid space. Laterally, seen in coronal section, the amygdala was bounded by white matter. These boundaries defined the total amygdala. The noncore amygdala was defined as the total amygdala minus the core amygdala.

Total cerebral volume. All brain tissue of the cerebral hemispheres, both gray and white matter, was included in the assessment of total cerebral volume. The midbrain superior to the pons was also included. The superior border of the pons was chosen as the point of demarcation because it is easily recognizable. This volume measurement was made using stereological methods as described above.

Cortisol levels. Blood samples were obtained to measure cortisol concentrations at 8:00 A.M. and 4:00 P.M. on the day before (baseline) and the day after oral administration of 1 mg dexamethasone at 11:00 P.M. (dexamethasone suppression test). Plasma was obtained within 1 hr of obtaining each sample by centrifuging the sample at ≅1000 × g for 15 min. All plasma samples were stored at −20°C until assay by fluorescence polarization immunoassay using the TDX analyzer and a commercially available kit (Abbott Laboratories).

Data analysis. Two-tailed paired t tests were used to compare post-depressed and control subjects on all demographic and MRI measures. The Pearson correlation was used to determine the significance of correlations among and between MRI measures and total cumulative duration of depression. Before using the Pearson correlation, variables were tested to determine whether they met criteria for normal distribution (Kolmogorov–Smirnov test). Pearson correlations were used to determine the correlation between age and hippocampal volumes separately in both the depressed and control samples, as well as in the total sample. A multiple regression with age and depression duration as independent variables was used to test these effects on hippocampal volumes. To examine the effect of age on hippocampal volumes, after removing the effect of depression duration, a regression analysis was conducted using age versus hippocampal volumes corrected for depression duration. This correction factor was derived from the multiple regression analysis with age and depression duration as independent variables and hippocampal volume as the dependent variable. In addition, to determine whether there was an interaction between age and depression status in predicting hippocampal volumes, these variables were combined into a new variable, and a multiple regression analysis was run using all three variables.

RESULTS

Demographic and cortisol data

Table 1 summarizes demographic and cortisol data for the 24 post-depressed subjects and their case-matched controls. The HAMD scores are consistent with the absence of acute current depression. Post-depressed subjects had a mean of 4.8 lifetime episodes of major depression (range 1–18) accounting for a lifetime mean of 1058 d depressed (range 21–3752; median, 624). Five subjects had received electroconvulsive therapy (ECT) previously during the course of their treatment and had elapsed times since last ECT treatment of 34, 30, and 14 years, and 7 and 11 months. Sixteen of the 24 post-depressed subjects were currently receiving antidepressants: selective serotonin reuptake inhibitors in four cases; tricyclic antidepressants in five cases; trazodone in two cases; and maprotiline, moclobemide, mirtazapine, nefazodone, and buproprion in one case each. Two post-depressed patients had previously been treated with neuroleptics: one with chlorpromazine and one with haloperidol. In both cases treatment duration was brief, and neither patient was psychotic at the time of treatment. Cortisol data were obtained from 17 of the total of 24 subject pairs. There was no difference between post-depressed and matched controls in either baseline cortisol levels (p = 0.56) or post-dexamethasone cortisol levels (p = 0.38) (Table 1), as would be expected in subjects who were not acutely depressed.

Table 2. Comparison of subjects with a history of major depression and matched controls on brain volumetric data

Variable	Depressed (n = 24) Mean	SD	Matched controls (n = 24) Mean	SD	Paired t test t	p
Hippocampal gray matter volume (mm^3)						
Left	2230	323	2482	305	−2.9	0.008
Right	2264	320	2468	309	−2.3	0.03
Total	4496	602	4951	601	−2.7	0.01
Amygdala gray matter volume (mm^3)						
Left core	531	93	610	106	3.3	0.004
Right core	514	97	585	102	2.8	0.009
Total core	1045	180	1196	202	3.2	0.004
Left noncore	1081	298	1111	253	−0.44	0.66
Right noncore	1147	341	1131	241	0.24	0.81
Total noncore	2228	610	2242	480	−0.11	0.91
Total cerebral volume ($mm^3 \times 10^3$)						
Whole brain	1075	170	1078	168	−0.08	0.94

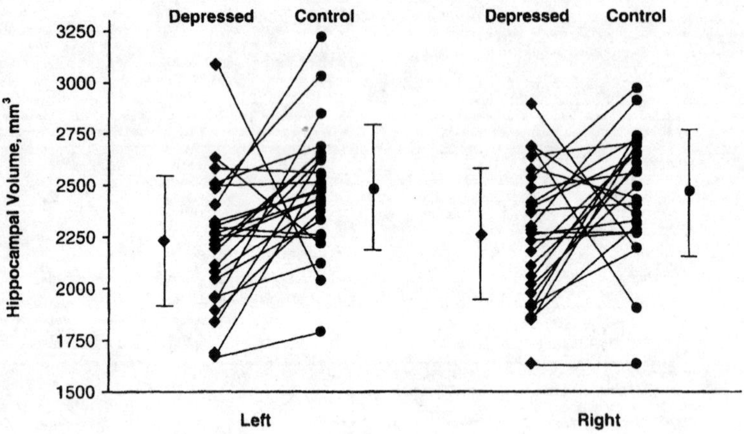

Figure 2. Left and right hippocampal gray matter volumes. The *lines* connect the hippocampal volumes for each subject pair consisting of subject with a history of major depression (post-depressed) and the age, gender, education, and height-matched case control; the mean and the SDs for each group are also shown.

In this sample, 26 women were postmenopausal and 22 were premenopausal. Of the 26 postmenopausal women, 14 were from the post-depressed group and 12 were controls (χ^2 p value = 0.67). In the total sample, 17 women were on hormone replacement therapy. Of women on hormone replacement therapy, 9/17 were post-depressed and 8/17 were controls (χ^2 p value = 0.85).

Brain volumetric data

Table 2 summarizes brain volumetric data for post-depressed subjects and matched controls. Mean total, left, and right hippocampal gray matter volumes were significantly smaller for post-depressed subjects than for controls. On average the differences were 9, 10, and 8% for the total, left, and right volumes, respectively (Fig. 2). Mean total, left, and right amygdala core nuclei volumes were significantly smaller in post-depressives than in control subjects; on average 13, 13, and 12% for total, left, and right volumes, respectively (Table 2), whereas amygdala noncore volumes, total amygdala volumes, and total cerebral volumes did not differ. Examining hormone replacement therapy alone as a predictor of total hippocampal volume, there was no statistically significant difference in volume between subjects on hormone

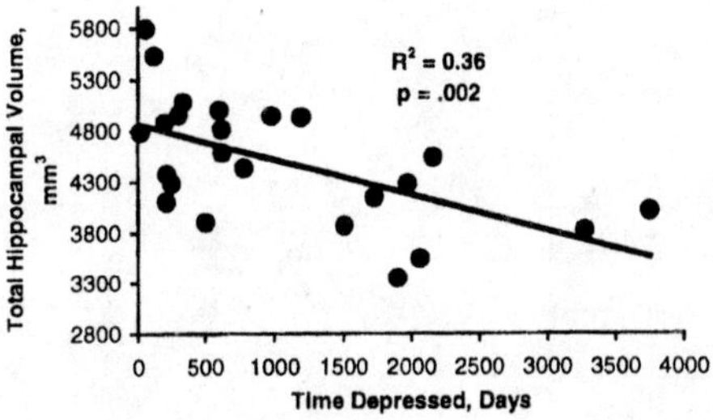

Figure 3. Correlation between duration of depression and hippocampal volume. The Pearson correlation between cumulative lifetime total days of major depression was derived from the Diagnostic Interview for Genetic Studies using the Post Life Charting Method (Post et al., 1988) and the total hippocampal gray matter volumes.

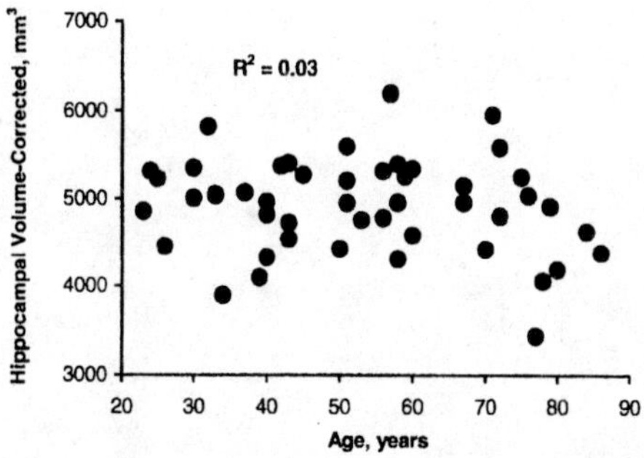

Figure 4. Correlation between age and total hippocampal gray matter volumes corrected for depression duration. The correction factor was derived from a multiple regression ANOVA using age and depression duration as independent variables and hippocampal gray matter volume as the dependent variable (see Materials and Methods).

replacement therapy (4699 mm^3) and those not on therapy (4780 mm^3) (p = 0.67). Postmenopausal status alone did not predict total hippocampal volume (4845 mm^3 premenopausal vs 4620 mm^3 postmenopausal; p = 0.23).

Correlations between hippocampal gray matter volumes, age, menopausal status, and total time depressed

In the total sample, the correlation between age and total hippocampal volume was $r = -0.19$ (p = 0.20). For post-depressed subjects the correlation between total hippocampal volume and age was $r = -0.32$ (p = 0.13). In control subjects the correlation between age and total gray matter hippocampal volume was $r = -0.08$ (p = 0.71). Analysis of interaction indicated that there was no interaction between age and depression status (p = 0.43). In contrast, there was a significant inverse correlation between total days depressed and total hippocampal gray matter volume ($r = -0.60$; p = 0.002) (Fig. 3). This was true for both left hippocampal gray matter volume ($r = -0.57$, p = 0.003) and right hippocampal gray matter volume ($r = -0.55$, p = 0.005).

To correct for a contribution of depression duration to the relationship between age and hippocampal volume, a regression analysis was conducted using age versus hippocampal volume corrected for depression duration. This analysis showed no significant correlation with age ($r = -0.17$, p = 0.26) (Fig. 4).

A multiple regression analysis did not find a significant relationship (p = 0.61) using hormone replacement therapy, postmenopausal status, and age as independent variables and total hippocampal volume as the dependent variable. Examination of left and right hippocampal volumes separately also did not yield significant relationships.

Correlations between hippocampal gray matter volumes and amygdala core nuclei volumes

The correlation between total hippocampal gray matter volume and total amygdala core nuclei volume for post-depressed subjects was r = 0.68, p = 0.0001 (Fig. 5), and this held for the left (r = 0.65, p = 0.0004) and right sides (r = 0.58, p = 0.002) as well. In control subjects these respective correlations were r = 0.50 (p = 0.01), r = 0.54 (p = 0.006), and r = 0.42 (p = 0.04). In contrast, the correlations in post-depressed subjects between total and both left and right hippocampal gray matter volumes and total ($r = -0.11$, p = 0.63) (Fig. 5), left (r = 0.15, p = 0.49), and right ($r = -0.02$, p = 0.93) amygdala noncore nuclei volumes, respectively, were not significant. The respective correlations in control subjects (r = 0.46, p = 0.02; r = 0.45, p = 0.03; and r = 0.42, p = 0.04) with amygdala noncore nuclei volumes were significant.

Neuropsychological data

As shown in Table 3, scores for list learning, total recall and list learning, long delay were significantly decreased in subjects with a history of depression compared with controls. Paragraph recall scores did not achieve significance. Trails A, Trails B, and WAIS information subscale scores were not significantly different between the groups. The WAIS block design subscale score was significantly less in subjects with a history of depression than in control subjects.

Effect of removing subjects who had received ECT

The data analyses comparing hippocampal gray matter volumes between post-depressed and control subjects were rerun after removal of the five subjects who had received ECT and their matched controls. There was still a significant difference in total ($t = -2.1$, p = 0.04) and left ($t = -2.4$, p = 0.03) hippocampal gray matter volumes and a trend toward a difference in right ($t = -1.8$, p = 0.08) hippocampal volumes between post-depressed and control subjects. In post-depressed subjects there was also a significant correlation between days depressed and both left ($r = -0.59$, p = 0.005) and right ($r = -0.53$, p = 0.01) hippocampal volumes.

DISCUSSION

The main findings of this study are the lack of a correlation between age and hippocampal volume in medically healthy subjects and the finding of smaller hippocampal volumes in subjects with a history of depression. These subjects also had evidence of poorer verbal memory performance, despite being in remission. Extending our pilot study (Sheline et al., 1996), we report that 24 women with a history of depression, but no medical comorbidity, had bilaterally smaller hippocampal volumes than age-matched controls. Findings of decreased hippocampal volumes have been reported in acutely depressed subjects (Narayan et al., 1998) and in patients suffering from post-traumatic stress disorder (Bremner et al., 1995). We show that post-depressed women exhibited

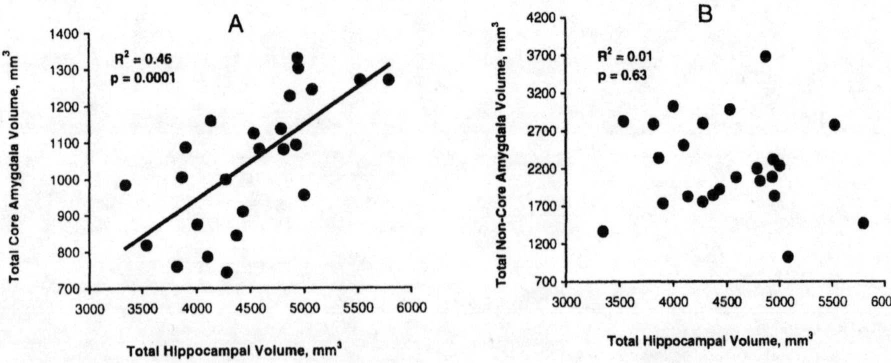

Figure 5. Correlations between hippocampal and amygdala volumes. *A*, The Pearson correlation between total hippocampal gray matter volume and the total amygdala core nuclei volume; *B*, the correlation between total hippocampal gray matter volume and total amygdala noncore volume in subjects with a history of major depression.

Table 3. Comparison of subjects with a history of major depression and matched controls on neuropsychological variables

	Depressed subjects (n = 24)		Matched controls (n = 24)		Paired t test	
Variable	Mean	SD	Mean	SD	t	p
List learning (total)	45.6	8.1	49.2	5.6	2.5	0.02
List learning (delayed)	9.4	2.4	10.6	1.6	2.5	0.02
Trails A	35.5	16.6	32.6	20.8	−0.70	0.49
Trails B	85.7	51.8	69.6	32.8	−1.6	0.12
Logical memory	25.1	9.0	27.2	6.6	1.0	0.31
WAIS information	21.4	4.9	21.6	4.1	0.17	0.87
WAIS block	29.9	10.4	33.9	10.0	2.4	0.03

abnormalities on a neuropsychological measure of hippocampal function, the AVLT, suggesting that their reduced hippocampal volumes were the result of functionally significant damage. Furthermore, hippocampal volumes correlated inversely with the cumulative lifetime duration of depression. In contrast to differences in hippocampal volumes and AVLT scores, post-depressed patients did not differ from control subjects in overall brain size or on general intellectual performance as assessed by the WAIS information subscale.

Given age- and depression-related increases in medical conditions, it is critical to know whether patients with changes in brain structure volumes had concurrent physical illnesses that could enhance neuronal vulnerability. In the present study, unlike most previous studies, we selected only subjects with no current or past medical or neurological conditions. An increased incidence of microinfarction has been linked to both chronic hypertension (Kobayashi et al., 1991) and diabetes (Aronson, 1973; Desmond et al., 1993). We excluded patients with any history of substance abuse because alcohol dependence can cause cerebral atrophy (Charness, 1993). Patients with a history of myocardial infarction were excluded because it is a cerebrovascular disease risk factor and produces a large independent increase in the incidence of depression (Carney et al., 1987).

Contrary to our initial hypothesis, there was not a significant age-related hippocampal volume loss in either post-depressed or control subjects. Some previous studies of hippocampal volume in "normal" aging found a decrease starting at age 50 (Jernigan et al., 1991), whereas others did not (Lim et al., 1990). Our sample showed slight (~1% per decade) nonsignificant decreases in hippocampal volumes with age, more so in the depressed population, although there was no interaction between age and depression status. It is possible that aging per se may not lead to neurodegeneration in the hippocampus but rather may increase vulnerability to other factors causing cell death, and these factors may have differed across study populations. It is possible that by selecting subjects without medical comorbidity we may have created a sample of "supernormals" who do not show a decrease in brain structure volumes with age.

One confounding variable is ECT. Although there has been no direct evidence demonstrating ECT-induced structural brain changes (Devanand et al., 1994), animal electroconvulsive stimulation (ECS) studies suggest that brief kindled seizures may induce selective hippocampal neuronal loss (Cavazos et al., 1994). ECS exposure sufficient to induce kindling, however, far exceeds the human equivalent ECT electrical doses. We did not exclude ECT-treated patients, because they had the most severe histories of depression. A *post hoc* analysis after removing the five ECT-treated subjects showed a significant difference in total hippocampal gray matter volume (p = 0.04) and a correlation between total days depressed and total hippocampal gray matter volume (p = 0.004). Another confound was ongoing antidepressant therapy in most post-depressed subjects, although there is no known evidence that therapeutic levels are neurotoxic or that antidepressant exposure reduces brain volumes.

Additional potentially confounding variables, which we examined *post hoc*, were menopausal status and hormone replacement therapy. The effects of estrogen on rat hippocampus dendritic spine density (Wooley et al., 1997) and on neuropsychological function in postmenopausal women in some studies (Resnick et al., 1998) make this an important variable to examine. We did not find any significant differences between the groups in either postmenopausal or hormone replacement status, making it unlikely that these factors could account for differences in brain volumes. When we examined the issue of whether there were differences in hippocampal volume between postmenopausal and premenopausal subjects and between subjects who had received hormone replacement therapy versus those who had not, we did not find significant differences. However, we have a small sample size, and it would be interesting to examine this question in a larger study prospectively with concurrent serum hormone level determination.

Our study found significant differences between post-depressed subjects and controls in a neuropsychological measure of hippocampal function, AVLT list learning, total score, and delayed score. In subjects with more severe hippocampal damage caused by mesial temporal sclerosis, the degree of left hippocampal atrophy in patients with left temporal lobe epilepsy was correlated with severity of verbal memory deficits as measured by AVLT total and delayed recall (Kilpatrick et al., 1997). In addition, in nondemented subjects who developed Alzheimer's disease during longitudinal followup (Tierney et al., 1996), the single biggest neuropsychological predictor was the AVLT score. Subjects in both groups had known hippocampal pathology that correlated with abnormalities in the AVLT. Our finding of abnormalities in AVLT in post-depressed subjects who also had hippocampal volume decreases appears to indicate hippocampal dysfunction. The groups did not differ, however, in logical memory test performance, another measure of hippocampal function (Squire, 1992). Depressed subjects did have lower WAIS block design subscale scores. Bremner et al. (1995) found that post-traumatic stress disorder patients performed more poorly on the Benton Visual Retention task, a test that reflects spatial memory and depends on right hippocampal integrity. Another possibility is that post-depressed subjects performed more poorly on timed tasks. However, both the WAIS block design and Trails A and B are timed tests; there was no difference in performance on Trails A and B between post-depressed and control subjects.

Although further study will be needed to fully elucidate the nature of the observed association between recurrent depression and volume reduction, evidence suggests that the link may be causal—that sustained depression in humans may cause hippocampal damage, resulting in a reduction of tissue volume and memory function. A limitation of the current study is that reliability of the Post Life Charting Method in determining retrospective measures of depression duration has not been established. There is no reason to believe that the data create a biased relationship between depression duration and hippocampal volumes, however, because volume data were obtained independently and blindly. The quantitative correlation between depression duration and hippocampal volume is explained most directly by such a causal relationship in that progressively more severe changes occur in the hippocampus as the length of time depressed, and presumably the length of time with abnormal GC levels, increases. Furthermore, in animals, repeated episodes of stress have been shown to damage the hippocampus. This appears to be mediated by GC-induced neurotoxicity (for review, see Sapolsky et al., 1986; Reagan and McEwen, 1997). In addition, there is evidence in normal elderly humans that long-term exposure to GCs predicts hippocampal atrophy and memory deficits (Lupien et al., 1998).

The relevance to depression of these studies showing that chronically elevated GC levels damage hippocampal neurons depends, however, on the assumption that depression is associated with dysregulation of the glucocorticoid system. Almost 40 years ago, excessive cortisol secretion during depression was first reported (Gibbons and McHugh, 1962). Hypercortisolism and insensitivity to feedback suppression during depression have been extensively investigated to determine the relative contributions of adrenal hypersensitivity to ACTH (Amsterdam et al., 1989), pituitary resistance to GC feedback (Holsboer et al., 1987), pituitary hypersensitivity to CRF and other hormones (Gold et al., 1984), and resistance at the hippocampus (Sapolsky et al., 1991; Young et al., 1991). Although we do not have cortisol levels from previous depressive episodes, many of our subjects had histories of hospitalization, ECT treatment, and multiple episodes, indicating relatively more severe major depression, a predictor of elevated cortisol and dexamethasone suppression test nonsuppression (Whiteford et al., 1987). Taken together, these findings suggest that HPA axis dysregulation in depression can produce repeated episodes of hypercortisolemia, which may result in hippocampal neurotoxicity.

The precise mechanisms whereby chronic glucocorticoid exposure leads to hippocampal cell death are not defined, but enhanced vulnerability to excitotoxicity may be a main factor (Armanini et al., 1990). We have shown a reduction in volumes of the core nuclei of the amygdala in recurrent major depression (Sheline et al., 1998) and now demonstrate a high correlation between hippocampal and amygdala core nuclei volume loss. Because glutamatergic pyramidal cells in the core nuclei of the amygdala are predominant and reciprocally connected with the hippocampus, it may be that overexcitation in one part of this circuit produces damage in connected structures. Furthermore, there was no difference in volumes of noncore amygdala nuclei, which contain primarily nonglutamatergic cells (Price et al., 1987).

In addition to glucocorticoid-induced neurotoxicity, other mechanisms consistent with hippocampal volume loss in recurrent depression include neurotoxic effects of corticotrophin-releasing factor (CRF) and a decrease in trophic factors such as brain-derived neurotrophic factor (BDNF). Elevated CRF levels have been described in both depressed humans (Nemeroff et al., 1984) and animal models of depression and have neurotoxic effects (Wong et al., 1995). Furthermore, CRF antagonists are neuroprotective against seizure-induced excitotoxicity (Maecker et al., 1997). Stress decreases the expression of BDNF (Duman et al., 1997), and BDNF is neuroprotective (Mamounas et al., 1995). These mechanisms—glucocorticoid toxicity, CRF neurotoxicity, and BDNF loss resulting in increased neuronal vulnerability—are not mutually exclusive and could all be operating to alter the vulnerability of hippocampal neurons in depression.

In summary, the present study shows an association between depression and structural changes in the hippocampus. It should be pointed out that volume changes cannot be equated with neuropathological studies directly performing cell counts; only the latter would provide direct evidence for cell loss. This gray matter hippocampal volume loss does not appear to be related to aging but could be related to factors commonly associated with aging, such as medical illnesses, which were not examined in this study. Depression-related volume loss does appear to be cumulative, suggesting that immediate recognition and treatment of depressive episodes is important in preventing cumulative damage that occurs with repeated episodes of depression.

REFERENCES

Aboitz F, Scheibel A, Zaidel E (1992) Morphometry of the Sylvian fissure and the corpus callosum, with emphasis on sex differences. Brain 115:1521–1541.

Amsterdam J, Maislin G, Berwish N, Phillips J, Winokur A (1989) Enhanced adrenocortical sensitivity to submaximal doses of cosyntropin in depressed patients. Arch Gen Psychiatry 46:550–554.

Andreasen NC, Flashman L, Flaum M, Arndt S, Swayzee V, O'Leary DS, Ehrhardt JC, Yuh WTC (1994) Regional brain abnormalities in schizophrenia measured with magnetic resonance imaging. JAMA 272:1763–1769.

Armanini MP, Hutchins C, Stein BA, RM Sapolsky (1990) Glucocorticoid endangerment of hippocampal neurons is NMDA-receptor dependent. Brain Res 532:7–12.

Aronson S (1973) J. Intracranial vascular lesions in patients with diabetes mellitus. Neuropathol Exp Neurol 32:183–196.

Bartzokis G, Mintz J, Marx P, Osborn D, Gutkind D, Chiang F, Phelan CK, Marder SR (1993) Reliability of in vivo volume measures of hippocampus and other brain structures using MRI. Magn Reson Imaging 11:993–1006.

Bremner J, Randall P, Scott T, Bronen R, Seibyl J, Southwick S, Delaney R, McCarthy G, Charney D, Innis R (1995) MRI-based measurement of hippocampal volume in patients with combat-related posttraumatic stress disorder. Am J Psychiatry 152:973–981.

Carney R, Rich M, teVelde A (1987) Major depressive disorder in coronary artery disease. Am J Cardiol 60:1273–1275.

Carroll R, Feinberg M, Greden J, Tarika J, Albala A, Haskett R, James M, Kronfol A, Lohr N, Steiner M, de Vigne J, Young E (1981) A specific laboratory test for the diagnosis of melancholia. Standardization, validation, and clinical utility. Arch Gen Psychiatry 38:15–22.

Cavazos JE, Das I, Sutula TP (1994) Neuronal loss induced in limbic pathways by kindling: evidence for induction of hippocampal sclerosis by repeated brief seizures. J Neurosci 14:3106–3121.

Charness ME (1993) Brain lesions in alcoholics. Alcohol Clin Exp Res 17:2–11.

Devanand DP, Dwork AJ, Hutchinson ER, Bolwig TG, Sackeim HA (1994) Does ECT alter brain structure? Am J Psychiatry 151:957–970.

Donald J, Marquardt W (1963) An algorithm for least-square estimation of nonlinear parameters. J Soc Indust Appl Math 11:431–441.

Duman RS, Heninger GR, Nestler EJ (1997) A molecular and cellular theory of depression. Arch Gen Psychiatry 54:597–606.

Duvernoy HM (1988) Human hippocampus: an atlas of applied anatomy. Munich: Bergmann Verlag.

Gibbons J, McHugh P (1962) Plasma cortisol in depressive illness. J Psychiatry Res 1:162–171.

Gold P, Chrousos G, Kellner C, Post R, Roy A, Avgerinos P, Schulte H, Oldfield E, Loriaux D (1984) Psychiatric implications of basic and clinical studies with CRF. Am J Psychiatry 141:619–627.

Gundersen HJG, Bendtsen TF, Korbo N (1988) Some new, simple and efficient stereological methods and their use in pathological research and diagnosis. Acta Pathol Microbiol Scand 96:379–394.

Holsboer F, Gerken A, Stalla G, Muller O (1987) Blunted aldosterone and ACTH release after human CRH administration in depressed patients. Am J Psychiatry 144:229–231.

Issa AM, Rowe W, Gauthier S, MJ Meaney (1990) Hypothalamic-pituitary-adrenal activity in aged, cognitively impaired and cognitively unimpaired rats. J Neurosci 10:3247–3254.

Jernigan TL, Archibald SL, Berhow MT, Sowell ER, Foster DS, JR Hesselink (1991) Cerebral structure on MRI, Part I: localization of age-related changes. Biol Psychiatry 29:55–67.

Kilpatrick C, Murrie V, Cook M, Andrews D, Desmond P, Hopper J (1997) Degree of left hippocampal atrophy correlates with severity of neuropsychological deficits. Seizure 6:213–218.

Kobayashi S, Okada K, Yamashita K (1991) Incidence of silent lacunar lesion in normal adults and its relation to cerebral blood flow and risk factors. Stroke 22:1379–1383.

Landfield PW, Baskin RK, Pitler TA (1981) Brain aging correlates: retardation by hormonal-pharmacological treatments. Science 214:581–584.

Lawrence MS, Sapolsky RM (1994) Glucocorticoids accelerate ATP loss following metabolic insults in cultured hippocampal neurons. Brain Res 646:303–306.

Lezak MD (1995) Neuropsychological assessment, Ed 3. New York: Oxford UP.

Lim KO, Zipursky RB, Murphy Jr GM, Pfefferbaum A (1990) In vivo quantification of the limbic system using MRI: effects of normal aging. Psychiatry Res 35:15–26.

Lupien SJ, de Leon M, deSanti S, Convit A, Tarshish C, Nair NPV, Thakur M, McEwen BS 1998 Cortisol levels during human aging predict hippocampal atrophy and memory deficits. Nat Neurosci 1: 69–73.

Maecker H, Desai A, Dash R, Rivier J, Vale W, Sapolsky R (1997) Astressin, a novel and potent CRF antagonist, is neuroprotective in the hippocampus when administered after a seizure. Brain Res 744:166–170.

Mamounas LA, Blue ME, Siuciak JA, Altar C (1995) BDNF promotes the survival and sprouting of serotonergic axons in the rat brain. J Neurosci 15:7929–7939.

Mayhew TM (1992) A review of recent advances in stereology for quantifying neural structure. J Neurocytol 21:313–328.

McEwen BS (1992) Re-examination of the glucocorticoid hypothesis of stress and aging. In: Progress in brain research (Swaab D, Hofman M, Mirmiran M, Ravid R, van Leeuwen F, eds), pp 356–383. New York: Elsevier.

McIntosh LJ, Sapolsky RM (1996) Glucocorticoids increase the accumulation of reactive oxygen species and enhance adriamycin-induced toxicity in neuronal culture. Exp Neurol 141:201–206.

Meaney MJ, Aitkin DH, van Berkel C Bhatnagar S, Sapolsky RM (1988) Effect of neonatal handling on age-related impairments associated with the hippocampus. Science 239:766–768.

Narayan M, Anderson E, Miller H, Staib L, Charney D, Bremner J (1998) Hippocampal volume in MDD. Abstract presented at the annual meeting of the American Psychiatric Association, May 1998, Toronto, Canada.

Nemeroff CB, Widerlov E, Walleus H, Karlsson I, Eklund K, Kilts CD, Loosen PT, Vale W (1984) Elevated concentrations of CSF corticotropin-releasing factor-like immunoreactivity in depressed patients. Science 226:1342–1344.

Nurnberger J, Blehar MC, Kaufmann CA, York-Cooler C, Simpson SG, Harkavy-Friedman J, Severe JB, Malaspina D, Reich T and collaborators from the NIMH Genetics Initiative (1993) Diagnostic interview for genetic studies. Rationale, unique features, and training. Arch Gen Psychiatry 11:849–859; 863–864.

Post RM, Roy-Byrne PP, Uhde T (1988) Graphic representation of the life course of illness in patients with affective disorder. Am J Psychiatry 145:844–848.

Price J, Russchen F, Amaral D (1987) The limbic region. II: The amygdaloid complex. In: Handbook of chemical neuroanatomy, Vol 5 (Bjorkland A, Hokfelt T, Swanson L, eds), pp 279–388. New York: Elsevier.

Rapp PR, Gallagher M (1996) Preserved neuron number in the hippocampus of aged rats with spatial learning deficits. Proc Natl Acad Sci USA 93:9926–9930.

Rasmussen T, Schliemann T, Sorensen JC, Zimmer J, West MJ (1996) Memory impaired aged rats: no loss of principal hippocampal and subicular neurons. Neurobiol Aging 17:143–147.

Reagan LP, McEwen BS (1997) Controversies surrounding glucocorticoid-mediated cell death in the hippocampus. J Chem Neuroanat 13:149–167.

Resnick S, Maki K, Golski S, Kraut M, Zonderman A (1998) Effects of estrogen replacement therapy on PET cerebral blood flow and neuropsychological performance. Horm Behav 34:171–182.

Rey A (1964) L'examen clinique en psychologie. Paris: Presses Universitaires de France.

Rice J, Endicott J, Knesevich M, Rochberg N (1987) The estimation of diagnostic sensitivity using stability data: an application to major depressive disorder. J Psychiat Res 21:337–345.

Robb RA (1990) A software system for interactive and quantitative analysis of biomedical images. In: 3D imaging in medicine, Vol F (Hohne KH, Fuchs M, Pizer SM, eds), pp 333–361. Nato ISI Series.

Sapolsky RM (1992) Is this relevant to the human? In: Stress, the aging brain and the mechanisms of neuron death, pp 305–339. Cambridge, MA: MIT.

Sapolsky RM, Krey LC, McEwen BS (1983) Corticosterone receptors decline in a site-specific manner in the aged rat brain. Brain Res 289:235–240.

Sapolsky RM, Krey LC, McEwen BS (1985) Prolonged glucocorticoid exposure reduces hippocampal neuron number: implications for aging. J Neurosci 5:1222–1227.

Sapolsky RM, Krey LC, McEwen BS (1986) The neuroendocrinology of stress and aging: the glucocorticoid cascade hypothesis. Endocrinol Rev 7:284–301.

Sapolsky RM, Uno H, Rebert CS, Finch CE (1990) Hippocampal damage associated with prolonged glucocorticoid exposure in primates. J Neurosci 10:2897–2902.

Sapolsky RM, Zola-Morgan S, Squire L (1991) Inhibition of glucocorticoid secretion by the hippocampal formation in the primate. J Neurosci 11:3695–3704.

Sheline YI, Wang PW, Gado MH, Csernansky JG, Vannier MW (1996) Hippocampal atrophy in recurrent major depression. Proc Natl Acad Sci USA 93:3908–3913.

Sheline YI, Gado M, Price JL (1998) Amygdala core nuclei volumes are decreased in recurrent major depression. NeuroReport 9:2023–2028.

Squire LR (1992) Declarative and nondeclarative memory: multiple brain systems supporting learning and memory. J Cognit Neurosci 4:232–243.

Tierney MC, Szalai JP, Snow WG, Fisher RH, Nores A, Nadon G, Dunn E, St. George-Hyslop PH (1996) Prediction of probable Alzheimer's disease in memory-impaired patients: a prospective longitudinal study. Neurology 46:661–665.

Tombaugh GC, Sapolsky RM (1992) Corticosterone accelerates hypoxia- and cyanide-induced ATP loss in cultured hippocampal astrocytes. Brain Res 588:154–158.

Watanabe Y, Gould E, McEwen BS (1992b) Stress induces atrophy of apical dendrites of hippocampal CA3 pyramidal neurons. Brain Res 588:341–345.

West MJ (1993) Regionally specific loss of neurons in the aging human hippocampus. Neurobiol Aging 14:287–293.

Wechsler D (1981) WAIS-R manual. New York: The Psychological Corporation.

Wechsler D (1987) Wechsler Memory Scale-Revised Manual. San Antonio, TX: The Psychological Corporation.

Whiteford H, Peabody C, Csernansky J, Warner M, Berger P (1987) Elevated baseline and postdexamethasone cortisol levels. A reflection of severity or endogeneity? J Affective Disord 12:199–202.

Wong M, Loddick S, Bongiorno P, Gold P, Rothwell N, Licinio J (1995) Focal cerebral ischemia induces CRH mRNA in rat cerebral cortex and amygdala. NeuroReport 6:1785–1788.

Wooley C, Weiland N, McEwen B, Schwartzkroin P (1997) Estradiol increases the sensitivity of hippocampal CA1 pyramidal cells to NMDA receptor-mediated synaptic input: correlation with dendritic spine density. J Neurosci 17:1848–1859.

Young EA, Haskett RF, Murphy-Weinberg V, Watson SJ, Akil H (1991) Loss of glucocorticoid fast feedback in depression. Arch Gen Psychiatry 48:693–698.

Annu. Rev. Med. 1999. 50:453–68

NATURAL HISTORY AND PREVENTATIVE TREATMENT OF RECURRENT MOOD DISORDERS

Ellen Frank, PhD and Michael E. Thase, MD
Department of Psychiatry, Western Psychiatric Institute and Clinic, University of Pittsburgh, School of Medicine, Pittsburgh, Pennsylvania 15213-2593; e-mail: franke@msx.upmc.edu

KEY WORDS: interpersonal psychotherapy (IPT), cognitive therapy, bipolar, unipolar depression, major depressive disorders

ABSTRACT

This chapter focuses on recent developments in our understanding of the etiology, epidemiology, and treatment of recurrent mood disorders. It addresses the changing relationship between endogenous and exogenous factors over time in the etiology of mood episodes. In the area of epidemiology, the chapter presents new information on the prevalence of various subtypes and male/female differences in lifetime risk. Complications of the mood disorders, such as suicide, and important comorbidities, including alcoholism and substance abuse, are discussed. In the area of treatment, the life-long nature of many of the mood disorders is described, as is the consequent role of the primary care physician in their management. The evidence for the efficacy of the depression-specific psychotherapies, cognitive therapy and interpersonal therapy, is reviewed. Current issues in the pharmacotherapy of mood disorders are discussed, including the relative efficacy of the older antidepressants versus the newer selective serotonin reuptake inhibitors (SSRIs) and the treatment of various subtypes of mood disorders, including dysthymia, chronic depression, and atypical depression. Finally, the chapter describes recent advances in the treatment of bipolar disorder.

INTRODUCTION

The mood disorders, including major depressive disorder, bipolar affective disorder, and their minor or subsyndromal variants, are common and potentially disabling conditions encountered by physicians in all areas of medical practice. The morbidity caused by these disorders is greatly underappreciated: A survey conducted by the World Health organization (WHO) revealed that the mood disorders currently rank as the world's fourth greatest cause of illness "burden" (a composite based on morbidity and mortality) (1). The WHO report further estimated that these disorders would rank second by the year 2020. Moreover, because the mood disorders cause less mortality than most other serious diseases, the proportion of illness burden associated with day-to-day disability is profound, and depression and bipolar disorder are thus already the world's leading cause of disability among adults (1). In the United States alone, these disorders cost society more than $70 billion each year (2, 3).

This article focuses on recent developments in the epidemiology and treatment of recurrent mood disorders. Fortunately, a large majority of mood disorders are treatable with modern forms of psychotherapy and antidepressant or mood-stabilizing medications, both singly (in the case of the depressive disorders) and in combination. The inherently good prognoses of most mood disorders may engender a false sense of complacency, however, and the risks of relapse, recurrence, and chronicity must be recognized and addressed specifically and vigorously. There is also some concern that effective short-term treatments may actually worsen the longer-term course of some forms of mood disorder, unless proper preventative or maintenance treatment is instituted for those at high risk for relapse or recurrent episodes (4, 5).

ETIOLOGY

The mood disorders illustrate the rich complexity of stress-diathesis models of human illness etiology. On the stress side of the equation, adversities such as the death of a loved one, romantic disappointment, or a vocational setback are common antecedents (6). On the diathesis side, both genetic (7) and certain acquired vulnerabilities (8) have been documented to increase lifetime risk. Bipolar disorders have the highest heritability rates (e.g. concordance rates for pairs of identical twins average at about 70%) (7), although the genetic contribution (probably from multiple loci) to the risk of major depressive disorder now appears considerable (9). Acquired vulnerabilities include both chronic and acute medical illnesses that affect well-being and/or brain function, as well as the enduring psychobiological sequelae of maltreatment during childhood, early parental loss, or severe trauma during adolescence or adult life (8).

The onset of new episodes of both recurrent depression and bipolar disorder appears to become more autonomous, or less tied to life stress, as the lifetime course of illness unfolds. Post (8) refers to this progressive change in vulnerability as kindling, and proposes that it results from the impact of repeated episodes of illness on brain functioning, perhaps in concert with the more normal changes that accompany aging. This process increases the incidence of objective signs of CNS dysfunction (e.g. increased rates of hypercortisolemia, abnormally low amounts of restful slow-wave sleep, and increased levels of affectively arousing phasic rapid eye movement or REM sleep) among those with recurrent disorders (10). Illness progression also probably accounts for the lower rates of spontaneous remission and placebo response observed in the recurrent mood disorders (10). It now appears virtually certain that the impact of states of depression and mania may be stored in neurons via changes in the activity of gene transcription factors and neuronal growth factors (11). Once a recurrent mood disorder is so "kindled," much lower degrees of stress or lifestyle disruption are necessary to trigger an episode of depression or mania (8). Such heightened vulnerability underscores the importance of vigilance and, often, the necessity of ongoing prophylactic treatment. At a more personal level, this uncoupling of normal stress-response relationships often adds to the patient's sense of powerlessness or of being out of control and may amplify hopelessness or suicidality.

EPIDEMIOLOGY

At least 12% of the adult population will suffer from a mood disorder at some point, with some surveys suggesting lifetime prevalence rates as high as 25% (12, 13). The cumulative risks of the specific major mood disorders are 10–18% for major depressive disorder and 1–3% for bipolar disorder (12, 13). Minor or subsyndromal forms of major depressive disorder include dysthymia (persistent, unremitting symptoms for at least two years), subsyndromal symptomatic depression (characterized by neither sufficient duration for dysthymia nor sufficient symptom severity for a major depressive episode), and adjustment disorders with depressive features (onset following a stressor; less severe and persistent than a major depressive episode). The lifetime risk of dysthymia is about 3–5% (12). A subsyndromal variation of bipolar disorder, called cyclothymia (lifetime prevalence 1–2%), is characterized by brief periods of hypomania and (usually) depression of insufficient duration and severity to warrant the major diagnosis (14).

Currently, the modal age of onset of bipolar disorder ranges between ages 15 and 25 (15). For major depressive disorder, the modal age of onset is about 10 years later (ages 25–35) (16). However, age of first onset of both disorders has decreased over the past four generations (17), and it appears that earlier onsets also are associated with greater lifetime incidence and higher rates of recurrence (16). Of course, an earlier modal age of onset does not diminish the importance of the depressive and bipolar syndromes that begin in late life.

Major depressive disorder and dysthymia are more common among women (morbid risk of 1.5- to 2.0-fold greater than that observed for men) (16). The role of reproductive hormones and cyclical hormonal patterns in this process cannot be discounted, although the impact of gender differences in economic power, social support, social role conflicts, threatening forms of life stress, and characteristic ways of coping also should not be minimized. The sex-ratio incidence of bipolar disorder, especially the classical form also known as manic depression (see below), is much closer to 1:1 (15). Rates of depression are typically higher in industrialized countries and, within such countries, rates are greater in urban than in rural locales (16).

For a fortunate minority (30–45%), a single lifetime episode of major depression may have few long-term sequelae. More often, major depressive episodes recur with increasing frequency. In fact, after a second lifetime episode, the risk of a third is at least 70% within 3 years (without prophylactic treatment) (18). The lifetime risk that someone with dysthymia will develop a major depressive episode similarly exceeds 70% (16). The average depressive episode lasts about 9 to 12 months without treatment, although about 20% run a chronic course of 2 years or longer. Once established, chronic episodes last an average of 5 to 8 years (16). Both more acute and chronic depressive episodes cause greater day-to-day impairment of quality of life than diabetes, high blood pressure, arthritis, or peptic ulcer disease (19), with dysthymia and the so-called "double" depressive syndrome (dysthymia plus a superimposed major depressive episode) associated with the most disability (20).The hallmark of bipolar disorders is a history of at least one manic or hypomanic (i.e. less severe and never psychotic) episode. Manic episodes are characteristically shorter in duration than depressions (1–6 months) and may be purely euphoric, mixed with depressive symptoms, and/or psychotic. Mixed and psychotic episodes tend to be more disabling and take longer to remit (15). The terms Type 1 or bipolar 1 are used to describe all bipolar disorders in which at least one full manic episode has occurred; the terms Type 2 or bipolar 2 describe those with a history of hypomania and at least one major depressive episode. About 10% of those with bipolar Type 1 disorder never suffer a major depressive episode (15). Over time, a subset of those with Type 2 disorders shift subtype diagnoses (because of the onset of mania) and, similarly, some cyclothymias shift to either major bipolar subtype (14). Nevertheless, bipolar Type 2 disorder and cyclothymia should not be viewed as simply formes früstes or transitional diagnoses, and most patients with these disorders do not develop full-blown bipolar Type 1 illness (14, 15).

The term rapid cycling is used when a patient with bipolar disorder suffers four or more episodes per year. Women are overrepresented among the bipolar 2 and rapid cycling subtypes (15, 21). Within the bipolar 1 grouping, women also tend to suffer a greater proportion of depressive episodes (15).

Major depressive disorder has several subforms of clinical import. As noted above, most people who suffer from one episode of depression will develop a recurrent (also known as unipolar) disorder. Early in the course of illness, it is not uncommon for an apparently unipolar disorder to switch to bipolar, especially when the onset of depression is before age 25 (22). After three or more depressive episodes, however, the onset of mania is much less likely (<5% incidence).

The three principal clinical subtypes of a depressive episode are melancholic, psychotic, and atypical. Melancholia, which tends to be more common after age 40, represents the more severe end of the spectrum and is characterized by signs and symptoms such as anhedonia (including diminished libido), loss of mood reactivity, psychomotor disturbances (retardation and/or agitation), sleep continuity disturbances and early morning awakenings, diminished appetite with weight loss, diurnal mood variation (worse in morning), and guilty ruminations (23). The more somatically focused nature of melancholia led to its former name of endogenous (i.e. arising from within) depression. However, this appellation proved too simplistic, minimizing both the role of psychosocial factors in more severe depressions and the importance of neurobiological factors in milder depressions.

Psychotic depressions are often melancholic and, unless part of a bipolar syndrome, also tend to be more common among older depressed patients (24). Delusions and, less commonly, auditory hallucinations tend to be mood-congruent, representing themes of guilt, sin, failure, punishment, disease, and nihilism.

The term atypical depression refers to a nonmelancholic, nonpsychotic depressive syndrome more common under age 50, characterized by "reverse" neurovegetative symptoms such as overeating, weight gain, and oversleeping (25). The descriptor atypical is now a misnomer because of the ubiquity of reverse neurovegetative symptoms among younger age groups. Like other nonmelancholic depressions, mood reactivity is usually preserved (i.e. a positive event can improve one's mood considerably), and many people with reverse neurovegetative features also experience the converse, rejection sensitivity (i.e. a crashing drop in subjective well-being following a rebuff or some other setback).

Beyond the somewhat arbitrary process of classification, the subtypes of major depressive episodes (bipolar, recurrent, melancholic, psychotic, and atypical) have specific treatment implications that, ultimately, reinforce their validity to clinicians.

Some recurrent depressive episodes follow a seasonal pattern, especially if they tend to begin in the fall or winter (26). Such depressions are more commonly nonmelancholic and often are characterized by one or more reverse neurovegetative symptom. Many, if not most, eventually meet criteria for bipolar disorder (more typically the Type 2 form), and there is some evidence that artificial manipulation of the photoperiod, either by moving to a more equatorial locale or by using bright white lights as phototherapy, may suppress an inherent seasonality.

COMPLICATIONS AND COMORBIDITIES

Suicide is the most dreaded complication of the mood disorders, and lifetime death rates of 10–15% are typically reported. Stated another way, the mood disorders account for about 60–75% of all deaths by suicide, which, in turn, ranks between the second and sixth most common cause of death across adult age groups (27). Suicide is more common among men, elders, individuals with more severe and/or psychotic symptoms, those with bipolar disorders, and those with more chronic or complicated syndromes. A prior attempt of severe intent, high levels of hopelessness, marked anxiety or insomnia, and complicating alcoholism or drug addiction are also associated with increased risk. Recent psychiatric hospitalization is another risk factor, perhaps because it denotes a high likelihood of suicidal ideations and other risk factors, as well as the possibility of treatment failure and the conveyance of a potential means of suicide in the form of prescribed tricyclic antidepressants (TCAs). It is a cruel irony that these robustly effective medications can be fatal if ingested in quantities as low as a 7- to 10-day supply (28).

People with alcoholism or drug addiction have profoundly increased lifetime rates of depression. Less commonly, substance abuse or dependence can develop as a form of self-medication in someone with a clear-cut history of antecedent mood disorder. Unless addressed therapeutically, concomitant substance abuse worsens the course of mood disorders. Other common comorbidities include anxiety disorders, general medical disorders (especially those with a more chronic course), and personality disorders. The mood disorders themselves may alter or "scar" personality development; conversely, people who have problems with excessive dependence on others, shyness or avoidance of emotionally charged circumstances, marked reactivity to or intolerance of normally stressful life events (e.g. aloneness, criticism, or romantic rejection), or excessive use of perfectionism as a means of coping may be more likely to develop a syndromal episode of depression. Less characteristically tied to personality, bipolar disorders nevertheless may have some forme früste expressions as traits of temperaments, such as mood lability, grandiosity, risk taking, sensation seeking, and self-centeredness.

TREATMENT

Background

At any moment, only about 60% of those with bipolar disorder and 40% with a depressive disorder are under the care of a professional for a mood disorder (29). The reasons for this woeful state of affairs include ignorance, stigma, and perceptions that efforts to receive treatment will be blocked by various barriers (29). Historically, the very notion of a "mental disorder" has elicited images of moral turpitude, incompetence, or weakness, and even today there is institutional discrimination against those with mood disorders in terms of health care benefits. Perhaps foremost, however, in delaying initiation of effective care is the failure to distinguish a mood disorder from more transient forms of symptomatic distress that will go away (without professional assistance) in time.

Primary care physicians thus have a critical role in the recognition and treatment of mood disorders. This role is particularly large because most people with mood disorders have primary care physicians and many are disproportionately heavy users of general medical services. Recent studies indicate that up to 20% of an average day's office visits are made by people with a mood disorder, and in some practices, proportions up to 40% are documented (30). In primary care, depressed patients are overrepresented among those receiving treatment for insomnia, "stress," chronic fatigue, headaches and unexplained pain, and gastrointestinal disturbances. A higher threshold of awareness and a relatively brief but standardized set of screening questions can routinely double the number of cases recognized (30).

In the treatment of the unipolar affective disorders, we focus on the efficacy of treatments and on new findings for specific subtypes of unipolar disorders. With respect to bipolar affective disorder or manic-depressive illness, we focus on the adequacy of dose in lithium maintenance treatment, on the use of anticonvulsants in the treatment of bipolar mood disorders, and finally on the previously unrecognized difficulty in treating bipolar depression.

Depression-Specific Psychotherapies

It is not mere coincidence that, roughly contemporaneous with the development of the Research Diagnostic Criteria (31), several short-term psychotherapeutic approaches to the treatment of major depression emerged in the United States. The move toward more specific categorization of nonpsychotic disorders facilitated the development of these "depression-specific" psychotherapies and provided the atmosphere in which these interventions could be tested empirically. The most prominent have been interpersonal psychotherapy (IPT) (32) and cognitive therapy (CT) (33).

There are a number of important commonalties between the two psychotherapies. Both were originally conceptualized as time-limited, acute interventions; both are clearly specified in treatment manuals; both use a present-oriented and pragmatic approach; and both are highly focused on the patient's depression and on the problems believed relevant to the onset and maintenance of the depressive episode.

INTERPERSONAL PSYCHOTHERAPY IPT examines the relationship between depression and interpersonal problems that may be causes or effects of the patient's current depressive episode. The techniques of IPT were developed to manage four basic interpersonal problem areas: (*a*) unresolved grief, (*b*) role transitions, (*c*) interpersonal role disputes (often marital disputes), and (*d*) interpersonal deficits. The major goals of IPT are achieved by ascertaining with the patient which of these four problems was associated with the onset of the current episode of depression and, subsequently, by working with the patient to renegotiate interpersonal difficulties associated with the primary problem area. Although maintenance interpersonal psychotherapy (IPT-M) (34) preserves the four distinctive problem areas and employs the strategies and techniques of IPT, it differs in that its primary goal is prevention of recurrence and it is conceptualized as a long-term rather than acute intervention.

The first acute-treatment study of IPT compared weekly IPT and amitriptyline, either alone or in combination, with a nonscheduled treatment-on-demand condition. Both active treatments were more effective than the control condition, and combined treatment was more effective than either treatment alone (35, 36).

The second acute-treatment study, the landmark NIMH Treatment of Depression Collaborative Research Program (37), compared imipramine plus clinical management therapy (a "minimally supportive therapy" provided by a psychiatrist), IPT, CT (33), or pill-placebo plus clinical management (PLA-CM). The primary analyses showed that at termination, patients in all treatments, including PLA-CM, evidenced significant reduction in depressive symptoms and improved functioning. When the study population was dichotomized according to baseline severity of depression, among more depressed subjects, IPT was comparable to imipramine in efficacy and both were superior to PLA-CM.

Two randomized controlled trials have demonstrated the efficacy of IPT as a prophylactic treatment for major depression. Klerman et al (38) conducted an eight-month study in female outpatients who had responded to 4–6 weeks of amitriptyline. Patients received weekly IPT, medication, both IPT and medication, or placebo and no therapy. Relapse rates were highest for patients receiving placebo alone (36%). Relapse rates in the other three active treatment groups were 12% on medication alone, 16.7% on IPT alone, and 12.5% on IPT combined with medication.

A second study, the Pittsburgh study of Maintenance Therapies in Recurrent Depression (39), contrasted IPT-M with maintenance pharmacotherapy (imipramine), combination pharmacotherapy/psychotherapy, and a control condition (placebo and no therapy) over a period of three years in depressed patients who had clear histories of recurrent depression and had been treated acutely with a combination of IPT and imipramine. Active medication provided the best prophylaxis; however, those who continued to receive IPT on a monthly basis following drug discontinuation remained well significantly longer ($p = 0.05$) than those assigned to medication clinic and placebo. Although IPT alone has not been tested adequately in the acute treatment of major depression in the elderly, one-year outcomes for maintenance treatment suggest that IPT-M alone is at least as efficacious as nortriptyline alone in elderly patients treated initially with the combination of nortriptyline and IPT (40).

COGNITIVE THERAPY Beck's model of cognitive therapy (CT) (33) posits that three types of cognition problems are involved in the genesis and/or maintenance of depression: (*a*) a disproportionate amount of time thinking gloomy or unpleasant thoughts; (*b*) errors in logic and information processing (41, 42); and (*c*) "deeper" cognitive structures, such as dysfunctional attitudes and depressogenic schema (41, 43, 44). In CT, both attitudes and schema are considered ultimately accessible through questioning techniques, as illustrated by the use of the Socratic method or guided discovery (33).

Beck's model of CT is the best-studied psychological treatment of major depression (45, 46). CT has been extensively compared with waiting-list control conditions and with other forms of psychotherapy, as well as pharmacotherapy; however, only a single trial has compared CT with a placebo–clinical-management condition (37).

In a meta-analysis by the Depression Guideline Panel of the Agency for Health Care Policy and Research (AHCPR) (45), CT had an overall efficacy rate of 46.6% (±6.9%), with an advantage of 30% (±22%) compared with waiting-list control conditions. Results of four studies indicate that CT is superior to low-contact or "treatment-as-usual" medication control conditions, whether CT is administered alone (47) or in combination with treatment-as-usual (48–50). Studies utilizing more rigorous pharmacotherapy conditions (37, 51–53) have yielded consistent evidence of parity between CT and antidepressant medication.

CT has not been as well studied as continuation- or maintenance-phase therapy. In the one controlled trial, monthly CT alone achieved the same level of prophylaxis over six months as did continuation pharmacotherapy (54). Two other studies, employing relatively small samples and a type of cognitive-behavior therapy not entirely consistent with Beck's model, failed to find any prophylactic value for continued "booster" therapy sessions after termination of acute treatment (55, 56).

Current Issues in the Pharmacotherapy of Depression

A key question on the minds of those involved in the treatment of unipolar disorders is the relative efficacy of the older tricyclic antidepressants (TCAs) versus the newer selective serotonin reuptake inhibitor antidepressants (SSRIs). Hundreds of studies document the efficacy of the TCAs. In the AHCPR's meta-analysis (45), the tricyclics had an overall, intent-to-treat efficacy rate of 55.5% in primary care settings, with an advantage of 15% compared with placebo control conditions (45a). The TCAs, however, have substantial side effects not typically observed with the newer SSRIs. A recent meta-analytic review (57) compared the efficacy of the SSRIs and TCAs in randomized controlled trials and found them equal. This kind of meta-analysis of short-term research studies, however, cannot take into account the SSRIs' greater acceptability to patients and ease of prescribing for physicians. Studies commissioned by the pharmaceutical industry analyzing formulary data suggest that patients are significantly more likely to refill SSRI than TCA prescriptions (J Fisher, personal communication), indicating that although efficacy in clinical trials may be equivalent for the two types of antidepressant treatments, effectiveness in naturalistic clinical settings may be greater for the SSRIs.

An unresolved question, however, is whether the SSRIs can equal the efficacy or effectiveness of the TCAs as long-term maintenance treatments. This is a critical question as epidemiologic data accumulate documenting that depression is recurrent in 80–90% of cases (58, 59). Clinical anecdotes of loss of efficacy with long-term use of SSRIs ("poop out") is yet to be documented in direct comparisons of TCAs and SSRIs. Our group's studies (39, 60) suggest that, for highly recurrent patients (median of four previous episodes) maintained on acute-dose TCA, the cumulative probability of remaining well for as long as five years is approximately 0.70–0.80. One maintenance study of an SSRI (61) showed only a 15% failure rate for paroxetine over an 18-month maintenance treatment when both recurrences and withdrawals for lack of efficacy were considered, as compared with a 57.4% failure rate for placebo. Such comparisons are suggestive of greater long-term efficacy of the TCAs; however, considering the greater difficulty of starting patients on these compounds, the overall benefits may not be greater.

Importance of Dose Adequacy in Mood Disorders

Keller and colleagues examining data from the NIMH Collaborative Study of the Psychobiology of Depression (62, 62a, 62b) have been in the forefront of demonstrating the importance of dose adequacy in the pharmacotherapy of unipolar disorders. An earlier study (63) documented the negative effects of underdosing in the acute treatment of unipolar depression, as well as the negative effects of stopping treatment too soon. A more recent paper focused on the importance of adequate dose in maintenance treatment (64). This analysis suggested that when patients were maintained on the same dose used to treat their acute episode, outcomes were comparable to those achieved in our randomized controlled trial (39). However, lower doses achieved relatively poor outcomes, as did a half-dose strategy in a controlled trial (65); the cumulative probability of remaining well with the half-dose strategy over a three-year period was less than 30%. Although data on the TCAs clearly indicate that a maximum tolerated dose strategy (generally equivalent to approximately 200 mg of imipramine) represents a highly effective acute and maintenance treatment, strategies for maximizing the efficacy of long-term maintenance treatment with SSRIs have yet to be developed.

Treatment of Various of Subtypes of Unipolar Depression

Among the important recent advances in the treatment of unipolar disorders has been the examination of treatment efficacy in specific subtypes, including minor or subsyndromal depression, dysthymia and chronic depression, and atypical depression.

The Wells et al (66) study described above provided a major impetus to examine the efficacy of treating depressive conditions that did not meet criteria for major depressive disorder. Recently reported results from a randomized trial comparing fluoxetine and placebo in the treatment of subsyndromal symptomatic depression (depressed mood or loss of interest and two additional depressive symptoms) provided evidence for the acute (67) and continuation treatment (68) efficacy of fluoxetine relative to placebo with respect to both symptomatic improvement and improvement in functioning.

Two groups have now demonstrated the efficacy of antidepressant pharmacotherapy in the treatment of more chronic forms of depression. Kocsis et al (69) showed that the TCA imipramine was superior to placebo in the treatment of chronic depression, while a series of multicenter collaborative studies demonstrated the efficacy of the SSRI sertraline in the treatment of dysthymia, "double" depression, and chronic major depression (70–72). Specifically, sertraline was as effective as imipramine and significantly better tolerated in all three chronic depressive subtypes (70–72). Moreover, sertraline showed significant prophylactic effects in an 18-month placebo-controlled maintenance phase study (70). Data from several other studies similarly support the tolerability advantage of the SSRIs for patients with chronic depressive disorders.

So-called atypical depression is generally defined by the presence of "reversed" vegetative symptoms (overeating, oversleeping), a complex of other symptoms that may include rejection sensitivity and "leaden" paralysis, and the absence of melancholia. Stewart et al (73) reviewed data from eight separate clinical trials conducted by his group and concluded that (*a*) the TCA imipramine was a poor treatment of atypical depression, just marginally superior to placebo, (*b*) the monoamine oxidase inhibitor (MAOI) phenelzine is significantly more effective than both imipramine and placebo, and (*c*) anxiety (included in some earlier definitions of atypicality) was not associated with differential medication response. Subsequently, Stewart et al (74) found that phenelzine, but not imipramine, had significant prophylactic effects for those with atypical depression.

Our own research group has focused on the treatment of the recurrent form of unipolar disorder, once considered a particular subtype of unipolar conditions. Recent epidemiological evidence (59, 60), however, suggests that this may be the predominant form of unipolar disorder. We have demonstrated that maintaining antidepressant treatment at acute dose levels can prevent new episodes in recurrent unipolar patients, both in midlife (39) and in late life (40). As implied above, in both the midlife and late life studies we also found a modest effect for monthly sessions of IPT.

Treatment of Bipolar Disorders

A controversy in the long-term treatment of bipolar disorder was the importance of treatment adequacy (as reflected in lithium blood level) in the protection against new bipolar episodes. Gelenberg et al (75) randomly assigned subjects to a high versus low dose strategy and found that patients maintained at a lithium level of 0.8 to 1.0 mEq/L had significantly better protection against new episodes than patients maintained at a level of 0.4 to 0.6 mEq/L. The value of this higher dose strategy, however, was somewhat mitigated by the fact that almost half of the high-dose group discontinued treatment, presumably because of intolerable side effects. An obvious challenge in lithium maintenance treatment is balancing side effects against therapeutic effects and helping patients manage the unpleasant side effects of this otherwise highly efficacious compound.

Although anticonvulsants have only recently been shown to be efficacious in randomized clinical trials of bipolar disorder (76, 77), they have been in clinical use as maintenance treatments since the first trials suggesting their efficacy as an acute treatment for mania. The tolerability of the anticonvulsants appears better than that of lithium; however, Baldessarini & Tondo (78) raise the question of whether anticonvulsants are as effective in protecting bipolar patients against suicide. They conclude that although the anticonvulsants are not appreciably less effective than lithium in protection against new episodes, lithium is clearly superior in protecting bipolar patients against suicide. These results, again, point to the need for the clinician to balance the relatively poorer tolerability of a compound against important prophylactic advantages when tolerated.

A final issue in the treatment of bipolar disorder is the relatively unrecognized difficulty in achieving adequate remission of bipolar depressive conditions. Our own group has found that time to a clear-cut remission of bipolar depression (defined as four weeks with an average Hamilton Depression Rating Scale score of ≤7) requires significantly longer than remission of manic episodes (79). Recent analyses from the acute treatment phase of our trial of maintenance therapies in bipolar disorder suggest that lithium alone leads to remission in less than 40% of bipolar depressed patients and that the addition of any antidepressant, including imipramine, an SSRI, or an MAOI, never leads to remission in more than 35% of patients who failed to remit on lithium (80).

Once thought of as a problem solved, bipolar disorder clearly presents a number of treatment challenges and dilemmas to the clinician. These include choice of compound for long-term prophylaxis, dose of that compound, and treatment of the less dramatic, but perhaps equally impairing, depressive side of manic-depressive illness.

Literature Cited

1. Murray CJL, Lopez AD. 1996. Evidence-based health policy—lessons from the Global Burden of Disease Study. *Science* 274:740
2. Greenberg PE, Stiglin LE, Finkelstein SN, Berndt ER. 1993. Economic burden of depression in 1990. *J. Clin. Psychiatry* 54:405–19
3. Wyatt RJ, Henter I. 1995. An economic evaluation of manic-depressive illness. *Soc. Psychiatry Psychiatr. Epidemiol.* 30: 213–19
4. Fava GA. 1994. Do antidepressants and antianxiety drugs increase chronicity in affective disorders? *Psychother. Psychosom.* 61:125–31
5. Thase ME, Kupfer DJ. 1996. Recent developments in the pharmacotherapy of mood disorders. *J. Consult. Clin. Psychol.* 64(4):1–14
6. Paykel ES, Cooper Z. 1992. Life events and social stress. In *Handbook of Affective Disorders*, ed. ES Paykel, pp. 149–70. New York: Guilford
7. Berrettini WH, Goldin LR, Gelernter J, et al. 1990. X-chromosome markers and manic-depressive illness: rejection of linkage to Xq28 in nine bipolar pedigrees. *Arch. Gen. Psychiatry* 47:366–73
8. Post RM. 1992. Transduction of psychosocial stress into the neurobiology of recurrent affective disorder. *Am. J. Psychiatry* 149(8):999–1010
9. Kendler KS. 1997. Social support: a genetic-epidemiologic analysis. *Am. J. Psychiatry* 154:1398–1404
10. Thase ME, Howland RH. 1995. Biological processes in depression: an updated review and integration. In *Handbook of Depression*, ed. EE Beckham, WR Leber, pp. 213–79. New York: Guilford
11. Duman RS, Heninger GR, Nestler EJ. 1997. A molecular and cellular theory of

depression. *Arch. Gen. Psychiatry* 54: 597–606
12. Kessler RC, McGonagle KA, Zhano S, et al. 1994. Lifetime and 12-month prevelence of DSM-III-R psychiatric disorders in the United States. Results from the National Comorbidity Survey. *Arch. Gen. Psychiatry* 51:8–19
13. Weissman MM, Bland RC, Canino GJ, et al. 1996. Cross-national epidemiology of major depression and bipolar disorder. *JAMA* 276(4):293–99
14. Howland RH, Thase ME. 1993. A comprehensive review of cyclothymic disorder. *J. Nerv. Ment. Dis.* 181:485–93
15. Goodwin FK, Jamison KR. 1990. *Manic-depressive Illness*. London/New York: Oxford Univ. Press
16. Smith AL, Weissman MM. 1992. Epidemiology. See Ref. 6, pp. 111–30
17. Klerman GL, Weissman MM. 1989. Increasing rates of depression. *JAMA* 261(15):2229–35
18. Frank E, Kupfer DJ, Perel JM, et al. 1990. Three-year outcomes for maintenance therapies in recurrent depression. *Arch. Gen. Psychiatry* 47:1093–99
19. Wells KB, Stewart A, Hays RD, et al. 1989. The functioning and well-being of depressed patients. Results from the medical outcomes study. *JAMA* 262(7): 914–19
20. Hays RD, Wells KB, Sherbourne CD, et al. 1995. Functioning and well-being outcomes of patients with depression compared with chronic general medical illness. *Arch. Gen. Psychiatry* 52:11–19
21. Bauer MS, Calabrese J, Dunner DL, et al. 1994. Multisite data reanalysis of the validity of rapid cycling as a course modifier for bipolar disorder in DSM-IV. *Am. J. Psychiatry* 151(4):506–15
22. Akiskal HS, Maser JD, Zeller PJ, et al. 1995. Switching from "unipolar" to bipolar II. An 11-year prospective study of clinical and temperamental predictors in 559 patients. *Arch. Gen. Psychiatry* 52: 114–23
23. Rush AJ, Weissenburger JE. 1994. Melancholic symptom features and DSM-IV. *Am. J. Psychiatry* 151(4):489–98
24. Schatzberg AF, Rothschild AJ. 1992. Psychotic (delusional) major depression: should it be included as a dictinct syndrome in DSM-IV? *Am. J. Psychiatry* 149:733–45
25. Quitkin FM, Stewart JW, McGrath PJ, et al. 1993. Columbia atypical depression. A subgroup of depressives with better response to MAOI than to tricyclic antidepressants or placebo. *Br. J. Psychiatry* 163(Suppl 21):30–34
26. Oren DA, Rosenthal NE. 1992. Seasonal affective disorders. See Ref. 6, pp. 551–68
27. Hawton K. 1992. Suicide and attempted suicide. See Ref. 6, pp. 635–50
28. Kapur S, Mieczkowski T, Mann JJ. 1992. Antidepressant medications and the relative risk of suicide attempt and suicide. *JAMA* 268:3441–45
29. Hirschfeld RMA, Keller MB, Panico S, et al. 1997. The National Depressive and Manic-Depressive Association consensus statement of depression. *JAMA* 277(4): 333–40
30. Freeling PR, Tylee A. 1992. Depression in general practice. See Ref. 6, pp. 651–66
31. Spitzer R, Endicott J, Robins E. 1978. Research diagnostic criteria: rationale and reliability. *Arch. Gen. Psychiatry* 35: 773–82
32. Klerman GL, Weissman MM, Rounsaville BJ, Chevron ES. 1984. *Interpersonal Psychotherapy of Depression*. New York: Basic Books
33. Beck AT, Rush AJ, Shaw BF. 1979. *Cognitive Therapy of Depression: A Treatment Manual*. New York: Guilford
34. Frank E. 1991. Interpersonal psychotherapy as a maintenance treatment for patients with recurrent depression. *Psychotherapy* 28:259–66
35. DiMascio A, Weissman MM, Prusoff BA, et al. 1979. Differential symptom reduction by drugs and psychotherapy in acute depression. *Arch. Gen. Psychiatry* 36:1450–56
36. Weissman MM, Prusoff BA, DiMascio A, et al. 1979. The efficacy of drugs and psychotherapy in the treatment of acute depressive episodes. *Am. J. Psychiatry* 136:555–58
37. Elkin I, Shea MT, Watkins JT, et al. 1989. NIMH Treatment of Depression Collaborative Research Program: 1. General effectiveness of treatments. *Arch. Gen. Psychiatry* 46:971–982
38. Klerman GL, DiMascio A, Weissman MM, Prusoff BA, Paykel ES. 1974. Treatment of depression by drugs and psychotherapy. *Am. J. Psychiatry* 131: 1186–191
39. Frank E, Kupfer DJ, Perel JM, et al. 1990. Three year outcomes for maintenance in therapies in recurrent depression. *Arch. Gen. Psychiatry* 47:1093–99
40. Reynolds III CF, Frank E, Houck PR, et al. 1997. Which elderly patients with remitted depression remain well with continued interpersonal psychotherapy after

discontinuation of antidepressant medication? *Am. J. Psychiatry* 154:958–62

41. Beck AT. 1976. *Cognitive Therapy and the Emotional Disorders*. New York: International Univ. Press
42. Burns D. 1980. *Feeling Good: The New Mood Therapy*. New York: William Morrow
43. Segal ZV. 1988. Appraisal of the self schema construct in cognitive models of depression. *Psychol. Bull.* 102:147–62
44. Young JE, Lindemann MD. 1992. An integrative schema-focused model for personality disorders. *J. Cogn. Psychother.* 6:11–23
45. *Depression Guideline Panel: Clinical Practice Guideline: Depression in Primary Care, Vol 2: Treatment of Major Depression (Clinical Practice Guideline No 5; AHCPR Publ. No 93-0551)*. 1993. Rockville, MD: US Dept. Health Hum. Serv. Public Health Serv. Agency Health Care Policy Res.

45a. Frank E, Karp JF, Rush AJ. 1993. Efficacy of treatments for major depression. *Psychopharmacol. Bull.* 29:457–75

46. Dobson KS. 1989. A meta-analysis of the efficacy of cognitive therapy for depression. *J. Consul. Clin. Psychol.* 57:414–19
47. Blackburn IM, Bishop S, Glen AIM. 1981. The efficacy of cognitive therapy in depression: a treatment trial using cognitive therapy and pharmacotherapy, each alone and in combination. *Br. J. Psychiatry* 139:181–89
48. Ross M, Scott M. 1985. An evaluation of the effectiveness of individual and group cognitive therapy in the treatment of depressed patients in an inner city health centre. *J. R. Coll. Gen. Pract.* 35:239–42
49. Scott MJ, Stradling SG. 1990. Group cognitive therapy for depression produces clinically significant reliable change in community-based settings. *Behav. Psychother.* 18.1–19
50. Teasdale JD, Fennell MJV, Hibbert GA, et al. 1984. Cognitive therapy for major depressive disorder in primary care. *Br. J. Psychiatry* 144:400–6
51. Hollon SD, DeRubeis RJ, Evans MD, et al. 1992. Cognitive therapy and pharmacotherapy for depression: singly and in combination. *Arch. Gen. Psychiatry* 49: 774–81
52. McKnight DL, Nelson-Gray RO, Barnhill J. 1992. Dexamethasone suppression test and response to cognitive therapy and antidepressant medication. *Behav. Ther.* 23: 99–111
53. Murphy GE, Simons AD, Wetzel RD, et al. 1984. Cognitive therapy and pharmacotherapy, singly and together in the treatment of depression. *Arch. Gen. Psychiatry* 41:33–41
54. Blackburn IM, Eunson KM, Bishop SA. 1986. A two-year naturalistic follow-up of depressed patients treated with cognitive therapy, pharmacotherapy and a combination of both. *J. Affect. Disord.* 10: 67–75
55. Baker AL, Wilson PH. 1985. Cognitive-behavior therapy for depression: the effects of booster sessions on relapse. *Behav. Ther.* 16:335–344
56. Kavanaugh DJ, Wilson PH. 1989. Prediction of outcome with group cognitive therapy for depression. *Behav. Res. Ther.* 27:333–43
57. Steffens DC, Krishnan KRR, Helms MJ. 1997. Are SSRIs better than TCAs? Comparison of SSRIs and TCAs: a meta-analysis. *Depression Anxiety* 6:10–18
58. Ernst C, Angst J. 1992. The Zurich Study XII. Sex differences in depression. Evidence from longitudinal epidemiological data. *Eur. Arch. Psychiatry Clin. Neurosci.* 241(4):222–30
59. Kessler RC, McGonagle KA, Swartz M, et al. 1993. Sex and depression in the National Comorbidity Survey. I: Lifetime prevalence, chronicity and recurrence. *J. Affect. Dis.* 29:85–96
60. Kupfer DJ, Frank E, Perel JM, et al. 1992. Five-year outcome for maintenance therapies in recurrent depression. *Arch. Gen. Psychiatry* 49:769–73
61. Pitts CD, Oakes R, Gergel IP. 1997. Paroxetine efficacy in the prevention of recurrent depression. Poster presented at Am. Coll. Neuropsychopharmacol. Meet., Kamuela, Hawaii
62. Keller MB, Klerman GL, Lavori PW, et al. 1982. Treatment received by depressed patients. *JAMA* 248:1848–55

62a. Katz MM, Secunda SK, Hirschfeld RMA, Koslow SH. 1979. NIMH clinical research branch collaborative program on the psychobiology of depression. *Arch. Gen. Psychiatry* 36:765–71

62b. Keller MB, Shapiro R. 1981. Major depressive disorder: initial results from a one-year prospective naturalistic follow-up study. *J. Nerv. Ment. Dis.* 169:761–68

63. Kupfer DJ, Freedman DX. 1986. Treatment for depression: 'standard' clinical practice as an unexamined topic. *Arch. Gen. Psychiatry* 43:509–11
64. Dawson R, Lavori PW, Coryell WH, et al. 1998. Maintenance strategies for unipolar depression: an observational study of levels of treatment and recurrence. *J. Affect. Dis.* 49:31–44

65. Frank E, Kupfer DJ, Perel JM, et al. 1993. Comparison of full dose versus half dose pharmacotherapy in the maintenance treatment of recurrent depression. *J. Affect. Dis.* 27:139–46
66. Wells KB, Burnam MA, Rogers W, et al. 1992. The course of depression in adult outpatients: results from the medical outcomes study. *Arch. Gen. Psychiatry* 49: 788–94
67. Judd LL. 1998. *Acute treatment outcomes with minor depression.* Presented at Annu. Meet. New Clin. Drug Eval. Unit Program, 38th, Boca Raton, Fla.
68. Rapaport MH. 1998. *The characterization of minor depression.* Presented at Annu. Meet. New Clin. Drug Eval. Unit Program, 38th, Boca Raton, Fla.
69. Kocsis JH, Voss C, Mann JJ, Frances A. 1986. Chronic depression: demographic and clinical characteristics. *Psychopharmacol. Bull.* 22:192–95
70. Keller MB, Kocsis JH, Thase ME, et al. 1998. Maintenance phase efficacy of sertraline for chronic depression: results of a double blind, placebo-controlled study. *JAMA*. In press
71. Thase ME, Fava M, Halbreigh U, et al. 1996. A placebo-controlled, randomized clinical trial comparing sertraline and imipramine for the treatment of dysthymia. *Arch. Gen. Psychiatry* 53(9): 777–84
72. Kocsis JH, Zisook S, Davidson J, et al. 1997. Double-blind comparison of sertraline, imipramine, and placebo in the treatment of dysthymia: psychosocial outcomes. *Am. J. Psychiatry* 154(3):390–95
73. Stewart JS, McGrath PJ, Rabkin JG, Quitkin FM. 1993. Atypical depression: a valid clinical entity? *Psychiatr. Clin. No. Am.* 16(3):479–95
74. Stewart JW, Tricamo E, McGrath PJ, Quitkin FM. 1997. Prophylactic efficacy of pheneizine and imipramine in chronic atypical depression: likelihood of recurrence on discontinuation after 6 months' remission. *Am. J. Psychiatry* 154(1): 31–36
75. Gelenberg AJ, Kane JM, Keller MB, et al. 1989. Comparison of standard and low serum levels of lithium for maintenance treatment of bipolar disorder. *N. Engl. J. Med.* 321:1489–93
76. Bowden CL, Brugger AM, Swann AC, et al; for the Depakote Mania Study Group. 1994. Efficacy of Divalproex vs lithium and placebo in the treatment of mania. *JAMA* 27:918–24
77. Bowden CL. 1996. Role of newer medications for bipolar disorder. *J. Clin. Psychopharmacol.* 16(2):48S–55S (Suppl. 1)
78. Baldessarini RJ, Tondo L. 1998. Recurrence risk in bipolar manic-depressive disorders after discontinuing lithium maintenance treatment: an overview. *Clin. Drug Invest.* 15(4):337–51
79. Hlastala SA, Frank E, Mallinger AG, et al. 1997. Bipolar depression: an underestimated treatment challenge. *Depression Anxiety* 5:73–83
80. Mallinger AG, Thase ME. 1997. Selected issues of bipolar disorder/best treatments for bipolar depression. Presented at Mental Health Clin. Res. Cent. Consult. Panel, Pittsburgh, PA

The New England Journal of Medicine

VOLUME 342 MAY 18, 2000 NUMBER 20

A COMPARISON OF NEFAZODONE, THE COGNITIVE BEHAVIORAL-ANALYSIS SYSTEM OF PSYCHOTHERAPY, AND THEIR COMBINATION FOR THE TREATMENT OF CHRONIC DEPRESSION

MARTIN B. KELLER, M.D., JAMES P. MCCULLOUGH, PH.D., DANIEL N. KLEIN, PH.D., BRUCE ARNOW, PH.D., DAVID L. DUNNER, M.D., ALAN J. GELENBERG, M.D., JOHN C. MARKOWITZ, M.D., CHARLES B. NEMEROFF, M.D., PH.D., JAMES M. RUSSELL, M.D., MICHAEL E. THASE, M.D., MADHUKAR H. TRIVEDI, M.D., AND JOHN ZAJECKA, M.D.

ABSTRACT

Background Patients with chronic forms of major depression are difficult to treat, and the relative efficacy of medications and psychotherapy is uncertain.

Methods We randomly assigned 681 adults with a chronic nonpsychotic major depressive disorder to 12 weeks of outpatient treatment with nefazodone (maximal dose, 600 mg per day), the cognitive behavioral-analysis system of psychotherapy (16 to 20 sessions), or both. At base line, all patients had scores of at least 20 on the 24-item Hamilton Rating Scale for Depression (indicating clinically significant depression). Remission was defined as a score of 8 or less at weeks 10 and 12. For patients who did not have remission, a satisfactory response was defined as a reduction in the score by at least 50 percent from base line and a score of 15 or less. Raters were unaware of the patients' treatment assignments.

Results Of the 681 patients, 662 attended at least one treatment session and were included in the analysis of response. The overall rate of response (both remission and satisfactory response) was 48 percent in both the nefazodone group and the psychotherapy group, as compared with 73 percent in the combined-treatment group ($P<0.001$ for both comparisons). Among the 519 subjects who completed the study, the rates of response were 55 percent in the nefazodone group and 52 percent in the psychotherapy group, as compared with 85 percent in the combined-treatment group ($P<0.001$ for both comparisons). The rates of withdrawal were similar in the three groups. Adverse events in the nefazodone group were consistent with the known side effects of the drug (e.g., headache, somnolence, dry mouth, nausea, and dizziness).

Conclusions Although about half of patients with chronic forms of major depression have a response to short-term treatment with either nefazodone or a cognitive behavioral-analysis system of psychotherapy, the combination of the two is significantly more efficacious than either treatment alone. (N Engl J Med 2000;342:1462-70.)

TRADITIONALLY thought of as an episodic, remitting illness, major depressive disorder often has a chronic course, with protracted episodes or incomplete remission between episodes.[1-3] At any given time, at least 3 percent of the U.S. population suffers from chronic depression.[4,5] Chronic forms of major depression are associated with more marked impairments in psychosocial function and work performance,[6-8] increased health care utilization,[5,9] and more frequent suicide attempts and hospitalization[10] than acute depression.

From the Department of Psychiatry, Brown University, Providence, R.I. (M.B.K.); the Unipolar Mood Disorders Institute, Department of Psychology, Virginia Commonwealth University, Richmond (J.P.M.); the Department of Psychology, State University of New York at Stony Brook, Stony Brook (D.N.K.); the Department of Psychiatry and Behavioral Sciences, Stanford University, Stanford, Calif. (B.A.); the Department of Psychiatry and Behavioral Sciences, University of Washington, Seattle (D.L.D.); the Department of Psychiatry, University of Arizona, Tucson (A.J.G.); the Department of Psychiatry, Cornell University Medical College, New York (J.C.M.); the Department of Psychiatry, Emory University School of Medicine, Atlanta (C.B.N.); the Department of Psychiatry and Behavioral Sciences, University of Texas Medical Branch at Galveston, Galveston (J.M.R.); the Department of Psychiatry, Western Psychiatric Institute and Clinic, University of Pittsburgh, Pittsburgh (M.E.T.); the Department of Psychiatry, University of Texas Southwestern Medical Center at Dallas, Dallas (M.H.T.); and the Department of Psychiatry, Rush–Presbyterian–St. Luke's Medical Center, Chicago (J.Z.). Address reprint requests to Dr. Keller at the Department of Psychiatry and Human Behavior, Brown University, 345 Blackstone Blvd., Providence, RI 02906.

Other authors were Janice A. Blalock, Ph.D. (M.D. Anderson Cancer Center, Houston); Frances E. Borian, R.N., and Darlene N. Jody, M.D. (Bristol-Myers Squibb, Plainsboro, N.J.); Charles DeBattista, D.M.H., M.D., Lorrin M. Koran, M.D., and Alan F. Schatzberg, M.D. (Stanford University, Stanford, Calif.); Jan Fawcett, M.D. (Rush–Presbyterian–St. Luke's Medical Ceñter, Chicago); Robert M.A. Hirschfeld, M.D. (University of Texas Medical Branch at Galveston, Galveston); Gabor Keitner, M.D., and Ivan Miller, Ph.D. (Brown University, Providence); James H. Kocsis, M.D. (Cornell University Medical College, New York); Susan G. Kornstein, M.D. (Virginia Commonwealth University, Richmond); Rachel Manber, Ph.D. (University of Arizona, Tucson); Philip T. Ninan, M.D., and Barbara Rothbaum, Ph.D. (Emory University School of Medicine, Atlanta); A. John Rush, M.D. (University of Texas Southwestern Medical Center at Dallas, Dallas); and Dina Vivian, Ph.D. (State University of New York at Stony Brook, Stony Brook).

Because they frequently begin early in life[11] and are often lifelong, chronic forms of major depression account for an inordinate proportion of the enormous burden of illness associated with depression.[12]

Several studies have demonstrated the efficacy of antidepressants as both initial[13-16] and maintenance[17,18] treatment for chronic forms of major depression, but controlled clinical trials of sufficient size to examine the efficacy of psychotherapy in chronic forms of major depression are lacking.[19] The combination of pharmacotherapy and psychotherapy has been recommended as the treatment of choice for depression by practice guidelines for psychiatrists[20] and as the treatment of choice for chronic forms of major depression in primary care practice.[21] However, the results of studies investigating whether combination treatment is superior to single treatments have been inconclusive.[22-24]

We present the main findings from the initial (12-week) phase of a long-term multicenter study comparing nefazodone alone, the cognitive behavioral-analysis system of psychotherapy alone,[25,26] or the two in combination with regard to efficacy in the treatment of patients with chronic forms of major depression. Nefazodone has had demonstrated efficacy in placebo-controlled trials and in numerous double-blind trials of short-term treatment of major depressive disorders,[27] as well as a demonstrated ability to prevent relapse after such treatment.[28]

The cognitive behavioral-analysis system of psychotherapy was developed specifically for the treatment of chronic forms of major depression and produced promising results in a small, open trial.[29] This approach draws on many behavioral, cognitive, and interpersonal techniques used in other forms of psychotherapy.[30-32] It teaches patients to focus on the consequences of their behavior and to use a social problem-solving algorithm to address interpersonal difficulties. It is more structured and directive than interpersonal psychotherapy[30] and differs from cognitive therapy[31] by focusing primarily on interpersonal interactions (including those with therapists). In this type of psychotherapy, patients learn how their cognitive and behavioral patterns produce and perpetuate their interpersonal problems and learn how to remedy maladaptive patterns of interpersonal behavior.

METHODS

Patients

We studied outpatients, recruited from 12 academic centers between June 1996 and December 1997, who fulfilled the criteria for a chronic major depressive disorder (at least two years' duration), a current major depressive disorder superimposed on a preexisting dysthymic disorder, or a recurrent major depressive disorder with incomplete remission between episodes in a patient with a current major depressive disorder and a total duration of continuous illness of at least two years. Diagnoses were based on the *Diagnostic and Statistical Manual of Mental Disorders,* fourth edition (DSM-IV),[33] and were obtained with use of the Structured Clinical Interview for Axis I DSM-IV Disorders.[34]

To be eligible for the study, the patients had to be between the ages of 18 and 75 years and to have had a score of at least 20 on the 24-item Hamilton Rating Scale for Depression (HRSD)[35] at screening and, after a two-week drug-free period, at base line. On this scale, higher scores indicate more severe depression. Laboratory tests, electrocardiography (if clinically indicated), and physical examinations were performed at the time of screening. Patients were required to discontinue taking monoamine oxidase inhibitors and fluoxetine at least four weeks before study entry, depot neuroleptic agents at least six months before entry, and other psychotropic medications at least two weeks before entry.

Patients were excluded from the study if they had any of the following: a history of seizures, abnormal findings on electroencephalography, severe head trauma, or stroke; evidence suggesting they were at high risk for suicide; a history of psychotic symptoms or schizophrenia; bipolar disorder, an eating disorder (if it had not been in remission for at least one year), obsessive–compulsive disorder, or dementia; antisocial, schizotypal, or severe borderline personality disorder; a principal diagnosis of panic, generalized anxiety, social phobia, or post-traumatic stress disorders or any substance-related abuse or dependence disorder (except those involving nicotine) within six months before the study began; absence of a response to a previous adequate trial of nefazodone or a cognitive behavioral-analysis system of psychotherapy; absence of a response to three previous adequate trials of at least two different classes of antidepressants or electroconvulsive therapy or to two previous adequate trials of empirical psychotherapy in the three years preceding the study; a serious, unstable medical condition; or a positive urine screen for drugs of abuse. Women of childbearing potential had to agree to use adequate contraception during the study. Patients were not allowed to take anxiolytic agents, sedatives, hypnotic agents, or any other types of sleep aids (pharmacologic or behavioral) during the study.

Study Design

The institutional review board at each center approved the study. All patients provided written informed consent. Patients who remained eligible at the end of the two-week evaluation period were randomly assigned, according to a central computerized randomization schedule, in a 1:1:1 ratio to receive nefazodone (Serzone, Bristol-Myers Squibb), psychotherapy, or a combination of nefazodone and psychotherapy. The Structured Clinical Interview for Axis I DSM-IV Disorders and the HRSD were administered by experienced clinical raters (study coordinators) certified to have a high rate of interrater reliability and level of procedural integrity. Each site implemented procedures to mask the patient's treatment assignment from the person who evaluated the results of the HRSD, and the degree of adherence to these procedures was monitored at each study visit. At all sites the rater was located at a separate physical location so that he or she could not see patients arriving for or departing from treatment sessions.

Among the patients who received nefazodone, the initial dose was 200 mg per day (100 mg twice a day) and was increased to 300 mg per day during the second week. Thereafter, the dose was increased weekly in increments of 100 mg per day to a maximum of 600 mg per day, to maximize the efficacy of the drug without producing intolerable side effects. To remain in the study, patients had to be receiving a dose of at least 300 mg per day by week 3.

Visits for medication were limited to 15 to 20 minutes. Psychopharmacologists followed a published manual[36] for clinical management (e.g., patients were questioned about the concomitant use of medications and symptoms, side effects, and illnesses they had had between visits). The psychopharmacologists were not allowed to make formal psychotherapeutic interventions (such as suggesting ways to cope with stressful life events).

The cognitive behavioral-analysis system of psychotherapy also followed a manual[37] specifying twice-weekly sessions during weeks 1 through 4 and weekly sessions during weeks 5 through 12. Twice-weekly sessions could be extended until week 8 if a patient was not adequately performing a learned social problem-solving procedure according to the criteria.

Psychotherapists (persons who had at least two years' experience after earning an M.D. or Ph.D. or at least five years' experience after earning an M.S.W.) attended a two-day training workshop and met the criteria for mastery of treatment procedures involved in the cognitive behavioral-analysis system of psychotherapy, as assessed by evaluation of their performance during two videotaped pilot cases. All psychotherapy sessions conducted during the study were videotaped, and supervisors reviewed the videotapes weekly to assess the psychotherapists' adherence to the treatment procedures.

Outcome Measures

The score on the 24-item HRSD was the primary outcome. The Global Assessment of Functioning Scale (Axis V in the DSM-IV) was administered at base line, and the results were evaluated by the same person who evaluated the HRSD results. Remission was defined a priori as an HRSD score of no more than 8 at both week 10 and week 12 for those who completed the 12-week protocol and at the time of withdrawal for those who did not complete the study. A satisfactory therapeutic response was defined as a reduction in the HRSD score by at least 50 percent from base line to week 10 and week 12, with a total score of 15 or less at these times but of more than 8 at week 10, week 12, or both for those who completed the study and at the time of departure for those who did not complete the study. The patients with these favorable outcomes were combined to form a single response group. All other patients were considered to have had no response.

Statistical Analysis

The base-line demographic and clinical characteristics of the treatment groups were compared with the use of analysis of variance for continuous variables and the Cochran–Mantel–Haenszel test for categorical variables, with site as the stratification variable. Preliminary paired t-tests were conducted separately for each treatment group to examine the significance of the changes in the HRSD scores from base line to the end point.

No outcome data were collected on patients who withdrew from the study after they withdrew, and a formal intention-to-treat analysis thus could not be performed. The primary analysis was a modified intention-to-treat analysis that included all patients who attended at least one treatment visit and who had at least one assessment after the base-line evaluation. Patients who underwent randomization but who did not return for a subsequent assessment were therefore not included in this analysis. Given this modified approach, the main efficacy analysis was a piecewise mixed-effects linear model that examined the relative differences between treatments with respect to the rate of change in the HRSD score (the linear slope) from base line to week 4 as one variable and from week 4 to week 12 (or the last visit) as a second variable. The a priori rationale for examining the first four weeks separately was that the earliest antidepressant effects of nefazodone are likely to occur at week 4 if a stable dosage has been achieved. Each model estimated fixed effects with respect to treatment and site, as well as the interactions between treatment and time. In addition, the models included a random intercept and a random slope. Interactions between treatment and site were not significant and therefore were not included in the models. The statistical significance of additional terms included in successive models was determined by the likelihood-ratio test. The error structure was specified as nonstationary autocorrelation in each model. There were no interim analyses of the data.

In addition to the mixed-model analysis, we examined response and remission rates that were based on the total HRSD score. We used the Cochran–Mantel–Haenszel test to analyze these rates in the modified intention-to-treat sample and among the patients who completed the study (with site as the stratification variable). We also performed an analysis of covariance of the change in total HRSD scores from base line to the end point, with base-line scores as the covariate, on these two samples. The model included treatment and site as the main effects. The interactions between treatment and site were again not significant and, hence, were not included in the model. We made pairwise comparisons of the means of the three treatment groups (adjusted for base-line values) using simple contrasts. Overall differences between treatments were evaluated with use of an alpha level of 0.05, whereas pairwise comparisons used an alpha level of 0.0167 (0.05 ÷ 3) with Bonferroni's correction.

We used Fisher's exact test to analyze the incidence of adverse events and rate of discontinuation of treatment in the three groups. All statistical tests were two-tailed. The data analysis was done by a biostatistical data-management company (Statprobe, Ann Arbor, Mich.), according to a plan devised by the authors. The company was selected and paid by Bristol-Myers Squibb.

Table 1. Status of the 681 Patients during the 12-Week Study, According to the Treatment Assignment.

Status	Nefazodone (N=226)	Psychotherapy (N=228)	Nefazodone and Psychotherapy (N=227)
	number (percent)		
Included in modified intention-to-treat sample*	220 (97)	216 (95)	226 (>99)
Completed the study	167 (74)	173 (76)	179 (79)
Withdrew from the study	59 (26)	55 (24)	48 (21)
Lack of efficacy	2 (1)	3 (1)	3 (1)
Adverse events	31 (14)	3 (1)	16 (7)
Withdrew consent	11 (5)	32 (14)	17 (7)
Protocol violation	2 (1)	2 (1)	0
Lost to follow-up	7 (3)	0	1 (<1)
Other reasons	6 (3)	15 (7)	11 (5)

*The modified intention-to-treat sample consisted of all randomized patients who attended at least one treatment visit and who had at least one efficacy assessment after the base-line evaluation.

RESULTS

Base-Line Clinical and Demographic Characteristics

A total of 1035 patients were screened for the study. Of the 354 who did not undergo randomization, 235 (66 percent) did not meet the study criteria, 47 (13 percent) withdrew their consent, and 72 (20 percent) were excluded for other reasons (e.g., failure to return for further evaluation or noncompliance). A total of 681 patients underwent randomization: 226 were assigned to receive nefazodone, 228 to receive psychotherapy, and 227 to receive combined treatment (Table 1). Randomization was not stratified according to site. At each site, approximately equal numbers of patients underwent randomization to the three groups. However, there were no significant differences among the groups with respect to base-line demographic and clinical characteristics (Table 2), either among the sites overall or within sites.

Treatment

For the modified intention-to-treat sample, the mean (±SD) final daily dose of nefazodone was 466±

TABLE 2. BASE-LINE CHARACTERISTICS OF THE PATIENTS.*

CHARACTERISTIC	NEFAZODONE (N=226)	PSYCHOTHERAPY (N=228)	NEFAZODONE AND PSYCHOTHERAPY (N=227)	ALL PATIENTS (N=681)
Female sex (%)	64.2	62.7	69.2	65.3
Age (yr)	42.2±11.0	43.2±10.8	44.4±10.3	43±10.7
White race (%)	87.2	91.7	92.5	90.5
Marital status (%)				
Married or cohabiting	42.9	41.6	43.6	42.7
Single	27.4	30.3	23.8	27.2
Widowed	2.7	1.3	2.2	2.1
Divorced or separated	27.0	26.8	30.4	28.0
Depression diagnosis (%)				
Chronic major depression	36.7	35.5	33.0	35.1
MDD with dysthymic disorder	42.9	39.9	44.1	42.3
Recurrent depression, with incomplete remission between episodes	20.4	24.6	22.9	22.6
Age at onset of MDD (yr)	25.6±13	27.5±13	27.1±13	26.7±13
Age at onset of dysthymia (yr)	17.8±13	19.7±14	20.3±14	19.3±14
Duration of current episode of MDD (yr)	7.5±9	7.8±10	8.0±9.5	7.8±9.6
Duration of current episode of dysthymia (yr)	22.3±15	22.5±15	24.2±16	23.0±15
History of anxiety disorder (%)	33.6	28.5	36.1	32.7
Diagnosis of coexisting personality disorder (%)	59.3	53.9	63.0	58.7
History of alcohol- or substance-abuse disorder (%)	34.5	33.3	31.7	33.2
Prior treatment with antidepressants (%)	57.5	59.5	63.6	60.2
Prior psychotherapy (%)	65.9	61.2	68.4	65.2
Prior treatment with both antidepressants and psychotherapy (%)	43.4	42.3	49.6	45.1
No prior treatment for depression (%)	19.9	22.0	17.1	19.7
Global Assessment of Functioning score†	53.8±5.4	53.9±5.7	53.6±5.6	54.0±5.6

*Plus–minus values are means ±SD. MDD denotes major depressive disorder.

†The score on the Global Assessment of Functioning Scale, which assesses the overall severity of psychiatric symptoms and functional impairment, can range from 1 to 100. Scores ranging from 1 to 20 indicate a patient who is a danger to others or to himself or herself. Scores ranging from 21 to 40 indicate a patient with moderate-to-severe impairments who should be hospitalized. Scores ranging from 41 to 60 indicate a patient with serious, nonpsychotic symptoms that impair function. Scores ranging from 61 to 80 indicate a patient with mild or transient symptoms who may require occasional counseling and psychotherapy. Scores ranging from 81 to 100 indicate a person with good functioning who does not require counseling.

144 mg in the nefazodone group (data available for 216 patients) and 460±139 mg in the combined-treatment group (221 patients). Among the patients who completed the study and for whom data on dose were available, the mean final daily dose of nefazodone was 520±100 mg among 92 patients with a response in the nefazodone group and 479±111 mg among the 152 patients with a response in the combined-treatment group. The dose was 491±125 mg among 73 patients without a response in the nefazodone group and 539±96 mg among the 27 patients without a response in the combined-treatment group.

For the modified intention-to-treat sample, the average number of psychotherapy sessions was 16.0±4.7 among 216 patients in the psychotherapy group and 16.2±4.8 among 226 patients in the combined-treatment group. Among those who completed the study, the 90 patients with a response in the psychotherapy group and the 152 such patients in the combined-treatment group attended a mean of 18.2±1.9 sessions, whereas the number was 17.7±1.9 among the 83 patients in the psychotherapy group who had no response and 17.9±1.4 among the 27 patients in the combined-treatment group who had no response.

Efficacy

Analyses revealed a significant improvement within patients in the HRSD scores from base line to week 12 in the group of patients who completed the study ($P<0.001$) and from base line to the last follow-up visit in the modified intention-to-treat sample ($P<0.001$) in all three groups. The mixed-effects piecewise linear regression examining the course of the scores during the 12 weeks of the trial (Fig. 1) showed that from base line through week 4, the average rate of improvement in the scores for patients in the combined-treatment group was not significantly different from the average rate of improvement in the scores for patients in the nefazodone group ($P=0.39$). However, the results of the analysis of the rate

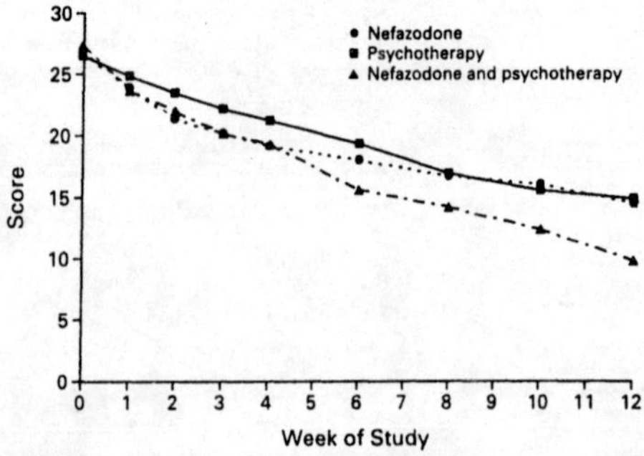

No. of Patients									
Nefazodone	220	202	195	194	188	181	164	160	153
Psychotherapy	216	180	190	185	190	174	168	166	156
Nefazodone and psychotherapy	226	210	212	206	201	197	184	182	173

Figure 1. Mean Scores on the Hamilton Rating Scale for Depression during the 12-Week Study.

The results of the analysis of the rate of improvement in the scores as a regression slope were as follows: for base line through week 4, $P<0.001$ for the comparison of combined treatment and psychotherapy, $P=0.004$ for the comparison of nefazodone and psychotherapy, and $P=0.39$ for the comparison of combined treatment and nefazodone; and for weeks 4 through 12, $P<0.001$ for the comparison of combined treatment and nefazodone and of psychotherapy and nefazodone and $P=0.06$ for the comparison of combined treatment and psychotherapy.

Table 3. Rates of Response and Remission.*

Group	Nefazodone	Psychotherapy	Nefazodone and Psychotherapy	P Value: Nefazodone vs. Psychotherapy	P Value: Nefazodone vs. Combined Treatment	P Value: Psychotherapy vs. Combined Treatment
	no. of patients (%)					
Modified intention-to-treat sample						
No. of patients	220	216	226			
Response	105 (48)	103 (48)	165 (73)	0.92	<0.001	<0.001
Remission	64 (29)	72 (33)	109 (48)	0.37	<0.001	<0.001
Satisfactory response	41 (19)	31 (14)	56 (25)	0.21	0.10	0.004
No response	113 (51)	113 (52)	57 (25)			
Patients who completed the study						
No. of patients	167	173	179			
Response	92 (55)	90 (52)	152 (85)	0.57	<0.001	<0.001
Remission	36 (22)	41 (24)	75 (42)	0.64	<0.001	<0.001
Satisfactory response	56 (34)	49 (28)	77 (43)	0.30	0.07	0.004
No response	73 (44)	83 (48)	27 (15)			

*The responses of two patients in the nefazodone group who completed the study could not be determined because no scores were available for the Hamilton Rating Scale for Depression at week 10 or 12. In the modified intention-to-treat sample, no post-randomization scores were available for two patients in the nefazodone group and four in the combined-treatment group. Remission was defined as a score of no more than 8 at both week 10 and week 12 for those who completed the 12-week protocol and when they left the trial for those who did not complete the study. A satisfactory response was defined as a reduction in the score by at least 50 percent from base line to week 10 and week 12, with a total score of 15 or less at these times but of more than 8 at week 10, week 12, or both for those who completed the study and at the time of departure for those who did not complete the study.

of improvement in the scores as a regression slope showed significant differences between the nefazodone group and the psychotherapy group (P=0.004) and between the combined-treatment group and the psychotherapy group (P<0.001). From week 4 through week 12, the average rate of improvement in the HRSD scores for patients in the combined-treatment group was significantly larger than the rate of improvement in scores for patients in the nefazodone group (P<0.001). There was also a significant difference in the rate of improvement in scores between the psychotherapy group and the nefazodone group (P<0.001) but not between the combined-treatment group and the psychotherapy group (P=0.06).

The overall rate of response was significantly higher in the combined-treatment group than in the nefazodone group or the psychotherapy group in both the modified intention-to-treat sample and the group of patients who completed the study (P<0.001 for all comparisons) (Table 3). For the modified intention-to-treat sample, the overall rates of response were 48 percent in the psychotherapy group (95 percent confidence interval, 41.5 to 54.8 percent), 48 percent in the nefazodone group (95 percent confidence interval, 41.0 to 54.3 percent), and 73 percent in the combined-treatment group (95 percent confidence interval, 68.6 to 80.1 percent) at the time of the last follow-up visit. Among the patients who completed the 12 weeks of treatment, the overall rates of response were 52 percent in the psychotherapy group (95 percent confidence interval, 44.6 to 59.6 percent), 55 percent in the nefazodone group (95 percent confidence interval, 47.5 to 62.6 percent), and 85 percent in the combined-treatment group (95 percent confidence interval, 79.7 to 90.2 percent). In both samples of patients, significantly more patients had a remission during combined treatment than during treatment with nefazodone or psychotherapy alone (P<0.001 for all comparisons) (Table 3). In the modified intention-to-treat sample, the remission rates were 33 percent in the psychotherapy group, 29 percent in the nefazodone group, and 48 percent in the combined-treatment group. The respective rates of remission among the patients who completed the study were 24 percent, 22 percent, and 42 percent.

An analysis of covariance revealed significant differences between treatment groups with respect to the final HRSD scores for both the modified intention-to-treat sample (Table 4) and in the patients who completed the study, with combined treatment more effective than either psychotherapy alone or nefazodone alone (P<0.001 for all comparisons). To examine the size of the differences between combined treatment and treatment with nefazodone or psychotherapy alone, we calculated effect sizes using Cohen's d (the difference between adjusted means divided by the pooled standard deviation). The effect sizes calculated for the group of patients who completed the study and for the modified intention-to-treat sample ranged from 0.54 to 0.64 for the comparison of combined treatment with the other two groups. There were no significant differences at end point between the nefazodone group and the psychotherapy group.

Rates of Discontinuation and Adverse Events

The rates of discontinuation were similar in the three groups (P=0.46) (Table 1), with 24 percent of

Table 4. Mean Scores on the Hamilton Rating Scale for Depression at Base Line, Week 12, and the Last Follow-up Visit.*

Variable	No. of Patients	Base Line	Week 12	Last Follow-up Visit
Score				
Nefazodone	220	26.8±0.32	14.7±0.70†	15.8±0.64†
Psychotherapy	216	26.4±0.33	15.1±0.69†	16.0±0.63†
Nefazodone and psychotherapy	226	27.4±0.32	9.7±0.65†	10.8±0.63†
P value for comparison between groups				
Nefazodone vs. psychotherapy			0.68	0.79
Nefazodone vs. combined treatment			<0.001	<0.001
Psychotherapy vs. combined treatment			<0.001	<0.001
Effect sizes (Cohen's d) for pairwise comparisons‡				
Nefazodone vs. psychotherapy			−0.05	−0.02
Nefazodone vs. combined treatment			0.59	0.54
Psychotherapy vs. combined treatment			0.64	0.56

*Plus–minus values are means ±SE. Higher scores on the 24-item test indicate more severe depression. Values for week 12 represent data from patients who completed the study, whereas values for the last follow-up visit represent data from the modified intention-to-treat sample.

†P<0.001 for the comparison with base-line score by the paired t-test.

‡The effect sizes were calculated as the difference between the adjusted means divided by the pooled standard deviation.

all patients not completing the 12-week study. The percentage of patients who dropped out because of lack of efficacy was low (1 percent in each group). The rate of discontinuation due to adverse events was 14 percent in the nefazodone group, 7 percent in the combined-treatment group, and 1 percent in the psychotherapy group. The most common reason for discontinuing psychotherapy was withdrawal of consent (in 14 percent of patients). Of the 32 patients who withdrew their consent, 5 did not want psychotherapy, 11 thought treatment was too time consuming, and 4 wanted medication. Seventy-two percent of the patients in the psychotherapy group who withdrew their consent did so within the first four weeks of treatment.

Table 5 lists the adverse events (whether or not they were thought to be related to treatment) that occurred in at least 10 percent of all patients. The adverse events in the groups receiving nefazodone were consistent with the known side effects of the medication, with headache, somnolence, dry mouth, nausea, and dizziness being the most common. Weight gain was rare, with no instances in the nefazodone or psychotherapy group and an incidence of 3.1 percent in the combined-treatment group. Sexual dysfunction (including impotence, psychosexual dysfunction, anorgasmia, and abnormal ejaculation) occurred in 3.5 percent of the patients in the nefazodone group, none of the patients in the psychotherapy group, and 3.5 percent of the patients in the combined-treatment group.

Table 5. Common Adverse Events.*

Adverse Event	Nefazodone (N=225)	Psychotherapy (N=221)	Nefazodone and Psychotherapy (N=226)	P Value†
		percent		
Headache	56	45	65	<0.001
Asthenia	17	6	20	<0.001
Pain	14	12	21	0.02
Abdominal pain	13	10	18	0.08
Infection	9	13	12	0.50
Back pain	8	10	12	0.23
Dry mouth	39	0	35	<0.001
Nausea	30	6	36	<0.001
Dyspepsia	21	12	19	0.02
Diarrhea	19	10	23	<0.001
Constipation	16	1	17	<0.001
Somnolence	40	1	36	<0.001
Dizziness	25	2	29	<0.001
Insomnia	19	8	19	0.004
Lightheadedness	12	<1	14	<0.001
Agitation	10	2	8	<0.001
Difficulty concentrating	9	1	10	<0.001
Pharyngitis	12	5	10	0.05
Sinusitis	12	11	10	0.89
Abnormal vision	15	<1	20	<0.001
Blurred vision	11	1	10	<0.001

*Adverse events that were reported by at least 10 percent of all patients are listed.

†Fisher's exact test was used to test for differences among the three groups.

DISCUSSION

We found that treatment with a combination of nefazodone and psychotherapy had significant advantages over treatment with nefazodone or psychotherapy alone. Despite the fact that the patients had had active depression for many years and that many had other psychiatric disorders as well, among the patients who completed the study, 85 percent of the patients in the combined-treatment group had a response to treatment by week 12, as compared with 55 percent of patients in the nefazodone group and 52 percent of patients in the psychotherapy group. The rates of response and remission in the combined-treatment group were substantially higher than those that might have been anticipated on the basis of the outcomes of previous trials in similar patients. By contrast, in the modified intention-to-treat sample, the rate of response of 48 percent in both the nefazodone group and the psychotherapy group was similar to the rates reported for treatment with sertraline (52 percent),[13] imipramine (51 percent),[13] and desipramine (51 percent)[18] in other studies of patients with chronic depression. The degree of superiority of combination therapy over monotherapy, as indicated by differences in the response rates and the sizes of the effects, suggests that combined treatment provides a clinically meaningful advantage. These results support previous recommendations,[21] based on clinical experience, for the use of both psychotherapy and medication to treat patients with chronic depression.

Nefazodone produced effects more rapidly than did psychotherapy, with significant advantages evident in the first four weeks, whereas psychotherapy had a greater effect during the second part of the trial. By week 12, the efficacy of the two approaches was similar. Although patients who were receiving nefazodone had higher frequencies of adverse events than those receiving psychotherapy, the rates of withdrawal from the study were similar in all three treatment groups. The fact that the efficacy of combined treatment and nefazodone was similar during the first four weeks of the study but that combined treatment was more efficacious later in the study suggests that when medication and psychotherapy are administered together, they continue to have independent rather than synergistic mechanisms of action.

A limitation of our study was the lack of a placebo control. However, a placebo-controlled study of patients with either a chronic major depressive disorder alone or a major depressive disorder plus dysthymia reported a relatively low rate of response to placebo (12 percent).[14] In a study on the treatment of chronic forms of depression, the use of a placebo control would most likely greatly decrease the number of patients willing to participate, thereby reducing the generalizability of the findings.[38]

Another limitation, common to all studies of psychotherapy, was our inability to mask patients and therapists in the psychotherapy groups. To counteract this limitation, we had persons who were unaware of the patients' treatment assignments administer the HRSD. However, the clinicians were obviously not unaware of the treatment that patients were receiving.

Further limitations of our study include the restrictive exclusion criteria, which also reduced the generalizability of the findings, and the rates of withdrawal in conjunction with the lack of further data on patients after they withdrew. The slightly lower rate of withdrawal in the combined-treatment group (21 percent) than in the nefazodone group (26 percent) or the psychotherapy group (24 percent) may have biased the outcome comparisons.

In summary, we found that the combination of pharmacotherapy (nefazodone) and the cognitive behavioral-analysis system of psychotherapy was significantly more efficacious than either treatment alone for outpatients with chronic forms of depression. The rates of response to either treatment alone were similar and were also similar to the rates reported in previous trials of antidepressants for the treatment of chronic forms of depression in outpatients, indicating that at least one form of psychotherapy is effective in treating such patients. Although similarly effective, nefazodone produced effects more rapidly than did psychotherapy.

Supported by Bristol-Myers Squibb.

We are indebted to Drs. Jack E. Carr, Pedro L. Delgado, Frank Dowling, Gregory Eaves, Robert H. Howland, and Carina Vocisano for assisting with the study.

Editor's note: Our policy requires authors of Original Articles to disclose all financial ties with companies that make the products under study or competing products. In this case, the large number of authors and their varied and extensive financial associations with relevant companies make a detailed listing here impractical. Readers should know, however, that all but 1 (B.A.) of the 12 principal authors have had financial associations with Bristol-Myers Squibb — which also sponsored the study — and, in most cases, with many other companies producing psychoactive pharmaceutical agents. The associations include consultancies, receipt of research grants and honorariums, and participation on advisory boards. Of the 17 other authors, 2 are employees of Bristol-Myers Squibb, 5 (L.M.K., G.K., I.M., R.M., D.V.) have no relevant additional financial ties, and the others have a variety of associations similar to those just mentioned. Details are included as part of the article on the *Journal*'s Web site (www.nejm.org) and are also available (as document no. 05552) from the National Auxiliary Publications Service, c/o Microfiche Publications, 248 Hempstead Tpk., West Hempstead, NY 11552.

REFERENCES

1. Judd LL, Akiskal HS, Paulus MP. The role and clinical significance of subsyndromal depressive symptoms (SSD) in unipolar major depressive disorder. J Affect Disord 1997;45:5-18.
2. Keller MB, Hanks DL, Klein DN. Summary of the DSM-IV mood disorders field trial and issue overview. Psychiatr Clin North Am 1996;19:1-28.
3. Kocsis JH, Klein DN, eds. Diagnosis and treatment of chronic depression. New York: Guilford Press, 1995.
4. Kessler RC, McGonagle KA, Zhao S, et al. Lifetime and 12-month prevalence of DSM-III-R psychiatric disorders in the United States: results from the National Comorbidity Survey. Arch Gen Psychiatry 1994;51:8-19.
5. Weissman MM, Leaf PJ, Bruce ML, Florio L. The epidemiology of dysthymia in five communities: rates, risks, comorbidity, and treatment. Am J Psychiatry 1988;145:815-9.
6. Wells KB, Burnam MA, Rogers W, Hays R, Camp P. The course of depression in adult outpatients: results from the Medical Outcomes Study. Arch Gen Psychiatry 1992;49:788-94.
7. Hays RD, Wells KB, Sherbourne CD, Rogers W, Spritzer K. Functioning and well-being outcomes of patients with depression compared with chronic general medical illnesses. Arch Gen Psychiatry 1995;52:11-9.
8. Miller IW, Keitner GI, Schatzberg AF, et al. The treatment of chronic depression. 3. Psychosocial functioning before and after treatment with sertraline or imipramine. J Clin Psychiatry 1998;59:608-19.
9. Howland RH. Chronic depression. Hosp Community Psychiatry 1993;44:633-9.
10. Klein DN, Norden KA, Ferro T, et al. Thirty-month naturalistic follow-up study of early-onset dysthymic disorder: course, diagnostic stability, and prediction of outcome. J Abnorm Psychol 1998;107:338-48.
11. Cassano GB, Akiskal HS, Perugi G, Musetti L, Savino M. The importance of measures of affective temperaments in genetic studies of mood disorders. J Psychiatr Res 1992;26:257-68.
12. Greenberg PE, Stiglin LE, Finkelstein SN, Berndt ER. The economic burden of depression in 1990. J Clin Psychiatry 1993;54:405-18.
13. Keller MB, Gelenberg AJ, Hirschfeld RMA, et al. The treatment of chronic depression. 2. A double-blind, randomized trial of sertraline and imipramine. J Clin Psychiatry 1998;59:598-607.
14. Kocsis JH, Frances AJ, Voss CB, Mann JJ, Mason BJ, Sweeney J. Imipramine treatment for chronic depression. Arch Gen Psychiatry 1988;45:253-7.
15. Harrison WM, Stewart JW. Pharmacotherapy of dysthymic disorder. In: Kocsis JH, Klein DN, eds. Diagnosis and treatment of chronic depression. New York: Guilford Press, 1995:124-45.
16. Thase ME, Fava M, Halbreich U, et al. A placebo-controlled, randomized clinical trial comparing sertraline and imipramine for the treatment of dysthymia. Arch Gen Psychiatry 1996;53:777-84.
17. Keller MB, Kocsis JH, Thase ME, et al. Maintenance phase efficacy of sertraline for chronic depression: a randomized controlled trial. JAMA 1998;280:1665-72.
18. Kocsis JH, Friedman RA, Markowitz JC, et al. Maintenance therapy for chronic depression: a controlled clinical trial of desipramine. Arch Gen Psychiatry 1996;53:769-76.
19. Markowitz JC. Psychotherapy of dysthymia. Am J Psychiatry 1994;151:1114-21.
20. American Psychiatric Association. Practice guidelines for major depressive disorder in adults. Am J Psychiatry 1993;150:Suppl:1-26.
21. Depression Guideline Panel. Depression in primary care. Vol. 2. Treatment of major depression. Clinical practice guideline, number 5. Rockville, Md.: Agency for Health Care Policy and Research. 1993. (AHCPR publication no. 93-0551.)
22. Rush AJ, Thase ME. Psychotherapies for depressive disorders. In: Maj M, Sartorius N, eds. World Psychiatric Association series on evidence and practice in psychiatry. Vol. 1. Depressive disorders. Chichester, England: John Wiley, 1999:161-206.
23. Roth A, Fonagy P. What works for whom? A critical review of psychotherapy research. New York: Guilford Press, 1996.
24. Conte HR, Plutchik R, Wild KV, Karasu TB. Combined psychotherapy and pharmacotherapy for depression: a systematic analysis of the evidence. Arch Gen Psychiatry 1986;43:471-9.
25. McCullough JP. Treatment for chronic depression: cognitive behavioral analysis system of psychotherapy. New York: Guilford Press, 2000.
26. *Idem.* Cognitive-behavioral analysis system of psychotherapy: an interactional treatment approach for dysthymic disorder. Psychiatry 1984;47:234-50.
27. Garlow SJ, Owens MJ, Nemeroff CB. Nefazodone. In: Sadock BJ, Sadock VA, eds. Kaplan & Sadock's comprehensive textbook of psychiatry. 7th ed. Vol. 2. Philadelphia: Lippincott Williams & Wilkins, 2000:2412-9.

28. Feiger AD, Bielski RJ, Bremner J, et al. Double-blind, placebo-substitution study of nefazodone in the prevention of relapse during continuation treatment of outpatients with major depression. Int Clin Psychopharmacol 1999;14:19-28.
29. McCullough JP. Psychotherapy for dysthymia: a naturalistic study of ten patients. J Nerv Ment Dis 1991;179:734-40.
30. Klerman GL, Weissman MM, Rounsaville BJ, Chevron ES. Interpersonal psychotherapy of depression. New York: Basic Books, 1984.
31. Beck AT, Rush AJ, Shaw BG, Emery G. Cognitive therapy of depression. New York: Guilford Press, 1979.
32. Lewinsohn PM. A behavioral approach to depression. In: Friedman RJ, Katz MM, eds. The psychology of depression: contemporary theory and research. Washington, D.C.: Hemisphere Publishing, 1974:157-78.
33. Diagnostic and statistical manual of mental disorders, 4th ed.: DSM-IV. Washington, D.C.: American Psychiatric Association, 1994.
34. First MB, Spitzer RL, Gibbon M, et al. Structured clinical interview for Axis-I DSM-IV disorders: patient edition (SCID-II, version 2.0). New York: New York State Psychiatric Institute Biometrics Research Department, 1994.
35. Hamilton M. Development of a rating scale for primary depressive illness. Br J Soc Clin Psychol 1967;6:278-96.
36. Fawcett J, Epstein P, Fiester SJ, Elkin I, Autry JH. Clinical management — imipramine/placebo administration manual: NIMH Treatment of Depression Collaboration Research Program. Psychopharmacol Bull 1987;23:309-24.
37. McCullough JP. Therapist manual for cognitive behavioral analysis system of psychotherapy. Richmond: Virginia Commonwealth University, 1995.
38. Rush AJ, Koran LM, Miller MB, et al. The treatment of chronic depression. 1. Study design and rationale for evaluating the comparative efficacy of sertraline and imipramine as acute, crossover, continuation, and maintenance phase therapies. J Clin Psychiatry 1998;59:589-97.

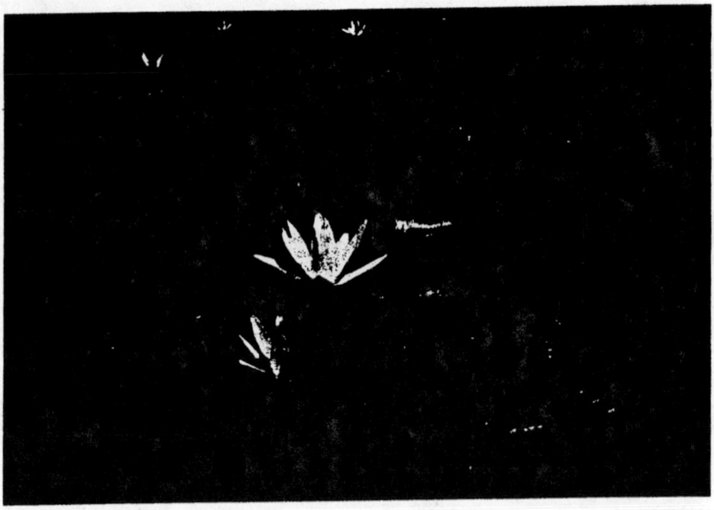

Okovanggo Delta, Botswana — Petros C. Karakousis, M.D.

ORIGINAL ARTICLE

Functioning and Utility for Current Health of Patients With Depression or Chronic Medical Conditions in Managed, Primary Care Practices

Kenneth B. Wells, MD, MPH; Cathy D. Sherbourne, PhD

Background: Health utility is the recommended outcome metric for medical cost-effectiveness studies. We compared health utility and quality of life for primary care patients with depression or chronic medical conditions.

Methods: Respondents were outpatients (N = 17 558) of primary care clinicians (N = 181) in 7 managed care organizations. Utility was assessed by time tradeoff, or the years of life that patients would exchange for perfect health, and standard gamble, or the required chance of success to accept a treatment that can cause immediate death or survival in perfect health. Probable 12-month depressive disorder and affective syndromes were assessed through self-report items from a diagnostic interview. Medical conditions were assessed with self-report. Quality of life was assessed by the 12-Item Short-Form Health Survey. Regression models were used to compare quality of life and utility for patients with depression vs chronic medical conditions.

Results: Patients with probable 12-month depressive disorder had worse mental health and role-emotional and social functioning and lower utility for their current health than patients with each chronic medical condition (for most comparisons, $P<.001$). Depressed patients had worse physical functioning than patients with 4 common chronic conditions but better physical functioning than patients with 4 other conditions (each $P<.001$). Patients with lifetime bipolar illness and 12-month double depression had the poorest quality of life and lowest utility.

Conclusions: Primary care patients with depressive conditions have poorer mental, role-emotional, and social functioning than patients with common chronic medical conditions, and physical functioning in the midrange. The low utility of depressed patients relative to patients with chronic medical conditions suggests that recovery from depression should be a high practice priority.

Arch Gen Psychiatry. 1999;56:897-904

DEPRESSION is associated with limitations in multiple domains of health-related quality of life (HRQOL), defined as perceptions of daily functioning and well-being in physical, social, and psychological domains, that equal or exceed those associated with most common chronic medical conditions, such as arthritis or diabetes.[1-4] Yet, levels of detection and treatment for depression in managed care, primary care settings remain moderate at best.[5-9] One factor that could contribute to low treatment rates is the perception of patients that recovery from depression is a relatively low priority relative to recovery from common medical conditions that are physically limiting. In this article, we compare both HRQOL and utility for current health of primary care patients with depression or chronic medical conditions.

Utility is defined as "the preference of the patient for a particular health outcome or health status."[9] A lower utility for a condition means a higher preference for recovery from that state. The ability to compare utility for diverse health states is a main reason why it is the recommended outcome for cost-effectiveness analyses.[9] Because of the low relative HRQOL of depressed patients, and because utility tends to be lower with more severe symptoms,[10,11] we hypothesize that utility for current health will also be at least as low for depressed patients as for those with chronic medical conditions. As a context for these comparisons, we also replicate previous comparisons by Wells et al[3] of depression and chronic medical conditions in mental and physical HRQOL.

Depression is a heterogeneous condition, and utility could also vary across different subtypes. Thus, we also explore differences in HRQOL and utility among subgroups of patients who screen positive for probable major depression, dysthymic disorder, subthreshold depressive symptoms, and bipolar disorder. We hypothesized that patients with more se-

From RAND, Santa Monica, Calif (Drs Wells and Sherbourne); and Department of Psychiatry and Behavioral Sciences, UCLA Neuropsychiatric Institute and Hospital, Los Angeles, Calif (Dr Wells).

METHODS

Data were gathered at the baseline assessment for Partners in Care, an experiment to evaluate the cost-effectiveness of improving quality of care for depression in primary care, managed care practices.[12]

SAMPLING

We selected 6 managed care organizations by purposive sampling from diverse geographic sites and included organizations with high enrollment of Hispanics. The organizations included staff-model health maintenance organizations, multispecialty group practices under a single prepaid health plan or a network of plans, and managed, public health clinics. Informed consent was obtained from clinicians. Of 183 eligible primary care clinicians, 181 agreed to participate. A consecutive sample of adult visitors was asked to complete a 10-minute self-report patient screener in Spanish or English. Informed consent was not obtained from patients because no identifiable information was collected, as approved by the Human Subjects Protection Committees of RAND, Santa Monica, Calif, and the organizations.

To enable the intervention study, the sample was restricted to patients with insurance that covered the mental health specialists fielding the interventions. In 4 organizations, virtually all patients were eligible. In one site, the study was limited to patients with prepaid plans, while in another it was restricted to those with prepaid plans and about 50% of those with fee-for-service plans. Across sites, staff approached 44 052 individuals, of whom 10 120 (23.0%) were ineligible, ie, younger than 18 years, ineligible insurance, or there for laboratory studies only or accompanying a patient. Of 33 932 eligible patients, 6600 (19.5%) refused the survey, and 27 332 agreed. This article excludes surveys completed in Spanish (n = 1754), because the items assessing utility were worded differently. The items used to measure utility were at the end of the survey, and 7211 English-speaking respondents (29.8%) did not complete them because they had to leave the clinic, so we excluded them, as well as an additional 809 patients (3.3%) who were missing data on age or depression. The analytic sample consisted of 17 558 patients. Persons who completed the items were younger and in better perceived general health ($P<.001$), more likely to be depressed ($P<.02$), and disproportionately from 2 sites. These factors explained only 5% of variance in response, however. We controlled for these factors in analyses and weighted the data for probability of participation and response.

MEASUREMENT OF HEALTH STATUS

Probable 12-month depressive disorder was assessed through self-report versions of stem items (E1, 2, 34) for *DSM-IV* major depressive and dysthymic disorder[13] of the 12-month Composite International Diagnostic Interview Version 2.1 (CIDI-12, 2.1).[14] These items ask whether there was a period of 2 weeks or more of daily sadness, depressed mood, or lack of interest in usual pleasurable activities in the past 12 months, or a 2-year or longer period of nearly daily depression or lack of interest extending into the last 12 months. In addition, we included 2 items to assess whether the respondent had had 1 week or more of daily depression or lack of interest in the past 30 days. We define *probable 12-month depressive disorder* as having a positive response on both a 12-month and a 30-day item. This criterion had a positive predictive value of 55% for 12-month major depressive or dysthymic disorder, based on 1485 study patients who, at the time of enrollment, completed the CIDI-12, 2.1 affective disorders section in person or by telephone.[14] Because the CIDI-12 requires a positive stem item to score disorder, the sensitivity of this criterion is by definition 100%. We conducted a methods study in which persons who scored positive on the 12-month items but negative on the 30-day items underwent a verbal repeat of the interview, and 10% at that step were positive. Thus, true sensitivity is somewhat below 100%.

We developed indicator variables defining probable affective syndromes, using the depression items and 2 stem items from the lifetime mania section of the lifetime version of the CIDI 2.1. We considered persons with any positive mania item to have probable lifetime bipolar disorder. Those who scored negative on mania but positive on the 12-month depression stem items were considered to have major depression only, dysthymia only, or double depression (concurrent major depression and dysthymia), depending on which stem items were positive. Those with all stem items negative but who reported

vere types, particularly bipolar disorder and concurrent major depression and dysthymic disorder, or double depression, will have the lowest utility for their current health.

RESULTS

The patients were diverse in age and ethnicity, eg, 16.9% were Hispanic (**Table 1**). The majority (62.0%) were women. The most common conditions were back problems (24.9%), arthritis (20.1%), hypertension (20.0%), and migraine (15.2%), while 16.5% had probable 12-month depressive disorder. The percentage with any affective syndrome was higher (33.5%) because it included persons with lifetime mania or either 12-month or 30-day symptoms. The most common syndrome was 12-month major depression only (19.8%). **Table 2** provides descriptive statistics for the HRQOL measures and for the TTO and SG for the whole sample and among those with less than the maximum utility, ie, greater than 0 on TTO or less than 100 on SG. Only 19.6% of patients were willing to trade any months of life for perfect health (by TTO), and these patients were on average willing to trade 39 days. Only 20.5% of patients were willing to accept anything less than a 100% chance of success to try a treatment that would offer either immediate death or cure (by SG), and on average these patients required a 74% chance of success to accept the treatment.

Table 3 describes HRQOL and utility of current health (unadjusted) for patients with depression only, both depression and a chronic medical condition, a medical condition only, or neither problem. On each HRQOL and utility measure, the differences among groups was highly statistically significant (each $P<.001$). By inspection of Table 3, mental HRQOL was poorest for those with depression and physical functioning was poorest for those

30-day symptoms were considered to have symptoms only. The remainder had no affective syndrome. Because we cannot directly test the validity of these screening measures, we consider the analyses to be exploratory.

We assessed current chronic medical conditions with a self-report checklist, derived from the Medical Outcomes Study.[5] The conditions were asthma, diabetes, hypertension, arthritis, migraine headaches, and chronic lung, neurologic, heart, gastrointestinal tract, vision, and back problems. The items assessed whether the individual currently had each condition. We assessed current HRQOL through the 12-Item Short-Form Health Survey (SF-12). We used the global mental and physical scales, which have excellent reliability and construct validity and account for more than 90% of the variance in longer-form measures.[15] These scales are standardized to a US adult general population mean of 50 and SD of 10 by means of norm-based scoring. Some physical items have a negative weight on the mental score, while psychological items have a negative weight on the physical score. As a result, the impact of depression on physical health may be underestimated while the impact of medical conditions on mental health may be underestimated.[16] Furthermore, some psychological items directly assess symptoms of depression, so it can be unclear whether an association with depression simply reflects the autocorrelation of depressive symptoms across measures. To avoid these problems, we also used the physical functioning items of the SF-12 (plus an additional item on vigorous activities from the SF-36) to create a physical functioning score (standardized on a 0-100 scale, with a higher score indicating better health), and the SF-12 social limitation and role-emotional limitation items to represent mental health (each standardized to a 0-100 scale, with a lower score indicating fewer limitations).

MEASUREMENT OF UTILITY

To assess utilities in a large sample at a reasonable cost, we opted for single-item measures of 2 standard approaches, the time tradeoff (TTO) (ie, years of life an individual is willing to give up for perfect health until death, relative to 10 years in a given health state) and the standard gamble (SG) (ie, the required chance for outcome success to accept a treatment that can result in either immediate death or perfect health, relative to living another 10 years in their current state of health).[17-19] One-day test-retest reliability on a different sample of 228 patients showed good reliability (Spearman correlation coefficients of 0.8 for TTO and 0.7 for SG).

For the TTO, patients were asked to imagine that there is a treatment that would permit them to live in perfect physical and mental health but that reduces life expectancy. Patients indicated how many months or years they would give up for a treatment that would allow them to live in perfect health, if they had 10 years to live. Maximum utility for current health is represented by a score of 0, and a higher TTO score indicates lower utility for current health. For the SG, patients were asked to imagine they had 10 years to live in their current state of health, both physical and mental, and that there was a treatment that could either give them perfect health or kill them immediately. Patients were asked to indicate what chance of success the treatment had to have before they would accept it. Maximum utility for current health is represented by 100, and a lower score on SG indicates lower utility.

ANALYSIS

To compare patients with depression or chronic medical conditions, we estimated multiple linear regression models. The dependent variables were the HRQOL and utility measures. The main independent variables were probable 12-month depressive disorder and the 11 chronic medical conditions. The covariates were patient demographics (age, sex, education, ethnic group, and site). In separate runs, we added the global physical and mental HRQOL scales as covariates to the TTO and SG analyses, to test whether depressed patients have lower utility than would be predicted from their HRQOL alone. We conducted parallel analyses using the affective syndrome indicators. Although individuals are clustered within providers and clinics, the intraclass correlations are less than 0.001, ie, trivial. We present results without adjustment for clustering.[20,21] We present adjusted means, controlling for all covariates in the regression. Because we report many significant findings in a consistent direction, a formal Bonferroni correction[22] for hypothesis testing is too conservative. We focus on results significant at .005 or better. All data are weighted to the characteristics of the full primary care patient population.

with a medical condition. Utility for current health was lowest, on both TTO and SG, for patients with both types of conditions, intermediate for patients with one type, and highest for patients with neither type.

Table 4 shows the adjusted mean HRQOL and utility for patients with and without each condition. The conditions can be grouped into (1) those associated with poorer HRQOL and lower utility across measures (depression; diabetes; chronic lung, neurologic, gastrointestinal tract, or back problems; or migraine); (2) those affecting physical HRQOL only (asthma, hypertension); and (3) those affecting HRQOL and utility, but not mental or role-emotional functioning (arthritis, heart disease, eye problems). This statement is based on the difference scores in Table 4 with $P<.001$.

Table 5 compares patients with depression and specific chronic conditions, adjusting for covariates. On global mental health, role-emotional, and social functioning, depressed patients had significantly worse HRQOL than did patients with each of the chronic medical conditions (each $P<.001$). The magnitude of the differences in global mental health, 13 to 15 points, was greater than 1 SD, a large effect. By the global physical scale, patients with 9 chronic conditions (all but asthma and hypertension) had worse physical HRQOL than depressed patients (each $P<.001$). However, patients with depression had worse physical functioning than did patients with asthma, hypertension, gastrointestinal tract problems, or migraines, while depressed patients had better physical function than patients with chronic lung, neurologic, heart, or back problems (each $P<.001$). The magnitude of the differences in physical functioning was 3 to 7 points, about one-fifth to one-tenth SD. A difference of 2 to 3 points on the parent instrument is often considered clinically meaningful. As shown in Table 5, depressed patients had lower utility for their current health by either TTO (a higher

Table 1. Characteristics of Primary Care Patients (Screened Sample With Utility Measures, N = 17 558)

	Actual No.	Weighted %
Age group, y		
17-24	1570	8.8
25-44	7512	42.7
45-54	3745	21.5
55-64	2128	12.3
65-69	1045	5.9
≥70	1558	8.8
Female sex	11 004	62.0
Ethnic groups (main)		
Hispanic	3071	16.9
African American	1352	7.9
Asian American	586	3.4
American Indian	560	3.2
European American	11 989	68.6
Education group, y		
<12	1329	7.5
12	4869	27.6
13-15	5513	31.3
≥16	5847	33.5
Current chronic condition		
Asthma	1550	8.8
Diabetes	1496	8.6
Hypertension	3492	20.0
Arthritis	3532	20.1
Chronic lung disease	695	4.0
Chronic neurologic disease	371	2.1
Heart disease	717	4.1
Chronic gastrointestinal tract disease	1517	8.7
Back problems	4378	24.9
Eye problems	1639	9.3
Migraines	2685	15.2
Probable depressive disorder	2896	16.5
Affective syndromes		
Lifetime bipolar (manic symptoms)	331	1.9
12-mo double depression	944	5.3
12-mo major depression	3479	19.8
12-mo dysthymia	151	0.9
1-mo symptoms only	987	5.6
No affective syndrome	11 666	66.5

score) or SG (a lower score) than did patients with each chronic medical condition. Most comparisons were highly significant, except neurologic conditions by TTO or SG and chronic lung or heart problems by SG.

When we added global mental and physical scales as covariates, depressive disorder retained a unique effect in predicting TTO (the depression coefficient had $t = 3.76$, $P<.001$). Furthermore, for SG (but not TTO), there were significant interaction terms between depression status and global mental and physical HRQOL (the pair of coefficients in the regression had $F_{2,45} = 5.42$; $P = .008$). Reductions in HRQOL lowered utility of current health more for depressed than for nondepressed patients. Stratified analyses indicate that for both depressed and nondepressed patients, those with worse mental and physical HRQOL had lower utility for their current health.

As shown in **Table 6**, patients with each of the affective syndromes had significantly worse physical functioning and global mental health and lower utility by TTO than did patients without an affective syndrome (each

Table 2. Health-Related Quality of Life and Utility of Primary Care Patients (N = 17 558)

	Weighted Mean (SD)	Range
Health-related quality of life		
Global physical*	48.0 (9.9)	11.0-67.9
Physical functioning*	74.3 (30.1)	0-100
Global mental*	50.2 (10.2)	9.0-71.0
Limited emotional role functioning†	19.8 (36.5)	0-100
Limited social functioning†	18.7 (27.9)	0-100
Utility		
Time tradeoff	7.7 (23.4)	0-120
Mean if >0‡	39.2 (39.4)	1-12
Standard gamble	94.6 (16.8)	0-100
Mean if <100§	73.9 (28.8)	0-99

*A high score represents good health.
†A high score represents poor health.
‡Included 19.6% (n = 3443).
§Included 20.5% (n = 3612).

$P<.001$). By SG, patients with dysthymia only or 30-day depressive symptoms only did not differ significantly in utility for their current health from patients with no affective syndrome. For HRQOL, the syndromes can roughly be ordered from worst to best health: 12-month double depression, lifetime bipolar, 12-month major depression only, 12-month dysthymia only, and 30-day symptoms only. Furthermore, utility for current health was significantly lower for patients with either 12-month double depression or lifetime bipolar disorder compared with patients with each of the other affective syndromes (data available from the authors).

COMMENT

We found that depressed patients place a lower utility on their current health than do patients with most common, chronic medical conditions, other factors being equal. This finding suggests that primary care practices should place a relatively high emphasis on helping patients recover from depression. This does not mean that patients will necessarily accept treatments, however. We did not directly measure patient preferences for treatments or resource allocation. Depressed patients could refuse treatments, for example, if they believe treatment is not efficacious, deny having depression, fear social stigma associated with treatment, or experience financial or other barriers to care.[1,5] Our finding of a relatively low utility for health states associated with depression is consistent with previous studies, based on data from patient or community samples with hypothetical case scenarios or vignettes, or ratings of current health.[10,11,23-25] What is new in our study is the availability of evidence from a large, consecutive sample of primary care patients from multiple managed care practices, and comparisons of both HRQOL and utility assessment across disease conditions.

Consistent with the previous work of Wells et al from the Medical Outcomes Study,[5] we found substantial decrements in physical and mental HRQOL associated with depression, equal to or often exceeding decrements as-

Table 3. Unadjusted Weighted Health and Utility by Depression and Chronic Condition Status for Primary Care Patients (N = 17 558)

	Probable Depression Only, Mean (SD) (n = 750)	Depression and Medical Condition, Mean (SD) (n = 2146)	Medical Condition Only, Mean (SD) (n = 8979)	Neither, Mean (SD) (n = 5683)	Overall Difference	
					$F_{3,17554}$	*P**
Health-related quality of life						
Physical functioning†	83.6 (24.8)	56.5 (34.3)	69.4 (30.3)	87.5 (22.1)	877.36	<.001
Global physical†	53.2 (8.7)	43.2 (11.5)	46.0 (10.0)	52.3 (6.7)	945.34	<.001
Global mental†	36.6 (11.2)	36.3 (10.6)	52.9 (7.9)	53.1 (7.2)	2041.31	<.001
Limited emotional role functioning‡	55.7 (44.4)	61.2 (30.2)	13.3 (30.6)	9.6 (26.5)	1101.98	<.001
Limited social functioning‡	36.6 (28.6)	47.1 (30.2)	16.0 (25.5)	10.8 (23.3)	859.27	<.001
Utility						
Time tradeoff	13.2 (29.9)	16.2 (31.9)	6.8 (21.9)	5.2 (19.8)	85.31	<.001
No. (%) >0	228 (30.5)	754 (35.0)	1620 (18.0)	841 (14.8)	. . .	
Mean if >0	43.3 (40.9)	46.1 (39.0)	37.6 (38.5)	35.1 (40.0)	. . .	
Standard gamble	94.2 (15.9)	90.0 (21.6)	94.8 (16.8)	96.3 (14.4)	54.26	<.001
No. (%) <100	192 (25.7)	701 (32.5)	1771 (19.7)	948 (16.7)	. . .	
Mean if <100	77.6 (25.0)	69.1 (28.1)	73.4 (29.2)	77.6 (28.6)	. . .	

**Ellipses indicate not applicable.*
†A high score represents good health.
‡A high score represents poor health.

sociated with common chronic medical conditions. Our conclusions about mental HRQOL are consistent across several measures, but our conclusions about physical HRQOL depended on the measure. The results for the global physical scale suggested that depressed patients had better physical HRQOL than patients with chronic medical conditions; on a pure physical limitations measure, however, depressed patients were in the midrange of the medical conditions. This difference may result from a methods effect, ie, the negative weighting of mental health items on the global scale, or from different results for different physical health items that contribute to the global scale. This is an important area for further research and scale development.

The HRQOL and utility described for depressed patients could also result from unmeasured comorbidities, particularly anxiety disorders. However, others have reported less marked effects on HRQOL for anxiety than depressive disorders.[2] In sensitivity analyses, we obtained the same results when controlling for comorbid alcohol abuse, assessed with an established screener.[25] The same criticism applies to findings for the medical conditions.

We also found that depressed patients had lower utility than nondepressed patients even after controlling for global mental and physical HRQOL scores. That is, the HRQOL scales did not fully account for the lower utility for current health of depressed patients. There may be something particularly aversive about severe affective states, such as fear of loss of control or social stigma, that is conceptually distinct from HRQOL, or the SF-12 measures may not be sufficiently comprehensive to capture the health states relevant to depressed patients.[16] This is an important area for further research given that the SF-12 is widely used and several investigators have proposed it as one efficient means for assessing utility in patient and community populations.[26,27] Another explanation could be that depressed patients may be especially prone cognitively to consider gambling with a chance of death to achieve perfect health on the SG item. However, we do not think that the low utility for current health of depressed patients can be explained by the negativistic cognition associated with depression,[28] because poor mental HRQOL was associated with lower utility for current health for both depressed and nondepressed patients.

Utility could differ for patients with depression and chronic medical conditions because of differences in acuteness of symptoms. Depressed patients had to have recent symptoms, but not patients with chronic medical conditions. However, this is also the nature of differences in conditions. Furthermore, the medical conditions reported were current, were associated with decrements in HRQOL, and thus were symptomatic. These self-report conditions are positively associated with clinician interview measures.[29] In addition, the relative order of utility for current health by TTO among patients with arthritis, diabetes, heart disease, and depression in our study was similar, despite different assessment and scoring methods, to those reported for a community sample.[23]

Using screening measures of affective syndromes, we found that patients with more severe syndromes, ie, 12-month double depression and lifetime bipolar illness, had worse HRQOL and lower utility for their current health than did patients with major depression, dysthymia, or depressive symptoms only. Patients with each syndrome had poorer HRQOL and lower utility for their current health than did patients without any affective syndrome. These findings emphasize the clinical importance of diverse affective states and suggest that even simple screening measures can help identify important impacts of affective conditions in large samples. It seems clinically reasonable that screens for lifetime bipolar illness and recent double depression would be associated with particularly adverse HRQOL and low utility, given the chronicity and recurrence associated with the full disorders.

Our study has limitations. We used brief screening measures of conditions. Rather than asking individuals

Table 4. Adjusted Profile of Health and Utility of Primary Care Patients With and Without Probable Depression and Specific Chronic Medical Conditions (N = 17 558)*

	Physical		Mental			Utility	
Health Condition	Global Physical†	Physical Functioning†	Global Mental†	Role-Emotional Functioning‡	Social Functioning‡	Time Tradeoff	Standard Gamble
Probable depression							
No	48.12 (0.08)	75.71 (0.24)	52.77 (0.06)	12.39 (0.25)	14.56 (0.21)	6.40 (0.18)	95.23 (0.14)
Yes	47.31 (0.19)	66.98 (0.57)	37.28 (0.20)	57.32 (0.83)	39.97 (0.56)	14.28 (0.58)	91.62 (0.38)
No − yes	−0.81 (0.20)	−8.73 (0.60)	−15.50 (0.22)	44.93 (0.88)	25.41 (0.60)	7.88 (0.61)	−3.61 (0.40)
t Test (*P*)	−4.07 (<.001)	−14.59 (<.001)	−71.65 (<.001)	51.15 (<.001)	42.24 (<.001)	12.91 (<.001)	−8.96 (<.001)
Asthma							
No	48.05 (0.08)	74.67 (0.24)	50.20 (0.08)	19.76 (0.29)	18.76 (0.22)	7.65 (0.19)	94.69 (0.13)
Yes	47.33 (0.23)	70.25 (0.71)	50.52 (0.23)	19.74 (0.89)	18.43 (0.70)	8.10 (0.65)	94.13 (0.48)
No − yes	−0.73 (0.24)	−4.42 (0.74)	0.31 (0.23)	−0.02 (0.93)	−0.32 (0.73)	0.45 (0.68)	−0.56 (0.50)
t Test (*P*)	−3.09 (.002)	−5.98 (<.001)	1.35 (.18)	−0.02 (.98)	−0.44 (.66)	0.65 (.51)	−1.11 (.27)
Diabetes							
No	48.26 (0.08)	74.93 (0.24)	50.29 (0.08)	19.59 (0.29)	18.47 (0.22)	7.50 (0.18)	94.92 (0.13)
Yes	45.07 (0.25)	67.30 (0.80)	49.65 (0.23)	21.62 (0.92)	21.48 (0.75)	9.71 (0.70)	91.58 (0.57)
No − yes	−3.19 (0.26)	−7.63 (0.83)	−0.64 (0.24)	2.03 (0.96)	3.01 (0.78)	2.21 (0.73)	−3.34 (0.60)
t Test (*P*)	−12.30 (<.001)	−9.20 (<.001)	−2.70 (.007)	2.12 (.03)	3.87 (<.001)	3.00 (.003)	−5.62 (<.001)
Hypertension							
No	48.17 (0.08)	74.92 (0.26)	50.27 (0.08)	19.52 (0.31)	18.73 (0.24)	7.72 (0.20)	94.67 (0.15)
Yes	47.25 (0.16)	71.73 (0.50)	50.07 (0.15)	20.71 (0.60)	18.73 (0.48)	7.59 (0.42)	94.53 (0.32)
No − yes	−0.93 (0.18)	−3.19 (0.56)	−0.21 (0.16)	1.19 (0.66)	0.01 (0.54)	−0.13 (0.47)	−0.14 (0.37)
t Test (*P*)	−5.16 (<.001)	−5.72 (<.001)	−1.28 (.20)	1.80 (.07)	0.02 (.99)	−0.27 (.79)	−0.38 (.71)
Arthritis							
No	48.86 (0.08)	76.36 (0.25)	50.22 (0.08)	19.44 (0.31)	18.32 (0.24)	7.37 (0.20)	94.88 (0.15)
Yes	44.54 (0.18)	66.00 (0.54)	50.28 (0.16)	21.02 (0.62)	20.35 (0.48)	8.96 (0.47)	93.68 (0.34)
No − yes	−4.32 (0.20)	−10.36 (0.60)	0.06 (0.17)	1.58 (0.69)	2.03 (0.55)	1.59 (0.52)	−1.20 (0.39)
t Test (*P*)	−21.38 (<.001)	−17.16 (<.001)	0.37 (.71)	2.30 (.02)	3.71 (<.001)	3.04 (.002)	−3.101 (.002)
Chronic lung disease							
No	48.19 (0.08)	74.88 (0.23)	50.29 (0.08)	19.55 (0.28)	18.47 (0.22)	7.65 (0.18)	94.74 (0.13)
Yes	43.12 (0.39)	59.76 (1.22)	48.85 (0.36)	24.76 (1.49)	25.08 (1.13)	8.77 (1.02)	92.24 (0.89)
No − yes	−5.07 (0.40)	−15.12 (1.25)	−1.44 (0.36)	5.21 (1.52)	6.61 (1.15)	1.12 (1.05)	−2.50 (0.90)
t Test (*P*)	−12.71 (<.001)	−12.15 (<.001)	−3.99 (<.001)	3.44 (.001)	5.75 (<.001)	1.07 (.29)	−2.76 (.006)
Chronic neurologic disease							
No	48.11 (0.08)	74.60 (0.23)	50.27 (0.08)	19.60 (0.28)	18.50 (0.21)	7.60 (0.18)	94.71 (0.13)
Yes	42.35 (0.54)	59.58 (1.72)	48.56 (0.48)	27.08 (1.93)	29.56 (1.53)	12.07 (1.64)	91.24 (1.20)
No − yes	−5.76 (0.54)	−15.02 (1.74)	−1.71 (0.48)	7.48 (1.95)	11.06 (1.55)	4.47 (1.65)	−3.47 (1.22)
t Test (*P*)	−10.63 (<.001)	−8.65 (<.001)	−3.57 (<.001)	3.84 (<.001)	7.15 (<.001)	2.71 (.007)	−2.86 (.004)
Heart disease							
No	48.17 (0.08)	74.86 (0.23)	50.24 (0.08)	19.68 (0.28)	18.55 (0.22)	7.69 (0.18)	94.75 (0.13)
Yes	43.67 (0.40)	60.73 (1.21)	49.97 (0.32)	21.67 (1.31)	22.86 (1.10)	7.80 (0.94)	91.99 (0.83)
No − yes	−4.50 (0.41)	−14.14 (1.23)	−0.28 (0.32)	2.00 (1.33)	4.30 (1.12)	0.11 (0.96)	−2.76 (0.85)
t Test (*P*)	−11.01 (<.001)	−11.46 (<.001)	−0.87 (.39)	1.50 (.14)	3.84 (<.001)	0.11 (.91)	−3.24 (.001)
Gastrointestinal tract disease							
No	48.18 (0.08)	74.65 (0.24)	50.37 (0.08)	19.41 (0.29)	18.24 (0.22)	7.35 (0.18)	94.71 (0.13)
Yes	46.01 (0.25)	70.39 (0.77)	48.81 (0.24)	23.43 (0.96)	23.90 (0.71)	11.33 (0.77)	93.87 (0.51)
No − yes	−2.17 (0.26)	−4.26 (0.79)	−1.56 (0.25)	4.02 (1.00)	5.66 (0.74)	3.98 (0.80)	−0.84 (0.53)
t Test (*P*)	−8.52 (<.001)	−5.37 (<.001)	−6.23 (<.001)	4.01 (<.001)	7.67 (<.001)	4.97 (<.001)	−1.58 (.11)
Back problems							
No	49.23 (0.08)	77.42 (0.25)	50.28 (0.09)	19.07 (0.31)	17.49 (0.24)	7.36 (0.20)	94.69 (0.15)
Yes	44.26 (0.15)	64.80 (0.45)	50.09 (0.14)	21.85 (0.55)	22.45 (0.42)	8.67 (0.38)	94.48 (0.26)
No − yes	−4.97 (0.17)	−12.63 (0.50)	−0.19 (0.15)	2.79 (0.61)	4.95 (0.47)	1.31 (0.43)	−0.22 (0.31)
t Test (*P*)	−29.18 (<.001)	−25.05 (<.001)	−1.25 (.21)	4.57 (<.001)	10.52 (<.001)	3.05 (.002)	−0.70 (.48)
Eye problems							
No	48.23 (0.08)	74.93 (0.24)	50.42 (0.08)	19.10 (0.29)	18.21 (0.22)	7.57 (0.19)	94.74 (0.14)
Yes	45.60 (0.25)	67.93 (0.74)	48.38 (0.23)	26.23 (0.96)	23.78 (0.71)	8.91 (0.68)	93.61 (0.49)
No − yes	−2.64 (0.26)	−7.00 (0.78)	−2.04 (0.24)	7.13 (1.00)	5.57 (0.75)	1.34 (0.72)	−1.14 (0.52)
t Test (*P*)	−10.29 (<.001)	−9.03 (<.001)	−8.46 (<.001)	7.13 (<.001)	7.48 (<.001)	1.87 (.06)	−2.20 (.03)
Migraine							
No	48.25 (0.08)	74.72 (0.24)	50.47 (0.08)	19.05 (0.30)	17.95 (0.23)	7.47 (0.19)	94.86 (0.14)
Yes	46.52 (0.18)	71.82 (0.55)	48.92 (0.18)	23.75 (0.72)	23.08 (0.53)	8.90 (0.51)	93.37 (0.36)
No − yes	−1.73 (0.19)	−2.90 (0.58)	−1.55 (0.19)	4.70 (0.78)	5.13 (0.57)	1.43 (0.56)	−1.49 (0.39)
t Test (*P*)	−9.04 (<.001)	−4.96 (<.001)	−8.06 (<.001)	6.04 (<.001)	8.94 (<.001)	2.57 (.01)	−3.83 (<.001)

*Unless otherwise indicated, data are given as mean (SE).
†A high score represents good health.
‡A high score represents poor health.

Table 5. Adjusted Difference in Health and Utility for Depression Relative to Specific Medical Chronic Conditions, Primary Care Patients (N = 17 558)*

	Physical		Mental			Utility	
Condition	Global Physical†	Physical Functioning†	Global Mental†	Role-Emotional Functioning‡	Social Functioning‡	Time Tradeoff	Standard Gamble
Asthma	-0.08 (0.31)	-4.32 (0.95)	-15.81 (0.32)	44.95 (1.29)	25.73 (0.94)	7.44 (0.94)	-3.06 (0.65)
t Test (*P*)	-0.27 (.79)	-4.56 (<.001)	-49.76 (<.001)	34.91 (<.001)	27.36 (<.001)	7.91 (<.001)	-4.73 (<.001)
Diabetes	2.39 (0.33)	-1.10 (1.04)	-14.86 (0.33)	42.90 (1.32)	22.40 (1.00)	5.68 (0.97)	-0.27 (0.71)
t Test (*P*)	7.15 (<.001)	-1.06 (.29)	-45.28 (<.001)	32.46 (<.001)	22.41 (<.001)	5.87 (<.001)	-0.38 (.70)
Hypertension	0.12 (0.27)	-5.55 (0.82)	-15.29 (0.27)	43.74 (1.11)	25.40 (0.81)	8.01 (0.79)	-3.48 (0.55)
t Test (*P*)	0.45 (.65)	-6.80 (<.001)	-55.90 (<.001)	39.42 (<.001)	31.51 (<.001)	10.20 (<.001)	-6.30 (<.001)
Arthritis	3.51 (0.29)	1.63 (0.87)	-15.56 (0.28)	43.35 (1.14)	23.38 (0.82)	6.29 (0.81)	-2.42 (0.57)
t Test (*P*)	12.12 (<.001)	1.88 (.06)	-55.03 (<.001)	38.07 (<.001)	28.41 (<.001)	7.81 (<.001)	-4.27 (<.001)
Chronic lung disease	4.26 (0.45)	6.39 (1.39)	-14.06 (0.43)	39.72 (1.79)	18.80 (1.31)	6.76 (1.23)	-1.12 (1.00)
t Test (*P*)	9.48 (<.001)	4.59 (<.001)	-32.70 (<.001)	22.21 (<.001)	14.38 (<.001)	5.52 (<.001)	-1.12 (.26)
Neurologic disease	4.96 (0.59)	6.29 (1.85)	-13.79 (0.54)	37.45 (2.20)	14.35 (1.69)	3.42 (1.76)	-0.14 (1.30)
t Test (*P*)	8.48 (<.001)	3.40 (.001)	-25.64 (<.001)	17.05 (<.001)	8.47 (<.001)	1.94 (.05)	-0.108 (.91)
Heart disease	3.69 (0.46)	5.40 (1.36)	-15.22 (0.39)	42.93 (1.61)	21.11 (1.28)	7.78 (1.15)	-0.85 (0.94)
t Test (*P*)	8.04 (<.001)	3.91 (<.001)	-38.96 (<.001)	26.69 (<.001)	16.46 (<.001)	6.76 (<.001)	-0.91 (.37)
Gastrointestinal tract disease	1.36 (0.34)	-4.47 (1.04)	-13.94 (0.34)	40.91 (1.39)	19.75 (0.99)	3.90 (1.03)	-2.77 (0.70)
t Test (*P*)	4.06 (<.001)	-4.32 (<.001)	-40.52 (<.001)	29.42 (<.001)	19.94 (<.001)	3.78 (<.001)	-3.95 (<.001)
Back problems	4.16 (0.27)	3.89 (0.81)	-15.31 (0.27)	42.14 (1.11)	20.46 (0.80)	6.58 (0.75)	-3.40 (0.51)
t Test (*P*)	15.27 (<.001)	4.84 (<.001)	-55.92 (<.001)	37.96 (<.001)	25.69 (<.001)	8.72 (<.001)	-6.70 (<.001)
Eye problems	1.83 (0.34)	-1.73 (1.02)	-13.46 (0.34)	37.79 (1.41)	19.84 (1.01)	6.54 (0.98)	-2.48 (0.68)
t Test (*P*)	5.37 (<.001)	-1.70 (.09)	-39.51 (<.001)	26.75 (<.001)	19.61 (<.001)	6.70 (<.001)	-3.64 (<.001)
Migraine	0.92 (0.29)	-5.84 (0.88)	-13.95 (0.31)	40.23 (1.24)	20.28 (0.87)	6.45 (0.85)	-2.12 (0.58)
t Test (*P*)	3.16 (.002)	-6.67 (<.001)	-45.49 (<.001)	32.36 (<.001)	23.24 (<.001)	7.59 (<.001)	-3.68 (<.001)

* Unless otherwise indicated, data are given as mean (SE).
†A high score represents good health.
‡A high score represents poor health.

Table 6. Adjusted Health and Utility for Primary Care Patients With Affective Syndrome (N = 17 558)*

	Physical		Mental			Utility	
Affective Syndromes	Global Physical†	Physical Functioning†	Global Mental†	Role-Emotional Functioning‡	Social Functioning‡	Time Tradeoff	Standard Gamble
None	48.26 (0.08)	76.60 (0.26)	54.18 (0.06)	8.16 (0.23)	12.61 (0.23)	5.49 (0.19)	95.48 (0.15)
Lifetime bipolar	40.70 (0.02)	00.40 (1.00)	41.07 (0.04)	40.10 (0.40)	07.10 (1.71)	10.00 (1.05)	00.40 (1.00)
t Test (*P*)	-2.87 (.004)	-4.76 (<.001)	-19.32 (<.001)	16.13 (<.001)	14.20 (<.001)	5.81 (<.001)	-4.59 (<.001)
Bipolar—none	-1.50 (0.52)	-8.11 (1.70)	-12.52 (0.65)	40.02 (2.48)	24.57 (1.73)	11.39 (1.96)	-6.02 (1.31)
t Test (*P*)	-2.87 (.004)	-4.76 (<.001)	-19.32 (<.001)	16.13 (<.001)	14.20 (<.001)	5.81 (<.001)	-4.59 (<.001)
12-mo Double depression	46.55 (0.33)	64.40 (1.01)	36.12 (0.36)	60.25 (1.42)	43.74 (0.99)	18.58 (1.17)	88.30 (0.79)
t Test (*P*)	-5.08 (<.001)	-11.74 (<.001)	-49.49 (<.001)	35.82 (<.001)	30.35 (<.001)	11.01 (<.001)	-8.89 (<.001)
Double—none	-1.71 (0.34)	-12.20 (1.04)	-18.07 (0.37)	52.09 (1.45)	31.13 (1.03)	13.09 (1.19)	-7.18 (0.81)
t Test (*P*)	-5.08 (<.001)	-11.74 (<.001)	-49.47 (<.001)	35.82 (<.001)	30.35 (<.001)	11.01 (<.001)	-8.89 (<.001)
12-mo Major depression only	47.63 (0.16)	70.24 (0.48)	42.75 (0.19)	41.93 (0.76)	29.62 (0.48)	10.68 (0.45)	93.96 (0.29)
t Test (*P*)	-3.63 (<.001)	-12.20 (<.001)	-57.42 (<.001)	42.23 (<.001)	31.84 (<.001)	10.46 (<.001)	-4.66 (<.001)
Major—none	-0.63 (0.17)	-6.36 (0.52)	-11.44 (0.20)	33.77 (0.80)	17.01 (0.53)	5.20 (0.50)	-1.52 (0.33)
t Test (*P*)	-3.63 (<.001)	-12.20 (<.001)	-57.42 (<.001)	42.33 (<.001)	31.84 (<.001)	10.46 (<.001)	-4.66 (<.001)
12-mo Dysthymia only	46.05 (0.75)	66.75 (2.26)	46.33 (0.80)	30.48 (3.23)	26.75 (2.30)	13.14 (2.72)	95.10 (1.16)
t Test (*P*)	-2.93 (.003)	-4.33 (<.001)	-9.75 (<.001)	6.89 (<.001)	6.12 (<.001)	2.81 (.005)	-0.32 (.75)
Dysthymia—none	-2.21 (0.76)	-9.85 (2.27)	-7.85 (0.81)	22.32 (3.24)	14.14 (2.31)	7.66 (2.72)	-0.38 (1.17)
t Test (*P*)	-2.93 (.003)	-4.33 (<.001)	-9.75 (<.001)	6.89 (<.001)	6.12 (<.001)	2.81 (.005)	-0.32 (.75)
30-d Symptoms only	48.12 (0.28)	73.48 (0.82)	46.66 (0.30)	29.44 (1.30)	21.69 (0.79)	8.97 (0.79)	94.77 (0.51)
t Test (*P*)	-0.50 (.62)	-3.70 (<.001)	-24.45 (<.001)	16.15 (<.001)	11.03 (<.001)	4.28 (<.001)	-1.32 (.19)
Symptoms—none	-0.14 (-0.29)	-3.13 (0.85)	-7.53 (0.31)	21.28 (1.32)	9.09 (0.82)	3.49 (0.82)	-0.70 (0.53)
t Test (*P*)	-0.50 (.62)	-3.70 (<.001)	-24.45 (<.001)	16.15 (<.001)	11.03 (<.001)	4.28 (<.001)	-1.32 (.19)

* Unless otherwise indicated, data are given as mean (SE).
†A high score represents good health.
‡A high score represents poor health.

to directly assess the value of hypothetical conditions, a common method applied to small patient samples with the use of sophisticated assessment technology,[10,24,30] we assessed the utility for their current health. The strength of our approach is the diversity and number of patients whose utilities were represented, rather than the depth in the assessment. The results might not apply to other managed, primary care practices. A consecutive patient sample overrepresents high utilizers and sicker individuals. Nonresponse on items that assessed utility was moderately high, but we weighted for nonresponse.

Overall, our findings emphasize the importance of attending to patient preferences for outcomes and suggest that depressed patients in managed, primary care practices have a strong desire to recover from depression, reinforcing the importance of quality improvement programs and patient education.

Accepted for publication June 29, 1999.

This work was supported by grant R01 HS08349 from the Agency for Health Care Policy and Research, Rockville, Md, and Research Scientist Award MH01170-05 and Research Center on Managed Care for Psychiatric Disorders grant P50 MH54623 from the National Institute of Mental Health, Bethesda, Md.

We acknowledge the contribution of Maureen Carney, MS, for coordinating the data implementation plan as well as the plan for test-retest data; Robert Bell, PhD, for his statistical advice on the analyses; Bernadette Benjamin, MS, for meticulous programming; and Roland Sturm, PhD, for developing the utility measures. We acknowledge the participating managed care organizations that provided access to their expertise and patients, implemented interventions, and provided in-kind resources: Allina Medical Group (Twin Cities, Minn), Patuxent Medical Group (Columbia, Md), Humana Health Care Plans (San Antonio, Tex), MedPartners (Los Angeles, Calif), PacifiCare of Texas (San Antonio), and Valley-Wide Health Services (San Luis Valley, Colo); and their internal behavioral health organizations and participating contract behavioral health organizations: Alamo Mental Health Group (San Antonio), San Luis Valley Mental Health/Colorado Health Networks (San Luis Valley), and GreenSpring Mental Health Services (Columbia).

Reprints: Kenneth B. Wells, MD, MPH, RAND, 1700 Main St, Santa Monica, CA 90407-2138 (e-mail: kenneth_wells@rand.org).

REFERENCES

1. Von Korff M, Ormel J, Katon W, Lin EE. Disability and depression among high utilizers of health care: a longitudinal analysis. *Arch Gen Psychiatry.* 1992;49:91-100.
2. Spitzer RL, Kroenke K, Linzer M, Hahn SR, Williams JB, deGruy FV III, Brody D, Davies M. Health-related quality of life in primary care patients with mental disorders: results from the PRIME-MD 1000 Study. *JAMA.* 1995;274:1511-1517.
3. Wells KB, Stewart A, Hays RD, Burnam MA, Rogers W, Daniels M, Berry S, Greenfield S, Ware J. The functioning and well-being of depressed patients: results from the Medical Outcomes Study. *JAMA.* 1989;262:914-919.
4. Hays RD, Wells KB, Sherbourne CD, Rogers W, Spritzer K. Functioning and well-being outcomes of patients with depression compared with chronic general medical illnesses. *Arch Gen Psychiatry.* 1995;52:11-19.
5. Wells KB, Sturm R, Sherbourne CD, Meredith L. *Caring for Depression.* Boston, Mass: Harvard University Press; 1996.
6. Wells K, Schoenbaum M, Unützer J, Lagomasino IT, Rubenstein LV. Quality of care for primary care patients with depression in managed care. *Arch Fam Med.* In press.
7. *Depression Guidelines Panel Depression in Primary Care, Volume I: Detection and Diagnosis.* Rockville, Md: US Dept of Health and Human Services, Public Health Service, Agency for Health Care Policy & Research; 1993. Publication 93-0550.
8. Üstun TB, Norman N, eds. *Mental Illness in General Health Care: An International Study.* New York, NY: John Wiley & Sons Inc; 1995.
9. Gold M, Siegel J, Russell L, Weinstein M. *Cost-Effectiveness in Health and Medicine.* New York, NY: Oxford University Press; 1966.
10. Revicki DA, Wood M. Patient-assigned health state utilities for depression-related outcomes: differences by depression severity and antidepressant medications. *J Affect Disord.* 1998;48:25-36.
11. Pyne JM, Patterson TL, Kaplan RM, Gillin JC, Koch WL, Grant I. Assessment of the quality of life of patients with major depression. *Psychiatr Serv.* 1997;48:224-230.
12. Wells KB. The design of Partners in Care: evaluating the cost-effectiveness of improving care for depression in primary care. *Soc Psychiatry Psychiatr Epidemiol.* 1999;34:20-29.
13. American Psychiatric Association. *Diagnostic and Statistical Manual of Mental Disorders, Fourth Edition.* Washington, DC: American Psychiatric Association; 1994.
14. World Health Organization. *Composite International Diagnostic Interview (CIDI) Core Version 2.1 Interviewer's Manual.* Geneva, Switzerland: World Health Organization; 1997.
15. Ware JE, Kosinski M, Keller SA. 12-Item Short-Form Health Survey: construction of scales and preliminary tests of reliability and validity. *Med Care.* 1996;34:220-233.
16. Simon GE, Revicki DA, Grothaus L, Vonkorff M. SF-36 summary scores: are physical and mental health truly distinct? *Med Care.* 1998;36:567-572.
17. Froberg DG, Kane RL. Methodology for measuring health-state preferences, I: measurement strategies. *J Clin Epidemiol.* 1989;42:345-354.
18. Froberg DG, Kane RL. Methodology for measuring health-state preferences, II: scaling methods. *J Clin Epidemiol.* 1989;42:459-471.
19. Torrance G. Measurement of health-state utilities for economic appraisal: a review. *J Health Econ.* 1986;5:1-30.
20. Searle SR. *Linear Models.* New York, NY: John Wiley & Sons Inc; 1971.
21. Huber PH. The behavior of maximum likelihood estimates under non-standard conditions. In: *Proceedings of the Fifth Berkeley Symposium on Mathematical Statistics and Probability.* Berkeley: University of California; 1967:221-233.
22. Feller W. *An Introduction to Probability Theory and Its Application.* New York, NY: John Wiley & Sons Inc; 1968.
23. Fryback DG, Dasbach EJ, Klein R, Klein BEK, Dorn N, Peterson K, Martin PA. The Beaver Dam Health Outcomes Study: initial catalog of health-state quality factors. *Med Decis Making.* 1993;13:89-102.
24. Sackett DL, Torrance GW. The utility of different health states as perceived by the general public. *J Chronic Dis.* 1978;31:697-704.
25. Rost K, Burnam MA, Smith RG. Development of screeners for depressive disorders and substance disorder history. *Med Care.* 1993;31:189-200.
26. Sherbourne CD, Keeler E, Unutzer J, Lenert L, Wells KB. Relationship between age and patients' current health state preferences. *Gerontologist.* 1999;39:271-278.
27. Lundberg L, Johannesson M, Isacson DGL, Borgquist L. The relationship between health-state utilities and the SF-12 in a general population. *Med Decis Making.* 1999;19:128-140.
28. Beck AT. *Cognitive Therapy and the Emotional Disorders.* New York, NY: International Universities Press Inc; 1976:116-119.
29. Wells KB, Manning WG, Burnam MA, Greenfield S, Ware JE Jr. How the medical comorbidity of depressed patients differs across health care settings: results from the Medical Outcomes Study. *Am J Psychiatry.* 1991;148:1688-1696.
30. Lenert LA, Morss S, Goldstein MK, Garber AM. Measurement of the validity of utility elicitations performed by computer interview. *Med Care.* 1997;35:915-920.

Acknowledgments

Blazer, D.G., Kessler, R.C., McGonagle, K.A., and Swartz, M.S. "The Prevalence and Distribution of Major Depression in a National Community Sample: The National Comorbidity Survey." *Am J Psychiatry* 151 (1994): 979–986. Copyright 1994, the American Psychiatric Association. Reprinted by permission.

Burke, K.C., Burke, J.D., Rae, D.S., and Regier, D.A. "Comparing Age at the Outset of Major Depression and Other Psychiatric Disorders by Birth Cohorts in Five U.S. Community Populations." *Arch Gen Psychiatry* 48 (1991): 789–795. Reprinted with the permission of American Medical Association.

Judd, L.L., Paulus M.P., Wells K.B., and Rapoport, M.H. "SocioeconomicBurden of Subsyndromal Depressive Symptoms and Major Depression in a Sample of the General Population." *Am J Psychiatry* 153 (1996): 1411–1417. Copyright 1996, the American Psychiatric Association. Reprinted by permission.

Kendler, K.S., and Gardner, C.O. "Boundaries of Major Depression: An Evaluation of DSM-IV Criteria." *Am J Psychiatry* 155 (1998): 172–177. Copyright 1998, the American Psychiatric Association. Reprinted by permission.

Kessler, R.C., Borges, G., and Walters, E.E. "Prevalence of and Risk Factors for Lifetime Suicide Attempts in the National Comorbidity Survey." *Arch Gen Psychiatry* 56 (1999): 617–626. Reprinted with the permission of American Medical Association.

Murphy, J.M., Laird, N.M., Monson, R.R., Sobol, A.M., and Leighton, A.H. "A 40-Year Perspective on the Prevalence of Depression." *Arch Gen Psychiatry* 57 (2000): 209–215. Reprinted with the permission of American Medical Association.

Bassuk, S.S., Berkman, L.F., and Wypij, D. "Depressive Symptomatology and Incident Cognitive Decline in an Elderly Community Sample." *Arch Gen Psychiatry* 55 (1998): 1073–1081. Reprinted with the permission of American Medical Association.

Berndt, E.R., Koran, L.M., Finkelstein, S.N., Gelenberg, A.J., et al. "Lost Human Capital from Early-Onset Chronic Depression." *Am J Psychiatry* 157 (2000): 940–947. Copyright 2000, the American Psychiatric Association. Reprinted by permission.

Kessler, R.C. "The Effects of Stressful Life Events on Depression." *Annu Rev Psychol* 48 (1997): 191–214. Reprinted with permission from the Annual Review of Psychology, Volume 48, ©1997, by Annual Reviews www.AnnualReviews.org.

Lewinsohn, P.M., Rohde, P., Seeley, J.R., Klein, D.N., and Gotlib, I.A. "Natural Course of Adolescent Major Depressive Disorder in a Community Sample: Predictors of Recurrence in Young Adults." *Am J Psychiatry* 157 (2000): 1584–1591. Copyright 2000, the American Psychiatric Association. Reprinted by permission.

Mueller, T.I., Leon, A.C., Keller, M.B., et al. "Recurrence after Recovery from Major Depressive Disorder during 15 Years of Observational Follow-up." *Am J Psychiatry* 156 (1999): 1000–1006. Copyright 1999, the American Psychiatric Association. Reprinted by permission.

Schulz, R., Beach, S.R., Ives, D.G., Martire, L.M., Ariyo, A.A., and Kop, W.J. "Association between Depression and Mortality in Older Adults." *Arch Intern Med* 160 (2000): 1761–1768. Reprinted with the permission of American Medical Association.

Krishnan, K.R., Hays, J.C., and Blazer, D.G. "MRI Defined Vascular Depression." *Am J Psychiatry* 154 (1997): 497–501. Copyright 1997, the American Psychiatric Association. Reprinted by permission.

Musselman, D.L., Evans, D.L., and Nemeroff, C.B. "The Relationship of Depression to Cardiovascular Disease: Epidemiology, Biology, and Treatment." *Arch Gen Psychiatry* 55 (1998): 580–592. Reprinted with the permission of American Medical Association.

Kendler, K.S., Heath, A.C., Martin, N.G., and Eaves, L.J. "Symptoms of Anxiety and Symptoms of Depression: Same Genes, Different Environments?" *Arch Gen Psychiatry* 44 (1987): 451–457. Reprinted with the permission of American Medical Association.

Kendler, K.S., Kessler, R.C., Walters, E.E., et al. "Stressful Life Events, Genetic Liability, and Onset of an Episode of Major Depression in Women." *Am J Psychiatry* 152 (1995): 833–842. Copyright 1994, the American Psychiatric Association. Reprinted by permission.

Malhi, G.S., Moore, J., and McGuffin, P. "The Genetics of Major Depressive Disorder." *Curr Psychiatry Rep* (2000): 165–169. Reprinted with the permission of Current Science Ltd.

Sullivan, P.F., Neale, M.C., and Kendler, K.S. "Genetic Epidemiology of Major Depression: Review and Meta-analysis." *Am J Psychiatry* 157 (2000): 1552–1562. Copyright 2000, the American Psychiatric Association. Reprinted by permission.

Weiss, E.L., Longhurst, J.G., and Mazure C. "Childhood Sexual Abuse as a Risk Factor for Depression in Women: Psychosocial and Neurobiological Correlates." *Am J Psychiatry* 156 (1999): 816–828. Copyright 1999, the American Psychiatric Association. Reprinted by permission.

Nesse, R.M. "Is Depression an Adaptation?" *Arch Gen Psychiatry* 57 (2000): 14–20. Reprinted with the permission of American Medical Association.

Drevets, W.C., Price, J.L., Simpson, J.R., Todd, R.D., Reich, T., Vannier, M., and Raichle, M.E. "Subgenual Prefrontal Cortex Abnormalities in Mood Disorders." *Nature* 386 (1997): 824–827. Reprinted by permission from Nature Vol. 386, pp. 824–827. Copyright © 1997 Macmillan Magazines Ltd.

Duman, R.S., Heninger, G.R., and Nestler, E.J. "A Molecular and Cellular Theory of Depression." *Arch Gen Psychiatry* 54 (1997): 597–606. Reprinted with the permission of American Medical Association.

Heim, C., and Nemeroff, C.B. "The Impact of Early Adverse Experiences on Brain Systems Involved in the Pathophysiology of Anxiety and Affective Disorders." *Biol Psychiatry* 46 (1999): 1509–1522. Reprinted with the permission of Elsevier Science.

Holsboer, F. "The Corticosteroid Receptor Hypothesis of Depression." *Neuropsychopharmacology* 23 (2000): 477–501. Reprinted by permission of Elsevier Science. Copyright 2000 by American College of Neuropsychopharmacology.

Mayberg, H.S., Liotti, M., Brannan, S.K., McGinnis, S., Mahurin, R.K., Jerabek, P.A., Silva, J.A., Tekell, J.L., Martin, C.C., Lancaster, J.L., and Fox, P.T. "Reciprocal Limbic-Cortical Function and Negative Mood: Converging PET Findings in Depression and Normal Sadness." *Am J Psychiatry* 156 (1999): 675–682. Copyright 1999, the American Psychiatric Association. Reprinted by permission.

Sheline, Y.I., Sanghavi, M., Mintun, M.A., and Gado, M.H. "Depression Duration but Not Age Predicts Hippocampal Volume Loss in Medically Healthy Women with Recurrent Major Depression." *J Neurosci* 19 (1999): 5034–5043. Copyright 1999 by the Society for Neuroscience.

Frank, E., and Thase, M.E. "Natural History and Preventative Treatment of Recurrent Mood Disorders." *Annu Rev Med* 50 (1999): 453–468. Reprinted with permission from the Annual Review of Neuroscience, Volume 50, ©1999, by Annual Reviews www.AnnualReviews.org.

Keller, M.B., McCullough, J.P., Klein, D.N., Arnow, B., Dunner, D.L., Gelenberg, A.J., Markowitz, J.C., Nemeroff, C.B., Russell, J.M., Thase, M.E., Trivedi, M.H., and Zajecka, J. "A Comparison of Nefazodone, the Cognitive Behavioral Analysis System of Psychotherapy, and Their Combination for the Treatment of Chronic Depression." *N Engl J Med* 342, 20 (2000): 1462–1470. Copyright © 2000 Massachusetts Medical Society. All rights reserved.

Wells, K.B., and Sherbourne, C.D. "Functioning and Utility for Current Health of Patients with Depression or Chronic Medical Conditions in Managed, Primary Care Practices." *Arch Gen Psychiatry* 56 (1999): 897–904. Reprinted with the permission of American Medical Association.